FRACTURES OF THE CERVICAL, THORACIC, AND LUMBAR SPINE

FRACTURES OF THE CERVICAL, THORACIC, AND LUMBAR SPINE

edited by
ALEXANDER R. VACCARO

Thomas Jefferson University Hospital
The Rothman Institute
Philadelphia, Pennsylvania

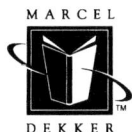

MARCEL DEKKER, INC.

NEW YORK · BASEL

MARCEL

DEKKER

2003

ISBN: 0-8247-0713-3

This book is printed on acid-free paper.

Headquarters
Marcel Dekker, Inc.
270 Madison Avenue, New York, NY 10016
tel: 212-696-9000; fax: 212-685-4540

Eastern Hemisphere Distribution
Marcel Dekker AG
Hutgasse 4, Postfach 812, CH-4001 Basel, Switzerland
tel: 41-61-260-6300; fax: 41-61-260-6333

World Wide Web
http://www.dekker.com

The publisher offers discounts on this book when ordered in bulk quantities. For more information, write to Special Sales/Professional Marketing at the headquarters address above.

Preface

Spinal trauma is a potentially devastating occurrence associated with significant morbidity and mortality. Fortunately, with improved "in-field" management protocols, "in-hospital" resuscitation measures, and further insight into the pathophysiology of spinal cord injury, progress is being made toward improving neurological function and quality of life for this patient population. In order to optimize postinjury intervention efforts by spinal care providers, a thorough understanding of all facets of spinal injury and spinal cord injury pathomechanics must be attained.

The medical literature is replete with generalized assessment and treatment guidelines for broad groups of spinal injuries; it lacks, however, a comprehensive and precise investigation into the particulars of various subgroups of traumatic pathology. Each fracture type has individualized assessment concerns, fracture subclassifications, immobilization techniques, nonoperative and operative indications, operative fixation strategies, and prognostic outlook. It is imperative that such vital information be included in any volume exploring contemporary spinal injury management. A comprehensive textbook that allows quick and easy reference to fracture subtypes, spinal injury management protocols, and aftercare is indispensable to the spinal care provider regardless of the level of academic training.

In an effort to develop a broad, in-depth but readable text on the comprehensive management of spinal injury, world-renowned experts were asked to focus on particular issues of spinal pathophysiology and fracture subtypes rather than on regional spinal pathology, as is often the case in other contemporary textbooks. This approach is invaluable when precise and current information is necessary to manage common and uncommon spinal traumatic pathology.

This book serves as an up-to-date review and a comprehensive resource. With a thorough understanding of the contemporary issues surrounding spinal trauma management, the spinal care provider can supply the best care and optimize the potential for gainful rehabilitation.

Alexander R. Vaccaro
Justin P. Kubeck

Contents

Contents

Contributors

Jean-Jacques Abitbol, M.D. California Spine Group, San Diego, California, U.S.A.

Todd J. Albert, M.D. Associate Professor, Department of Orthopaedic Surgery, Thomas Jefferson University Hospital and the Rothman Institute, Philadelphia, Pennsylvania, U.S.A.

Glenn M. Amundson, M.D. Assistant Professor, Department of Orthopedic Surgery, University of Kansas Medical Center, Kansas City, Kansas, U.S.A.

Howard S. An, M.D. Department of Orthopedic Surgery, Rush-Presbyterian-St. Luke's Medical Center, Chicago, Illinois, U.S.A.

D. Greg Anderson Department of Orthopaedic Surgery, University of Virginia School of Medicine, Charlottesville, Virginia, U.S.A.

Paul A. Anderson, M.D. Clinical Associate Professor, Department of Orthopaedic Surgery, University of Washington, Seattle, Washington, U.S.A.

David Andreychik, M.D. Associate, Department of Orthopaedic Surgery, Geisinger Medical Center, Danville, Pennsylvania, U.S.A.

Juan Bartolomei, M.D. Assistant Professor, Department of Neurosurgery, Yale University School of Medicine, New Haven, Connecticut, U.S.A.

Hugh L. Bassewitz, M.D.   William Beaumont Hospital, Royal Oak, Michigan, U.S.A.

Edward C. Benzel, M.D., F.A.C.S.   Director, Spinal Disorders, Department of Neurosurgery, The Cleveland Clinic Foundation, Cleveland, Ohio, U.S.A.

James Bicos, M.D.   Department of Orthopaedic Surgery, Rush Medical College, Rush Presbyterian St. Luke's Medical Center, Chicago, Illinois, U.S.A.

Oren G. Blam, M.D.   Clinical Instructor and Chief Resident, Department of Orthopaedic Surgery, Thomas Jefferson University Hospital, Philadelphia, Pennsylvania, U.S.A.

Michael J. Bolesta, M.D.   Associate Professor, Department of Orthopaedic Surgery, University of Texas Southwestern Medical Center, Dallas, Texas, U.S.A.

Christopher M. Bono, M.D.   Clinical Instructor, Department of Orthopaedic Surgery, University of California at San Diego, San Diego, California, U.S.A.

Robert H. Boyce, M.D.   Department of Orthopaedics and Rehabilitation, Vanderbilt University Medical Center, Nashville, Tennessee, U.S.A.

Russ Brummett   University of Pennsylvania, Philadelphia, Pennsylvania, U.S.A.

Douglas C. Burton   University of Kansas Medical Center, Kansas City, Kansas, U.S.A.

Rocco R. Calderone, M.D.   Vice Chairman, Department of Surgery, St. John's Regional Medical Center, Oxnard, California, U.S.A.

Frank P. Cammisa, Jr., M.D.   Chief, Spinal Surgical Service and Associate Professor of Surgery, Department of Orthopedics, Hospital for Special Surgery, Weill Medical College of Cornell University, New York, New York, U.S.A.

John J. Carbone, M.D.   Johns Hopkins Bayview Hospital, Baltimore, Maryland, U.S.A.

Daniel A. Capen, M.D.   University of Southern California, Los Angeles, California, U.S.A.

Jens Chapman, M.D.   Harborview Medical Center, Seattle, Washington, U.S.A.

Aaron A. Cohen-Gadol, M.D.   Department of Neurological Surgery, Mayo Clinic and Mayo Foundation, Rochester, Minnesota, U.S.A.

Mark Dekutoski, M.D.   Assistant Professor, Department of Orthopedic Surgery, Mayo Clinic and Mayo Foundation, Rochester, Minnesota, U.S.A.

Rick B. Delamarter, M.D. Medical Director, The Spine Institute at St. John's Health Center, Santa Monica, and Associate Clinical Professor, Department of Orthopaedic Surgery, UCLA School of Medicine, Los Angeles, California, U.S.A.

Francis Denis, M.D. Clinical Professor, Twin Cities Spine Center, Minneapolis, Minnesota, U.S.A.

Christopher J. DeWald, M.D. Assistant Professor, Department of Orthopaedic Surgery, Rush Medical College, Rush Presbyterian St. Luke's Medical Center, and Chief, Section of Spine Surgery, Division of Orthopedic Surgery, Cook County Hospital, Chicago, Illinois, U.S.A.

John F. Ditunno, Jr., M.D. Professor of Rehabilitation Medicine and Project Director, Regional Spinal Cord Injury Center of the Delaware Valley, Thomas Jefferson University, Philadelphia, Pennsylvania, U.S.A.

Douglas M. Ehrler, M.D. Omni Orthopaedics, Canton, Ohio, U.S.A.

Frank J. Eismont, M.D. Professor and Vice Chairman, Department of Orthopaedics and Rehabilitation, University of Miami School of Medicine, Miami, Florida, U.S.A.

Jeffrey S. Fischgrund, M.D. Private practice, Southfield, Michigan, U.S.A.

Christopher S. Formal, M.D. Magee Rehabilitation Hospital, Philadelphia, Pennsylvania, U.S.A.

Steven R. Garfin, M.D. Department of Orthopaedics, University of California, San Diego, San Diego, California, U.S.A.

Stanley D. Gertzbein, M.D., F.R.C.S.(C) Professor, Department of Orthopedics, Baylor College of Medicine, Houston, Texas, U.S.A.

Alexander J. Ghanayem, M.D. Associate Professor and Chief, Division of Spine Surgery, Department of Orthopaedic Surgery and Rehabilitation, Loyola University of Chicago, Maywood, Illinois, U.S.A.

Federico P. Girardi, M.D. Clinical Instructor, Department of Orthopedics, Hospital for Special Surgery, Weill Medical College of Cornell University, New York, New York, U.S.A.

Jonathan N. Grauer, M.D. Department of Orthopaedics and Rehabilitation, Yale University School of Medicine, New Haven, Connecticut, U.S.A.

Stephen M. Hankins, M.D. Department of Orthopaedic Surgery, Medical College of Pennsylvania, Hahnemann University Hospital, Philadelphia, Pennsylvania, U.S.A.

Mitchel B. Harris, M.D., F.A.C.S. Professor, Department of Orthopaedics, Wake Forest University, Bowman Gray School of Medicine, Winston-Salem, North Carolina, U.S.A.

James S. Harrop, M.D.   Jefferson Medical College, Philadelphia, Pennsylvania, U.S.A.

Robert F. Heary, M.D.   Associate Professor, Department of Neurological Surgery, UMDNJ–New Jersey Medical School, Newark, New Jersey, U.S.A.

Jeffrey S. Henn, M.D.   Division of Neurological Surgery, Barrow Neurological Institute, Phoenix, Arizona, U.S.A.

Harry N. Herkowitz, M.D.   Chairman, Department of Orthopaedic Surgery, William Beaumont Hospital, Royal Oak, Michigan, U.S.A.

Alan S. Hilibrand, M.D.   Assistant Professor and Director of Medical Education, Department of Orthopaedics, Thomas Jefferson University Hospital and the Rothman Institute, Philadelphia, Pennsylvania, U.S.A.

John P. Kostuik, M.D., F.R.C.S. (C)   Professor and Chief, Spine Surgery, Department of Orthopaedics, Johns Hopkins University Medical Center, Baltimore, Maryland, U.S.A.

Robert J. Kowalski, M.D.   Department of Neurosurgery, The Cleveland Clinic Foundation, Cleveland, Ohio, U.S.A.

Justin P. Kubeck   Thomas Jefferson University Hospital and the Rothman Institute, Philadelphia, Pennsylvania, U.S.A.

Anh X. Le, M.D.   Alpine Orthopaedic Medical Group, Inc., Stockton, and Clinical Instructor, Orthopedic Surgery, University of California, Davis, Sacramento, California, U.S.A.

G. Michael Lemole, Jr., M.D.   Department of Neurosurgery, Barrow Neurological Institute, Phoenix, Arizona, U.S.A.

Ellen Leppek   University of Southern California, Los Angeles, California, U.S.A.

Steven C. Ludwig, M.D.   Assistant Professor, Department of Orthopaedic Surgery, Milton S. Hershey Medical Center of The Pennsylvania State University College of Medicine, Hershey, Pennsylvania, U.S.A.

Dante G. Marchesi, M.D.   Associate Professor, Division of Orthopaedic Surgery, McGill University, Montreal, Quebec, Canada

Rex A. W. Marco   University of Texas M.D. Anderson Cancer Center, Houston, Texas, U.S.A.

Ralph J. Marino, M.D.   Clinical Associate Professor, Department of Rehabilitation Medicine, Mount Sinai School of Medicine, New York, New York, U.S.A.

W. R. Marsh, M.D.   Department of Neurological Surgery, Mayo Clinic and Mayo Foundation, Rochester, Minnesota, U.S.A.

Robert A. McGuire, M.D.   Professor, Department of Orthopedics, University of Mississippi Medical Center, Jackson, Mississippi, U.S.A.

Robert F. McLain, M.D.   Director, Spine Fellowship Program, Department of Orthopaedic Surgery, The Cleveland Clinic Foundation, Cleveland, Ohio, U.S.A.

R. Alden Milam IV   University of Pennsylvania, Philadelphia, Pennsylvania, U.S.A.

William Mitchell, M.D.   Jefferson Medical College, Philadelphia, Pennsylvania, U.S.A.

John Noack   University of Kansas Medical Center, Kansas City, Kansas, U.S.A.

Manohar M. Panjabi, Ph.D.   Professor, Department of Orthopaedics and Rehabilitation, Yale University School of Medicine, New Haven, Connecticut, U.S.A.

Tushar Ch. Patel, M.D.   Clinical Assistant Professor, Department of Orthopaedics and Rehabilitation, Yale University School of Medicine, New Haven, Connecticut, U.S.A.

Gregory J. Przybylski, M.D.   Associate Professor, Department of Neurological Surgery, Northwestern University, Chicago, Illinois, U.S.A.

Thomas J. Puschak, M.D.   Private practice, Seattle, Washington, U.S.A.

Louis G. Quartararo, M.D.   Assistant Professor, Department of Orthopaedic Surgery, Thomas Jefferson University Hospital and the Rothman Institute, Philadelphia, Pennsylvania, U.S.A.

Wolfgang Rauschning, M.D., Ph.D.   Professor, Department of Orthopedic Surgery, Uppsala University, Uppsala, Sweden

Bernard A. Rawlins, M.D.   Associate Professor, Department of Orthopaedics, Hospital for Special Surgery, Weill Medical College of Cornell University, New York, New York, U.S.A.

Afshin E. Razi, M.D.   Department of Orthopedic Surgery, New York University–Hospital for Joint Diseases, New York, New York, U.S.A.

Glenn R. Rechtine, M.D.   Professor, Department of Orthopaedics and Rehabilitation, University of Florida, Gainesville, Florida, U.S.A.

Paul T. Rubery, M.D.   Thomas Jefferson University Hospital and the Rothman Institute, Philadelphia, Pennsylvania, U.S.A.

Mustasim N. Rumi, M.D.   Department of Orthopaedic Surgery, Milton S. Hershey Medical Center of The Pennsylvania State University College of Medicine, Hershey, Pennsylvania, U.S.A.

Scott Rushton   University of Pennsylvania, Philadelphia, Pennsylvania, U.S.A.

Michael F. Saulino, M.D., Ph.D.   Assistant Professor, Department of Rehabilitation Medicine, Thomas Jefferson University, Philadelphia, Pennsylvania, U.S.A.

Rick C. Sasso, M.D.   Clinical Instructor, Department of Orthopaedic Surgery, Indiana University School of Medicine, Indianapolis, Indiana, U.S.A.

Arjun Saxena   Jefferson Medical College, Philadelphia, Pennsylvania, U.S.A.

Paul E. Savas, M.D.   Clinical Instructor, Department of Orthopedic Surgery, Medical College of Virginia, and MidAtlantic Spine Specialists, Richmond, Virginia, U.S.A.

Daniel M. Schwartz, Ph.D., D.A.B.N.M.   President and CEO, Surgical Monitoring Associates, Bala Cynwyd, Pennsylvania, U.S.A.

Kanwaldeep S. Sidhu, M.D.   St. Clair Orthopaedics and Sports Medicine, Detroit, Michigan, U.S.A.

Jeff S. Silber   Thomas Jefferson University Hospital and the Rothman Institute, Philadelphia, Pennsylvania, U.S.A.

Marco T. Silva, M.D.   Thomas Jefferson University Hospital and the Rothman Institute, Philadelphia, Pennsylvania, U.S.A.

Volker K. H. Sonntag, M.D.   Vice Chairman, Division of Neurological Surgery, and Director, Residency Program, Barrow Neurological Institute, Phoenix, Arizona, U.S.A.

Jeffrey M. Spivak, M.D.   Director, Hospital for Joint Diseases Spine Center, and Department of Orthopedic Surgery, New York University–Hospital for Joint Diseases, New York, New York, U.S.A.

Rajiv Taliwal, M.D.   Department of Orthopaedics, Hospital for Special Surgery, Weill Medical College of Cornell University, New York, New York, U.S.A.

Bobby Tay, M.D.   Assistant Professor, Department of Orthopaedics, University of California, San Francisco, School of Medicine, and Division of Orthopaedics, San Francisco General Hospital, San Francisco, California, U.S.A.

Alexander R. Vaccaro, M.D.   Professor, Department of Orthopaedic Surgery, Thomas Jefferson University Hospital and the Rothman Institute, Philadelphia, Pennsylvania, U.S.A.

Michael J. Vives, M.D.   Assistant Professor of Clinical Orthopedics, Department of Orthopedic Surgery, University of Medicine and Dentistry of New Jersey, Newark, New Jersey, U.S.A.

Kirkham B. Wood, M.D.   Associate Professor, Department of Orthopedic Surgery, University of Minnesota, Minneapolis, Minnesota, U.S.A.

Paulino Yanez, M.D.   Department of Neurological Surgery, Mayo Clinic and Mayo Foundation, Rochester, Minnesota, U.S.A.

Seth M. Zeidman, M.D.   Chief, Complex Spinal Surgery, Department of Neurological Surgery, University of Rochester, Rochester, New York, U.S.A.

FRACTURES OF THE CERVICAL, THORACIC, AND LUMBAR SPINE

1

Spinal Injury: Etiology, Demographics, and Outcomes

RALPH J. MARINO

Mount Sinai School of Medicine, New York, New York, U.S.A.

I INCIDENCE AND PREVALENCE

The incidence of spinal cord injury (SCI) has been estimated to be between 30 and 40 cases per million per year, or about 10,000 new cases annually (1). A recent report from a state-based registry found an incidence rate of 59 cases per million for patients in hospitals, and 77 per million including prehospital fatalities (2). There is not sufficient reporting of SCI in the United States to determine whether the incidence has changed in recent years. Prevalence of SCI has been estimated to be between 721 and 906 persons per million population, or about 183,000 to 230,000 persons in the United States (1).

II DEMOGRAPHICS

The information regarding the demographics and case descriptions of spinal cord injury patients in this chapter comes from the Model Spinal Cord Injury Systems of care funded by the National Institute on Disability and Rehabilitation Research, Office of Special Education and Rehabilitative Services, Department of Education. The Model SCI Systems program has been funded since 1970, and data collected in a national SCI database (the Database) since 1973. Over the years, the number and geographical spread of centers have varied. The Database is not population-based, so it cannot be used to determine incidence and prevalence. Demographic data represent an incidence series of cases admitted to the Model SCI Systems, which may differ from prevalence data. The Model SCI System, the Database, and limitations of the Database have been described elsewhere (3,4). Where relevant, information

1

from the Database is supplemented by data from state registries of SCI and other sources.

A   Age at Injury

Data from the Database indicate that the mean age at injury is 32.3 years [standard deviation (sd) = 15.8 years], and the median age at injury is 27 years (4). The highest incidence occurs in the 16- to 30-year-old range, with 54% of all injuries (Fig. 1) (4). The percentage of individuals over age 60 sustaining a SCI has been climbing steadily in the Database, from 4.5% during the 1973 to 1977 period to 11.5% during the 1994 to 1998 period (4). This trend reflects the aging in the general population over the same time.

B   Sex

Males sustain SCI more frequently than females by a 4:1 ratio. In the Database, 81.5% of the sample is male (4). This is a slightly higher proportion than that reported by most state registries. The proportion of males in state registries ranges from a low of 69% in Louisiana (5) to a high of 80.4% in Arkansas (6).

C   Race/Ethnicity

Of those entered in the Database since 1990, 58.1% are White, 28% are African-American, 8.4% are Hispanic, 0.4% are Native American, and 2.1% are Asian (7). These proportions are significantly different from the proportions in the general population, where 80.3% are White (8). State registries also demonstrate this disproportionate inclusion of minorities. The incidence of SCI among African-Americans is nearly twice that for Whites in Louisiana (5) and Virginia (9), while the rates were found to be similar in Mississippi (2). Where rates for minorities are increased, much of the increase has been due to greater rates of violence as a cause of SCI (6,10).

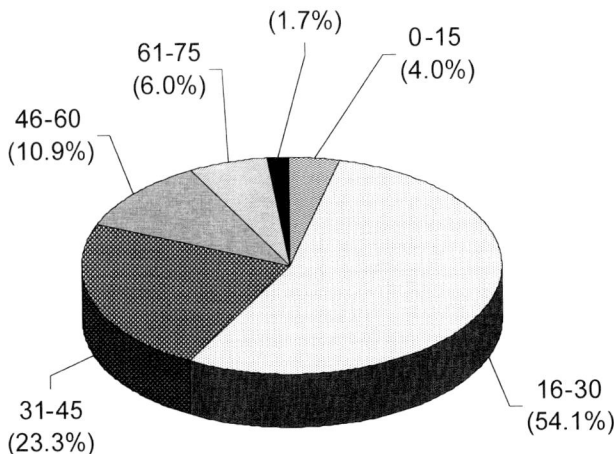

Figure 1   Age at injury. (From Ref. 4.)

III ETIOLOGY

Since 1990, the most frequent cause of SCI in the Database has been motor vehicle crash (37.4%), followed by violence (25.9%) and falls (21.5%) (Fig. 2) (7). Over time, there has been an increase in the proportion of injuries due to violence and falls and a decrease in the proportion due to motor vehicle crashes (7). Due to limitations of the Database, it is not clear whether these changing proportions are due to changes in incidence rates or other factors, such as a change in the centers that contribute to the Database or changing referral patterns. However, others have noted an increasing proportion of admissions due to violence-related SCI (11).

Etiology of SCI is influenced by age, gender, and race/ethnicity. Vehicular crash is the leading cause of SCI up to age 45, after which falls become the most common etiology (Fig. 3) (1). The proportion of injuries due to violence and sports decreases with age, while that due to falls increases. According to the Database, the leading causes of SCI for both males and females are auto accidents, falls, and gunshot wounds. However, auto accidents account for a higher proportion of injuries in females than males (51.5 vs. 31.4%) and gunshot wounds for a higher proportion in males than females (18.3 vs. 11.3%) (4). Males are more likely than females to sustain SCI as a result of diving (8.0 vs. 3.2%) and motorcycle accidents (6.1 vs. 1.7%) (4). Etiology of SCI by race is shown in Fig. 4 (4). Vehicular crash is the leading cause of injury for Whites, Native Americans, and Asians, while violence is the leading cause of injury for African-Americans and Hispanics (4).

IV SEVERITY OF INJURY

There are approximately equal proportions of people with complete and incomplete injuries in the Database, with a slightly higher percentage of persons with tetraplegia than paraplegia. Based on neurological status at discharge, SCI is classified as complete tetraplegia in 23.3%, incomplete tetraplegia in 30.2%, complete paraplegia in 26.1%, and incomplete paraplegia in 19.7% (4). The severity of injury is dependent upon etiology (Fig. 5) (4). Vehicular crash results in incomplete tetraplegia in about

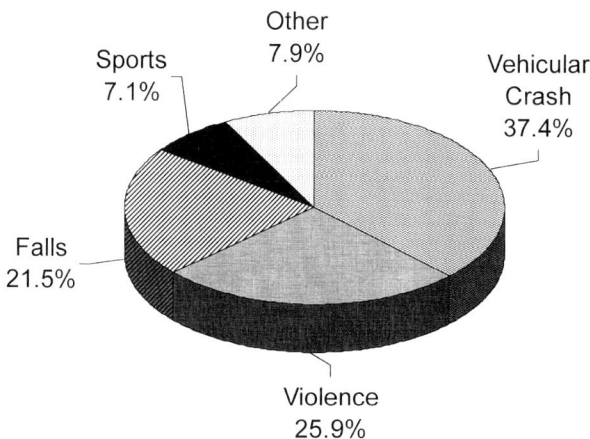

Figure 2   Etiology of SCI since 1990. (From Ref. 7.)

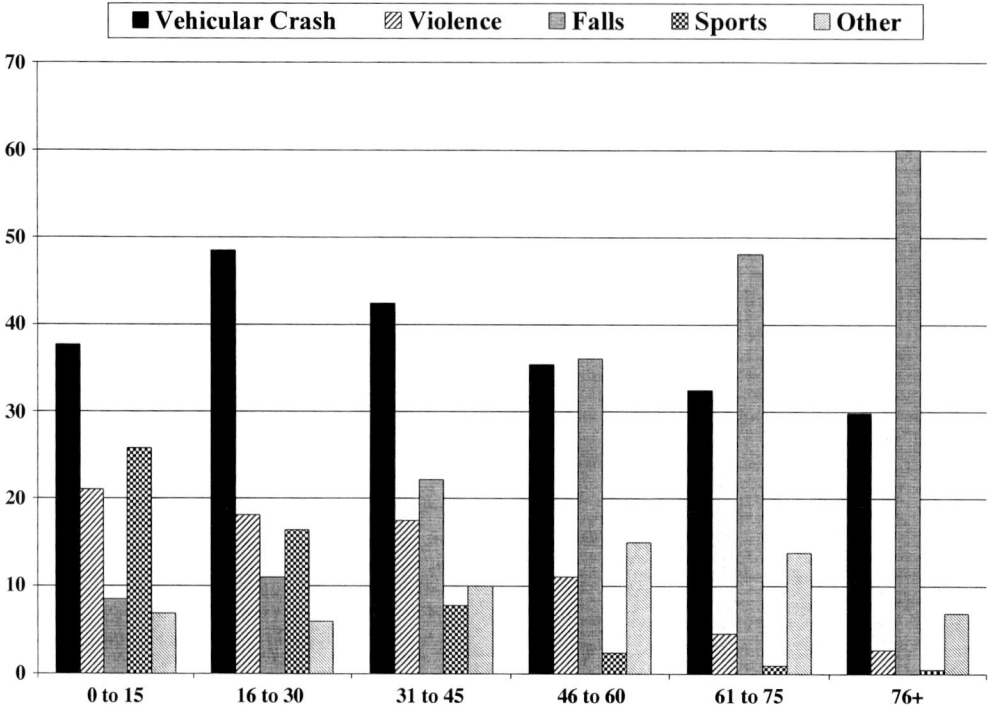

Figure 3   Etiology of SCI by age group. (Adapted from Ref. 1.)

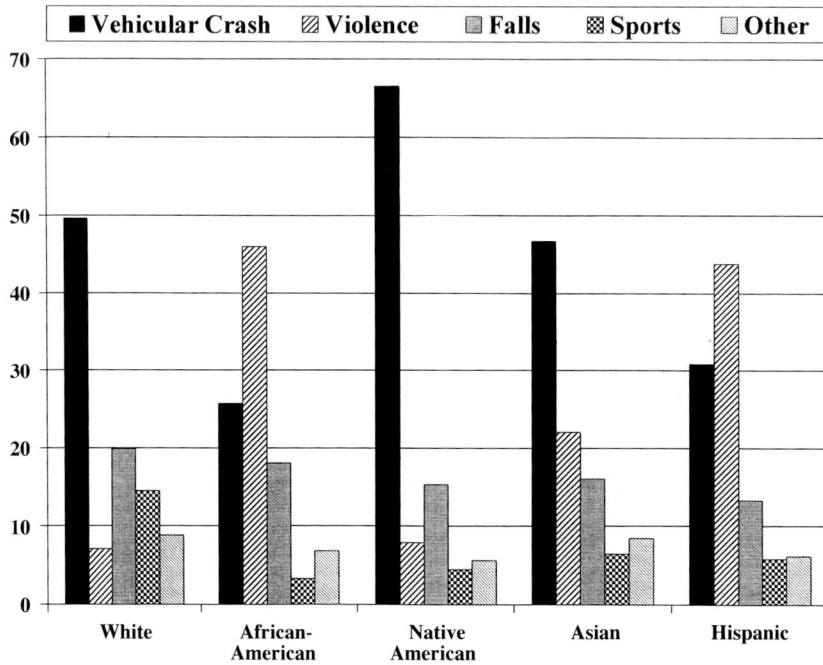

Figure 4   Etiology of SCI by racial/ethnic group. (Adapted from Ref. 4.)

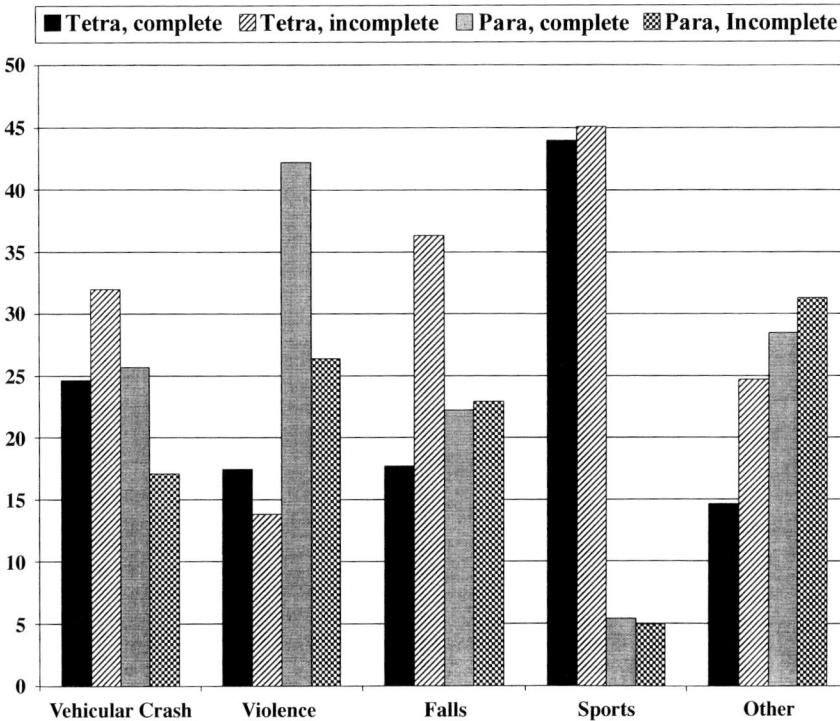

Figure 5   Severity of SCI by etiology. (Adapted from Ref. 4.)

one-third of cases, and in complete tetraplegia or complete paraplegia in 25% of cases each. Acts of violence are more likely to result in paraplegia (68% paraplegia: 42% complete, 26% incomplete), while sports injuries largely result in tetraplegia (89% tetraplegia: 44% complete, 45% incomplete) (4). Compared to nonviolent injuries, SCI caused by violence is more likely to be complete at admission and to remain complete at discharge (12).

V   COSTS

Based on 10,000 new cases of SCI yearly, the total direct cost for all causes of SCI in the United States has been estimated at $7.736 billion (13). This estimate does not include indirect costs such as lost wages, fringe benefits, and productivity, which can account for up to 65% of total aggregate costs (14). Lifetime costs vary by severity of injury and age at injury (Table 1). Higher costs are associated with more severe injuries and with younger age at injury. These data, derived from the Model Systems, may overestimate costs for incomplete SCI because they include only those individuals who required inpatient rehabilitation. Johnson et al. (15) used a state-based registry to examine costs of all SCI in Colorado (15). They found that 30% of individuals with SCI received no inpatient rehabilitation services. This is reflected in the lower average first-year cost for those with motor functional injuries, only $60,267 in 1992 dollars (15).

Table 1 Direct Costs of SCI by Severity of Injury (in 1999 dollars)

Severity of injury	Average cost first year	Average cost each subsequent year	Lifetime cost if age 25 at injury	Lifetime cost if age 50 at injury
High tetraplegia (C1-C4)	$549,800	$98,483	$2,100,185	$1,236,390
Low tetraplegia (C5-C8)	$355,037	$40,341	$1,187,507	$752,019
Paraplegia (all levels)	$200,897	$20,442	$701,716	$478,614
Motor functional (any level)	$162,032	$11,355	$468,097	$339,239

Source: National Spinal Cord Injury Statistical Center. Spinal Cord Injury: Facts and Figures at a Glance. Birmingham, AL: University of Alabama at Birmingham, 2000.

VI MORTALITY

Although life expectancy has been increasing for individuals with SCI, it still lags that of the general population, even for the least severe injuries (motor functional). Life expectancy is shorter as severity of injury and age increase, and is shortest for ventilator-dependent individuals (Table 2) (7). Individuals aged 60 and older who are ventilator-dependent have a life expectancy of only 1.2 years. Mortality is greater during the first year postinjury than in subsequent years, so that life expectancy is greater in those who survive 1 year after SCI (Table 3) (7). One-year mortality has steadily decreased since the 1970s, according to the Database. Compared to the 1973 to 1977 period, the odds of dying by 1 year postinjury for persons injured during 1993 to 1998 dropped by 67% (16).

During the first year postinjury, respiratory and cardiac-related causes account for over half of all deaths. After the first year, no single cause accounts for more than 20% of deaths. The top three causes of death after 1 year are heart disease (18.8%), external causes (18.3%), and respiratory complications (18.0%) (16). The only significant trend over time has been a decrease in deaths from urinary causes (16).

Table 2 Life Expectancy for Persons Who Survive the First 24 Hours After SCI

Age at injury (years)	No SCI	Motor functional (any level)	Para	Low-tetra (C5–C8)	High-tetra (C1–C4)	Ventilator-dependent (any level)
20	57.2	51.6	45.2	39.4	33.8	16.2
40	38.4	33.5	27.8	23.0	18.7	7.2
60	21.2	17.5	13.0	9.6	6.8	1.2

Source: National Spinal Cord Injury Statistical Center. Spinal Cord Injury: Facts and Figures at a Glance. Birmingham, AL: University of Alabama at Birmingham, 2000.

Table 3 Life Expectancy for Persons Who Survive at Least 1 Year Postinjury

Age at injury (years)	No SCI	Motor functional (any level)	Para	Low-tetra (C5–C8)	High-tetra (C1–C4)	Ventilator-dependent (any level)
20	57.2	52.5	46.2	41.2	37.1	26.8
40	38.4	34.3	28.7	24.5	21.2	13.7
60	21.2	18.1	13.7	10.6	8.4	4.0

Source: National Spinal Cord Injury Statistical Center. Spinal Cord Injury: Facts and Figures at a Glance. Birmingham, AL: University of Alabama at Birmingham, 2000.

VII SUMMARY

There are between 183,000 and 230,000 people in the United States with traumatic SCI, with about 10,000 new cases annually. While relatively infrequent, costs of SCI are high, with lifetime costs for new injuries estimated at $7.736 billion. SCI occurs predominantly in males and in the young (<30 years of age). Compared to younger individuals, older individuals are more likely to sustain SCI as a result of falls, and less likely as a result of violence or sports. African-American and Hispanic minority groups have a higher incidence of violence-related SCI than Whites. Severity of injury is influenced by etiology. Mortality is decreasing, but life expectancy continues to lag that of the general population, particularly in more severe injuries.

REFERENCES

1. Go BK, DeVivo MJ, Richards JS. The epidemiology of spinal cord injury. In: Stover SL, Delisa JA, Whiteneck GG, editors. Spinal cord injury: clinical outcomes from the Model Systems. Gaithersburg, MD: Aspen Publishers, Inc., 1995: 21–55.
2. Surkin J, Gilbert BJ, Harkey HL, Sniezek J, Currier M. Spinal cord injury in Mississippi. Findings and evaluation, 1992–1994. Spine 2000; 25:716–721.
3. Stover SL, DeVivo MJ, Go BK. History, implementation, and current status of the National Spinal Cord Injury Database. Arch Phys Med Rehabil 1999; 80:1365–1371.
4. Nobunaga AI, Go BK, Karunas RB. Recent demographic and injury trends in people served by the Model Spinal Cord Injury Care Systems. Arch Phys Med Rehabil 1999; 80:1372–1382.
5. Bayackly AR, Lawrence AW. Spinal cord injury in Louisiana. New Orleans, LA. Louisiana Office of Public Health, 1991 Annual Report. 1992.
6. Acton PA, Farley T, Freni LW, Ilegbodu VA, Sniezek JE, Wohlleb JC. Traumatic spinal cord injury in Arkansas, 1980 to 1989. Arch Phys Med Rehabil 1993; 74:1035–1040.
7. National Spinal Cord Injury Statistical Center. Spinal Cord Injury: Facts and Figures at a Glance. Birmingham, AL: University of Alabama at Birmingham, 2000.
8. U.S. Bureau of Census. Statistical abstract of the United States: 1997, 117th ed. Washington, D.C.: U.S. Department of Commerce, 1997.
9. Hickman JK. Spinal cord injury in Virginia: a statistical fact sheet. Fishersville, VA. Virginia Department of Rehabilitative Services, 1993.
10. Price C, Makintubee S, Herndon W, Istre GR. Epidemiology of traumatic spinal cord injury and acute hospitalization and rehabilitation charges for spinal cord injuries in Oklahoma, 1988–1990. Am J Epidemiol 1994; 139:37–47.

11. Farmer JC, Vaccaro AR, Balderston RA, Albert TJ, Cotler J. The changing nature of admissions to a spinal cord injury center: violence on the rise. J Spinal Disord 1998; 11:400–403.
12. Marino RJ, Ditunno JFJ, Donovan WH, Maynard FJ. Neurologic recovery after traumatic spinal cord injury: data from the Model Spinal Cord Injury Systems. Arch Phys Med Rehabil 1999; 80:1391–1396.
13. DeVivo MJ. Causes and costs of spinal cord injury in the United States. Spinal Cord 1997; 35:809–813.
14. Berkowitz M, Harvey C, Greene CG, Wilson SE. The Economic Consequences of Traumatic Spinal Cord Injury. New York: Demos Publications, 1992.
15. Johnson RL, Brooks CA, Whiteneck GG. Cost of traumatic spinal cord injury in a population-based registry. Spinal Cord 1996; 34:470–480.
16. DeVivo MJ, Krause JS, Lammertse DP. Recent trends in mortality and causes of death among persons with spinal cord injury. Arch Phys Med Rehabil 1999; 80:1411–1419.

2

Anatomy and Pathophysiology of Traumatic Spinal Cord Injury

OREN G. BLAM

Thomas Jefferson University Hospital, Philadelphia, Pennsylvania, U.S.A.

DOUGLAS M. EHRLER

Omni Orthopaedics, Canton, Ohio, U.S.A.

WOLFGANG RAUSCHNING

Uppsala University, Uppsala, Sweden

ALEXANDER R. VACCARO

Thomas Jefferson University Hospital and the Rothman Institute, Philadelphia, Pennsylvania, U.S.A.

I GROSS ANATOMY

The spinal cord extends from the foramen magnum to approximately the L1–L2 disc space. It is continuous with the medulla oblongata and terminates in the conus medullaris. Below this level the nerve roots running inferiorly are collectively called the cauda equina (Fig. 1A–D). The cauda equina runs within the spinal canal, which is bordered anteriorly by the vertebral bodies and posteriorly by the dorsal bony arch. The spinal canal measures approximately 45 cm in length in males and 42 cm in females (1). There are two enlargements in the spinal cord that run from C4 to T1 and from L2 to S3. These enlargements correspond to areas of upper and lower extremity innervation. In all there are 31 nerve roots that branch from the spinal cord (8 cervical, 12 thoracic, 5 lumbar, 5 sacral, and 1 coccygeal). In cross-section the cord is slightly flatter in the AP plane. It reaches its maximum transverse diameter between C3 and C6, which is approximately 13 to 14 mm (2).

Membranous layers covering the spinal cord are referred to as the meninges (3). The meninges consist of three layers—the dura, arachnoid, and pia mater. The dura is attached anteriorly to the posterior longitudinal ligament. The pia mater is composed of a superficial layer (epi-pia) and a deep layer (pia-glia). This pia mater

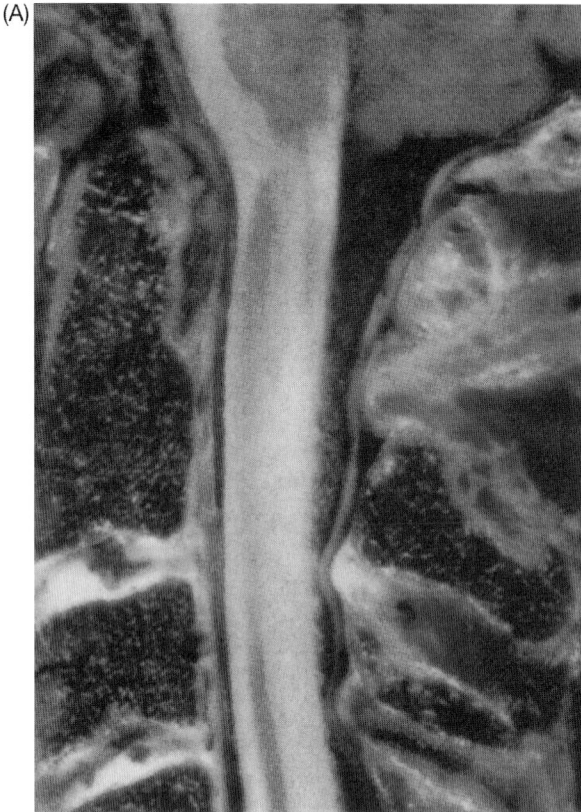

Figure 1   (A) Midsagittal section through the upper cervical spine of a 34-year-old man. The odontoid process is the most prominent structure. The synovial joint between the anterior arch of the atlas and the dens shows signs of slight degeneration. Note also the transverse portion of the cruciate ligament which holds the odontoid process posteriorly. The transverse ligament is covered by the tectorial membrane which constitutes a reinforcement of a parietal blade of the dura mater and which is continuous with the dura mater of the skull. In addition, the thin apical ligament of the dens directly anchors the tip of the dens to the clivus portion of the foramen magnum. Posteriorly, the thin atlanto-occipital membrane connects the posterior arch of the atlas with the rim of the foramen magnum.

invests the spinal cord. A small thread of the pia mater extends from the distal end of the spinal cord as the filum terminale, which connects the conus medullaris to the periosteum of the first coccygeal vertebrae.

Topographically there are six distinct grooves in the spinal cord (4) (Fig. 2). Posteriorly there is a posterior median sulcus and two posterior lateral sulci. These two posterior lateral sulci correspond to the regions of entrance for the posterior rootlets. They are referred to as the dorsal root entry zones (DREZ). Anteriorly in the midline there is an anterior median fissure in which the anterior spinal artery runs. There are two ventral lateral sulci that correspond to the exit zones for the anterior rootlets. They are referred to as the anterior root exit zones (AREZ) (5).

(B)

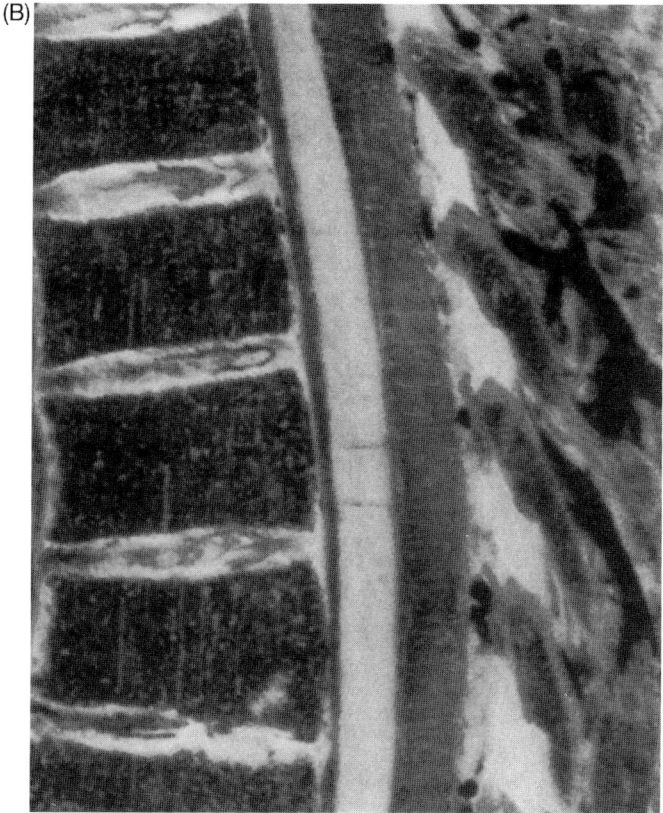

Figure 1 (B) Midsagittal section through the midthoracic spine of a 64-year old female. Due to the supine position of the cadaver, there is engorgement of the deep posterior veins. All disks show degenerative changes. The disk between T9 and T10 is completely resorbed and the cartilaginous end plates have fused. On the most spondylitic segments, the anterior longitudinal ligament is thicker than in the less degenerated segments. Normally thoracic disks have a perfectly straight posterior margin. Of note is the relationship of the laminae to the intervening ligamentum flavum. The long slender spinous processes as well as the flat wide laminae overlap like obliquely sloping shingles, completely hiding the ligamentum flavum. The latter attaches to the adjacent laminae in a consistent fashion: in the anterior surface of the lamina above and in the upper rim of the lamina below. Viewed from the spinal canal (anteriorly), only a narrow band of bone is visible; the posterior wall of the spinal canal thus is predominantly elastic-ligamentous, yet shielded by the "hidden" lamina portion. Note that the veins behind the dura (belonging to the posterior internal venous plexus) are invariably located at the level of the bony lamina, not the ligamentum flavum.

II MICROSCOPIC ANATOMY

Internally the spinal cord is divided into gray and white matter (Fig. 2). The gray matter is roughly in the shape of the letter "H" (6). It is composed of nerve cell bodies of efferent and interneural neurons arranged into distinct vertical columns, connective tissue, and vascular components. This gray matter extends the entire

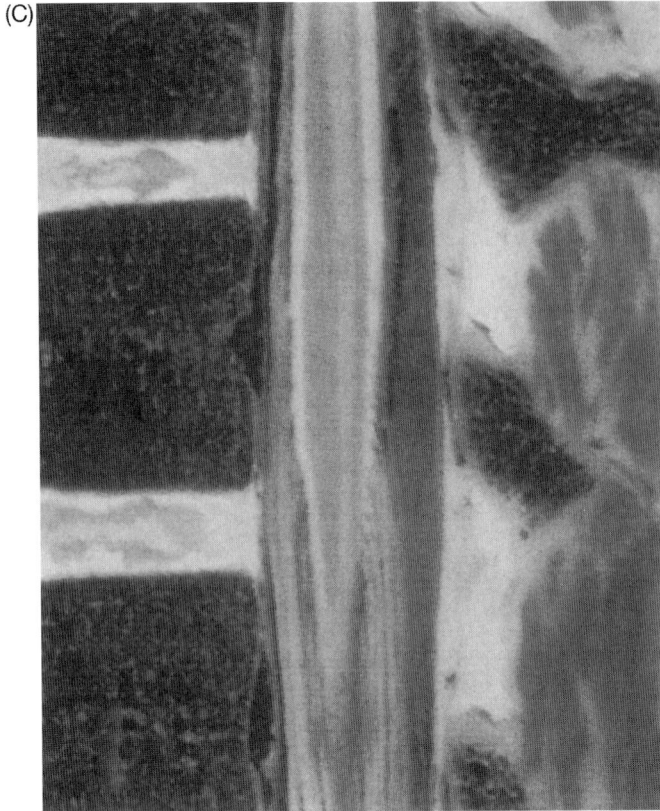

Figure 1 (C) Sagittal section in the midline through the thoracolumbar spine of a young female adult. The conus medullaris typically terminates at the L1-L2 disk level. This specimen also shows the caudal extension of the conus, the filum terminale, and also outlines the central canal of the spinal cord. The upper two vertebrae show vascular venous outlet foramina (Batson) through which the veins in the vertebral body communicate with the anterior epidural veins. Note the marked increase in disk height from the lower thoracic to the upper lumbar spine. The posterior annulus of all disks is straight, rendering the anterior wall of the spinal canal straight. The conus medullaris is surrounded by bundles of thick cauda equina roots, motor anterolaterally and sensor dorsolaterally. The intrathecal reserve space is much smaller than in the thoracic and cervical spine.

length of the spinal cord. Surrounding the gray matter is the white matter, which is composed of ascending and descending fibers in distinct tracts. The gray matter is divided into three horns, posterior, intermediate, and anterior (7). The posterior horn is composed of somatosensory neurons, interneurons, and tract cells. This posterior horn is further subdivided into three main segments. The substantia gelatinosa relays information regarding pain, temperature, and touch (7). The nucleus proprius relays information concerning proprioception, two-point discrimination, and body movement. Both of these run the entire length of the spinal cord. The nucleus dorsalis relays proprioceptive information and runs from C8 to L3.

(D)

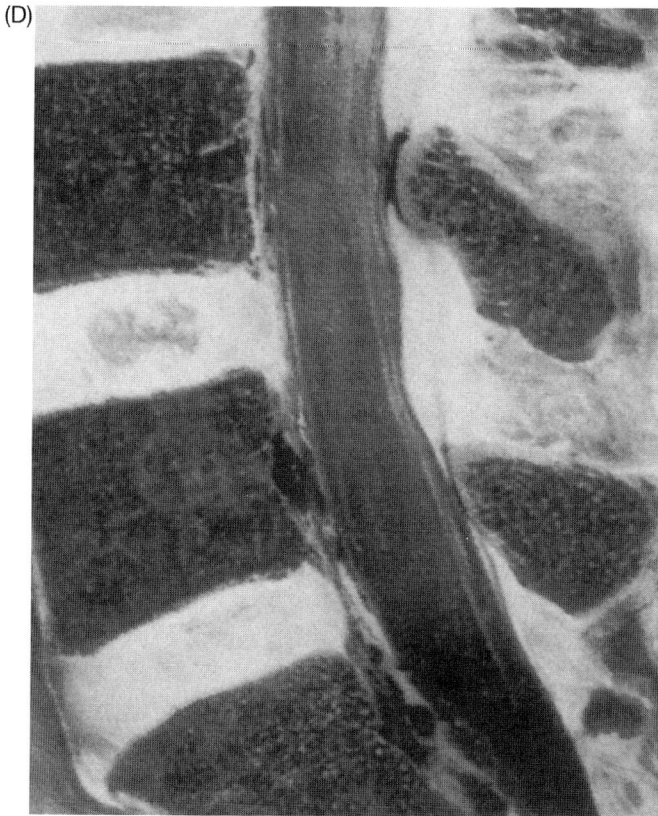

Figure 1 (D) Sagittal section through a normal lower lumbar spine and upper sacrum of a young female through the lateral portion of the thecal sac. The segmental root bundles converge toward each intervertebral foramen. The L3, L4, and L5 disks all display a slight posterior convexity, and the outermost layers of the annulus fibrosus attach beyond the apophyseal ring. The vertebral bodies typically have a concave posterior contour. In the midportion of the posterior vertebral wall at L5 a large venous vascular foramen (outlet foramen of the Batson plexus) exists through which veins traversing the vertebral bodies communicate with the ventral internal venous plexus. The laminae have a characteristic shape: toward the spinal canal only a narrow vertical band of cortical bone is exposed, superiorly the laminae have a sharp ridge, and from behind the laminae slope postero-inferiorly. The ligamentum flavum attaches superiorly to the laminae's inferior posteriorly receding surface. At the infra-adjacent lamina the ligamentum flavum attaches to the sharp upper ridge and a small area behind it. Note that the ligamentum flavum at the lumbosacral level is much thinner than at levels above.

The intermediate gray matter is composed of cells of the preganglionic sympathetic neurons from T1 to L2 (6). It also contains preganglionic parasympathetic fibers from S2 through S4.

The anterior horn gray matter contains somatomotor neurons. It is subdivided into medial, lateral, and central columns (7). All of them function to innervate muscle units (1). The medial column innervates axial, abdominal, spinal, and intercostal

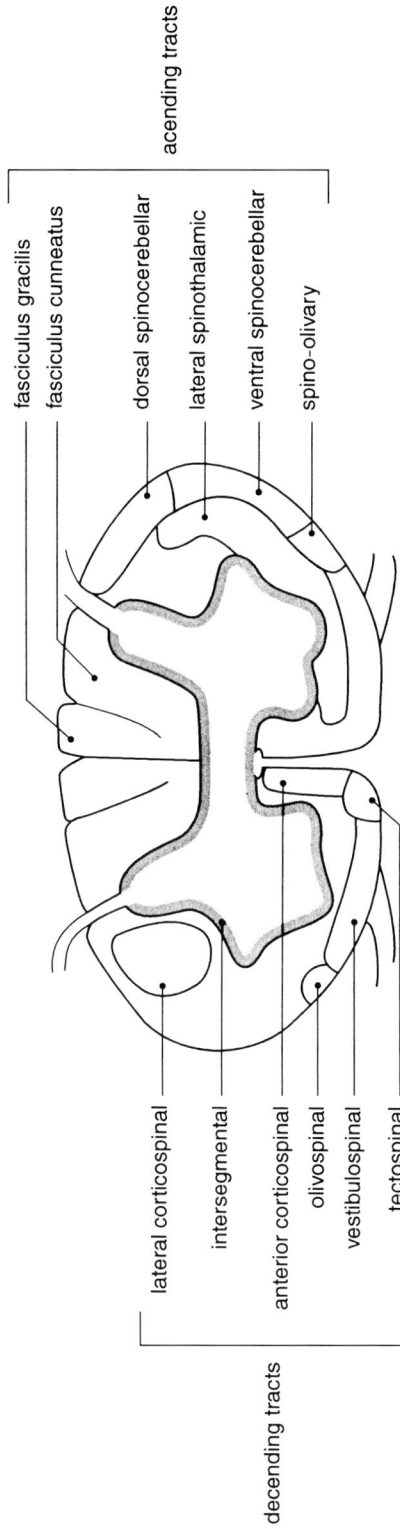

Figure 2 Cross-sectional depiction of the spinal cord. Sensory nerve roots enter posteriorly at the dorsal root entry zones, and motor nerve roots exit anteriorly at the ventral root exit zones. An anterior median fissure communicates the anterior spinal artery while a posterior median sulcus provides for a dorsal vascular channel. The H-shaped gray matter is composed mainly of neuronal cell bodies. The white matter is divided into dorsal, lateral, and ventral columns transmitting ascending and descending neuronal axons that are grouped into tracts: (1) fasciculus gracilis, (2) fasciculus cunneatus, (3) dorsal spinocerebellar, (4) ventral spinocerebellar tract, (5) lateral spinothalamic tract, (6) spino-olivary tract, (7) anterior corticospinal tract, (8) tectospinal tract, (9) vestibulospinal tract, (10) olivo-spinal tract, (11) intersegmental or propriospinal tract, (12) lateral corticospinal tract.

muscles. The central portion innervates the diaphragm. The lateral portion innervates the appendicular skeleton and is present only in the cervical and lumbosacral regions.

The white matter of the spinal cord is composed of motor and sensory nerve tracts, connective tissue, and vascular tissue (Fig. 2). These ascending and descending fibers are organized into distinct tracts. The white matter is divided into posterior, lateral, and anterior columns (1).

The posterior column lies between the posterior horns of the gray matter. It is divided centrally by the posterior median septum. Below T6 it is composed of the fasciculus gracilis and above this level it is joined by the fasciculus cuneatus (6). These two tracts are separated by the posterior intermediate sulcus on each side. They carry proprioception, vibratory, and tactile information from the lower and upper extremities, respectively (8).

The lateral column is located between the anterior and posterior root entry zones (4). It contains both ascending and descending tracts. The lateral corticospinal tract is a descending pathway relaying voluntary motor function. This is a crossed tract. The fibers are arranged so that more caudad motor fibers are located laterally. The posterior spinocerebellar tract is an ascending uncrossed tract that relays pain as well as proprioception, touch, and pressure. The anterior spinocerebellar tract is similar, only its fibers are crossed. The lateral spinothalamic tract is an ascending crossed tract relaying pain and temperature sensations. The spinotectal tract is an ascending crossed pathway relaying information of pain, temperature, and tactile sense to visual reflexes. The spinoreticular tract carries sensory input from the skin, joints, and muscles. The spino-olivary tract relays cutaneous and proprioceptive input. This area of the spinal cord also carries autonomic fibers of a descending nature to regulate visceral functions.

The anterior column lies between the two anterior root entry zones. The anterior corticospinal tract carries 10 to 15% (6) of the uncrossed pyramidal tract fibers that did not become part of the lateral corticospinal tract. The anterior spinothalamic tract carries ascending fibers relaying information regarding light touch. The tectospinal tract is a crossed tract relaying information to control reflexes in response to visual stimuli. It terminates in the upper thoracic cord. The medial and lateral vestibulo-spinal tracts are descending fibers relaying information regarding muscle control and equilibrium from inner ear and cerebellum.

III PATHOPHYSIOLOGY

Neurological dysfunction following traumatic spinal cord injury is a result of both an initial mechanical insult and ongoing processes that disrupt normal cord anatomy and function. The primary traumatic insult may cause cord transection, compression, or distraction that disrupt neuronal and glial architecture. The amount of energy applied to the cord, the specific mechanism of injury, the level of injury to the spinal cord, and patient factors including the preinjury space available for the cord and medical comorbidities all help determine the pattern and degree of neurological deficit following this primary insult (9). The secondary cascade of events then exacerbates injury to the cord and may propagate the spinal cord injury caudally or rostrally, which explains why some patients with acute spinal cord injury may experience neurological deterioration in the acute postinjury period. While the primary traumatic insult can be addressed by clinicians only through developing and implementing preventative measures, understanding the secondary processes of spinal cord injury may afford an opportunity for therapeutic intervention.

The secondary cascade was first suggested almost a century ago by Allen (10), who highlighted the deleterious effects of ongoing hemorrhage, edema, and ischemia. Secondary mechanisms have since been found to involve vascular dysfunction leading to ischemia and hemorrhage, inflammation with cellular and molecular mechanisms of continued neuronal and glial destruction, and other modes of injury including excitotoxicity and apoptosis (Fig. 3). In paralleling the discovery of these processes, it is useful to examine the pathophysiology of spinal cord injury first on a histopathological level and then on a molecular level. Agents that may intervene in some of these secondary processes give further insight into the pathophysiology of spinal cord injury.

IV HISTOPATHOLOGICAL CHANGES FOLLOWING SPINAL CORD INJURY

The first changes evident in spinal cord anatomy following traumatic injury are punctate hemorrhages in the gray and white matter within 15 min of injury. Disruption of thin-walled capillary or postcapillary venules causes bleeding, and red-cell diapedesis into the substance of the cord may result from inflammatory second messenger effects on blood vessel endothelium (11). The area involved in bleeding appears to progress centrifugally, with hemorrhagic lesions found predominantly in the gray matter but also in the white matter 3 to 5 days postinjury (12).

An edematous reaction also begins within this central area of hemorrhage and progresses outward. Presumably from inflammatory changes in endothelial leakiness, the interstitial swelling develops at first as a nonproteinacious edema. With further cell breakdown and intracellular/extracellular osmotic imbalance, the interstitial space becomes engorged with protein-rich fluid. The swelling obliterates the subarachnoid and subdural spaces. The edema and hemorrhage progress outwardly both at the level of injury as well as rostrally and caudally, which may be evident as soon as 4 h after the trauma (13).

Occlusion of small intramedullary and pial arteries and veins has been documented within 20 min of injury. Larger vessels, including the anterior and posterior spinal arteries and sulcal arteries, appear to be spared (12). The smaller vessels that do get occluded undergo a process of thrombosis and fibrinoid necrosis. The resultant ischemia helps to propagate spinal cord injury, especially in remote areas of the posterior columns where infarction may be evidenced months after the injury (12). Release of cord compression early after spinal cord injury results in a reperfusion hyperemia response. In an experimental study, longer compression times led to less hyperemia (14).

Inflammatory cells become evident in the zone of injury within several hours. Leukocytes infiltrate the site of trauma, including systemically derived inflammatory cells and local microglial-derived macrophages (15). In one study, depletion of peripheral macrophages after spinal cord injury in rats improved functional outcome, suggesting the central role of hematogenously derived inflammatory cells (16).

Cell death and dysfunction become apparent with evidence of axonal disruption, cell fragmentation, and myelin breakdown occurring within several hours of injury. Cell ultrastructural integrity and intracellular transport are disrupted, so a

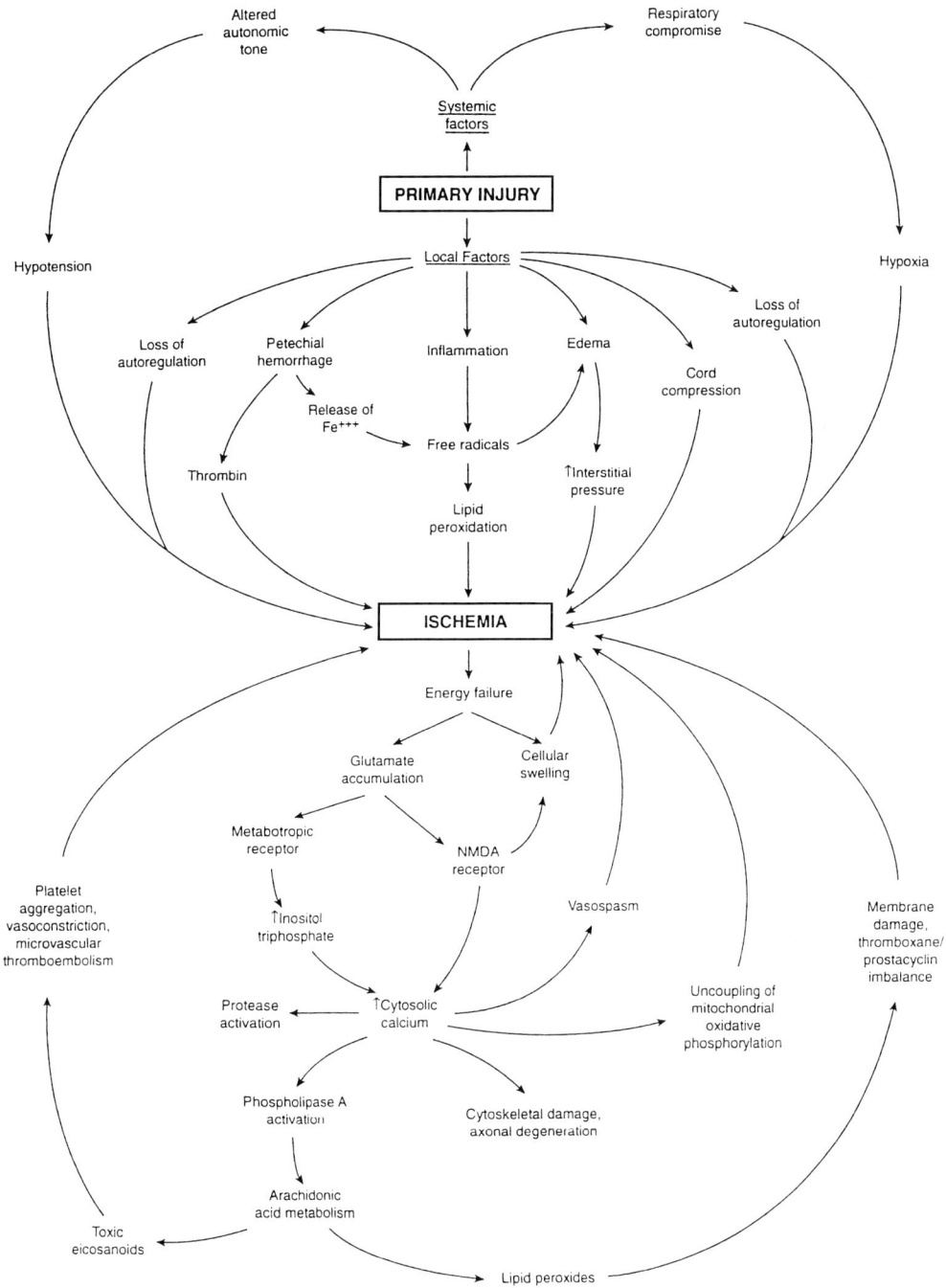

Figure 3 Schematic representation of key mechanisms, molecular species, and interrelations underlying the pathogenesis of acute SCI. Principal pathways of secondary injury that converge upon ischemia are emphasized, and others have been omitted for simplicity. These pathogenetic determinants represent the logical targets for therapeutic modulation. (Reproduced with permission from Ref. 9.)

buildup of multiple organelles is seen in axonal processes (17). Demyelination and Wallerian degeneration of long fiber tracts distant from the primary zone of injury may be observed.

These acute changes in spinal cord histopathology last from approximately 48 h to 1 week after the injury. Afterward, a decrease in interstitial edema and a resorption of cellular debris and hemorrhage occurs. As degenerated tissue is absorbed, cavitation of the cord begins centrally. In the months to years following the traumatic injury, cystic areas may coalesce to form macroscopic syrinxes filled with cerebrospinal fluid, which occur more frequently in patients with greater degrees of neurological deficit (18). Vessels occluded by clot gradually are replaced first by intimal hyperplasia and then, to a variable degree, by recanalization (19). Also, the degenerated gray and white matter are replaced with scar tissue, either from surviving astrocytes surrounding the zone of injury or from systemic fibroblast cells. The fibrous scar tissue includes the damaged spinal cord, the surrounding leptomeninges, and the contiguous vertebral periosteum. This scar tissue formation yields a sclerotic and adherent cord with obliterated subarachnoid and subdural spaces.

V MOLECULAR EVENTS FOLLOWING SPINAL CORD INJURY

Traumatic spinal cord injury induces metabolic dysregulation in neuronal, axonal, and glial tissue. Ischemia leads to energy store depletion, and ATP-dependent ion pumps fail (9). Within 5 min of severe spinal cord injury, intracellular sodium begins to increase while potassium and magnesium concentrations decrease, correlating with a decrease in axonal compound action potential transmission (a measure of axonal function). Calcium concentration and water content seem to follow the increase in intracellular sodium within 15 min of injury, leading to axonal swelling. These ionic shifts can be attenuated or arrested by sodium channel blockade with tetrodotoxin in vitro, suggesting the sodium channel as a major effector of spinal cord injury (20). Certain potassium channels also exhibit altered behavior shortly after spinal cord injury, with "fast" potassium channel blockade by 4-aminopyridine improving axonal compound axon potentials in vitro (21). The elevated extracellular potassium concentration may impede axonal signal conduction, leading to early neurological dysfunction and possibly being the etiology of spinal shock. The increased intracellular calcium may have myriad deleterious effects on calcium-dependent enzymatic pathways, including the uncoupling of mitochondrial oxidative phosphorylation thereby depleting energy stores, disrupting intracellular transport, degrading cell membranes, and generating free radicals (22). Furthermore, intracellular calcium concentration has been found to be directly proportional to the degree of tension experienced by the injured axon (23).

Expression of the inflammatory cytokine tumor necrosis factor-alpha (TNF-α) has been found to be upregulated in the spinal cord following acute spinal cord injury (24). Permeability to TNF-α across the blood–brain and blood–cord barrier increases after spinal cord injury. This increase in TNF-α transport occurs diffusely —even in the brain following a lumbar spinal cord injury—and remains saturable in experimental studies (25). Therefore, there is a diffuse upregulation of TNF-α transport rather than a local mechanical disruption of the blood–brain/cord barrier. A major effect of TNF-α is to activate the proinflammatory transcription factor NF-

κB, which upregulates various genes coding for cytokines, adhesins, and other in-flammatory agents (26).

Inhibition of TNF-α may improve functional recovery, providing evidence that TNF-α plays a central role in the inflammatory response to spinal cord injuy. Systemic administration of the anti-inflammatory cytokine IL-10 30 min after spinal cord injury can decrease TNF-α expression and improve functional recovery of injured axons in a murine model (24). Another study showed a decrease in lesion volume following systemic IL-10 administration 3 days following simulated spinal cord injury (27). Infusion of basic fibroblast growth factor, another anti-inflammatory cytokine, diminished the zone of injury following spinal cord injury; while IL-4, ciliary neurotrophic factor, and nerve growth factor showed nonstatistical trends toward reducing the zone of injury (28).

The success of anti-inflammatory steroids in improving functional recovery following spinal cord injury yields further insight into the molecular mechanisms of neurological damage. To date, only methylprednisolone treatment has been shown to be clinically effective in large multicenter, double-blinded, randomized trials (29). Progesterone administration was also neuroprotective in an experimental study (30). The proposed mechanisms by which steroids prevent neurological deterioration include decreasing the area of ischemia in the cord (31); reducing TNF-α expression and NF-κB binding activity (32); decreasing free radical oxidation and thereby stabilizing cell and lysosomal membranes; checking calcium influx into damaged cells; and reducing cord edema (9).

Stimulation of receptor-mediated enzyme pathways such as the phospholipase A2 and phospholipase C/diacylglycerol lipase systems can lead to membrane phospholipid degradation (33). Excitatory amino acid receptors may be responsible for initiating lipase and phospholipase activity as well as facilitating calcium ion disequilibrium (34); and levels of norepinephrine, epinephrine, and dopamine are increased in the zone of injury following spinal cord injury (31). Certain glutamate receptors are also involved in mediating spinal cord injury, with evidence implicating both N-methyl D-aspartate (NMDA)-sensitive (35) and non-NMDA, kainate-sensitive glutamate receptors (36).

Free radical formation within the traumatized spinal cord may further intracellular damage. Free radicals are extremely reactive and cause lipid peroxidation, structural protein oxidation, and membrane destabilization (33). Hypoxia from disrupted microcirculation may promote free radical formation, as can calcium-mediated enzyme reactions, iron ion release from red blood cell degradation, and leukocyte-mediated cytotoxicity(22).

Another recently discovered mechanism of cell death following spinal cord injury is apoptosis in the white matter. Apoptotic glial cells may be noted over a wide distribution of vertebral levels following spinal cord injury (37). Biochemical signals from injured axons, inflammatory cells, or the surrounding vasogenic edema may lead to glial autodestruction. The loss of oligodendrocytes through apoptosis is a further mechanism for axonal demyelination, thereby contributing to neurological deterioration.

Spinal cord injury is therefore an ongoing process following acute injury. Research into intervention in this secondary cascade is yielding new potential treatments for patients with spinal cord injuries.

REFERENCES

1. Nolte J. Spinal cord. In: Nolte A, ed. The Human Brain. St. Louis: Mosby-Yearbook, 1988:114–145.
2. Lang J. Clinical Anatomy of the Cervical Spine. New York: Thieme Medical Publishers, 1993.
3. Vaccaro A. Spine anatomy. In: Garfin S, Vaccaro A, eds. Orthopaedic Knowledge Update Spine. Rosemont: American Academy of Orthopaedic Surgeons, 1997:11–12.
4. Heller J, Pedlow F. Anatomy of the cervical spine. In: Clark C, ed. The Cervical Spine. Philadelphia: Lippincott-Raven, 1998:12–14.
5. Kubo Y, Waga S, Kojima T. Microsurgical anatomy of the lower cervical spine and cord. Neurosurgery 1994; 34:895–902.
6. Vaccaro A, Ahmad S, Rausching W, Garfin S. Anatomy and pathophysiology of spinal cord injury with APSCI. In: Levine A, ed. Spine Trauma. Philadelphia: WB Saunders, 1998:75–86.
7. Snell R. Clinical Neuro Anatomy for Medical Students, 3rd ed. Boston: Little Brown, 1992.
8. Gilman S, Newman S. Manter and Gatz's Essentials of Clinical Neuro-Anatomy and Neurophysiology, 8th ed. Philadelphia: FA Davis, 1992:54–97.
9. Amar AP, Levy MC. Pathogenesis and pharmacological strategies for mitigating secondary damage in acute spinal cord injury. Neurosurgery 1999; 44:1027–1040.
10. Allen AR. Surgery of experimental lesion of spinal cord equivalent to crush injury of fracture dislocation of spinal column: a preliminary report. JAMA 1911; 57:878–880.
11. Long JB, Kinney RC, Malcolm DS, et al. Intrathecal dynorphin A (1–13) and dynorphin A (3–13) reduce rat spinal cord blood flow by non-opioid mechanisms. Brain Res 1987; 436:374–379.
12. Tator CH, Koyanagi I. Vascular mechanisms in the pathophysiology of human spinal cord injury. J Neurosurg 1997; 86:483–492.
13. McVeigh JF. Experimental cord crushes with special references to the mechanical factors involved and subsequent changes in the areas affected. Arch Surg 1923; 7:573–600.
14. Carlson GD, Minato Y, Okada A, Gorden CD, Warden KE, Barbeau JM, Biro CC, Bahnuik E, Bohlman HH, Lamanna JC. Early time-dependent decompression for spinal cord injury: vascular mechanisms of recovery. J Neurotrauma 1997; 14:951–962.
15. Blight AR. Macrophages and inflammatory damage in spinal cord injury. J Neurotrauma 1992; 9:S83–S91.
16. Popovich PG, Guan Z, Wei P, Huitinga I, van Rooijen N, Stokes BT. Depletion of hematogenous macrophages promotes partial hindlimb recovery and neuroanatomical repair after experimental spinal cord injury. Exp Neurol 1999; 158:351–365.
17. Bresnahan JC, King JS, Martin GF, Yashon D. A neuroanatomical analysis of spinal cord injury in the rhesus monkey. J Neurol Sci 1976; 28:521–542.
18. Curati WL, Kingsley DP, Kendall BE, Moseley IF. MRI in chronic spinal cord trauma. Neuroradiol 1992; 35:30–35.
19. Wolfman L. The disturbances of circulation in traumatic paraplegia in acute and late stages. Paraplegia 1965; 2:231–236.
20. LoPachin RM, Gaughan CL, Lehning EJ, Kaneko Y, Kelly TM, Blight A. Experimental spinal cord injury: spatiotemporal characterization of elemental concentrations and water contents in axons and neuroglia. J Neurophysiol 1999; 82:2143–2153.
21. Fehlings MG, Nashmi R. Changes in pharmacological sensitivity of the spinal cord to potassium channel blockers following acute spinal cord injury. Brain Res 1996; 736:135–145.
22. Slucky AV. Pathomechanics of spinal cord injury. Spine: State Art Rev 1999; 13:409–417.

23. Torg JS, Thibault L, Scnnet B, Pavlov H. The pathomechanics and pathophysiology of cervical spinal cord injury. Clin Orthop 1995; 321:259–269.

24. Bethea JR, Nagashima H, Acosta MC, Briceno C, Gomez F, Marcillo AE, Loor K, Green J, Dietrich WD. Systemically administered interleukin-10 reduces tumor necrosis factor-alpha production and significantly improves functional recovery following traumatic spinal cord injury in rats. J Neurotrauma 1999; 16:851–863.

25. Pan W, Kustin AJ, Bell RL, Olson RD. Upregulation of tumor necrosis factor alpha transport across the blood-brain barrier after acute compressive spinal cord injury. J Neurosci 1999; 19:3649–3655.

26. Bethea JR, Castro M, Keane RW, Lee TT, Dietrich WD, Yezierski RP. Traumatic spinal cord injury induces nuclear factor kappa B activation. J Neurosci 1998; 18:3251–3260.

27. Brewer KL, Bethea JR, Yezierski RP. Neuroprotective effects of interleukin-10 following excitotoxic spinal cord injury. Exp Neurol 1999; 159:484–493.

28. Lee TT, Green BA, Dietrich WD, Yezierski RP. Neuroprotective effects of basic fibroblast growth factor following spinal cord contusion injury in the rat. J Neurotrauma 1999; 16:347–356.

29. Bracken MB, Shepard MJ, Holford TR, Leo-Summers L, Aldrich EF, Fazl M, Fehlings MG, Herr DL, Hitchon PW, Marshall LF, Nockels RP, Pascale V, Perot PL, Piepmeier J, Sonntag VK, Wagner F, Wilberger JE, Winn HR, Young W. Administration of methylprednisolone for 24 or 48 hours or tirilzad mesylate for 48 hours in the treatment of acute spinal cord injury: results of the third National Acute Spinal Cord Injury Randomized Controlled Trial. JAMA 1997; 277:1597–1604.

30. Thomas AJ, Nockels RP, Pan HQ, Shaffrey CI, Chopp M. Progesterone is neuroprotective after experimental spinal cord trauma in rats. Spine 1999; 24:2134–2138.

31. Daneyemez M. Silicone rubber microangiography of inured acute spinal cord after treatment with methylprednisolone and vitamin E in rats. Spine 1999; 24:2201–2205.

32. Xu J, Fan G, Chen S, Wu Y, Xu XM, Hsu CY. Methylprednisolone inhibition of TNF-alpha expression and NF-kB activation after spinal injury in rats. Brain Res Mol Brain Res 1998; 59:135–142.

33. Farooqui AA, Horrocks LA. Lipid peroxides in the free radical pathophysiology of brain diseases. Cell Mol Neurobiol 1998; 18:599–608.

34. Haghigi SS, Johnson GC, de Vergel CF, Vergel-Rivas BJ. Pretreatment with NMDA receptor antagonist MK801 improves neurophysiological outcome after an acute spinal cord injury. Neurol Res 1996; 18:509–515.

35. Yanase M, Sakov T, Fukuda T. Role of N-methyl-D-aspartate receptor in acute spinal cord injury. J Neurosurg 1995; 83:884–888.

36. Agrawal SK, Fehlings MG. Role of NMDA and non-NMDA ionotropic glutamate receptors an traumatic spinal cord axonal injury. J Neurosci 1997; 17:1055–1063.

37. Li GL, Farooque M, Holtz A, Olsson Y. Apoptosis of oligodendrocytes occurs for long distances away from the primary injury after compression trauma to rat spinal cord. Acta Neuropathol 1999; 98:473–480.

3

Biomechanics of the Injured Cervical Spine

PAUL E. SAVAS

Medical College of Virginia and MidAtlantic Spine Specialists, Richmond, Virginia, U.S.A.

I INTRODUCTION

Cervical spine injuries account for numerous disabilities and deaths in the United States annually (1). Most of the catastrophic cervical spine injuries result from head impacts when the head stops and the moving neck is forced to stop the moving torso. The forces generated are complex and can lead to a variety of cervical spine injury patterns.

To understand the mechanisms of injury and the methods of treatment for the various cervical spine injury patterns, knowledge of the functional anatomy and the physiological motion of the cervical spine is necessary.

II FUNCTIONAL SPINAL ANATOMY

The cervical spine consists of seven vertebrae with unique morphometry aligned normally in lordosis. The cervical vertebrae can function as a unit through complex interactions to provide support for the cranium, to protect vital neural structures, and to provide a wide range of motions (2).

The cervical spine may be divided into an upper cervical region, the occipitoatlantoaxial region (occiput-C1–C2), and a lower cervical region, the subaxial region (C3–C7).

The occipitoatlantoaxial complex serves as a transitional zone between the cranium and the spine. It is one of the most complex articulations in the body. The unique anatomy of the first and second vertebrae contribute to the versatile flexibility of the occipitoatlantoaxial complex.

The first cervical vertebra, atlas or C1, is a modified ring of bone. By virtue of embryological development, C1 has no central body, and has a thin posterior neural arch just posterior to the facet joints (3). This thin area of the ring is a frequent area for fractures, and is a result of a depression in the superior aspect of the ring that accommodates the vertebral artery as this artery passes between the ring of C1 and the occiput. The large lateral masses of C1 contain the concave elliptical superior articulating facets that accommodate the convex occipital condyles, and provide the only weight-bearing articulations between the skull and the spinal column. The stability of the occipitoatlantal motion segment is significantly reduced after 50% or more resection of a unilateral occipital condyle. At the occipital-cervical junction, significant hypermobility occurs during flexion/extension after a 25% unilateral condlectomy, during axial rotation after a 75% unilateral condlectomy, and during lateral bending after a 100% unilateral condlectomy (4). The inferior facets of the atlas and the superior facets of the axis are slightly convex; this allows significant flexibility at the expense of stability (5).

The second cervical vertebra, the axis or C2, more typically resembles the other cervical vertebrae. Posteriorly, the axis contains a bifid spinous process and anteriorly, the odontoid process or dens. The dens projects vertically from the superior aspect of the body of the axis and articulates with the posterior aspect of the anterior arch of the atlas.

The atlantoaxial articulation is heavily dependent on ligamentous interconnections, which collectively are referred to as the cruciate complex (6–10). As no intervertebral disk is present between the occiput and C1, nor between C1 and C2, in normal circumstances, stability is maintained in part by the ligaments of the cruciate complex. Anteriorly, the atlanto-occipital ligament or membrane, appearing as a continuation of the anterior longitudinal ligament, attaches to the anterior aspect of the body of C2. The anterior longitudinal ligament is stronger at C1-C2 than at any other level in the spine (11). Posteriorly, the posterior atlanto-occipital ligament connects the posterior ring of C1 to the posterior aspect of the foramen magnum.

The apical and alar ligaments contribute to the stability of the atlantoaxial and the atlanto-occipital joints (12,13). The apical ligament extends from the tip of the odontoid to the anterior lip of the foramen magnum. The alar ligaments consist of atlanto and occipital fibers that connect the dens to the occipital condyles and to the lateral masses of the atlas. The alar ligaments are primary restraints to axial rotation and to lateral bending in the occipitoatlantoaxial complex (6,7).

The transverse atlanto ligament is the primary restraint to anterior atlantoaxial subluxation. The tensile strength of the transverse ligament is greater than that of the alar ligaments (8).

In the lower cervical spine (C3–C7), the subaxial vertebrae have a similar appearance. Dorsal lateral superior projections of the vertebral body, called the uncinate processes, help prevent lateral displacement (14).

The facet joints in the lower cervical spine arise from the superior and inferior aspects of the pedicle. The facets tilt upward approximately 45 degrees from the horizontal. This characteristic inclination allows for flexion/extension and for lateral bending. Lateral bending is coupled with rotation (15). Any rotation of the lower cervical spine is accompanied by lateral bending in the same direction (16–18).

The facets can act as important stabilizing structures to absorb compression forces and to limit flexion. In normal motion, the facets may absorb approximately

20 to 30% of compression loads (19). In addition to resisting hyperflexion, the intact facets may resist shear forces. In experimental studies, a cervical facetectomy of more than 50% significantly compromised the shear strength of the cervical motion segment (20–22).

As in the occipitoatlantoaxial complex, stability in the lower cervical spine is enhanced by the circumferential attachments of the anterior longitudinal ligament, the posterior longitudinal ligament, and the interspinous ligaments.

A role of the cervical musculature is the production of physiological motion of the cervical spine. Several groups of muscles may be activated simultaneously to create coupled motion patterns. The musculature may resist excessive forces and may provide a neutralizing and stabilizing effect; however, the precise role of the musculature in maintaining spinal stability is not exactly clear (23,24).

III SPINAL STABILITY

The three-column theory of spinal anatomy, as in the thoracolumbar spine (25), helps to define factors associated with spinal stability.

The anatomical structures of the anterior column include the anterior longitudinal ligament, the anterior half of the annulus fibrosis, and the anterior half of the vertebral body. The middle column contains the posterior half of the annulus fibrosis and vertebral body, and the posterior longitudinal ligament. The posterior column consists of all structures posterior to the posterior longitudinal ligament.

The anatomical structures that contribute the most resistance to compressive forces are the vertebral centrum and the intervertebral disk. Biomechanical studies of the vertebral body have demonstrated compression failure occurring more consistently at the end plates (26).

The cervical disk may resist compressive and other pathological loads more effectively than do the vertebrae (19). In laboratory testing with forces evenly distributed, cervical vertebral endplate failure preceded disk failure (27,28). The cervical intervertebral disc is relatively resistant to direct shear loading, and it might provide the greatest resistance during horizontal translation. However, during all but direct compression, a portion of the disk is subjected to tensile forces (29).

In the middle column, compressive forces are transmitted through the posterior vertebral body wall to the uncovertebral joints. The uncovertebral joints can reduce primary and coupling motions, especially in response to axial rotation and lateral bending loads (30).

In a study to quantify the extent of injury to the distinct anatomical structures and spinal columns, it was observed that flexion instability correlated best with injury to the interspinous/supraspinous ligaments and the ligamentum flavum; extension instability correlated best with anterior longitudinal ligament and pedicle injury; axial rotation instability correlated best with anterior disk/endplate and capsular ligament injuries; lateral bending instability correlated best with posterior disk/endplate injuries; anterior column injuries correlated best with extension, axial rotation, and lateral bending instabilities; and posterior column injuries correlated best with flexion instability (31,32).

The complexity of the cervical vertebral interactions makes the formation of an unequivocally acceptable and standardized definition and classification of spinal stability difficult. The integrity of the anatomical and neural elements and the characteristics of spinal motion must be carefully considered. A classification system proposed by Panjabi (33) appears most comprehensive and contains parameters that may be useful for other systems of classification. Parameters and guidelines vary from region to region within the cervical spine and at each level.

In the upper cervical spine (occipitoatlantal complex) clinical instability is suggested by axial rotation to one side greater than 8 degrees, and translation of greater than 1 mm between the basion of the occiput and the top of the dens with flexion/extension. At C1–C2, instability is suggested by a lateral overhang of C1 on C2 of greater than 7 mm total, unilateral C1–C2 axial rotation of greater than 45 degrees, C1–C2 translation of greater than 4 mm between the anterior border of the dens and the posterior border of the anterior ring of C1, and less than 13 mm of space between the posterior body of C2 and the posterior ring of C1.

In the lower cervical spine, criteria for instability include anterior and/or posterior column element disruption, abnormal disk narrowing, spinal cord damage and/or nerve root damage, a developmentally narrow spinal canal (sagittal diameter less than 13 mm or Pavlov's ratio less than 0.8), sagittal plane translation greater than 3.5 mm or 20%, and/or sagittal plane rotation greater than 20 degrees on dynamic flexion/extension lateral cervical radiographs, or sagittal plane translation greater than 3.5 mm or 20%, and sagittal plane angulation greater than 11 degrees on resting cervical lateral radiographs.

Establishing the integrity of the osseous structures is simpler, since bony fractures can be demonstrated on plain x-rays or CT scans. Anterior column failure and instability may occur when there is greater than 25% loss of vertebral body height. This degree of compression can be associated with ligamentous rupture (34). Instability may also occur with bony injury to the anterior column when at least 20% of the vertebral body is sheared off in compression, as in a teardrop-type fracture (35).

Ligamentous injury cannot always be reliably detected. The extent of injury can be inferred from radiographs by the presence of abnormal angulation, translation, and separation. The annulus fibrosis and the posterior longitudinal ligament play a crucial role in providing stability. Experimentally, it can be demonstrated that the cervical spine can resist flexion forces despite sectioning of the interspinous, supraspinous, and facet capsule attachments. Not until sectioning of the posterior longitudinal ligament did sudden angulation of at least 11 degrees or translation of at least 3.5 mm occur in the cervical motion segment. This also occurred when the ligamentous complexes were sectioned from anterior to posterior under extension forces (35).

IV   DESIGNATION AND ANALYSIS OF INJURY USING FORCE VECTORS

It is difficult to clinically determine the precise force vectors that create a specific cervical injury. The primary force vector of the acute cervical spinal injury can only be inferred, since the condition of the injury mechanism is not controlled and is usually not directly observed. Soft tissue trauma to the head may be misleading, and may occur from secondary impact after spinal cord injury. Furthermore, cervical spinal cord injury has been demonstrated without craniocervical impact (36,37), and in the absence of radiographic evidence (38). For these reasons, a universally accepted classification for cervical spine fractures and dislocations does not exist.

Controlled laboratory experiments have demonstrated that isolated force vectors such as flexion, extension, vertical compression, lateral flexion, rotation, and/or a combination of these can produce isolated injuries specific to the force vector (39–42). Most likely, the injury results from multiple simultaneous forces that are resolved into a predominant vector, rather than by a single isolated injury force. Classifications of injury based on a predominant injury force vector have been established (43) and can in part be explained using a three-dimensional coordinate system with sagittal, horizontal, and frontal axes (44,45).

The column concept of the spine is valuable in understanding the pathophysiology and mechanistic action of the force vectors producing the cervical spine injuries. A predominant flexion force vector causes compression of the vertebral body and disc (anterior and middle columns) and simultaneous distraction of the posterior elements (posterior column). Conversely, a hyperextension force vector causes simultaneous distraction of the anterior column and simultaneous compression of the posterior column. This indicates a dynamic and reciprocal action that involves all the columns of the spine. Despite this, however, a single force vector, such as flexion, may cause different types of injuries that may be grouped together. It should also be reasonably noted that a direct relationship between the magnitude of a causative force and the type of injury may be present (i.e., the greater the force, the more severe the injury) (46).

V CLINICAL BIOMECHANICS OF SPECIFIC CERVICAL SPINE INJURIES

A Flexion Injuries

Flexion injuries are caused by a predominant force vector exerted axially primarily in the region of the anterior elements. Forward translation and/or rotation of the cervical vertebrae may occur in the sagittal plane. Simultaneous compression of the anterior column and distraction of the posterior column of the spine occur (47).

B Simple Wedge Compression Fractures

A hyperflexion force sufficient to cause impaction of one vertebra against an adjacent vertebra may cause this type of fracture. Minimal deformations suggest a midline, axially directed force of low magnitude (48). A compression fracture with central depression probably results from a greater force in which the intervertebral disk, as a wedge, is driven through the end plate into the vertebral body (49). During axial compression testing, 88% of the applied load passed through the disk, and maximum intradiskal pressure occurred in flexion with axial compression (50).

C Clay-Shoveler's Fractures

A clay-shoveler's fracture is an avulsion fracture of the spinous process. It occurs most commonly at C7 (51). This fracture develops when the head and upper cervical spine are forced into flexion and overcome the opposing action of the interspinous ligaments.

D   Anterior Subluxation (Ligamentous Hyperflexion Strain)

Hyperflexion and simultaneous distractive forces during rapid head acceleration or deceleration can cause tensile failure of the posterior osseous-ligamentous structures. Progressive ligamentous injury can occur from posterior to anterior and can contribute up to a 30 to 50% incidence of delayed instability (52). Minor sprains may be painful but have minimal long-term consequence. Major ligamentous injuries are highly unstable; their diagnosis may be initially missed or frequently delayed, because initial radiographs are interpreted as negative. Plain radiographs may show only subtle signs of instability: local kyphosis, angulation of adjacent endplates at a single level, or interspinous widening. A supine cross-table lateral x-ray may not reveal injury, because the supine position places the neck in extension which may reduce the deformity. Dynamic flexion/extension radiographs should be avoided, as they may cause dislocation and spinal cord injury. CT with sagittal reconstruction and MRI with fat suppression techniques may be useful in identifying posterior ligamentous injuries (53).

E   Teardrop Fractures

The major injury forces in the teardrop fracture appear to be acute flexion and compression with the spine in an attitude of flexion (54–58). In contradistinction, strong vertical forces applied to the neck in a straightened position create burst-type fractures. Shearing forces across the intervertebral disk and retrolisthesis of the vertebral body into the spinal canal can occur (59). Tensile failure of the posterior osseous-ligamentous structures can cause interspinous separation and fracturing of the lamina and spinous processes. The posterior longitudinal ligament usually is preserved and it may guide realignment during fracture reduction.

Stages of this type of compression-flexion injury have been proposed (54). Stage I injuries consist of blunting of the anterior superior vertebral margin of the vertebral body with no evidence of failure of the posterior ligaments. Stage II injuries show changes as seen in Stage I and, in addition, wedging of the anterior vertebral body and loss of height of the anterior centrum. A "beak" appearance of the anterior inferior vertebral body results. In Stage III lesions, the beak is fractured, and a fracture line passes obliquely from the anterior surface of the vertebral body through the inferior subchondral endplate. With further force, a Stage IV lesion develops having less than 3 mm of displacement of the posteroinferior margin into the spinal canal. In Stage V injuries, there is evidence of posterior ligament disruption and more significant retropulsion into the spinal canal. The higher stages represent unstable injuries and are frequently associated with spinal cord injuries. Complete spinal cord injury has been observed in 25% of Stage III injuries, 38% of Stage IV injuries, and 91% of Stage V injuries (54).

Compression-flexion teardrop injuries should be differentiated from an avulsion fracture of the anterior inferior corner of the vertebral body caused by hyperextension. The avulsion-type teardrop fracture is usually stable and should not be confused with the highly unstable flexion teardrop fracture.

F   Flexion-Distraction Injuries

Flexion-distraction injuries represent a continuum of ligamentous injuries. They range from sprains or minor tears of the interspinous ligaments and the facet capsules, to more severe, unstable injuries that involve complete disruption of the ligamentous structures and disk and result in subluxations, dislocations, and fracture/dislocations of the facets and posterior elements.

Bilateral facet subluxation results from a flexion distraction force, usually without a rotational component; it results in a sprain of the posterior cervical ligaments. There may be a partial disruption of the interspinous ligaments as well as a partial disruption of the facet capsules. Widening between the spinous processes locally may be detected on a flexion radiograph. The facet joints may be subluxated superiorly and anteriorly, and may result in slight kyphosis of less than 10 degrees on a lateral radiograph (60).

The next stage of injury is the bilateral "perched" facet. This injury represents a progression of the previous flexion-distraction mechanism. The inferior articular process translates superiorly and anteriorly until the inferior tip of the facet comes to rest on the top of the superior facet below. A local segmental kyphosis results, a complete rupture of the facet capsules and the interspinous ligaments occurs, and there may be partial disruption of the ligamentum flavum and posterior annulus. The force between the tips of the perched facets is usually considerable, and little motion is detected on dynamic flexion extension radiographs.

Bilateral facet dislocation injuries represent the terminal progression of the predominant hyperflexion force vector. Considerable tensile loading of the posterior elements causes significant ligamentous disruption all through the functional spinal unit. This causes the facets to ride up and be displaced superiorly and anteriorly. In approximately 30 to 50% of these cases, an associated traumatic disk herniation develops (61,62). The disk disruption creates an anterior column flexion instability that must be considered when reconstruction of the posterior tension band is performed to resist flexion. Any significant asymmetrical forces can contribute to lateral bending and to axial rotation; this creates a more dominant unilateral injury rather than a bilateral dislocation. Fractures of the posterior elements, such as laminar fractures, spinous process fractures, and facet fractures may be observed in more than 50% of cases. Vertebral artery injury and occlusion have been detected by angiography in approximately 50 to 60% of patients with facet dislocation (63). When enough force is present to create translation of greater than 50%, patients are at increased risk of having spinal cord injury and/or progression of their neurological deficits.

G Flexion-Rotation

A flexion-rotation mechanism more commonly leads to unilateral ligamentous injuries that are less common than bilateral ligamentous hyperflexion distraction-type injuries. They differ from their bilateral counterparts since a rotational force vector is present. The degree of rotational deformity increases proportionately with the amount of disruption and translation of the facet. That is, with less rotational force, subluxation results rather than a unilateral dislocation.

H Unilateral Facet Dislocations

A unilateral facet dislocation results from an exaggeration of the physiological coupling motion of the cervical spine. In normal circumstances, lateral bending is coupled with axial rotation. During injury, an exaggeration of flexion, lateral bending, and axial rotation results in a unilateral subluxation or dislocation. The combination of simultaneous flexion-distraction and rotational forces, when most severe, can cause complete disruption of the facet capsule, attenuation of the interspinous ligaments, and partial disruption of the posterolateral corner of the disc and uncinate process. Translation is approximately 25% and, in general, is less than that observed in bilateral facet dislocations.

When significant shear and/or vertical compression force components are added to the predominant flexion-rotation injury vector, unilateral facet fractures, bilateral facet fractures, unilateral fracture dislocations, and fracture-separation of the lateral mass may occur (64).

I Bilateral Facet Fractures

Unlike the ligamentous injuries involving the cervical facets and lateral masses, facet fractures do not represent a continuum of the injury mechanisms. Fractures may occur bilaterally involving the superior articular processes, the inferior articular processes, or a combination of the two (65). These fractures develop from a mechanism of injury involving slight flexion and translation. If the shearing action is severe, disruption of the posterior longitudinal ligament and disk may occur. Bilateral inferior facet fractures occur more commonly with lesser shear forces as compared with bilateral superior facet fractures. In both types of fractures, the interspinous ligaments are stretched but not completely disrupted. Tensile loading of the posterior elements during the flexion force may lead to disruption of the ligamentum flavum, to spinous process fractures, or to laminar fractures (66). Unlike the facet dislocations resulting from ligamentous injury, the facet capsule in general is not disrupted, and the instability occurs through the bony fracture margins of the facet complex. The resulting instability patterns are in bidirectional rotation and anterior translation.

J Unilateral Facet Fractures

Unilateral facet fractures are distinct types of injuries, with slightly different mechanisms of injury. Inferior, superior, and/or lateral mass separation-type fractures may occur.

1 Superior Facet Fracture

A superior facet fracture is the most common type of facet fracture (64). The mechanism of injury is predominantly rotation in slight flexion. The capsule of the injured facet is usually intact and, as a result, may carry a displaced fragment into the neural foramen. Disruption of the posterior superior corner of the intervertebral disk may also occur. The capsule of the contralateral noninjured facet remains intact, and there may be stretching of the interspinous ligaments.

2 Inferior Facet Fracture

An inferior facet fracture is also a flexion-rotation injury. The involved facet capsule is usually disrupted, and a posterior greenstick fracture of the facet develops. The resulting instability is predominantly rotational with a minimal flexion component (64).

3 Fracture Separation of the Lateral Mass

The mechanism of injury in this type of fracture, unlike the other two types of facet fractures, is usually extension-rotation. The predominant injury force is rotational. The rotational movement can produce instability at more than one level (65). Most of the instability occurs at the level of the fracture or at the level below the fracture separation (60). A pedicle fracture, and a vertical laminar fracture with associated injury to the facet capsules develop. A true dislocation at one level or at two levels may result, and a free-floating lateral mass can be observed. Various combinations of injury patterns may develop: two-level fracture separations of the lateral mass, two-level unilateral facet fractures, or alternate-level injuries.

K Flexion-Lateral Bending

Rarely does a cervical spine injury result from a predominant lateral flexion or lateral bending injury force vector. Because of the physiological coupling motion in the cervical spine, a lateral flexion force vector is usually accompanied by a rotational force vector, and acts as a modifying injury force rather than as a primary injury force. An uncinate process fracture may be the only discrete fracture resulting from lateral flexion of the cervical spine (57). In cases where lateral displacement occurs, as in a Jefferson fracture, the lateral displacement may be attributable to a simultaneous vertical compression force.

L Hyperextension Injuries

Hyperextension injuries of the cervical spine are not uncommon (66,67). Forced hyperextension is the common mechanism of injury. The predominant injury force vector is usually a direct frontal blow to the head, or through an acceleration/deceleration mechanism.

During hyperextension, the posterior spinal elements experience compressive forces. Distractive tensile forces coupled with shearing forces cause disruption of the anterior longitudinal ligament, separation of the intervertebral disc at the vertebral end-plate junction, disruption of the posterior longitudinal ligament, fracture or dislocation of the facets, and posterior displacement of the vertebral centrum (54). When the injury develops primarily through the soft tissue structures, the overall residual deformity may have a normal or near-normal appearance (68). This may increase the chance of not detecting a serious and unstable spinal injury.

Neurological injury is not uncommon in hyperextension injuries (69). In patients with congenital spinal stenosis and/or cervical spondylosis, spinal cord compression can occur during hyperextension. During hyperextension, the area of the spinal canal is decreased, the spinal cord is shortened, and direct pressure is placed on the spinal cord by encroaching degenerative osteophytes, a posterior bulging disc, and an invaginating ligamentum flavum. Spinal cord necrosis may occur and may lead to a central cord syndrome (70).

M Atlas Fractures

When the predominant injury force vector is hyperextension, fractures of the posterior arch of C1 may occur (71). During hyperextension at the C1–C2 articulation, the anterior arch of C1 is compressed against the dens. The posterior arch of C1 is compressed between the impinging occiput and the posterior elements of C2. The bending moment applied to the atlas increases the tensile forces through the ring, and fractures develop at the areas of least resistance—the thin bone of the bilateral groove for the vertebral artery. This mechanism of injury may also result in associated injuries such as a traumatic spondylolisthesis of the axis and an anterior teardrop fracture of C2. A hyperextension avulsion fracture of the anterior arch of C1 may occur as tensile forces are increased at the insertion site on C1 of the longus colli and the anterior longitudinal ligament (71).

When lateral bending and axial rotation force vectors simultaneously overpower the hyperextension force, asymmetrical injuries of the atlas, such as a lateral mass fracture, may develop. These combined forces may cause displacement of the lateral mass without displacement of the entire ring of C1. Other types of C1 fractures that may develop from these combined injury forces include an ipsilateral anterior and posterior arch fracture, a unilateral anterior arch fracture, a simple and/or comminuted lateral mass fracture, and a transverse process fracture (72–74) (Fig. 1).

When predominantly vertical axial compression forces are applied to the atlas, a burst fracture, the Jefferson fracture, occurs.

N   Hyperextension Teardrop Fractures

Hyperextension teardrop fractures can be confused with the more common flexion teardrop fracture. Radiographically, a small bony fragment appears displaced from the anterior vertebral body endplate. The avulsion is thought to occur through the fibrous attachments of the annulus to the end plate. Associated posterior element fractures may occur, but the midsagittal body fracture of the flexion teardrop fracture is absent (75).

O   Axis Fracture (Hangman's Fracture)

The pathogenesis of traumatic spondylolisthesis of the axis, a fracture through the C2 pars interarticularis, has been studied extensively.

Experimental and clinical studies have demonstrated that the initial injurious force is predominantly hyperextension with axial loading (76). During injury, tensile forces through the anterior longitudinal ligament, the intervertebral disk, and the posterior longitudinal ligament are balanced by compression forces through the posterior elements. When the hyperextension and axial loading forces overcome this balance, shearing forces produce fractures through the C2 pars interarticularis, the weakest and most susceptible region to fatigue failure in this instance. If a significant

Figure 1   An illustration of various types of fractures of the atlas. (A) An axial projection of the atlantoaxial complex illustrating certain ligamentous and bony structures. (B) A fracture through the posterior arch, bilaterally. (C) A four-part burst fracture. (D) An avulsion fracture of the anterior inferior arch resulting from hyperextension. (E) A comminuted lateral mass fracture. (F) An ipsilateral fracture of the anterior and posterior arches. (G) An isolated unilateral anterior arch fracture. (H) A simple unilateral fracture of the lateral mass. (I) An ipsilateral transverse process fracture. (From Ref. 74a.)

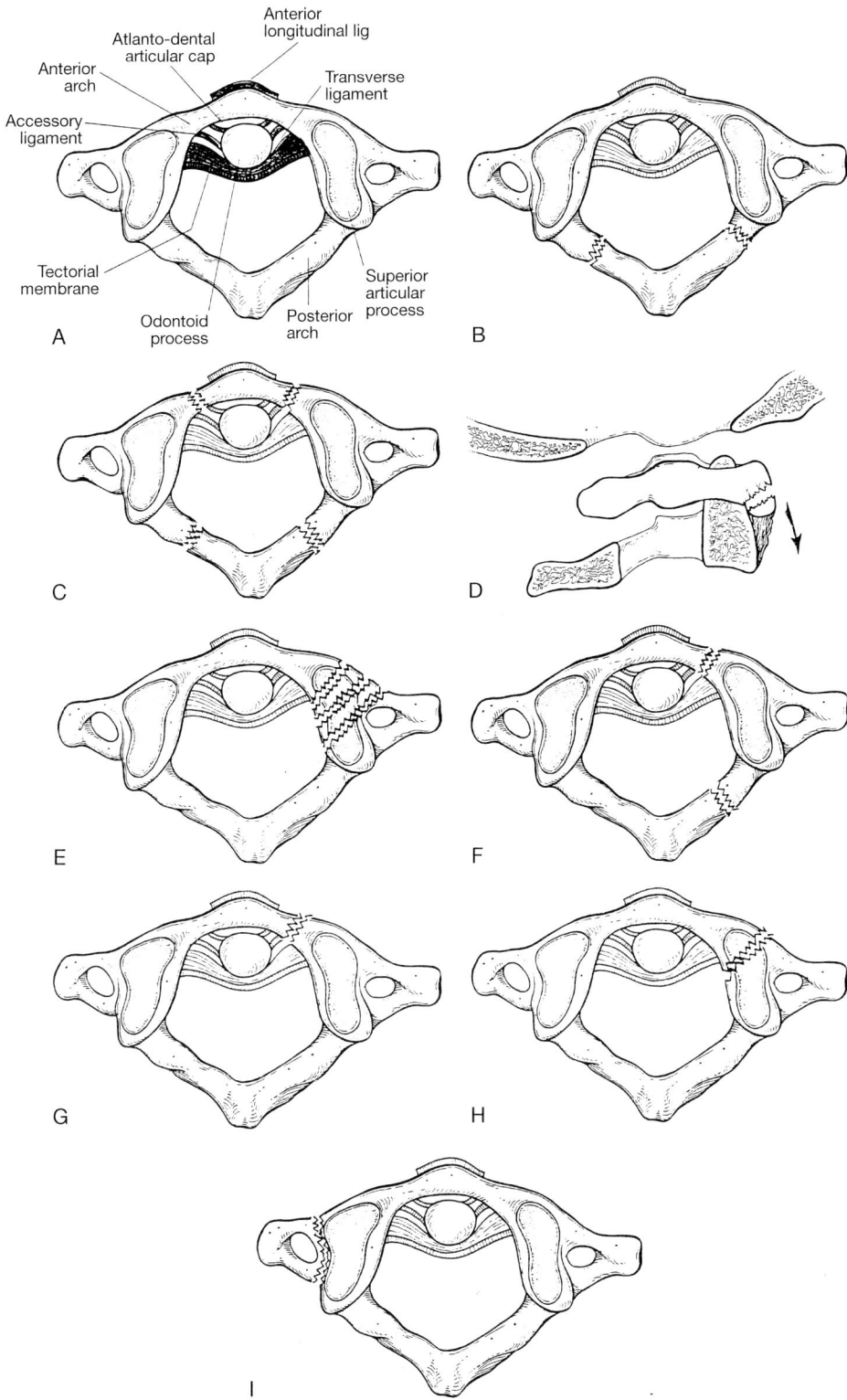

A Anterior arch, Anterior longitudinal lig, Atlanto-dental articular cap, Transverse ligament, Accessory ligament, Tectorial membrane, Odontoid process, Posterior arch, Superior articular process

lateral bending force component is present, an asymmetrical unilateral neural-arch fracture may develop. In the case of bilateral fractures, an uncommon oblique fracture may propagate through the vertebral body of C2 sparing injury to the ipsilateral neural arch. Angulation and translation result from flexion or distraction that follows the hyperextension force that caused the fracture. This propagating flexion-distraction mechanism, from a posterior to anterior direction, can cause disruption of the annulus fibrosis (77). The anterior longitudinal ligament may rupture from tensile forces propagated by the hyperextension force.

Various combinations of associated fracture patterns involving the facets and pedicles can occur. The most common variation is a bipedicular fracture with bilateral facet dislocation. Most likely, a flexion-distraction force produces the bilateral facet dislocation, and the hyperextension force causes the pars interarticularis fractures. A useful classification (72,73) describes the injured anatomical structures, the mechanism of injury, the sequence of injury, and provides guidance for management options (Fig. 2).

Traumatic spondylolisthesis of C2 on C3 may be caused not only by a Hangman's fracture but by other fractures, such as bilateral facet or laminar fractures. These fractures usually result from flexion-distraction or shear forces, and may be associated with ligamentous injuries as well as other fractures.

P   Whiplash

Whiplash injuries, or acceleration-deceleration injuries of the cervical spine, represent a syndrome of various clinical circumstances and abnormalities that may not be obvious at initial or follow-up examinations. Classically, the clinical history is of a rear-end vehicular accident.

The exact mechanism of whiplash injury is not clear and numerous factors influence the extent of injury (78). At impact, it appears that the head moves first into flexion and then, within 0.2 s, into extension (79). However, this initial pattern of head motion during injury is debated (80). During impact, the cervical spine and the remainder of the body are accelerated forward while the head remains behind, held in its resting position by its own inertia (81). The sudden forward pull by the trunk creates shear forces through the neck and the lower cranium "whipping" the head forcefully backward and causing extension of the cervical spine. Likewise, with sudden deceleration of the body, the head moves into a forward or anterior position and then recoils into extension (82).

Motion analysis from simulated testing of the cervical vertebrae during whiplash reveals distinct patterns of vertebral motion during impact. C6 rotates into extension and the upper cervical spine moves into initial flexion. Maximum rotation of C6 induces C5 to extend. With the upper cervical motion segments in flexion and the lower segments in extension, the cervical spine assumes an S-shaped posture, and C5–C6 exhibits an open-book motion with an upward-shifted instantaneous axis of rotation (83).

Injuries to capsular and spinal ligaments may be part of the mechanism contributing to the whiplash symptom complex. During whiplash simulation testing, peak strains of the capsular ligaments occurred at the C6–C7 level (84).

Motion of the head and the loads causing whiplash can be affected by preventive safety factors. An appropriately constructed and positioned headrest at the levels

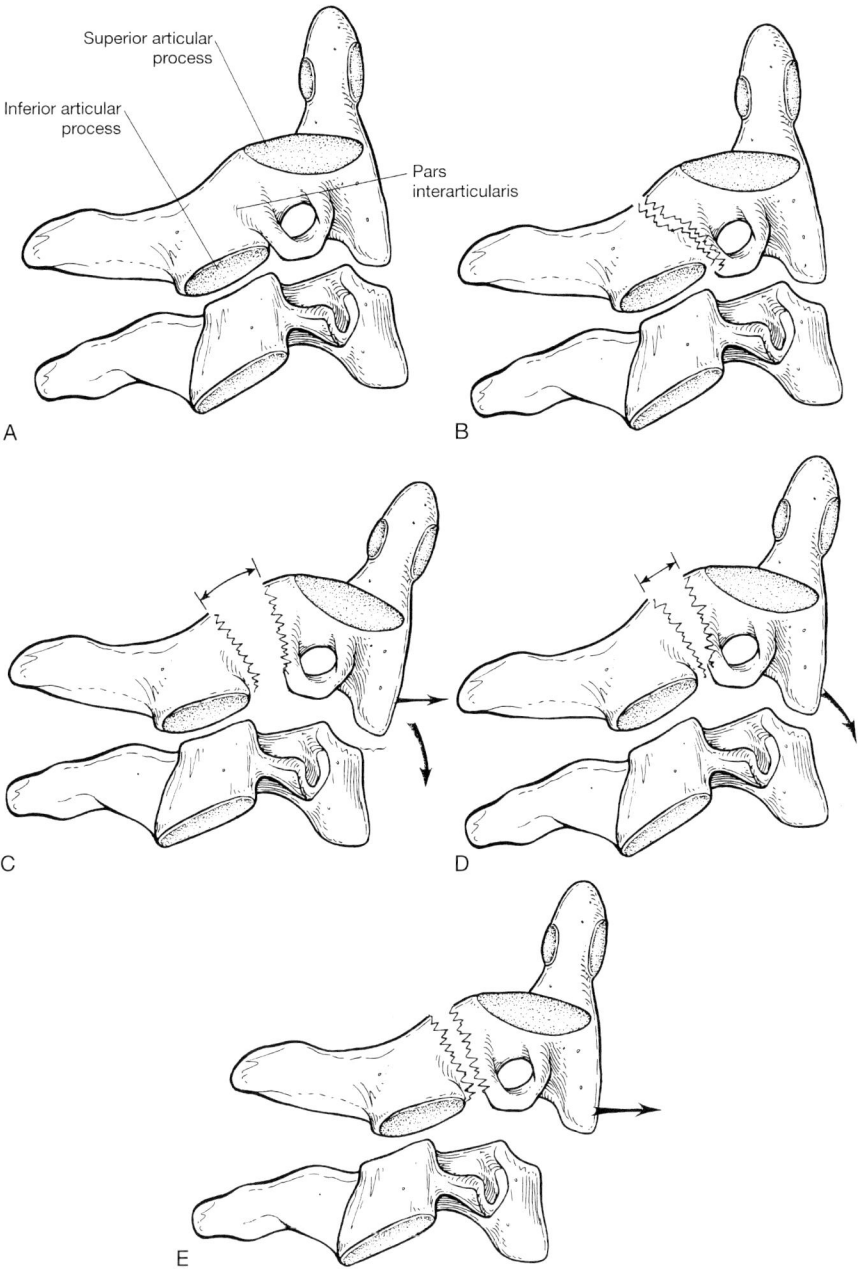

Figure 2 An illustration of different types of atlas fractures that may lead to traumatic spondylolisthesis. (A) Normal anatomical relationships of the atlas to C3. (B) A fracture through the pars interarticularis, bilaterally, without angulation and/or anterior translation. (C) A pars interarticularis fracture with anterior displacement and significant angulation. (D) A pars interarticularis fracture with significant angulation without anterior translation. (E) A pars interarticularis fracture with anterior translation leading to a unilateral or bilateral facet dislocation of C2 on C3. (From Ref. 72.)

of the ears can limit extension. A seat-belt shoulder strap can restrain and decrease the acceleration forces of the torso, thereby decreasing the inertial forces on the cervical spine. A stiffer car seat can also decrease the acceleration of the torso; this minimizes the shear forces and the bending stresses in the neck (82).

An airbag restraint system may reduce fatalities in frontal vehicular crashes. Few data exist to document specific fracture patterns after airbag deployment. In a small study (85), it was found that non-seat-belted drivers demonstrated flexion injuries of the cervical and thoracic spine and direct impaction fractures to the face and sternum. One lap-shoulder-belted driver demonstrated an extension injury of the upper cervical spine.

Q   Odontoid Fractures

High-energy trauma and motor vehicle accidents are the most common causes of adult odontoid fractures (86,87). The odontoid fracture might not be diagnosed during the initial emergency room evaluation because of diverting factors such as facial trauma, altered mental status, head injury, and other associated injuries of high-energy trauma. Low-velocity falls may more commonly cause odontoid fractures in children and the elderly. In the elderly, myelopathic symptoms may be caused by an occult odontoid fracture (88).

Concomitant cervical spine injuries, such as a Jefferson fracture, may occur in approximately 18% of patients with odontoid fractures (89).

Various mechanisms have been suggested for odontoid fractures, such as hyperflexion, hyperextension, axial compression, rotation, shear, and lateral bending (90–92). From experimental studies, it appears that the predominant mechanism is a combination of axial compression and horizontal shear (93).

Anterior displacement of the odontoid occurs more frequently than posterior displacement, except in the elderly. When a hyperflexion force is present, an intact transverse ligament may be involved in translating the odontoid anteriorly; when hyperextension is present, the anterior ring of the atlas may displace the odontoid posteriorly (8).

When rotational forces are applied, an avulsion fracture of the odontoid tip may occur. This type of odontoid fracture represents an avulsion injury to the alar ligaments and cranial cervical ligamentous complex rather than a direct injury to the tip of the odontoid (94). An oblique odontoid tip avulsion fracture is a relatively uncommon odontoid injury, and it most likely results from injury to the alar ligament rather than to the apical ligament. This fracture can be confused with the rare ossiculum terminale, the secondary center of ossification.

The most common odontoid fracture develops at the waist of the odontoid just superior to the body of the axis. This fracture has the highest rate of nonunion for odontoid fractures. The high rate of nonunion and poor prognosis may be related to the age of the patient, to a delay in diagnosis (greater than 7 days), to the direction of displacement (posterior greater than anterior), to the degree of translation (greater than 2 mm), and to the degree of comminution injuring the extraosseous and intraosseous anastomotic vasculature (95,96).

Another type of odontoid fracture is one that propagates through the body of C2. Contrasted with the waist-type dens fracture, a larger fracture surface area of bleeding cancellous bone with this type of fracture accounts for the relatively higher rates of union (97).

When an odontoid fracture develops, strong simultaneous additional forces to vertical compression and horizontal shear may lead to associated injuries such as fractures of the ring of C1, traumatic spondylolisthesis of C2, and traumatic atlantoaxial (C1–C2) subluxations and dislocations.

R   Atlantoaxial Subluxations and Dislocations

The mechanism of these types of injuries is related to any pathological process that compromises the C1–C2 ligamentous structures and causes an abnormal relationship between the ring of C1 and the ring of C2. The main causes are trauma or inflammation.

In traumatic cases, either anterior or posterior abnormal displacement of C1 in relation to C2 may occur, with or without an associated rotary subluxation/dislocation of C1 on C2. The type of injury is related in part to the predominant injury force vector.

For an anterior dislocation of C1 from C2, the predominant injury force vector is hyperflexion. In this case, the force pattern is similar to that of an odontoid fracture. If the force is severe enough, continuation of the injury leads to the displacement of the ring of C1. With hyperextension, a posterior displacement of C1 in relation to C2 occurs. In this case as well, a posteriorly displaced dens fracture may occur, as the progressive horizontal compression of the anterior ring of C1 shears and breaks the dens. In two cases, a posterior dislocation of C1 on C2 occurred in which the dens was not fractured and the ring of C1 was lifted over the dens (98,99). In these instances, a strong vertical distractive force combined with hyperextension contributed to the injury.

Rotary subluxation, which may lead to a dislocation or to a fixed rotational deformity, occurs when the predominant injury force vector is at an angle to the sagittal plane and is sufficiently off-center enough to develop a torque on C1 (100).

The transverse ligament acts as the primary restraint to anterior atlantoaxial translation. The alar ligaments act as the primary restraint to excessive rotation of the atlas in relation to the axis, and they act as secondary restraints to anterior displacement of the atlas. When the transverse ligament is incompetent, the alar ligaments cannot fully prevent further displacement of the atlas when the injury force is sustained (8).

Continued rotatory subluxation may occur when the secondary restraints to rotation (the tectorial membrane, the accessory atlantoaxial ligaments, and the facet capsules) become compromised (101). A rotary dislocation of C1 from C2 may develop as rotation progresses to approximately 63 to 65 degrees. If the transverse ligament is disrupted and anterior translation of C1 exceeds 5 mm, rotatory dislocation of C1 on C2 may develop as rotation progresses to approximately 45 degrees (102).

Lateral tilt of the head may occur when a lateral flexion force combined with rotation exceeds the physiological coupling movement of C1 on C2. During lateral flexion, the opposite alar ligament tightens. On the side of flexion, the concave inferior facet shifts inferiorly and posteriorly as the contralateral superior facet shifts anteriorly and superiorly. With further lateral bending, rotation of the dens tightens the opposite alar ligament, and motion is inhibited. In this rotated, flexed position, the alar ligaments are most taut and are at greatest risk for rupture (103). Radiographically, this may be demonstrated on open-mouth views that indicate an overlap of the lateral mass of C1 in relation to the superior articular facet of C2. Abnormal anterior displacement of the posterior wall of the anterior ring of C1 from the anterior surface of the dens may be observed on the lateral x-ray view (104).

In nontraumatic cases, chronic subluxation may lead to a fixed atlantoaxial rotational deformity. The pathophysiology for this condition is not well defined. Various hypotheses have been proposed concerning the dynamic effects on the soft tissue structures of the neck that are created from pathological inflammatory changes (105,106). Spasm and inflammation of the sternocleidomastoid muscle may lead to contracture of that muscle and to a gradual restrained posture of the neck. Effusion and synovitis of the C1–C2 facet joints and capsules may lead to attenuation and excessive laxity of the capsules. As rotation and stretching of the capsules and ligamentous structures progresses, invaginated inflamed synovial folds may prevent the reduction of the displaced facet joints. If reduction is not obtained and deformity persists, secondary contractures may develop that lead to fixation of the atlantoaxial rotational deformity.

S   Compression Burst Fracture

A burst fracture of the ring of C1 results from forceful axial compression, usually a direct blow to the head (107). The caudally driven occipital condyles act like a wedge to compress the ring of C1 between the condyles and the ring of C2. Although classically described as a four-part Jefferson fracture, a two-part or three-part fracture occurs more frequently (91,108) (Fig. 1). On open-mouth radiographs, splaying and bilateral lateral displacement of the lateral masses of the ring of C1 in relation to C2 may be observed. A total of ≥7 mm of displacement indicates instability.

When axially loaded, the straightened cervical spine acts as a segmented column (109,110). When the neck is partially flexed, the cervical spine is in fact straightened. In the straightened cervical spine, the axial load is transmitted with greater force from the head to the thoracic spine compared to when the cervical spine is in the normal lordotic posture (111,112). When the cervical spine is not straight, the load-carrying capacity is reduced and the segmental spinal column may buckle (113,114). Compression of the vertebral body may cause varying degrees of retropulsion of the posterior vertebral wall into the spinal canal (115). Positioning a cervical burst fracture into either extension or compression can significantly increase canal occlusion as compared with canal occlusion in the neutral position (116).

T   Occipital Condyle Fractures

Fractures of the occipital condyle are rare. They may be associated with other fractures of the spine (117).

Occipital condyle fractures may be classified as impacted fractures, fractures associated with a basilar skull fracture, or an avulsion fracture (82). Impacted fractures and fractures associated with a basilar skull fracture are usually the result of a forceful axial compression force. This force coupled with a rotation or shear can lead to an avulsion fracture of the occipital condyle (118). In the avulsion-type fracture, the restraint and stabilizing effect of the alar ligament is compromised, and significant instability may occur.

U   Occipitoatlantal Dislocations

The exact mechanism of this often fatal injury is not definitive. The injury might not be recognized unless specifically looked for. From postmortem examinations, it has been suggested that the primary injury force vector is hyperflexion (119); others suggest hyperextension (120,121). In either case, there is displacement and translation of the occipital condyles away from the C1 articular surfaces, as the stout stabilizing craniocervical ligaments and articular capsule are ruptured.

V   Spinal Cord Injury Without Radiographic Abnormality (SCIWORA)

In a child with a spinal cord injury and the absence of any abnormal findings on plain radiographs, a hyperextension injury to the cervical spine should be suspected. Several large studies have provided insight into this interesting spinal injury (38,122). It appears that the unique anatomical and biomechanical characteristics of the skeletally immature spine account for the normal radiographic appearance of the cervical spine despite a high-energy injury with neurological impairment. Failure was found to occur through the weak physeal or the cartilaginous endplate (123). Hyperextension appeared to be the predominant mechanism of injury. A high index of suspicion is recommended, since lack of recognition most often leads to an error in diagnosis of this injury (124).

VI   CONCLUSION

The response of the cervical spine to impact loading during injury is complex. Various cervical injury patterns can be produced from specific force vectors. An understanding of the mechanisms of injury and the pathological forces acting on the cervical spine can guide the treating physician to an accurate diagnosis and effective treatment of these injuries.

REFERENCES

1. Sances A Jr, Mykleburst JB, Weber RD, Larson SJ, Cusick JF, Walsh PR. Bioengineering analysis of head and spine injuries. CRC Crit Rev Bioeng 1981; 5(2):79–122.
2. Voo LM, Pintar FA, Yoganandan N, Liu YK. Static and dynamic bending responses of the human cervical spine. J Biomech Eng 1998; 120(6):693–696.
3. Sherk HH, Parke WW. Developmental anatomy. In: Bailey RW, Sherk HH, eds. The Cervical Spine, 2nd ed. Philadelphia: Lippincott, 1989:1–7.
4. Vishteh AG, Crawford NR, Melton MS. Stability of the craniovertebral junction after unilateral occipital condyle resection: a biomechanical study. J Neurosurg 1999; 90(suppl 1):91–98.
5. Fielding JW. Cineroentgenography of the normal cervical spine. J Bone Joint Surg Am 1957; 39:1280.
6. Dvorak J, Panjabi MM. Functional anatomy of the alar ligaments. Spine 1987; 12:183.
7. Dvorak J, Schiender E, Saldinger P. Biomechanics of the craniocervical region: The alar ligaments. J Orthop Res 1988; 6:452.
8. Fielding JW, Cochran GVB, Lawsing JF III. Tears of the transverse ligament of the atlas. J Bone Joint Surg Am 1974; 56:1683.
9. Goel VK, Winterbottom JM, Schulte KR. Ligamentous laxity across C0-C1-C2 complex: Axial torque rotation characteristics until failure. Spine 1990; 15:990.

10. Panjabi MM, Oxland TR, Parks EH. Quantitative anatomy of cervical spine ligaments. Part I. Upper cervical spine. J Spinal Disord 1991; 4(3):270–276.
11. Mykleburst JB, Pintar F, Yoganandan N. Tensile strength of spinal ligaments. Spine 1988; 13:526–531.
12. Panjabi M, Dvorak J, Crisco J III, Oda T, Hilibrand A, Grob D. Flexion, extension, and lateral bending of the upper cervical spine in response to alar ligament transections. J Spinal Disord 1991; 4(2):157–167.
13. Panjabi M, Dvorak J, Crisco JJ, III, Oda T, Wang P, Grob D. Effects of alar ligament transection on upper cervical spine rotation. J Orthop Res 1991; 9(4):584–593.
14. Clausen JD, Goel VK, Traynelis VC, Scifet J. Uncinate process and Luschka joints influence the biomechanics of the cervical spine: quantification using a finite element model of the C5-C6 segment. J Orthop Res 1997; 15(3):342–347.
15. Panjabi M, Oda T, Crisco JJ, III, Dvorak J, Grob D. Posture affects motion coupling of the upper cervical spine. J Orthop Res 1993; 11(4):525–536.
16. Panjabi MM, Summers DJ, Pelker RR. Three-dimensional load displacement curves of the cervical spine. J Orthop Res 1986; 4:152.
17. Moroney SP, Schultz AB, Miller AA. Load displacement properties of lower cervical spine motion segments. J Biomech 1998; 21(9):769.
18. Maurel N, Lavaste F, Skalli W. A three-dimensional parameterized finite element model of the lower cervical spine. Study of the influence of the posterior articular facets. J Biomech 1997; 30(9):921–931.
19. Maiman DJ, Sances A Jr, Mykleburst JB. Compression injuries of the cervical spine. Neurosurgery 1983; 13:254–260.
20. Raynor RB, Pugh J, Shapiro I. Cervical facetectomy and its effect on spine strength. J Neurosurg 1985; 63:278–282.
21. Raynor RB, Moskovich R, Zidel P, Pugh J. Alterations in primary and coupled motions after facetectomy. Neurosurgery 1987; 21:681–687.
22. Kumaresan S, Yoganandan N, Pintar FA. Finite element modeling of cervical laminectomy with graded facetectomy. J Spinal Disord 1997; 10(1):40–46.
23. Gebhard JS, Donaldson DH, Brown CW. Soft-tissue injuries of the cervical spine. Orthop Rev 1994; 5(suppl):9–17.
24. Yoganandan N, Sances A Jr, Maiman DJ. Experimental spinal injuries with vertical impact. Spine 1986; 11:855–860.
25. Denis F. Spinal instability as defined by the three column spine concept in acute spinal trauma. Clin Orthop Rel Res 1983; 189:65–76.
26. Sances A Jr, Mykleburst JB, Maiman DJ. The biomechanics of spinal injuries. CRC Crit Rev Bioeng 1984; 11:1–76.
27. Maiman DJ, Yoganandan N. Biomechanics of cervical spine trauma. Clin Neurosurg 1991; 37:543–570.
28. Brown T, Hanson R, Yorra A. Some mechanical tests on the cervical spine with particular reference to the intervertebral discs. J Bone Joint Surg 1957; 39:1135–1141.
29. Mouradian WH, Fietti VG, Cochran GV, Fielding JW. Fractures of the odontoid process: A laboratory and clinical study of mechanisms. Orthop Clin North Am 1978; 9: 985–1001.
30. Zdeblic TA, Abitbol JJ, Kunz D. Cervical stability after sequential capsule resection. J Spinal Disord 1993; 18:2005–2008.
31. Panjabi MM, White AA, Johnson RM. Cervical spine mechanics as function of transection of components. J Biomech 1975; 8:327–336.
32. Panjabi MM, Oxland TR, Parks EH. Quantitative anatomy of cervical spine ligaments. Part II. Middle and lower cervical spine. J Spinal Disord 1991; 4(3):277–285.
33. White AA, Panjabi MM. Clinical Biomechanics of the Spine, 2nd ed. Philadelphia: Lippincott, 1990.

34. Mazur JM, Stauffer ES. Unrecognized spinal instability associated with seemingly "simple" cervical compression fractures. Spine 1983; 8:687–692.

35. White AA, Panjabi MM. Update on the evaluation of instability of the lower cervical spine. Instr Course Lect 1987; 36:499–520.

36. Huelke DR, O'Day J, Mendelsohn RA. Cervical injuries suffered in automobile crashes. J Neurosurg 1981; 54:316–322.

37. Sances A Jr, Mykleburst J, Cusick JF. Experimental studies of brain and neck injury. In: 25th Stapp Car Crash Conference Proceedings, Society of Automotive Engineers, Warrendale, Pennsylvania, 1981:149–194.

38. Pang D, Wilberger JE. Spinal cord injury without radiographic abnormalities in children. J Neurosurg 1982; 57:114–129.

39. Panjabi MM, Duranceau JS, Oxland TR, Bowen CE. Multidirectional instabilities of traumatic cervical spine injuries in a porcine model. Spine 1989; 14(10):1111–1115.

40. Chen IH, Vasavada A, Panjabi MM. Kinematics of the cervical spine: changes with sagittal plane loads. J Spinal Disord 1994; 7(2):93–101.

41. Dvorak J, Panjabi MM, Novotny JE, Antinnes JA. In vivo flexion/extension of the normal cervical spine. J Orthop Res 1991; 9(6):828–834.

42. Oda T, Panjabi MM, Crisco JJ, III. Three-dimensional translational movements of the upper cervical spine. J Spinal Disord 1991; 4(4):411–419.

43. Panjabi MM. Cervical spine models for biomechanical research. Spine 1998; 23(24): 2684–2700.

44. Roaf R. International classification of spinal injuries. Paraplegia 1972; 10:78.

45. White AA, Panjabi MM, Brand RA. A system for defining position and motion of the human body parts. Med Biol Eng 1975; 13:261.

46. Zhu Q, Ouyang J, Lu W. Traumatic instabilities of the cervical spine caused by high-speed axial compression in a human model. An in vitro biomechanical study. Spine 1999; 24(5):440–444.

47. Shono Y, McAfee PC, Cunningham BW. The pathomechanics of compression injuries in the cervical spine. Nondestructive and destructive investigate methods. Spine 1993; 18(14):2009–2019.

48. Schaaf RE, Gehweiler JA, Miller MD. Lateral hyperflexion injuries of the spine. Skeletal Radiol 1978; 3:73.

49. Crowell RR, Shea M, Edwards WT, Clothiaux PL, White AA. Cervical injuries under flexion and compression loading. J Spinal Disord 1993; 6(2):175–181.

50. Goel VK, Clausen JD. Prediction of load sharing among spinal components of a C5-C6 motion segment using the finite element approach. Spine 1998; 23(6):684–691.

51. Cancelmo JJ Jr. Clay shoveler's fracture: A helpful diagnostic sign. AJR 1972; 115: 540–541.

52. Southern EP, Pelker RR, Crisco JJ, III, Panjabi MM. Posterior element strength six months postinjury in the canine cervical spine. J Spinal Disord 1993; 6(2):155–161.

53. Vaccaro AR, Falatyn SP, Flanders AE, Balderston RA, Northrup BE, Cotler JM. Magnetic resonance evaluation of the intervertbral disc, spinal ligaments, and spinal cord before and after closed traction reduction of cervical spine dislocations. Spine 1991; 24(12):1210–1217.

54. Allen BL, Ferguson RL, Lehmann TR. A mechanistic classification of closed, indirect fractures and dislocations of the lower cervical spine. Spine 1982; 7:1–27.

55. Bozic KJ, Keyak JH, Skinner HB. Three-dimensional finite element modeling of a cervical vertebra: An investigation of burst fracture mechanism. J Spinal Disord 1994; 7:102–110.

56. Harris JH, Edeiken-Monroe B, Kopaniky DR. A practical classification of acute cervical spine injuries. Orthop Clin North Am 1986;17:15–30.

57. Lee C, Kim KS, Rogers LF. Triangular cervical vertebral body fractures: Diagnostic significance. AJR 1982; 138:1123–1132.
58. Torg JS, Pavlov H, O'Neill MJ, Nichols CE Jr, Sennett B. The axial load teardrop fracture. A biomechanical, clinical and roentenographic analysis. Am J Sports Med 1991; 19(4):355–364.
59. Chang DG, Tencer AF, Ching RP. Geometric changes in the cervical spinal canal during impact. Spine 1994; 19:973–980.
60. Levine AM. Facet Fractures and Dislocations. In: Levine AM, Eismont FJ, Garfin SR, Zigler JE, eds. Spine Trauma. Philadelphia: W.B. Saunders Company, 1998:331–366.
61. Doran SE, Papadopoulos SM, Ducker TB. Magnetic resonance imaging documentation of coexistent traumatic locked facets of the cervical spine and disk herniation. J Neurosurg 1993; 79:341–345.
62. Eismont FJ, Arena MJ, Green BA. Extrusion of an intervertbral disc associated with traumatic subluxation or dislocation of cervical facets. J Bone Joint Surg Am 1991; 73:1555–1560.
63. Willis BK, Greiner F, Orrison WW. The incidence of vertebral injury after midcervical spine fracture or subluxation. Neurosurg 1994; 34(3):435–441.
64. Levine AM. Facet injuries in the cervical spine. In: Camins MB, O'Leary PF, eds. Disorders of the Cervical Spine. Baltimore: Williams & Wilkins, 1992:289–302.
65. Shanmuganathan K, Mirvis SE, Levine AM. Rotational injury of cervical facets: CT analysis of fracture patterns with implications for management and neurologic outcome. AJR 1994; 163:1165–1169.
66. Yoganandan N, Pintar FA, Maiman DJ, Cusick JF, Sances A Jr, Walsh PR. Human head-neck biomechanics under axial tension. Med Eng Phys 1996; 18(4):289–294.
67. Johnson G. Hyperextension soft tissue injuries of the cervical spine: a review. J Accid Emerg Med 1996; 13(1):3–8.
68. Forsythe HF. Extension injuries of the cervical spine. J Bone Joint Surg Am 1964; 46: 1792.
69. Bohlman HH. Acute fractures and dislocations of the cervical spine. J Bone Joint Surg Am 1979; 61:1119–1142.
70. Johnson RM, Crelin ES, White AA, Panjabi MM. Some new observations on the functional anatomy of the lower cervical spine. Clin Orthop 1975; 111:192.
71. White AA, Panjabi MM. The clinical biomechanics of the occipitoatlantoaxial complex. Orthop Clin North Am 1978; 9:867–878.
72. Levine AM, Edwards CC. Fractures of the atlas. J Bone Joint Surg Am 1991; 73:680–691.
73. Levine AM, Edwards CC. The management of traumatic spondylolisthesis of the axis. J Bone Joint Surg Am 1985; 67:217–226.
74. Landells CD, Peteghem PKV. Fractures of the atlas: classification, treatment and morbidity. Spine 1987; 13:450–452.
74a. Vaccaro AR, Cottler JM. Upper cervical spine injuries in the adult. In: An HS, ed. Principles and Technologies of Spine Surgery. Philadelphia: Williams & Wilkins, 1998: 336–337.
75. Levine AM, Lutz B. Extension teardrop injuries of the cervical spine. 20th Annual Meeting of the Cervical Spine Research Society, Palm Desert, California, December 3–5, 1992, abstr. No. 49.
76. Levine AM, Rhyne AL. Traumatic spondylolisthesis of the axis. Semin Spine Surg 1991; 3:47–60.
77. Cornish BL. Traumatic spondylolisthesis of the axis. J Bone Joint Surg Br 1968; 50: 31.
78. Yoganandan N, Pintar FA, Kleinberger M. Cervical spine vertebral and facet joint kinematics under whiplash. J Biomech Eng 1998; 120(2):305–307.

79. McKenzie JA, Williams JF. The dynamic behavior of the head and cervical spine during "whiplash." J Biomech 1971; 4:477.
80. Gay JR, Abbott KH. Common whiplash injuries of the neck. JAMA 1953; 152:1698.
81. Yoganandan N, Pintar FA. Inertial loading of the human cervical spine. J Biomech Eng 1997; 119(3):237–240.
82. Hodgson VR, Thomas LM. Mechanisms of cervical spine injury during impact to the protected head. In: 24th Stapp Car Crash Conference Proceedings, Society of Automotive Engineers, Warrendale, Pennsylvania, 1980.
83. Kaneoka K, Ono K, Inami S, Hayashi K. Motion analysis of cervical vertebrae during whiplash loading. Spine 1999; 24(8):763–769.
84. Panjabi MM, Cholewicki J, Nibu K, Grauer J, Vahldiek M. Capsular ligament stretches during in vitro whiplash simulations. J Spinal Disord 1998; 11(3):227–232.
85. Blacksin MF. Patterns of fracture after air bag deployment. J Trauma 1993; 35(6):840–843.
86. Ackerson TT, Patzakis MJ, Moore TM. Fractures of the odontoid: A ten-year retrospective study. Contemp Orthop 1982; 4:54–67.
87. Anderson LD, Clark CR. Fractures of the odontoid process of the axis. In: Cervical Spine Research Society Editors Committee, eds. The Cervical Spine, 2nd ed. Philadelphia: Lippincott, 1989:325–343.
88. Crockard HA, Heilman AE, Stevens JM. Progressive myelopathy secondary to odontoid fractures: Clinical, radiological, and surgical features. J Neurosurg 1993; 78:579.
89. Hadley MN, Browner C, Sonntag VK. Axis fractures: A comprehensive review of management and treatment of 107 cases. Neurosurgery 1985; 17:281.
90. Amyes EW, Anderson FM. Fracture of the odontoid process. Arch Surg 1956; 72:377.
91. Jefferson G. Fracture of the atlas vertebra. Br J Surg 1920; 7:407.
92. Pederson AK, Kostuik JP. Complete fracture-dislocation of the atlantoaxial complex: case report and recommendations for a new classification of dens fractures. J Spinal Disord 1994; 7:350–355.
93. Atloff, B. Fracture of the odontoid process. An experimental study. Acta Orthop Scand 1979(Suppl):177.
94. Scott EW, Haid RW, Peace D. Type I fractures of the odontoid process: implications for atlanto-occipital instability. J Neurosurg 1990; 72:488–492.
95. Shatzker J, Rorabeck CH, Waddell JP. Non-union of the odontoid process: an experimental investigation. Clin Orthop 1975; 108:127–137.
96. Schiff DCM, Parke WW. The arterial supply of the odontoid process. J Bone Joint Surg Am 1973; 55:1450–1456.
97. Hanssen AD, Cabenela ME. Fractures of the atlas in adult patients. J Trauma 1987; 27:928.
98. Harolson RH III, Boyd HB. Posterior dislocation of the atlas on the axis without fracture. Report of a case. J Bone Joint Surg Am 1969; 51:561.
99. Patzakis MJ. Posterior dislocation of the atlas on the axis: a case report. J Bone Joint Surg Am 1974; 56:1260.
100. Meyers BS, McElhaney JH, Doherty BJ, Paver JG, Gray L. The role of torsion in cervical spine trauma. Spine 1991; 16(8):870–874.
101. Dvorak J, Panjabi M, Gerber M. CT-functional diagnostics of the rotatory instability of the upper cervical spine: I. An experimental study on cadavers. Spine 1987; 12:197.
102. Fielding JW, Hawkins RJ. Atlanto-axial rotatory fixation. J Bone Joint Surg Am 1977; 59:37.
103. Panjabi MM, Dvorak J, Crisco JJ, III. Flexion, extension, and lateral bending of the upper cervical spine in response to alar ligament transection. J Spinal Disord 1991; 4:157.

104. Shapiro R, Youngberg AS, Rothman SLG. The differential diagnosis of traumatic lesions of the occipito-atlanto-axial segment. Radiol Clin North Am 1973; 11:505.
105. Hess JH, Bronstein IP, Abelson SM. Atlanto-axial dislocations: unassociated with trauma and secondary to inflammatory foci in the neck. Am J Dis Child 1935; 49: 1137.
106. Kawabe N, Hirotani H, Tanaka O. Pathomechanism of atlantoaxial rotatory fixation in children. J Pediatr Orthop 1989; 9:569.
107. Nightingale RW, McElhaney JH, Richardson WJ, Myers BS. Dynamic responses of the head and cervical spine to axial impact loading. J Biomech 1996; 29(3):307–318.
108. Alker GJ, Oh YS, Leslie EV. Post mortem radiology of head and neck injuries in fatal traffic accidents. Radiology 1975; 114:611.
109. Torg JS, Sennett B, Vegso JJ, Pavlov H. Axial loading injuries to the middle cervical spine segment. An analysis and classification of twenty-five cases. Am J Sports Med 1991; 19(1):6–20.
110. Ordway NR, Seymour RJ, Donelson RG, Hojnowski LS, Edwards WT. Cervical flexion, extension, protrusion, and retraction. A radiographic segmental analysis. Spine 1999; 24(3):240–247.
111. Torg J, Truex R, Marshall J, Hodgson V, Quedenfeld T, Spealman A, Nichols C. Spinal injury at the level of the third and fourth cervical vertebra from football. J Bone Joint Surg Am 1977; 59:1015–1019.
112. Torg J, Quedenfeld T, Burstein A, Spealman A, Nichols C. National football head and neck injury registry: report on cervical quadriplegia, 1971 to 1975. Am J Sports Med 1979; 7:127–132.
113. Nusholtz GS, Huelke DF, Lux P, Alem, Montalvo F. Cervical spine injury mechanisms. In: 27th Stapp Car Crash Conference Proceedings. Society of Automotive Engineers, Warrendale, Pennsylvania, 1983:179–198.
114. Yoganandan N, Kumaresan S, Voo L, Pintar FA. Finite element model of the human lower cervical spine: parametric analysis of the C4-C6 unit. J Biomech Eng 1997; 119(1):87–92.
115. Chang DG, Tencer AF, Ching RP, Treece B, Senft D, Anderson PA. Geometric changes in the cervical canal during impact. Spine 1994; 19(8):973–980.
116. Ching RP, Watson NA, Carter JW, Tencer AF. The effect of post-injury spinal position on canal occlusion in a cervical spine burst fracture model. Spine 1997; 22(15):1710–1715.
117. Spencer JA, Yeakley JW, Kaufman HH. Fracture of the occipital condyle. J Neurosurg 1984; 15:101–103.
118. Bozboga M, Unal F, Hepgul K. Fracture of the occipital condyle. Case report. Spine 1992; 17:1119–1121.
119. Alker GJ, Oh YS, Leslie EV. High cervical spine and craniocervical junction injuries in fatal traffic accidents. Orthop Clin North Am 1978; 9:1003–1010.
120. Bucholz RW, Burkhead WZ. The pathologic anatomy of fatal atlanto-occipital dislocation. J Bone Joint Surg Am 1979; 61:248–250.
121. Eismont FJ, Bohlman HH. Posterior atlanto-occipital dislocation with fractures of the atlas and odontoid process. J Bone Joint Surg Am 1978; 60:397.
122. Ruge JR, Sinson GP, McLone, et al. Pediatric spinal injury: the very young. J Neurosurg 1988; 68:25–30.
123. Aufdermaur M. Spinal injuries in juveniles. J Bone Joint Surg Br 1974; 56:512–519.
124. Orenstein JB, Klein BL, Ochsenschlager DW. Delayed diagnosis of pediatric cervical spine injury. Pediatrics 1992; 89:1185–1188.

4

Emergency Management of Spine Trauma

DANIEL A. CAPEN and ELLEN LEPPEK

University of Southern California, Los Angeles, California, U.S.A.

Spinal trauma and its cost in health-care dollars continue to increase, especially in developed countries where high-speed transportation and high-speed recreation are on the increase. In first-, second-, and third-world countries, violence also contributes heavily to the spine trauma population. Trauma remains a disease that represents a leading cause of death in the first four decades of life. Trauma also permanently disables many members of society at an estimated cost of 100 billion dollars annually. Emergency treatment of spine and multiple traumas represents the first opportunity to successfully impact ultimate outcomes of the injury.

In a large percentage of severe high-energy trauma cases, death occurs instantly. The emergency medical transport system in the United States and similarly developed countries allows an increased rate of survivability. However, in the best of circumstances, 30% succumb in the earlier, initial phases of care and an additional 20% succumb to later problems in the initial weeks and months following the trauma. Most often, these causes of death relate to infection or multiple organ failure, including the chronic manifestations of head trauma, hemorrhagic shock and spinal cord injury (1).

Isolated spine trauma most frequently results from sports-related injuries, falls, and some low-velocity gunshot wounds (2). This represents approximately half of the cases seen in the major spinal cord injury centers. Multisystem involvement must be addressed early in the treatment of these low-energy injuries, but early attention to the spine is usually possible without risk of hemorrhage, head trauma, or other injury that often delays spine surgery in high-energy injury (3–5).

The trauma associated with a spine injury in the remaining group is most frequently associated with high-energy vehicular trauma, falls from heights, and some violence. The breakdown of associated trauma with spinal cord injury includes fractures of the trunk (18%); long bone fractures (14%); head and facial trauma (14%); and chest and abdominal injury (18%) (6,7).

I INITIAL MANAGEMENT

Initial management of the multiple trauma or isolated spinal trauma patient is done by emergency medical technicians, doctors in the field, paraprofessionals in the field, and even "good samaritan" citizens trained in CPR. This initial care is often instrumental in allowing the patient to survive with a minimum of injury and with some reduction in the likelihood of complete paralysis. Enhancement of recovery begins with this care (1,8). The actual delivery of field care from emergency medical technicians and paramedics can often be instrumental in survivability. The Emergency Medical Services Act of 1973 established guidelines for this care. Since the advent of that system, steady improvement in emergency services has been noted in the United States and other developed countries.

Toscano (1) cited an incidence of severe complications associated with transfer, but in the past 10 years significant improvement from the sited 26% neurological complication rate has been noted. During patient transport, the emphasis has been placed on the ABCs of life support together with splinting of all fractures, establishment of intravenous lines, and administration of initial fluid done by the field technicians, sometimes under the guidance of emergency room physicians. Universal teaching on splinting the spine with bed board, orthotic devices, and some traction apparatus have permitted early immobilization or reduction before the patient reaches the hospital. Attending sports physicians are well versed in contact sports injuries, including support of the spine, logrolling, and immediate bracing of the spine (9). Some traction devices are available to some emergency technicians. Inboard traction devices are also available to immobilize cervical spine fractures during transportation. All uncontrolled motion of the spine must be avoided to preserve as much neurological function as possible. It has been emphasized that any unconscious or semiconscious patient must be assumed to have a spinal cord injury until proven otherwise.

Assessment of the airway and cardiovascular status is also done in the field. Field emergency personnel initialize protection of vital functions, maintaining airway, supporting and assisting respiratory efforts, and assessing most phases of bodily function. In rural areas, fix-winged airplane and helicopter transportation are also available so that transportation to a major trauma center can take place.

Nasal tracheal, oral tracheal, and even sometimes surgical tracheal intubation are required, especially in maxillofacial trauma. Patients are often in severe distress and clearing the airway to establish gas exchange is critical. Attention to the hemodynamic system is also essential. Establishing of intravenous lines and fluid flow in the field is often instrumental in preventing or providing early treatment of shock, as well as protecting the spinal cord itself from hypovolemia.

A physician or health paraprofessional often supervises athletic events in the United States. Contact sports, in particular, have a relatively high incidence of potential for spinal trauma. Athletic competition becomes secondary when there is potential for spinal cord injury. Temporary loss of consciousness, temporary neurological extremity injury, or any suggestion that the central nervous system or spinal cord has been damaged necessitates immediate cessation of the activity, transportation for evaluation, and communication between the health-care professional and the coach, parents, and injured athlete.

II   EMERGENCY TREATMENT

Once the patient is transported to the emergency room, the emergency physician and trauma team are called upon to triage as well as evaluate and begin treatment of all injuries (10–12). Life-threatening injuries are treated first. Intoxication can complicate the initial evaluation. Establishing of basic life support methods includes evaluation of the patient for the presence of coma. The Glasgow Coma Scale (Table 1) is frequently utilized to assess neurological status. In the conscious patient, full cooperation for a neurological exam is facilitated. In the presence of severe maxillofacial or other trauma (as noted on the Glasgow Coma Scale) spinal cord evaluation is made much more difficult. The oral tracheal and endotracheal system can be injured in high-energy trauma with maxillofacial fractures, blood in the nares, and, occasionally, even tracheal injury. Establishing an airway, even if it requires surgical tracheotomy, is essential to survival.

Large lines may need to be established to support the cardiovascular system. Hemodynamic stability is essential to avoid shock and multiorgan failure, and to preserve spinal cord function when the cord is injured.

Basic trauma treatment frequently involves the attempt to triage secondary injuries but provide some emergency treatment (13). Obviously, spinal deformity and spinal support can be established while life-threatening injuries are treated. The early phases of management require obvious efforts to attempt to diagnose any spinal cord injury.

Table 1   Glasgow Coma Scale

Eye opening
  Spontaneous
    To voice
    To pain
    None
Verbal response
  Oriented
  Confused
    Inapposite
    Incomprehensible
    None
Motor response
  Obeys commands
    Localizes pain
    Withdrawal (pain)
    Flexion (pain)
    Extension (pain)
    None

Early treatment of spinal cord injury has been enhanced over the years by administration of methylprednisolone. Investigators for the Third National Acute Spinal Cord Injury Study concluded that methylprednisolone improves neurological recovery after the first 24 to 48 h. Tirilazad mesylate can be used for 48 h after acute spinal cord injury. Bracken and coworkers have clearly defined the benefits in this national research, randomized, double-blind group (14–16). The National Acute Spinal Cord Injury Study Group documented with 16 acute spinal cord injury centers in North America that the effect of the 48-h methylprednisolone regimen was significant at 6 weeks and 6 months. Patients who received the 48-h regimen and who started treatment at 3 to 8 h were more likely to improve one full neurological grade. The 48-h group was also reported to experience greater sepsis and severe pneumonia than patients in the 24-h methylprednisolone and tirilazad groups, but other complications were similar.

Tirilazad is a lazeroid in the drug class of lipid peroxidase inhibitors. In addition, it exhibits neuroprotective effects by a variety of other mechanisms, such as improving spinal cord blood flow and membrane stabilization. Because lazeroids have none of the glucocorticoid properties of methylprednisolone, tirilazad may have fewer side effects (12). Except for gunshot trauma to the spine, the corticosteroid protocol, when implemented immediately, is very effective at reducing cord swelling and establishing the optimum environment for recovery. The dosage profile described in the study involves a loading intravenous dose of 30 mg/kg of methylprednisolone for 15 to 30 min, followed by 5.4 mg/kg/h for 23 h. The incidence of stress ulceration and other systemic complications exists, but there is definitive, positive, documented effect on recovery. This treatment must be administered and is considered standard of care. It cannot be used in children under the age of 13, during pregnancy, or in patients with diabetes or infection.

Table 2 describes several common multiple trauma problems that require triage through the interaction of the general surgeon and the emergency physician. Intra-

Table 2 Life-Threatening Complications of Common Injuries

Injury complication contributing factor
Pneumothorax
Tension pneumothorax
Positive pressure ventilation
Blunt chest trauma
Arrhythmia
Pericardial tamponade
Myocardial contusion
Atrial rupture
Tracheal
Airway obstruction
Hemorrhage, edema
Subcapsular hematoma (spleen, liver)
Massive hemorrhage
Delay in diagnosis

abdominal and intrathoracic hemorrhage, as well as extremity hemorrhage, must be immediately controlled. Large volumes of fluid plus blood replacement and use of plasma expanders are all modalities to reduce the period of time the patient has severe hypoperfusion. The general surgeon must be able to recognize, diagnose, and treat severe liver lacerations, the effects of blunt chest trauma causing pericardial tamponade, and spleen rupture or avulsion of intestines, all of which represent severe, potentially life-threatening disorders. Emergency abdominal surgery may be required while temporizing measures are instituted for the spine trauma. Once life-threatening chest and abdominal injuries are treated or ruled out, attention can be given to the spine.

In the polytrauma patient with a spinal cord injury, there is an additional diagnostic dilemma. Hypotension can be a direct result of hypovolemia. However, hypotension can also be due to neurogenic problems associated with loss of vascular tone and increased vascular capacitance if bradycardia is present in these patients with neurogenic shock (17).

Soderstrom documented systemic blood pressure less than 100 in 69% of patients reviewed with cervical spine injury (3). Obvious recognition of this problem, as well as ruling out potential intra-abdominal trauma, is essential. The treatment for neurogenic shock includes limited volume replacement with use of vasopressors; overinfusion can result in fatal pulmonary edema.

Vasopressors in the face of hypovolemic hypotension or cardiogenic causes can present the physician with life-threatening complications. If intra-abdominal injuries and long bone fractures are ruled out, treatment of neurogenic shock should be instituted if cord injury is present. Table 3 delineates a reasonable protocol for the essentials of initial treatment of a multitrauma patient, whether it is from gun violence or high-speed, high-energy trauma.

III SPINAL EVALUATION

Once life-threatening injuries have been treated, hemodynamic status is established, and after clear documentation of cerebral function, assessment of the spine and spinal cord must be made. Initially, evaluation of the spine must include radiographs of the entire spine. Numerous studies have clearly documented that missile injuries do not destabilize the spine, except in extremely rare occurrences (2). However, fractures can be missed in high-energy trauma because reduction may have taken place spontaneously or can have been achieved by the emergency technicians. Any pretracheal edema on cervical spine films is an obvious clue. Slight angulations or slight facet incongruity, as well as small anterior vertebral fractures or spinous process fractures can also be clues.

In the thoracic spine, it is critical not to accept AP and lateral chest x-rays as being diagnostic of spine stability. Thoracic spine instability can be suspected in multiple rib fractures, first rib fractures, or any trauma where a direct blow is evidenced in the posterior upper thoracic spine. Otherwise, the thoracic spine is usually stable. In the thoracolumbar spine and lumbar spine, fractures must be ruled out in the presence of pelvic instability or in the presence of significant transverse process fractures. Pedicle widening on the AP film is also considered a hallmark of spinal fractures. The literature is replete with information on late diagnoses of peripheral fractures. It is also evident that multiple traumas have an association with multiple

Table 3 Basic Trauma Treatment

1. Contact and consult with field team.
2. Prepare emergency area for victim.
3. Establish airway and begin respiratory support, if needed.
4. Establish fluid replacement to restore circulation; treat shock.
5. Evaluate and reevaluate physical status:
    neurological
    chest
    abdomen
    extremities
6. Foley catheter for drainage and monitoring.
7. Chest tube (prn):
    abdominal tap (prn)
    nasogastric tube
8. Evaluate:
    CNS
    spine
    long bones
9. Spinal protection:
    skeletal traction
    neck bracing
10. Methylprednisolone for spinal cord injury.
11. In coma, everything is injured or fractured until proved otherwise.
12. Plan appropriate treatment for spine injury.

noncontiguous spinal fractures (18–20). Finding one spinal fracture does not assure the physician that no other fractures exist. Up to 15% of patients have noncontiguous spinal fractures. In the event of some plain radiographic suggestion of spinal instability, CT and MRI scanning may be employed early on to further delineate the problem. Emergency information from diagnostic MRI and CT scanning has proven valuable, especially when ligamentous or disk injury is present and accompanies instability. Emery eloquently described a black stripe sign indicative of posterior torn ligaments (20). Others have also described the value of early CT and MRI imaging. Reference 21 provides useful information to assist the physician in interpretation of subtle signs of instability.

Table 4 Acute Management of Spinal Cord Injury

1. Maintenance of perfusion systolic blood pressure >90 mmHg.
2. 100% O_2 saturation via nasal cannula.
3. Early diagnosis by plain radiography.
4. Methylprednisolone therapy (loading dose 30 mg/kg followed by infusion at rate of 5.4 mg/kg/h for 23 to 48 h).
5. Immediate traction reduction for cervical fracture and dislocation.
6. Spinal imaging (MR imaging and/or computed tomography).
7. Surgery, if indicated, for residual cord compression or fracture instability.

Source: Ref. 12.

One of the other absolute essentials in dealing with emergency management of the spinal cord and spinal trauma patient is to thoroughly evaluate and reevaluate neurological status. Unfortunately, the presence of head trauma and intoxication can initially delay or distort neurological evaluation and makes the evaluation extremely difficult.

IV LEVEL OF CONSCIOUSNESS

Making certain the patient has an acceptable level of consciousness and documenting neurological function are essential. Serial evaluations of functional physical activity and the patient's neuromotor skills are assessed. The ASIA motor index form is a detailed evaluation of motor function. The Frankel scale is a generic scale addressing function, but is nonspecific with respect to the gradation and exact level of function.

Focal tenderness that is elicited from the patient creates an index of suspicion of a ligamentous injury. Transitory sensory deficit that is not present at the time of the examination (Lhermitte's sign) also creates a high index of suspicion with regard to the possibility of spinal instability. The diagnoses of any motor or sensory loss are also heavily relied upon to determine the presence of spinal instability. If a totally normal neurological evaluation is present, there is much more justification for motion studies to determine the nature and extent of any potential instability. The presence of a neurological deficit mandates CT or MRI scanning to fully assess the spine. In larger individuals, when C7–T1 is not visualized on the lateral view, a CT scan of that region can be important.

Radiographic hints regarding the presence of instability include (1) abnormal relationship between the anterior margins of the posterior bony structures in the foramen magnum and the anterior margin of the spinous process of C1 and C2; (2) prevertebral edema in the cervical spine; (3) widening of spinous process relationships when compared to other segments; and (4) pedicular widening on the AP in the lumbar spine. All of these signs and others are described in Reference 21. The extent of evaluation accuracy when a patient has a depressed level of consciousness (Glasgow Coma score of less than 10) is difficult for the practitioner. Many major skeletal injuries are overlooked because of decreased pain response and because the brain injury takes immediate precedence. In a large series, Mackersie et al. (4) described a 14% incidence of axial spine fractures in the setting of head trauma. Obviously, in any obtunded or unconscious patient, complete study of the spine is imperative.

Accurate assessment of the extent of spinal trauma and instability is imperative. There can be a determination of the need for treatment based upon the extent of the spine trauma. The American Spine Injury Assessment (ASIA) impairment scale (Table 5) can serve as a guide for appropriate treatment and for expected outcomes. Initial evaluation must include an assessment of sensorimotor function and bowel and bladder innervation. Performance of a rectal exam is essential if any question exists regarding neurological loss. Obvious sensory deficits or subtle loss of sharp–dull discrimination, temperature, and light touch are key. Manual muscle testing is graded by a standard system: Grade 0—no function; Grade 1—trace or palpable contraction without the ability to move the joint; Grade 2—poor joint range of motion with gravity eliminated; Grade 3—fair joint motion against gravity; Grade 4—some ability to resist gravity and some manual resistance; Grade 5—normal range of motion against significant resistance. This represents one of the key factors

Table 5 ASIA Impairment Scale

A = Complete: No motor or sensory function is preserved in the sacral segments S4–S5.
B = Incomplete: Sensory but not motor function is preserved below the neurological level
    and extends through the sacral segments S4–S5.
C = Incomplete: Motor function is preserved below the neurological level, and the majority
    of key muscles below the neurological level have a muscle grade less than 3.
D = Incomplete: Motor function is preserved below the neurological level, and the majority
    of key muscles below the neurological level have a muscle grade greater than or equal
    to 3.
E = Normal: Motor and sensory function is normal.

in the ASIA motor index rating system, but also complies with grading systems in guidelines described for physical examination.

If a neurological disorder exists, establishing the lowest level, where complete function, both motor and sensory, exists is important. Damage to specific areas of the spinal cord creates specific syndromes. The anterior cord involves damage to the anterior two-thirds of the cord and is heralded by complete loss of motor and sharp–dull sensation. The posterior columns are spared, which allows crude sensation. This syndrome offers a poor prognosis. Central cord syndromes are heralded by damage and dysfunction primarily in the hand, with little loss in the lower extremities, although a spastic gait often is retained. Fine motor use of the upper extremities is often the last to recover. Brown Sequard–type syndromes, which are rare in high trauma but common in missile or stab injuries, are characterized by the loss of ipsilateral motor function and contralateral pain. Posterior cord syndromes are rare and associated with direct trauma; they involve loss of proprioception and position sense. Isolated root injuries can also occur from unilateral facet translation, dislocation, or traumatic instability with disk injury. Once a neurological evaluation has been established, maintenance and reevaluation to diagnose either improvement or decline is essential. Multiple serial neurological examinations by a standardized approach are essential to provide feedback for the patient. Loss of neurological function occurs in unrecognized instability, cord edema, and ascending hematoma. These conditions must be treated immediately or they can preclude recovery. No clear evidence exists to establish that emergency surgery is beneficial beyond 8 h from the time of trauma. In most university settings, early decompression is accepted, but has not been documented to provide superior functional outcome.

In emergency treatment of spinal trauma, if any suspicion of spinal cord trauma exists it is imperative to implement the methylprednisolone regimen. When it is clear that spine stability has been established, secondary care to long bone fractures and conservative care to non-destabilizing spine fractures can be given. In any circumstance, it cannot be overemphasized that serial neurological evaluations must be performed in the first 24 to 48 h in any polytrauma patient. If discharge from the emergency setting is contemplated, several factors must be considered. First and foremost, absolutely no neurological symptomatology has existed at any time during the trauma. Second, the entire spine has been radiographed and evaluated completely and successfully. Third, other than musculoskeletal pain, no significant or severe symptomatology exists. Fourth, no other system injury can be present. Fifth and final, the patient must be able to interact completely on his own, without having had any periodic or transitory functional loss.

V ANESTHESIA IN MULTISYSTEM TRAUMA

If spinal trauma is present together with life-threatening cardiovascular, abdominal, or cranial injuries, the spinal surgeon must be involved in the surgical team. This must be considered a part of the emergency care in spine trauma, as nonspinal surgery is often required prior to complete spine evaluation.

Spinal personnel must assure safe transport to and from the operating room, along with maintenance of spinal alignment during the procedure. Most trauma centers deal with multiple trauma and spine trauma, and multiple personnel are often available. However, in hospitals where the problem is less frequently seen, the orthopedic or spinal surgeon must be prepared for hands-on management.

Reestablishing reasonable blood pressure, blood flow, and oxygenization for cord benefit, realignment of the spine, and maintenance of alignment are all imperative to assure good outcomes and are the responsibility of the spinal surgeon. The anesthiologist must also be aware that cervical, thoracic, and lumbar trauma may accompany maxillofacial trauma, head trauma, and multisystem injury. The spinal surgeon must also provide information during the resuscitation period regarding avoidance of overdose of glucose in trauma as described in Refence 22.

VI REDUCTION AND ALIGNMENT OF THE SPINE IN THE EMERGENCY SETTING

Many cases of multiple traumas are present with spinal fractures. Realignment or establishment of external stabilization can be performed in the emergency room or in the first 12 to 24 h. The procedures can be accomplished with minimal sedation and analgesia so that continuous neurological evaluation can take place.

Failure to maintain patient contact can lead to serious complications. Tongs and traction or halo traction can result in disaster if continuous monitoring is not performed. Increasing traction and leaving the patient unattended can be fraught with risk due to the presence of partial ligamentous injury. Once the traction exceeds the ligamentous tolerance, over distraction can occur, resulting in severe neurological abnormality. In the presence of C-arm fluoroscopic visualization or with continuous monitoring, distraction can be avoided. A gentle amount of sedation that is reversible together with muscle relaxation can assist in the procedure. General anesthesia to permit reduction is fraught with complications, although Vaccaro has described safe emergent cervical reductions with awake intravenous sedation. With closed reduction, as with surgery, there is a window of safe surgical and nonsurgical intervention. Increased risk of neurological complication due to cord edema does occur after the first 24 to 48 h. After that, some physicians wait up to 7 days before they manipulate the spinal elements, especially in the presence of spinal instability.

Accurate assessment and early supervision of the spine in multiple trauma helps to reduce complications, achieve the desired results, and maximize outcomes. Rapid reestablishment of spinal alignment also creates the environment for maximum cord recovery. Once the spine has been realigned in the face of deteriorating neurological function, surgery on an urgent basis can be contemplated.

VII   SUMMARY

Initial contact with trauma victims is the initial step to recovery. Life-threatening injury may delay spinal surgery but must not delay urgent measures to reduce or stabilize the spine and to optimize recovery of the cord by medical treatment.

REFERENCES

1. Toscano J. Prevention of neurologic deterioration before admission to spinal cord injury unit. Paraplegia 1988; 26(3):143–150.
2. Kane T, Capen DA, Waters R, et al. Spinal cord injury from civilian gunshot wounds: The Rancho experience 1980–1988. J Spinal Disord 1991; 4:306–311.
3. Soderstrom CA, McCordle DQ, Duder TB, et al. The diagnosis of intra-abdominal injury in patients with cervical cord trauma. J Trauma 1983; 23:1061–1065.
4. Mackersie RC, Shackford SR, Garfin SR, et al. Major skeletal injuries in the obtunded blunt trauma patient: A case for routine radiologic surgery. J Trauma 1988; 28:1450.
5. Blauth M, Knop C, Bastian L, Krettek C, Lange U. Complex injuries of the spine. (Komplexe Verletzungen der Wirbelsaule.) Orthopade 1998; 27:17–31.
6. Injury in America, a Continuing Public Health Problem. Washington, DC: National Academy Press, 1985:18.
7. Trunkey DD, Federle M, Cello J. Special diagnostic procedures. In: Blaisdell FW, Trunkey DD, eds. Trauma Management. Vol. 1: Abdominal Trauma. City: Thieme-Strattoin, 1982:19–43.
8. Kish DL. Prehospital management of spinal trauma: an evolution. Crit Care Nurs Q 1999; 22:36–43.
9. McGuire RA, Neville S, Green BA, et al. Spinal instability and the logrolling maneuver. J Trauma 1987; 27:525–531.
10. Grundy D, Swain A, Russell J. ABC of spinal cord injury. Early management and complications. Br Med J 1986; 292:44–47.
11. Water RL, Meyer PR Jr, Adkins RH, Felton D. Emergency, acute and surgical management of spine trauma. Arch Phys Med Rehabil 1999; 80:1383–1390.
12. Delamarter RB, Coyle J. Acute management of spinal cord injury. J Am Acad Orthop Surg 1999; 7:166–175.
13. Kienlen J, de La Coussaye JE. Management of multiple trauma in the emergency room. J Chir (Paris) 1999; 136:240–251.
14. Bracken MB. Administration of methylprednisolone for 24 or 48 hours or tirilazad mesylate for 48 hours in the treatment of acute spinal cord injury. Results of the Third National Acute Spinal Cord Injury Randomized Controlled Trial. National Acute Spinal Cord Injury Study. JAMA 1997; 277:1597–1604.
15. Bracken MB, Aldrich EF, Herr DL, Hitchon PW, Holford TR, Marshall LF. Clinical measurement, statistical analysis, and risk-benefit: controversies form trial of spinal injury. J Trauma 2000; 48:558–561.
16. Seidl EC. Promising pharmacological agents in the management of acute spinal cord injury. Crit Care Nurs Q 1999; 22:44–50.
17. Teasell RW, Arnold JM, Krassioukov A, Delaney GA. Cardiovascular consequence of loss of supra spinal control of the sympatheric nervous system after spinal cord injury. Arch Phys Med Rehabil 2000; 81:506–516.
18. Calenoff L, Chessara JW, Rogers LF, et al. Multiple level spinal injuries; the importance of early recognition. Am J Roentgen 1978; 130:665–669.
19. Keenen TL, Antony J, Benson, BR. Non-contiguous spinal fractures. J Trauma 1990; 30(4):489–491.

20.   Emery SE, Pathrial MN, Wilbur RG, et al. Magnetic resonance imaging of post-traumatic spinal ligament injury. J Spin Disord 1989; 2(4):229–233.
21.   Capen DA. Comprehensive management of spine trauma. St Louis: Mosby, 1998.
22.   Drummond JC, Moore SS. The influence of dextrose administration on neurologic outcome after temporary spinal cord ischemia in the rabbit. Anesthesiology 1989; 70:64.

5

Timing of Surgery Following Spinal Cord Injury

MICHAEL J. VIVES

University of Medicine and Dentistry of New Jersey, Newark, New Jersey, U.S.A.

STEVEN R. GARFIN

University of California, San Diego, San Diego, California, U.S.A.

JEAN-JACQUES ABITBOL

California Spine Group, San Diego, California, U.S.A.

ALEXANDER R. VACCARO

Thomas Jefferson University Hospital and the Rothman Institute, Philadelphia, Pennsylvania, U.S.A.

I TIMING OF SURGERY IN SPINAL CORD INJURY

As many as 10,000 people a year sustain and survive spinal cord injury (SCI) and approximately 200,000 people live with some degree of SCI in the United States today. Many of the recent medical developments in the treatment of SCI have been related to injury prevention and rehabilitation. Advances in pharmacological therapy have been shown to have a positive effect on preventing progression and even improving neurological function following SCI.

Evidence to support surgical management of SCI due to fractures or dislocations of the spine is substantial. What remains controversial, however, is the optimal timing of surgical intervention. Timing of surgery should be analyzed in terms of a risk/benefit ratio in regard to the potential for neural recovery, associated systemic medical complications, as well as cost to society.

II PATHOPHYSIOLOGY OF SPINAL CORD INJURY

The initial injury to the spinal cord may involve a contusion, laceration, blast effect, ischemic event, or transient or ongoing compression. Neural injury usually occurs when the energy of the trauma overwhelms the ability of the spinal column to dissipate the energy of impact. Energy is then directly imparted on the spinal cord (1). The primary mechanical insult to the cord may be a result of one or a combination of vector forces, such as hyperflexion, extension, rotation, or axial loading. Impact is often transient. Persistent neural compression may occur by displaced bone fragments or disk elements.

In response to the primary injury, a set of acute-phase interactions involving a cascade of complex biochemical events is triggered, which leads to secondary injury. Acutely, hemorrhage and edema in the cord are compounded by autonomic dysfunction and bradycardia, potentially increasing the degree of ischemia to the cord. At the cellular level, hypoxia is accompanied by an uncoupling of oxidative phosphorylation and aerobic glycolysis with abrupt shifts in the level of ions and water content across cell membranes (2). Histologically, central cord gray matter necrosis occurs within the first few hours of injury, followed by cystic degeneration and scar tissue formation along axonal long tracts (3). There are various mechanisms of secondary neuronal injury that may involve accumulation of free radicals (4,5), abnormal influx of calcium ions, endorphin interactions with central opiate receptors (6,7), and tissue damage initiated by inflammatory mediators (8). The understanding that secondary injury occurring shortly following the initial trauma alters to varying degree the patient's ultimate potential for neurological recovery has led to the concept of a "window of opportunity" where spinal cord injury–reducing intervention may be possible.

A Pharmacological Intervention

Pharmacological intervention, aimed at interruption of the secondary injury cascade in the early postinjury period, continues to evolve. The addition of high-dose steroids administered intravenously within 8 h of injury has been demonstrated in Phase II of the National Acute Spinal Cord Injury Study, to decrease the extent of neurological deficit in some patients (through primarily root level preservation) (9,10). Another study has shown that high-dose steroids given for 48 h is more effective than a 24-h treatment regimen if it is instituted between 3 and 8 h following spinal injury (10); however, complications may be higher. The beneficial influence of the timing of early administration of specific pharmacological agents following spinal cord injury adds further support to the concept of the secondary injury process and the potential for modulation through timely intervention.

B Necessity for Surgical Treatment

Experimental data exist to support the efficacy of surgical decompression of specific cases of spinal cord injury. Rabinowitz and colleagues (11) studied this in a canine model. In this study, the distal spinal cord (L4 level) of each of the beagles was constricted by 60% of its original value with nylon ties. One group received methylprednisolone and no surgery; one group received methylprednisolone and was decompressed surgically at 6 h; and the third group was surgically decompressed at 6 h without concomitant steroids. The authors demonstrated that surgical decompression, with or without methylprednisolone, resulted in significantly better neurological recovery than methylprednisolone alone.

Despite evidence from animal experiments it has been difficult to establish definitively the efficacy of operative decompression in human clinical studies. In the majority of reports, variables such as age, type and severity of injury, and the nature and timing of surgical intervention have not been controlled. Only the study by Vaccaro et al. has been prospectively randomized (12). Furthermore, since many patients with partial or complete cord injury improve somewhat over time by natural history, it is difficult to attribute neurological improvement definitely to the effects of operative decompression.

In the setting of complete sensorimotor loss below the injury level, surgical decompression aims to improve function of compressed nerve roots and preserve function in compressed, but potentially viable, long tracts (13). Older studies in this patient population cast doubts about the role of surgery in this setting. Several dated publications have taken the position that patients treated without surgery fared better than those who were managed with surgery (14–17). Most of the patients in those series, however, were treated with laminectomy, which has since been shown to be suboptimal (if not contraindicated as a stand-alone procedure), with a predilection for late instability, progressive deformity, and neurological deficit (18). Anterior decompression, in contrast, is often more effective in decompressing the cord and nerve roots in the setting of trauma. In 1992, Anderson and Bohlman reported the outcome of 51 patients undergoing late anterior decompression and stabilization following a cervical fracture or dislocation. All patients exhibited complete motor tetraplegia and were treated at a mean of 15 months (range 1 month to 13 years) after injury. While only one patient demonstrated improved long tract function, 31 of 51 patients had significant improvement in root function (19).

In the setting of an incomplete spinal cord injury, the preservation of some function below the level of injury implies that some long tracts are viable. In patients with incomplete injuries to the cervical spinal cord, Bohlman and Anderson (20) reported on the outcome of 58 patients who underwent an anterior decompression and fusion at a mean of 13 months. Fifty percent of the patients displayed marked improvement in their preexisting ambulatory status. The improvement in patients who had grade 1 or 2 lower extremity motor function was particularly notable. In these initially nonambulatory patients, more than 50% percent were ambulatory postoperatively. Patients with incomplete thoracic spinal cord injuries also appear to improve after decompression and stabilization (21). Controlled studies are lacking and may be difficult to perform because of ethical concerns.

III   TIMING OF SURGERY

The benefits of surgical decompression in a patient with an incomplete spinal cord injury and mechanical compression or gross instability are not currently argued. However, the need to operate early, compared to the potential benefits of delay, is a controversial area. It seems intuitive that the sooner persistent spinal cord compression is relieved, especially in the setting of incomplete sensorimotor loss, the better the chance for neurological recovery. However, some studies have shown that an acutely injured and inflamed spinal cord might be more susceptible to further injury during surgical manipulation. No definitive study has been done in human patients to clearly demonstrate the superiority of one approach over the other (early versus late surgery).

A   Experimental Evidence

In the 1950s a number of laboratory research studies were conducted to explore the relationship of the duration of spinal cord compression to the potential for neurological recovery. Using epidural balloons, Tarlov (22) developed a model of graded spinal cord compression in dogs. He demonstrated that the time course for the development of paralysis and the duration of spinal cord compression after production of total paralysis influenced the degree of functional neurological recovery. If paralysis was produced rapidly, functional motor recovery did not occur if decompression was delayed more than 9 h. If paralysis was produced slowly, however, motor recovery could occur even when the decompression was delayed up to 1 week.

More recently, Carlson et al. (23) studied the timing and efficacy of early decompression in 21 beagles. The dogs' spinal cords were traumatically loaded dorsally at T13 until somatosensory-evoked potential amplitudes were reduced by 50%. Spinal cord displacement was continued for either 30 min (seven dogs), 60 min (eight dogs), or 180 min (six dogs), followed by a 3-h monitoring period. Regional spinal cord blood flow was determined by tracing fluorescent microspheres immediately after laminectomy (baseline), immediately after cessation of cord compression, and at 5, 15, and 180 min after decompression. Evoked potentials continued to be absent 5 min after cessation of compression in all dogs. Somatosensory-evoked potential recovery was observed in six of seven dogs in the 30-min compression group, five of eight dogs in the 60-min compression group, and none of the six dogs in the 180-min compression group. The authors emphasized the degree of early reperfusion hyperemia after decompression as an important element in neural recovery. They concluded the degree of early reperfusion hyperemia was inversely proportional to the duration of spinal cord compression and proportional to electrophysiological recovery. The critical time period for decompression seemed to be from 1 to 3 h.

Delamarter and colleagues (24) studied the effects of immediate and delayed spinal cord decompression in 30 dogs. All of the dogs underwent fourth lumbar laminectomy with compression of the caudal spinal cord to one-half the diameter of the spinal canal. The dogs were divided into five groups, which were decompressed at increasing intervals: group I, immediately; group II, after 1 h; group III, after 6 h; group IV, at 24 h; and group V, at 1 week. Neurological testing, somatosensory-evoked potentials, and histological examinations were performed. They found that neurological recovery was inversely proportional to the duration of compression, while histological changes progressed with the duration of compression. In their study, decompression in 1 h or less provided the best chance for recovery, while after 6 h little chance for recovery was observed. The authors suggested that the initial event was not solely responsible for all neurological changes and that there was a window of time during which cord injury could be reversed.

While these experimental models offer insight into the pathophysiology involved in traumatic spinal cord compression, they do not adequately simulate the pathomechanics involved following an actual spinal cord injury. Noting that these injuries in humans involve an initial impact followed by sustained compression by bone or soft tissue, Guha et al. (25). developed a biphasic clip compression model to produce injury. Clips with varying initial compression forces were applied to the spinal cord. The duration of compression was graded up to 4 h. Their results suggested that the major determinant of recovery was the amount of force imparted to the cord through the initial clip compression. The length of the sustained compression also influenced recovery, but only for animals injured with smaller initial compression forces. If the initial injury force was small, decompression was beneficial even after prolonged compression. The implications of these findings have relevance to the spectrum of outcomes seen after human spinal cord injury. When the initial injury is severe enough to cause shear injury to the long tracts, resulting in complete sensorimotor loss distally, the timing of decompression may not affect functional neurological outcome. In patients with less severe initial injury, with potentially viable neural pathways and incomplete sensorimotor loss, continued compression may propagate secondary injury, converting reversible neural deficits into irreversible ones (13).

B Clinical Studies

Outside the controlled setting of the research laboratory, investigations into the effect of the timing of decompression after spinal cord injury are more difficult to interpret. Arguments in favor of early and delayed decompression can be analyzed on multiple levels, including prospects for neurological recovery, relationship to systemic complications, and economics.

C Neurological Recovery

Proponents of delayed surgery have cited the risk for neurological worsening associated with early decompression and stabilization of an acutely injured spine. Marshall (26) examined this issue in a multicenter, multispecialty study. After reviewing close to 300 cases, they determined that the small percentage of patients who experienced neurological (and other systemic physiological) deterioration had all undergone surgery in less than 5 days. A similar conclusion had been reached earlier by Heiden et al. (27).

These findings could be partially accounted for, however, by the small rate of spontaneous neurological worsening seen even in the absence of surgery (17). Indeed, multiple authors have retrospectively reported no difference in the neurological outcome in patients treated with early surgery versus those treated on a delayed basis. In a retrospective study involving 106 patients, 49 of which underwent surgical decompression in less than 8 h, Petitjean (28) reported that early surgery had no influence on neurological outcome. The extent of the spinal injury (complete versus incomplete) was the only predictor of outcome. Levi and colleagues (29) retrospectively reviewed 103 consecutive cervical spine injuries to determine the influence of timing of surgery on neurological outcome. Patients were divided into complete and incomplete injury groups; these groups were subdivided into those decompressed in less than 24 h and those operated on after 24 h. No statistically significant difference in neurological outcome was found between the early and delayed surgery groups. The groups, however, were not matched for preoperative neurological grade. Additionally, those patients who underwent delayed surgery did so for logistical reasons.

Likewise, Wolf and coworkers (30) examined this issue in 103 patients with cervical spine injuries. Fifty-three of these patients were treated operatively, 35 in less than 24 h after injury, and 18 at greater than 24 h. The neurological outcome between the two groups did not differ significantly. While these studies demonstrated no risk for neurological worsening with early surgery, such data are generally cited by advocates of delayed surgery since they also fail to demonstrate neurological improvement with early decompression.

In contrast, there have been several other retrospective series reporting a notably improved neurological outcome in patients treated with early surgery. A retrospective study by Mirza et al. (31) involving 43 patients compared patients undergoing surgery earlier than (average 1.8 days) or later than (average 14.1 days) 72 h after acute injury of the cervical spinal cord. There was no significant difference in age, sex, procedure types, steroid use, injury severity score, Glasgow Coma Score, or preoperative ASIA motor index. Postoperatively, neurological improvement was significantly higher in the early surgery group.

Using 72 h as a cutoff between early and late surgery, Levi et al. (29) also retrospectively reported improved neurological outcomes with early surgery. Hadley and colleagues (32) retrospectively reviewed their experience with operative management of facet fracture dislocations. In their study, all 10 patients who made a significant neurological recovery had surgery within 8 h of injury, with six having surgery within 5 h. Likewise, Ducker (33) and Aebi (34) independently reported improved neurological outcomes in patients decompressed within 6 h of injury compared with those delayed beyond that point.

In a controlled, prospective study analyzing the optimal timing of surgery in spinal cord injury, Vaccaro and colleagues (12) studied 123 patients with subaxial cervical spine injuries. The patients ranged in age from 15 to 75 years and were neurologically classified as ASIA class A through D. Patients with worsening neurological function or with significant epidural hematoma were excluded. Patients were randomized into two admission-matched groups (by age, sex, and motor score). In one group, patients underwent surgery less than 72 h after injury. In the late group, patients were operated on more than 5 days after injury. In this study, there was no statistically significant difference in neurological outcome between patients undergoing surgery within 72 h or 5 days from injury. The authors postulated that the lack of significant difference in outcome may be related to their selection of time frames.

The clinical literature on the optimal timing of surgical decompression in spinal cord injury is deficient in well-designed prospective studies to definitively address this issue. An increased understanding of the pathophysiology of secondary injury pathways and compelling evidence from studies in the animal laboratory strongly suggest that timing does influence neurological outcome following some spinal cord injuries. It has been speculated that the "early" time frames utilized in clinical studies may be outside the "window of opportunity" for meaningful intervention to alter neurological outcome (12,35). The most rapid progression of pathological changes in neural tissue seems to occur over the first 8 h (9,36). Realistically, however, decompression within this time from injury is often logistically difficult.

D Systemic Complications

Patients with spinal injuries are predisposed to a number of complications related to physiological changes due to injury, side effects from pharmacological agents, and extended recumbence and immobilization. Urinary tract infections are one of the most common complications seen in the initial months after spinal cord injury and are a frequent cause of fever, chills, and sepsis (37). Gastrointestinal bleeding frequently occurs in the early period after spinal cord injury. While imbalanced parasympathetic and sympathetic innervation to the gastrointestinal tract and trauma-related stress play a role, high-dose intravenous steroids increase the risk considerably (9). Complications related to immobilization include pressure sores, especially over the sacrum. Venous thromboembolism has historically been associated with spinal cord injury in high numbers. While some early studies reported a prevalence of over 50%, with current prophylactic strategies the prevalence is probably less than 5% (38). Tetraplegics are at risk for atelectasis and pneumonia due to decreased vital capacity and impaired cough resulting from abdominal and intercostal paralysis. Higher level tetraplegics (C4–C5) are at particular risk for such respiratory morbidity (39).

Theoretically, some of these complications can be reduced by early mobilization after spinal stability has been achieved. As such, another area of debate surrounding the optimal timing of surgical intervention involves the risk for medical complications. The contemporary trend for management of multitrauma patients with nonspinal injuries has been for earlier surgical intervention. This rationale has been driven by the concept of the "golden hour," the initial period after injury before complications in multiple organ systems develop. Presumably, patients are in better physiological condition soon after the initial trauma than a few days later due to the medical sequelae of trauma and immobilization such as atelectasis, pneumonia, deep vein thrombosis, and renal insufficiency.

Some retrospective studies performed 15 to 20 years ago argued against this notion in the case of spinal injuries. Heiden and colleagues (27) reported a near 20% increase in pulmonary complications in patients surgically decompressed in the first week compared to those operated on beyond that point. Sonntag and Francis (40) recently reviewed a series of studies recommending delayed surgery based on increased perioperative morbidity and mortality in patients undergoing early surgery. Many of the studies supporting their argument, however, had been done over 15 years ago.

More recent data from centers with extensive experience in the surgical management of spinal injuries suggest that early operation is not detrimental and actually decreases systemic complications. Wilberger (41) compared the complication rate in patients undergoing surgery within the first 24 h after injury with those stabilized beyond that point. The early surgery group had lower rates of thrombophlebitits, pulmonary embolism, pneumonia, and decubiti. Hadley and colleagues (32) addressed this issue in a retrospective study of patients undergoing early surgery after facet-fracture dislocations. In this study, in addition to improved neurological outcomes, the authors also demonstrated no difference in the rate of systemic complications. Krengel et al. (42) and Levi and coworkers (29) reported a substantial reduction in complications such as atelectasis, pneumonia, and thrombophlebitis in patients undergoing surgery acutely after their injuries. McBroom and colleagues (43) studied systemic complications in a group of patients surgically stabilized within 24 h of injury compared with a group stabilized at greater than 60 h after injury. The study group involved 38 patients undergoing thoracic or lumbar stabilization.

Patients who were surgically stabilized within the first 24 h had a statistically significant decrease in pulmonary and total complications.

In a retrospective study previously mentioned, Mirza and colleagues (31) compared treatment at one institution within 72 h with treatment at another institution where surgery was performed at an average of 14 days after injury. Aside from the philosophical differences in the timing of surgery at the two institutions (Harborview Medical Center and the State University of New York), patients were treated in a similar fashion. Patients at both institutions underwent immediate indirect neurological decompression by closed reduction. Medical records were reviewed for pulmonary, neurological, thrombotic, wound, pressure-sore- or infection-related complications during the acute hospitalization. Complications that increased the acute care stay were classified as major; those that did not affect the length of acute care hospitalization were classified as minor. The number of total complications was greater in the group of patients who underwent late surgery. This difference, however, was not statistically significant with the numbers available.

E Economics

Cost issues associated with the timing of intervention are related to overall length of stay and amount of time utilizing intensive care resources. The increasing financial pressures on hospitals in today's evolving healthcare industry have made cost reduction through decreased length of stay and consumption of resources an issue of paramount importance. While the studies addressing this issue are uniformly retrospective, there is general consensus that early surgery is probably beneficial in terms of cost containment (assuming complications are not increased).

Campagnolo and associates (44) retrospectively examined the length of acute hospital stay in 64 patients with cervical, thoracolumbar, or cauda equina injuries. Patients were divided into two groups based on whether they underwent spinal stabilization earlier or later than 24 h after injury. The difference in the average length of stay was statistically significant: 37.5 days for the early group versus 54.7 days for the late group. McBroom's data (43) support these findings. Fractures of the thoracic or lumbar spine were divided into two groups: those stabilized within 24 h of injury versus those stabilized at greater than 60 h. Earlier stabilization led to earlier rehabilitation for the patient and a decrease in length of acute hospital stay, intensive care unit stay, and time requiring mechanical ventilation. Levi's study (29) analyzing 103 consecutive patients with cervical spine trauma reached similar conclusions. Patients were divided into those undergoing surgery in less than 24 h compared to those stabilized beyond that point. The early group had shorter length of stay, decreased expenses, earlier transfer to rehabilitation, and easier patient care.

A large retrospective study involving 156 polytrauma patients undergoing surgery for spinal cord injury examined this issue in detail (45). The patients were separated into two groups: those undergoing surgery in less than 48 h and those undergoing surgery beyond that point. The groups were matched for Glasgow Coma Score, injury severity score, and abbreviated injury severity score. Those patients who had an injury severity score of 18 or greater and who underwent early surgery had fewer intensive care days, fewer acute hospital days, and lower overall charges than the late surgery group. Patients with a lower injury severity score also benefited in the above-mentioned categories, but the differences were less pronounced.

IV SUMMARY

The timing of surgery after spinal cord injury continues to be controversial. Our increased understanding of the pathophysiology of secondary injury pathways along with data from animal experimentation suggest a narrow window of opportunity exists where decompression may influence neurological outcome, depending on the extent of the initial injury to the cord. Clinically, however, achieving surgical decompression in such a narrow time frame is logistically difficult. This may contribute to the lack of clear-cut evidence to support the laboratory studies. From the standpoint of systemic complications and cost containment, recent data from centers with extensive experience demonstrate clear benefit from "early" surgery. Future developments in pharmacological modalities may alter the opportunity for neurological improvement (with or without surgery). Additional research into the specific timing of early intervention will continue to be necessary to clarify the treatment window for pharmacological and surgical interventions.

REFERENCES

1. Slucky AV, Eismont FJ. Treatment of acute injury of the cervical spine. J Bone Joint Surg [Am] 1994; 76:982–986.
2. Jannsen L, Hansebout R. Pathogenesis of spinal cord injury and newer treatments: a review. Spine 1989; 14:23–32.
3. Bernbeck J, Delamarter R. Pathophysiology and initial treatment of acute spinal cord injuries. In: Cotler JM, Simpson JM, An HS, Silveri CP, eds. Surgery of Spinal Trauma. Philadelphia: Lippincott, Williams & Wilkins, 2000:49–51.
4. Demopoulos HB, Flamm ES, Pietronigro DD, Seligman MD, Tomasula J, DeCrescito V. The free radical pathology and the microcirculation in the major central nervous system disorders. Acta Physiol Scand 1980; 492(suppl):91–119.
5. Hall ED, Braughler JM, McCall JM. New pharmacologic treatment of acute spinal cord trauma. J Neurotrauma 1988; 5:81–89.
6. Faden AI. Opioid and nonopioid action mechanisms may contribute to dynophin's pathophysiological actions in spinal cord injury. Ann Neurol 1990; 24:67–74.
7. Hall ED, Wolf DL, Althaus JS, Von Voightlander PF. Beneficial effects of the kappa opoid receptor agonist U-50488H in experimental acute brain and spinal cord injury. Brain Res 1987; 435:174–180.
8. Young W, Huang P, Kume-Kick J. Cellular ionic and biomolecular mechanisms of the injury process. In: Benzel E, Tator C, eds. Contemporary Management of Spinal Cord Injury. City: American Association of Neurological Surgeons, 1995:28–31.
9. Bracken MB, Shepard MJ, Collins WF, Holford TR, Young W, Baskin DS. A randomized, controlled trial of methylprednisolone or naloxone in the treatment of acute spinal-cord injury. N Engl J Med 1990; 322:1405–1411.
10. Bracken MB, Shepard MJ, Holford TR, Leo-Summers L, Aldrich EF, Fazl M, Fehlings M, Herr DL, Hitchon PW, Marshall LF, Nockels RP, Pascale V, Perot PL Jr. Administration of methylprednisolone for 24 or 48 hours or trialazid mesylate for 48 hours in the treatment of acute spinal cord injury: results of the Third National Acute Spinal Cord Injury Randomized Controlled trial. National Acute Spinal Cord Injury Study. JAMA 1997; 277(20):1597–1694.
11. Rabinowitz RS, Currier BL, Jimenez MA. The effect of urgent surgical decompression, decompression and methylprednisolone, and methylprednisolone alone on the outcome of spinal cord injury: a blinded, prospective, randomized trial in beagles. Presented at

the American Academy of Orthopaedic Surgeons Annual Meeting, February 1996, Atlanta, Georgia: paper #514.

12. Vaccaro AR, Daugherty RJ, Sheehan TP, Dante SJ, Cotler JM, Balderston RA, Herbison GJ, Northrup BE. Neurologic outcome of early versus late surgery for cervical spinal cord injury. Spine 1997; 22:2609–2613.

13. Cooper PR. Injuries of the cervical spine: surgical treatment. In: Clarke CR, Ducker TB, Dvorak J, Garfin SR, Herkowitz HN, Levine AM, Pizzutillo PD, Sherk HH, Ullrich CG, Zeidman SM, eds. The Cervical Spine, 3rd ed. Philadelphia: Lippincott-Raven, 1998: 551–555.

14. Guttman L. The conservative management of closed injuries of the vertebral column resulting in quadriplegia. In: Harris JH, ed. The Radiology of Acute Cervical Spine Trauma. Baltimore: Williams and Wilkins, 1978:1534–1551.

15. Bedbrook GM. Spinal injuries with tetraplegia and paraplegia. J Bone Joint Surg [Br] 1979; 61:267–284.

16. Wilmot CB, Hall KM. Evaluation of the acute management of tetraplegia: conservative versus surgical treatment. Paraplegia 1986; 24:148–153.

17. Frankel HL, Hancock DO, Hyslop G, Melzak J, Michaelis LS, Ungar GH, Vernon JD, Walsh JJ. The value of postural reduction in the management of closed injuries of the spine with paraplegia and tetraplegia—Part 1. Paraplegia 1969; 7:179–192.

18. Bohlman HH. Acute fractures and dislocations of the cervical spine: an analysis of three hundred hospitalized patients and review of the literature. J Bone Joint Surg [Am] 1979; 61:1119–1142.

19. Anderson PA, Bohlman HH. Anterior decompression and arthrodesis of the cervical spine: long-term motor improvement. Part II: Improvement in complete traumatic quadriplegia. J Bone Joint Surg [Am] 1992; 74:683–692.

20. Bohlman HH, Anderson PA. Anterior decompression and arthrodesis of the cervical spine: long-term motor improvement. Part I. Improvement in incomplete traumatic quadriparesis. J Bone Joint Surg [Am] 1992; 74:671–682.

21. Maiman DJ, Larson SJ, Benzel EC. Neurological improvement associated with late decompression of the thoracolumbar spinal cord. Neurosurgery 1984; 14:302–307.

22. Tarlov IM. Spinal cord compression studies. III. Time limits for recovery after gradual compression in dogs. Arch Neurol Psych 1954; 71:588–597.

23. Carlson GD, Minato Y, Okada A, Gorden CD, Warden KE, Barbeau JM, Biro CL, Bahnuik E, Bohlman HH, Lamanna JC. Early time-dependent decompression for spinal cord injury: vascular mechanisms of recovery. J Neurotrauma 1997; 14(12):951–962.

24. Delamarter RB, Sherman J, Carr JB. Pathophysiology of spinal cord injury: recovery after immediate and delayed decompression. J Bone Joint Surg [Am] 1995; 77:1042–1049.

25. Guha A, Tator CH, Endrenyi L, Piper I. Decompression of the spinal cord improves recovery after acute experimental spinal cord compression injury. Paraplegia 1987; 25: 324–339.

26. Marshall LF, Knowlton S, Garfin SR, Klauber MR, Eisenberg HM, Kopaniky D, Miner ME, Tabbador K, Clifton GL. Deterioration following spinal cord injury. J Neurosurg 1987; 66:400–404.

27. Heiden JS, Weiss MH, Rosenberg AW, Apuzzo ML, Kurze T. Management of cervical spinal cord trauma in Southern California. J Neurosurg 1975; 43:732–736.

28. Frankel HL, Hancock DO, Hyslop G, et al. The value of postural reduction in the initial management of closed injuries of the spine with paraplegia and tetraplegia. Part I. Paraplegia 1969; 7:179–192.

29. Petitjean ME, Pointillart V, Dixmerias F, Wiart L, Sztark F, Lassie P, Thicoipe M, Dabadre P. Medical treatment of spinal cord injury in the acute stage. Ann Fr Anesth Reanim 1998; 17(2):114–122.

30. Levi L, Wolf A, Rigamonti A, Ragheb J, Mirvis S, Robinson WL. Anterior decompression in cervical spine trauma: does the timing of surgery affect the outcome. Neurosurgery 1991; 29:216–222.
31. Wolf A, Levi L, Mirvis S, Ragheb J, Huhn S, Rigamonti D, Robinson WL. Operative management of bilateral facet dislocation. J Neurosurg 1991; 75:883–890.
32. Mirza SK, Krengel WF III, Chapman JR, Anderson PA, Bailey JC, Grady MS, Yuan HA. Early versus delayed surgery for acute cervical spinal cord injury. Clin Orthop 1999; 359:104–114.
33. Hadley MN, Fitzpatrick BC, Sonntag VKH, Browner CM. Facet fracture-dislocation injuries of the cervical spine. Neurosurgery 1992; 30:661–666.
34. Ducker TB, Bellegarrigue R, Salcman M, et al. Timing of operative care in cervical spinal cord injury. Spine 1984; 9:525–531.
35. Aebi M, Mohler J, Zach GA, Morsher E. Indication, surgical technoque and results of 100 surgically treated fractures and fracture-dislocation of the cervical spine. Clin Orthop 1986; 203:244–257.
36. Vaccaro AR, Singh K. Pharmacologic treatment and surgical timing for spinal cord injury. Current Opinion Orthop 1999; 10:112–116.
37. Tator CH, Fehlings MG. Review of the secondary injury theory of spinal cord trauma with emphasis on vascular mechanisms. J Neurosurg 1991; 75:15–26.
38. National Institute on Disability and Rehabilitation Research Consensus Statement. The prevention and management of urinary tract infections among people with spinal cord injuries. J Am Paraplegia Soc 1992; 15:194–204.
39. Naso F. Cardiovascular problems in patients with spinal cord injury. Phys Med Rehabil Clin North Am 1992; 3:741–749.
40. Fishburn MJ, Marino RJ, Ditunno JF. Atelectasis and pneumonia in acute spinal cord injury. Arch Phys Med Rehabil 1990; 71:197–200.
41. Sonntag VKH, Francis PM. Patient selection and timing of surgery. In: Benzel EC, Tator CH, eds. Contemporary Management of Spinal Cord Injury. Park Ridge, IL: American Association of Neurologic Surgeons, 1995:97–108.
42. Wilberger JE. Diagnosis and management of spinal cord trauma. J Neurotrauma 1991; 8:21–30.
43. Krengel WF III, Anderson PA, Henley MB. Early stabilization and decompression for incomplete paraplegia due to a thoracic-level spinal cord injury. Spine 1993; 18:2080–2087.
44. McBroom RJ, Tucker WS, Waddell JP. Early versus delayed fixation of the thoraco-lumbar spine in polytrauma patients. Orthop Trans 1995; 19:149.
45. Campagnolo DI, Esquieres RE, Kopacz KJ. Effect of timing of stabilization on length of stay and medical complications following spinal cord injury. J Spinal Cord Med 1997; 20(3):331–334.
46. Fellrath RF Jr, Hanley EN Jr. Spinal injury and polytrauma: influence of surgical timing. Orthop Trans 1995; 19:149.

6

Physical Examination: ASIA Motor/Sensory Examination and Spinal Cord Injury Syndromes

BOBBY TAY

University of California, San Francisco, School of Medicine and San Francisco General Hospital, San Francisco, California, U.S.A.

FRANK J. EISMONT

University of Miami School of Medicine, Miami, Florida, U.S.A.

I INTRODUCTION

Traumatic spinal cord injury afflicts more than 8000 new patients per year (1). This figure will tend to increase over time as improved methods of transportation, life-support, and trauma care will allow for greater survival rates from high-energy trauma. The evaluation and management of patients with spinal injury are often complicated because it typically occurs in the context of polytrauma. In addition, the level of complexity in rehabilitating these patients is increased by the functional limitations placed upon the patient as a result of neurological injury. The most important part of the treatment of a patient with spinal cord injury begins with the initial assessment. The careful evaluation and clear documentation of the patient's neurological status will allow the treating physician to best decide the appropriate initial treatment as well as to determine the prognosis for functional recovery and the long-term rehabilitation goals for each individual. This chapter will focus on the physical examination of the patient with spinal cord injury, with emphasis on the recommendations made by the American Spinal Injury Association (ASIA). It will also describe the various spinal cord syndromes that may be encountered by the treating physician.

II GENERAL PHYSICAL EXAMINATION

After the initial resuscitation has been performed, the secondary survey involves a careful physical examination of the patient. This involves removal of all clothing and a systematic evaluation of the entire body for abrasions, contusions, lacerations, and limb asymmetry suggesting underlying injury. The extremities should be palpated for the presence of instability or crepitus. The peripheral pulses should be palpated and any absence or differences in the strength of the pulses should incite an investigation for the cause. The abdomen should be assessed for peritoneal signs or contusions. The chest is auscultated for the presence of normal, symmetric breath sounds and palpated for crepitus and abnormal motion.

Once the general physical examination is complete, the spine can be palpated in a systematic fashion from occiput to sacrum. In a comatose patient, the cervical spine must be cleared radiographically before removal of the cervical collar since 3 to 5% of these patients will have an associated neck injury. The patient is carefully rolled just enough to palpate each of the spinous processes and the intervening interspinous spaces in order to determine the presence of any localized tenderness, step-off, crepitation, or interspinous widening. Areas of ecchymosis are noted as they may indicate severe spinal column injury.

III NEUROLOGICAL ASSESSMENT

The neurological assessment of a patient with spinal cord injury requires an understanding of the basic anatomy of the spinal cord, its ascending and descending tracts, and the exiting nerve roots (2).

The spinal cord is composed of central gray matter (neuronal cell bodies) surrounded by white matter (axons). Within a cross-section of the cord, several important anatomical structures can be identified. These include the lateral spinothalamic tracts that are responsible for transmitting pain and temperature sensation, the lateral corticospinal tracts that are responsible for the motor function, and the posterior columns that transmit position sense, vibratory sensation, and deep pressure sensation. The spinothalamic tracts cross to the opposite side of the spinal cord within three levels of entering the cord. In contrast, the corticospinal tracts and the posterior columns innervate myotomes and dermatomes at the same levels that they exit the spinal column. These tracts carry a specific topographical organization; the most central portions represent the function of the more proximal areas of the body and the more peripheral portions represent the function of the distal areas of the body (Fig. 1).

The spinal roots exit the vertebral column through the intervertebral foramina. In the cervical spine, the C1 root exits above the C1 body, the C2 root exits below the C1 body, and the C8 root exits below the C7 body. In the thoracic and lumbar spine, each root exits under the pedicle of the same number.

A Definitions

Understanding the terminology used in the description of patients with spinal cord injury is essential for their classification and in communicating the degree of injury to physicians and therapists. These definitions are given as described in the International Standards for Neurological and Functional Classification of Spinal Cord Injury (3).

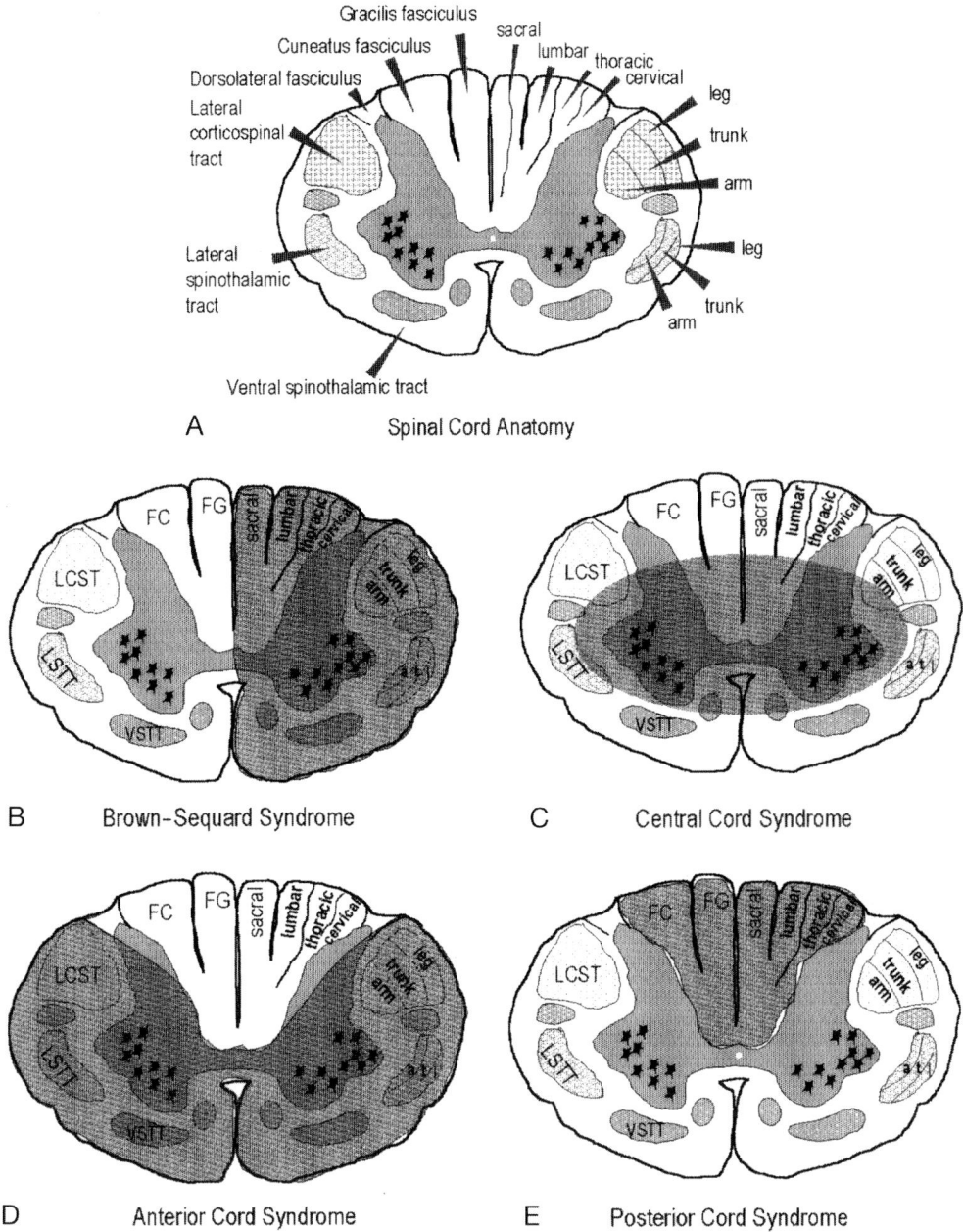

Figure 1 (A) Cross-section through cervical spinal cord showing specific motor and sensory tracts as well as the topographical organization of the motor and sensory tracts. (B) Brown-Sequard syndrome with hemisection of cord (red). (C) Central cord syndrome with injuries to the central portion of the spinal cord affecting the arms more than the legs. (D) Anterior cord syndrome with sparing of only the posterior columns of the spinal cord. (E) Posterior cord syndrome affects only the posterior columns.

1. Tetraplegia/quadriplegia—refers to the impairment or loss of motor/sensory function in the cervical segments of the cord due to damage of neural elements within the spinal canal. This leads to impairment of the function of the arms, trunk, legs, and pelvic organs.
2. Paraplegia—refers to the impairment or loss of motor/sensory function in the thoracic, lumbar, or sacral segments of the spinal cord. Arm function is spared.
3. Dermatome—refers to the area of skin innervated by the sensory axons within each segmental nerve.
4. Myotome—refers to the collection of muscle fibers innervated by the motor axons within each segmental nerve.
5. Neurological level:
   a. Sensory level—the most caudal segment of the spinal cord with normal sensation. This may differ from side to side.
   b. Motor level—the most caudal segment of the spinal cord with normal motor function. This may also differ from side to side. Because many of the muscles tested are innervated by more than one root level, if a muscle has at least grade 3 (antigravity) strength, it is considered to have intact innervation by the more rostral of the innervating segments as long as the next most rostral key muscle has full strength.
6. Skeletal level—refers to the level of greatest vertebral damage.
7. Incomplete injury—this term is used to describe a patient who has partial preservation of sensory and/or motor function found below the neurological level and must include the lowest sacral segment (normal perianal sensation and rectal tone). Any evidence of sacral sparing which is manifested by the presence of perianal sensation, sensitivity to sharp and dull pin prick, toe flexion, or anal sphincter control indicates an incomplete injury that carries a significantly better prognosis for functional return (2).
8. Complete injury—this term describes the patient who has absence of sensory and motor function below the neurological level, including the lowest sacral segment.
9. Zone of partial preservation—these are dermatomes and myotomes caudal to the neurological level that remain partially innervated.
10. Spinal shock—this term describes the period of time (usually the initial 24–48 h after injury) during which there is cessation of all reflex, motor, and sensory function below the level of injury. Spinal shock is caused by metabolic derangements in the neurons within the cord that prevents the conduction of action potentials. The end of spinal shock is marked by the return of the bulbocavernosus reflex, a local reflex arc at the S2–S4 levels. In Stauffer's series, 99% of his patients had return of their bulbocavernosus reflex within 24 h from the time of injury. The anal wink also returns at the end of spinal shock but is not as easily demonstrated as the bulbocavernosus reflex (2).

IV ASIA MOTOR AND SENSORY EXAMINATION

The motor and sensory examination outlined by ASIA is the most widely accepted and utilized system to assess the impact of spinal cord injury on the patient. It involves the use of a grading system to evaluate the remaining sensory and motor function. The system allows the patients to be assessed through scales of impairment and functional independence.

A   Determination of Sensory Levels

The sensory level is determined by the patient's ability to perceive pinprick (using a disposable needle or safety pin) and light touch (using a cotton ball). Testing of a key point in each of the 28 dermatomes on the right and the left sides of the body as well as evaluation of perianal sensation is required (Figs. 2 and 3). The variability in sensation for each individual stimulus is graded on a three-point scale: 0 = absent; 1 = impaired; 2 = normal; NT = not testable.

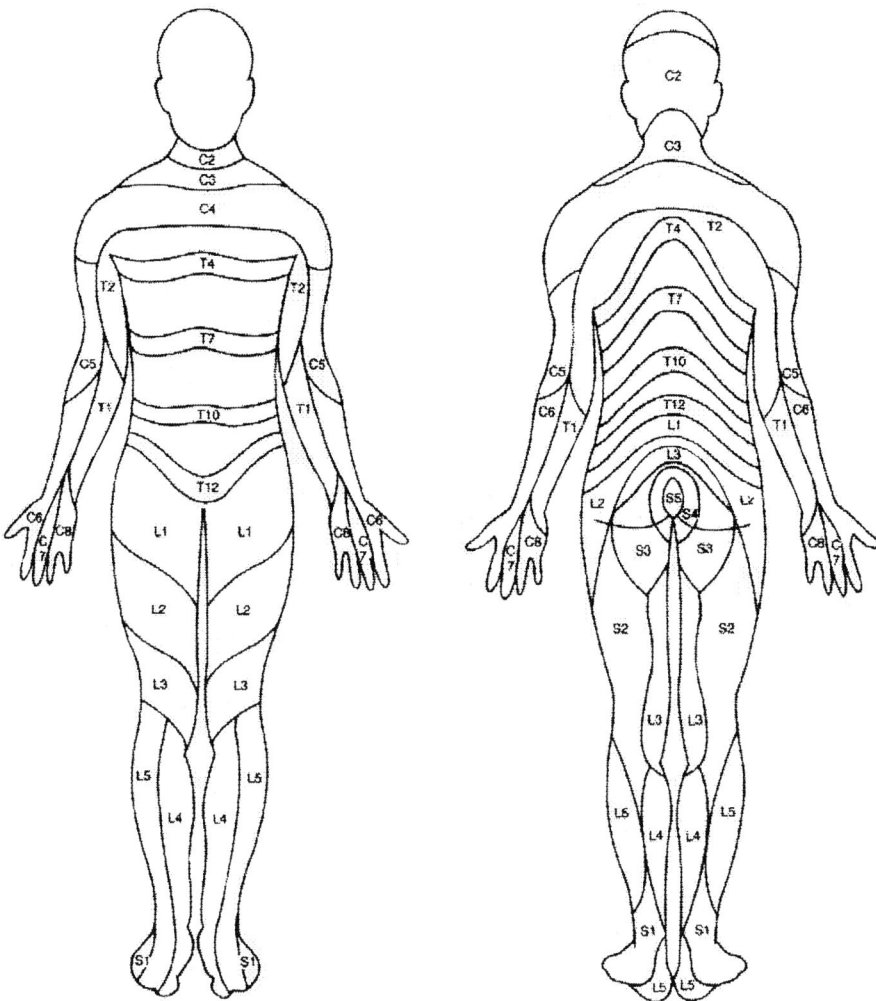

Figure 2   Dermatomal map showing distribution of sensory levels over the body.

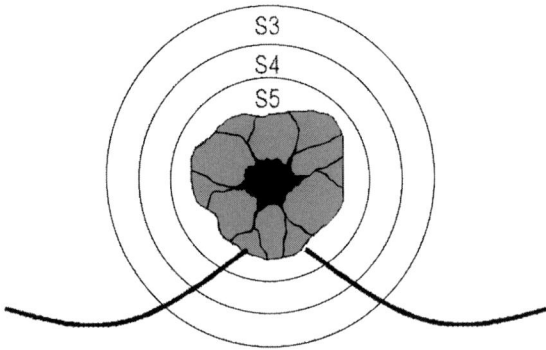

Figure 3 Dermatomal map around the anus showing the sensory levels tested using light touch and pinprick.

In the cervical spine, the C3 and C4 nerve roots supply sensation to the entire upper neck and chest in a capelike distribution from the tip of the acromion to just above the nipple line. The next adjacent sensory level is the T2 dermatome. The brachial plexus, C5–T1, supplies the upper extremities.

ASIA also recommends testing of pain and deep pressure sensation in the same dermatomes as well as an evaluation of proprioception by testing the position sense of the index fingers and great toes on each side.

B   Determination of Motor Levels

The motor level is determined (3) by manual testing of a key muscle in the 10 paired myotomes from rostral to caudal (Fig. 4). The strength of each muscle is graded on a six-point scale: 0=total paralysis; 1=palpable or visible contraction; 2=full range of motion of the joint powered by the muscle with gravity eliminated; 3=full range of motion of the joint powered by the muscle against gravity; 4=active movement with full range of motion against moderate resistance; 5=normal strength; and NT = not testable. For myotomes that are not clinically testable by manual muscle evaluation, the motor level is presumed to be the same as the sensory level (C1–C4, T2–L1, S2–S5).

ASIA also recommends evaluation of diaphragmatic function (via fluoroscopy, C4 level) and the abdominal musculature (via Beevor's sign, which is the upward migration of the umbilicus from upper abdominal contraction in the absence of lower abdominal contraction due to paralysis at the T10 level). Evaluation of medial hamstring and hip adductor strength is also recommended but not required.

C   ASIA Impairment Scale

Once spinal shock has resolved, the motor and sensory examination allows the patient to be graded on a scale of functional impairment (3). The grading system used is a modification of the Frankel classification system.

> ASIA A (complete): No sensory or motor function is preserved below the level of injury, including the sacral segments S4–S5.

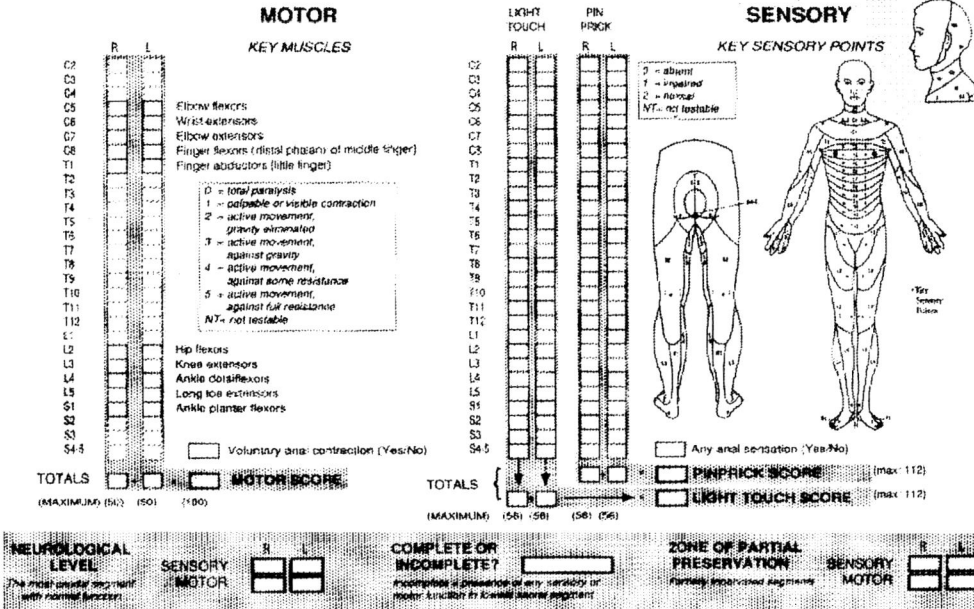

Figure 4   ASIA motor and sensory scoring form.

ASIA B (incomplete): Sensory function is spared, but there is no motor function below the level of injury except for the preservation of sacral segments S4–S5.

ASIA C (incomplete): Motor function is preserved below the neurological level and more than half of the key muscles below the neurological level have a muscle strength less than grade 3.

ASIA D (incomplete): Motor function is preserved below the neurological level and at least half of the muscles below the neurological level have a muscle strength of at least grade 3.

ASIA E (Normal).

D   ASIA Functional Independence Measure

The functionality of an individual with spinal cord injury is dependent on multiple factors including age, body habitus, overall fitness, and motivation (3). In addition, patients with complete spinal cord injuries will often regain one root level of function on each side over the ensuing 6 months following injury. Despite the individual variability, some generalizations can be made on the useful function that a person can attain after suffering an injury at a specific neurological level (Fig. 5). Patients with C5-level tetraplegia will require assistance to transfer, groom, and feed themselves. C6-level tetraplegic patients should be able to dress and feed themselves independently after functional splinting or tendon transfers. If they are young, thin, and strong, about 50% of them should be able to transfer independently. Patients with C7-level tetraplegia will have active finger motion and should be independent

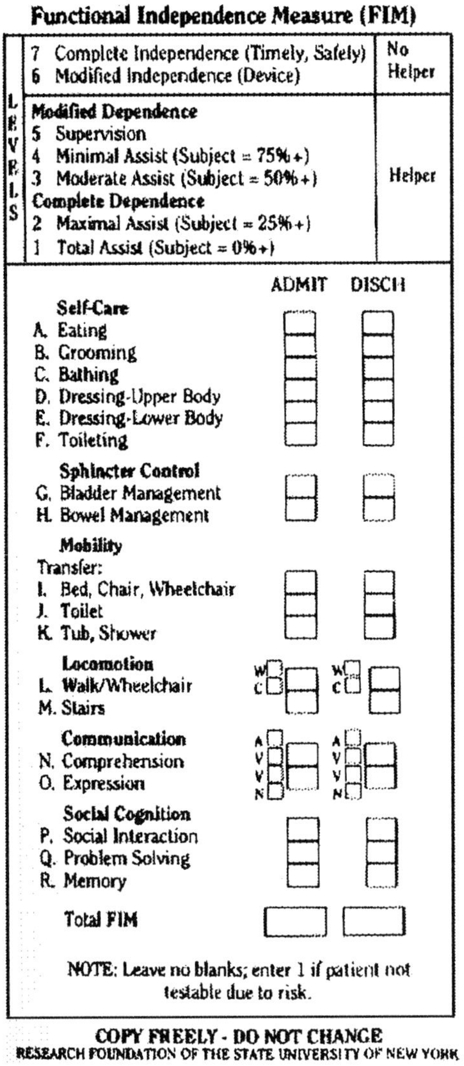

Functional Independence Measure (FIM)

7 Complete Independence (Timely, Safely) 6 Modified Independence (Device)	No Helper
Modified Dependence 5 Supervision 4 Minimal Assist (Subject = 75%+) 3 Moderate Assist (Subject = 50%+) **Complete Dependence** 2 Maximal Assist (Subject = 25%+) 1 Total Assist (Subject = 0%+)	Helper

L E V E L S (vertical label at left)

ADMIT   DISCH

Self-Care
A. Eating
B. Grooming
C. Bathing
D. Dressing-Upper Body
E. Dressing-Lower Body
F. Toileting

Sphincter Control
G. Bladder Management
H. Bowel Management

Mobility
Transfer:
I. Bed, Chair, Wheelchair
J. Toilet
K. Tub, Shower

Locomotion
L. Walk/Wheelchair   W / C
M. Stairs

Communication
N. Comprehension   A / V
O. Expression   V / N

Social Cognition
P. Social Interaction
Q. Problem Solving
R. Memory

Total FIM

NOTE: Leave no blanks; enter 1 if patient not
testable due to risk.

Figure 5   ASIA functional independence measure.

in transfers, grooming, and self-feeding. Patients with neurological levels of C6 and below will be able to drive an automobile with hand controls. Although ambulation with bracing is theoretically possible for T1–T12 paraplegics, practically all of these people will be wheelchair-bound because of the tremendously high-energy cost of ambulation with bracing. L1–L3-level paraplegics will be household ambulators with functional bracing. L4- and L5-level paraplegics will be community ambulators. In general, trauma that results in a complete spinal cord injury will also cause injury to the spinal roots exiting at the same level. These roots suffer a peripheral nerve injury because they originate from normal spinal cord just proximal to the level of damage. Thus we would expect the function of the root to return within 6 months. Sixty-six to 80% of patients can be expected to recover at least one nerve root level of function following a complete cord injury (4). This must be clearly distinguished from return of cord function (2).

The ASIA guidelines provide an instrument to evaluate and measure objectively the impact of spinal cord injury on the patient. This instrument, the Functional Independence Measure, is also a widely accepted and utilized approach to evaluate the progress or lack of progress of a patient over time or after a specific treatment. It assesses six areas of functionality with two or more points of evaluation within each area. These areas include self-care, sphincter control, mobility, locomotion, communication, and social cognition. The levels of functionality are graded on a seven-point scale (total assist=1 and complete independence=7).

E   Evaluation of Reflexes and Muscle Tone

Although the ASIA neurological examination stresses the importance of motor and sensory evaluation, a complete neurological examination is often necessary to understand the exact nature of the spinal injury. The other key components of the neurological examination include the assessment of the patient's reflexes and muscle tone. Assessment of reflexes and muscle tone gives clues to the possibility of cord injury, especially in comatose or seemingly uncooperative patients.

F   Stretch Reflex

The stretch reflex is a basic mechanism to maintain tone in the muscles. The reflex is mediated by Group Ia afferent neurons which monosynaptically stimulate the alpha motor neurons of the stretched muscle and postsynaptically inhibit its antagonist muscles. The reflex arc is modulated by the cerebral cortex that prevents excessive reaction with stimulation. The most common stretch reflexes are described here: biceps reflex—C5; brachioradialis—C6; triceps—C7; knee jerk—L4; posterior tibial—L5; and Achilles—S1.

Several important reflexes are mediated through the central nervous system via cutaneous stimulation. These include the abdominal reflex, the cremasteric reflex, the anal wink, and the bulbocavernosus reflex. The abdominal reflex can be subcategorized into the upper abdominal reflex that tests the T7–T10 levels and the lower abdominal reflex that tests the T10–T12 levels. The reflex is elicited by stroking the skin in each quadrant of the abdomen and noting whether the umbilicus is drawn toward the stimulated area. An asymmetry in the abdominal reflex may indicate the presence of a lower motor neuron lesion. The bulbocavernosus reflex evaluates the local reflex arc involving the S2–S4 roots. The cremasteric reflex tests levels from T12–L2 and is elicited by stroking the skin of the inner thigh. In a normal reflex, the scrotum is drawn upward by the ipsilateral cremasteric muscle. Bilateral absence of a cremasteric reflex is indicative of an upper motor neuron lesion while unilateral absence is suggestive of a lower motor neuron lesion. The anal wink tests the integrity of the S4 and S5 levels. Stimulation of the skin around the anal sphincter should normally elicit a reflex contraction.

In addition to the evaluation of these normal reflexes, any pathological reflexes should be sought. The Babinski sign describes the extension of the great toe and splaying of the remaining toes when the lateral plantar surface is stroked by a sharp object. The presence of a Babinski sign is a strong indicator of a disorder of the corticospinal tract. The Oppenheim reflex is the demonstration of the Babinski sign upon stroking the ipsilateral tibial crest. Hoffman's sign is demonstrated by flicking the nail of the patient's middle finger. When the sign is positive, this maneuver will lead to a prompt adduction of the thumb and flexion of the index finger. This reflex is commonly associated with injury to the corticospinal tracts above C6.

Muscle tone refers to the resistance that the examiner perceives when passively manipulating the limbs of the patient. During normal circumstances, the examiner will encounter a certain amount of resistance as the muscle is brought through a range of motion. In pathological states, two abnormalities of tone may exist: hypotonia or hypertonia. The state of hypotonia refers to a decrease in the normal resistance encountered during passive manipulation of the limbs. Muscles will be hypotonic if their ventral roots are cut or damaged, if there is a transection of the dorsal roots that carry afferent information from the muscle, or if there are lesions in the cerebellum. Hypertonia refers to an increase in resistance to passive manipulation of the limbs. This state presents in two forms: rigidity and spasticity. Spasticity is a "clasp-knife" type of resistance in which there is an increase in resistance to passive manipulation occurring at the initial portions of the manipulation. As the manipulation proceeds, however, the resistance suddenly decreases and disappears. Rigidity is a "cogwheel" type of resistance to passive manipulation.

V CLINICAL SYNDROMES IN SPINAL CORD INJURY

A General

In general, greater recovery of function can be expected in cases where there is more initial sparing of motor and sensory function distal to the level of injury and when recovery of function is rapid. Ninety percent of incomplete injuries can be classified into either Brown-Sequard syndrome, central cord syndrome, and anterior cord syndrome (5–7) (Fig. 1).

B Brown-Sequard Syndrome

The pattern of neurological deficit seen in Brown-Sequard syndrome (Fig. 1B) is typically caused by hemisection of the spinal cord from a penetrating injury such as a gunshot or a stabbing. The pattern of neurological deficit is best understood by reviewing the local spinal anatomy at the level of injury. The corticospinal tracts (motor) and the posterior columns (proprioception, deep pressure) decussate at the craniocervical levels while the spinothalamic tracts (pain and temperature) cross to the opposite side of the cord within two to three levels of entering the spinal cord. Thus, unilateral lateral column damage results in ipsilateral muscle paralysis below the level of injury with spasticity, hyperreflexia, clonus, loss of superficial reflexes, and a positive Babinski sign. Injury to the dorsal column results in an ipsilateral loss of joint position sense, vibratory sense, and tactile discrimination below the level of injury. Damage to the lateral spinothalamic tracts results in loss of pain and temperature sensation on the contralateral side of the body beginning one or two dermatome levels below the level of injury. It is important to realize that concurrent root injury may superimpose radicular symptoms over the classic Brown-Sequard pattern of neurological deficit. This type of injury carries the best prognosis for recovery of neural function, bowel and bladder function, and ambulatory capacity.

In his series of 60 patients, Bosch found that 90% of his patients showed neurological improvement (5).

C Central Cord Syndrome

As its name implies, central cord syndrome (Fig. 1C) results from injury to the central portions of the spinal cord. This pattern is most often associated with an extension injury of the cervical spine causing a "pinching" of the spinal cord at the affected level. Typically, the patients are elderly and have preexisting cervical stenosis. Patients with central cord syndrome present with minimal to no motor and sensory function in the upper extremities and the proximal leg muscles. Distal motor function in the lower limbs is spared. This pattern reflects the unique topographical organization of the spinal cord in which proximal motor function is represented at the more central portions of the cord while the distal musculature is represented in the more peripheral portions of the spinal cord. Perianal sensation and rectal tone are preserved. Central cord syndrome carries the second best prognosis for recovery of ambulatory capacity and bowel and bladder function with 50% of patients showing functional improvement (5).

D Anterior Cord Syndrome

Anterior cord syndrome (Fig. 1D) is the result of damage to the anterior two-thirds of the spinal cord. This area classically receives its blood supply from the anterior spinal artery. The posterior columns are preserved. The classic mechanism of injury involves a flexion compression force on the cervical spine. Patients will have minimal, if any, distal motor function because of damage to the lateral corticospinal tracts. Muscle groups at the level of injury will exhibit flaccid paralysis and fasciculations while the muscle groups below the level of injury will exhibit spastic paralysis. Bilateral injury to the lateral spinothalamic tracts leads to a loss of sensitivity to pain and temperature. Anterior cord syndrome carries the poorest prognosis for functional recovery, with 16% of patients showing neurological improvement (5).

E Posterior Cord Syndrome

Posterior cord syndrome (Fig. 1E) is a very rare injury isolated to the posterior columns, with sparing of the anterior two-thirds of the spinal cord. Patients lose their ability to discern deep pressure and vibration and joint position. Ambulation is only possible with visual feedback.

F Conus Medullaris Syndrome

This syndrome is caused by damage to the tip of the spinal cord. The injury typically occurs after fractures at the T12–L1 level. With a pure conus medullaris injury, patients will have isolated bowel and bladder dysfunction. However, because the spinal roots also emerge from the spinal cord in this area, trauma at this level will typically result in deficits reflecting both cord and root components. There is better hope for recovery/improvement of the functions controlled by the L1–L4 roots that have already left the spinal cord above the level of injury. The L5–S1 innervated dermatomes and myotomes have a poorer prognosis for recovery since they are still within spinal cord tissue at this level. In addition, patients who show persistent loss of bowel, bladder, and sexual function for more than several weeks after the injury have a poor prognosis for further improvement.

G   Cauda Equina Syndrome

Cauda equina syndrome is caused by injury to the spinal rootlets below the level of the spinal cord (typically below the L1–L2 level). Roots are more difficult to injure and have a better ability to recover from injury than spinal cord tissue. The patients will present with bowel and bladder dysfunction, motor deficits, and radicular symptoms from lower motor neuron damage.

H   Discussion

The neurological examination and classification schemes promoted by the American Spinal Injury Association have provided a standard method by which we assess the impact of spinal cord injury on the individual patient. Because of its wide acceptance and utilization, the grading scales have also given us a powerful tool with which we can compare new "improved" treatments for spinal cord injury to the standards of the past. Only through this systematic and objective method of assessing these patients can we find ways to improve their functional outcomes.

REFERENCES

1. Fine PR, Kuhlemeier KV, DeVivo MJ, Stover SL. Spinal cord injury: an epidemiologic perspective. Paraplegia 1979;17:237–250.
2. Stauffer ES. Diagnosis and prognosis of acute cervical spinal cord injury. Clin Orthop 1975:9–15.
3. Maynard FMJ. International Standards for Neurological and Functional Classification of Spinal Cord Injury. Chicago: American Spinal Injury Association, 1996:26.
4. Stauffer ES. Neurologic recovery following injuries to the cervical spinal cord and nerve roots. Spine 1984;9:532–534.
5. Bosch A, Stauffer ES, Nickel VL. Incomplete traumatic quadriplegia. A ten-year review. JAMA 1971;216:473–478.
6. Schneider RC. The syndrome of acute central cervical spinal cord injury. J Neurosurg 1955;12:95.
7. Schneider RC CG, Pantek H. The syndrome of acute central cervical spinal cord injury. J Neurosurg 1954;11:546.

7

Imaging in Spinal Trauma

RUSS BRUMMETT and SCOTT RUSHTON

University of Pennsylvania, Philadelphia, Pennsylvania, U.S.A.

ALEXANDER R. VACCARO

Thomas Jefferson University Hospital and the Rothman Institute, Philadelphia, Pennsylvania, U.S.A.

I INTRODUCTION

Evaluation and examination of acutely injured spinal patients is a complex multi-factoral process that begins with specific in-field management protocols and culminates in a well-organized and individualized treatment pathway. Trauma to the spinal column and spinal cord can be a devastating, life-altering injury that can have major debilitating, long-term effects. Thus it is critically important that a thorough and accurate evaluation be conducted in order that appropriate measures be taken in a timely manner so as to minimize permanent disability. This task can be exceptionally difficult in the acute trauma setting secondary to factors such as altered mental status, combativeness, and uncooperative behavior that may be the result of an associated head injury or substance abuse. It is for this reason that imaging of the spine plays such a crucial role in the initial evaluation of the traumatic spine-injured patient.

Plain x-rays have long been the standard for the initial evaluation of the spine in trauma patients. Recommendations of what films are necessary initially have varied over the years and the majority of the debate has centered on screening films of the cervical spine. Some authors believe that most cervical spine fractures can be reliably diagnosed on a single cross-table lateral radiograph (1) (Fig. 1). In contrast, other authors have recommended the use of additional views including AP, odontoid, and oblique views (2–4). This has not been universally accepted and the current recommendations for spine-injury screening include the cross-table lateral, antero-posterior, and open mouth odontoid views (5–7). Obviously the mechanism of injury,

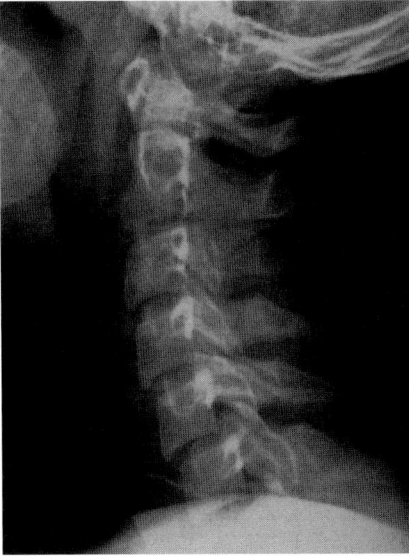

Figure 1 Lateral cervical spine plain radiograph of a 17-year-old male following a high-speed MVA. Note the evidence of cervical subluxation at the C4–C5, C5–C6 levels indicative of potential cervical instability. The possibility of a unilateral facet complex disruption at these levels must be excluded.

physical examination, and other associated injuries will serve as the ultimate guide for imaging studies, but overall these recommended views will detect the vast majority of spinal abnormalities.

More detailed evaluation of known or suspected abnormalities found on plain x-rays may be better carried out with the use of computed tomography (CT) (8–16) and magnetic resonance imaging (MRI) (17–22). In the past, conventional tomography was used more frequently, but with the development and much wider availability of CT and MRI scans, conventional tomography is now utilized less often. In contrast to conventional tomography, CT evaluation involves a significantly decreased amount of radiation exposure as well as better spatial and contrast resolution. However, in instances in which CT scanning is not available, conventional tomography of the lateral spine is still effective in detecting subtle injuries to the cervical spine. Specifically, it has a role in delineating minimally displaced fractures or fractures involving the vertebral body or posterior elements that lie in the axial plane (23). With the advent of faster state-of-the-art spiral CT scanners, CT is now playing a much more prominent role in the evaluation of spine-injured patients.

The development of magnetic resonance imaging has revolutionized the evaluation of organ systems and its application to the assessment of spinal trauma is ever increasing. While plain films are useful in the initial assessment and for establishing the presence of bony injury, they are severely limited in their ability to detect ligamentous, spinal cord, and other soft tissue injury. CT scans may demonstrate the presence of a disk herniation or hematoma and, in combination with myelography, may detect cord compression, but this combination (myelography/CT) has a relatively limited application in the routine management of spinal cord injury. It is for

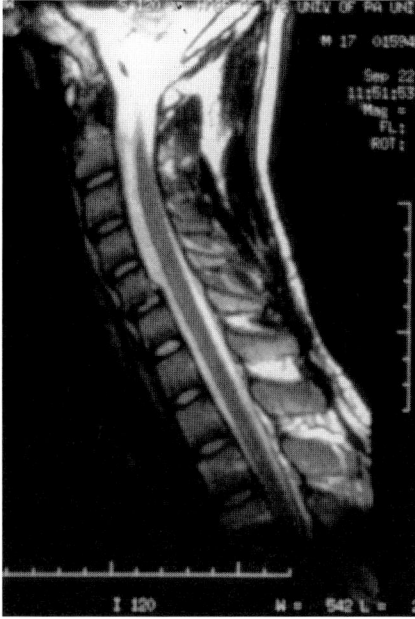

Figure 2 Sagittal T2-weighted MRI following a traumatic C5–C6 fracture subluxation. Note the listhesis present at the C5–C6 level and the absence of extradural compression at the level of injury. This injury was operatively stabilized with a posterior-only approach due to the lack of compressive anterior pathology from an extruded intervertebral disk fragment.

this reason that MRI has assumed a critical role in evaluating the spinal cord for direct pathology such as the presence of a contusion, hematoma, or edema. MRI scans are also crucial for investigating acute intervertebral disk pathology or ligamentous injuries, which may imply spinal instability (Fig. 2). Further improvements in MRI technique and resolution have led to an ever-increasing role of imaging in spinal fractures.

II PLAIN X-RAYS

In general, it has been agreed that trauma patients with high-energy injuries should have three views of the cervical spine. Subsequent x-rays should be tailored to physical and neurological examination findings. Once an injury is identified, further focused x-rays of the region may be obtained or additional studies may be indicated (i.e., CT, MRI). Also, once an injury is identified, complete spine radiographs should be obtained to include the cervical, thoracic, and lumbar spine. The importance of complete spine x-rays in the presence of a known spinal injury has been underscored by several studies (24–26). Delayed neurological deterioration is noted to occur in as many as 5% (27) of spine-injured patients and is particularly noted with previously unrecognized lesions. Missed lesions are especially common in double-level fractures, head-injured patients, upper cervical spine injuries, and cervicothoracic injuries (25,28,29). One study (24) found that 30 of 69 patients with burst fractures of the thoracic and lumbar spine had associated fractures at other levels. Of these, 14 were located greater than two levels from the primary burst injury. Vaccaro et al. (25) found that approximately 11% of 327 spine-injured patients had other noncontiguous spinal fractures. Delayed identification of noncontiguous injuries may lead to further instability and neurological deterioration. Therefore, in the setting of a known spinal injury, a careful search for injuries at other levels should be performed at the very least by obtaining orthogonal radiography of the entire spinal column.

Plain x-rays will demonstrate the majority of bony abnormalities involving the vertebral bodies as well as the posterior elements. Ligamentous instability may also be inferred by specific findings (i.e., subluxation) on plain radiography. Indicators of cervical spine instability on plain films include displacement of a vertebral body of greater than 3.5 mm and angulation of greater than 11 degrees relative to adjacent vertebrae. Associated findings include disk-space widening and splaying of the posterior spinous processes. These findings may indicate posterior ligamentous injury (30–35) and associated spinal instability and warrant further workup.

It is critically important that the plain film evaluation of the cervical spine include all seven cervical vertebrae (36,37). In certain patient habituses, this may be difficult. A swimmer's view or caudal traction on the shoulders may assist in visualizing the cervicothoracic junction (28,38). Initial evaluation of the lateral view may demonstrate a loss of the normal gentle lordosis, which may be due to muscular spasm or injury or may simply be the result of the trauma patient being immobilized in a cervical collar. There may also be evidence of soft-tissue injury and edema illustrated by deviation of the trachea or prevertebral soft-tissue swelling. The evaluation of soft-tissue swelling has historically been regarded as an important part of the radiographic evaluation of the trauma patient. Prevertebral thickening, however, may be the result of a multitude of factors, including radiological technique, positioning, and patient habitus. It is widely felt that a prevertebral soft tissue of more than 10 mm at C1, greater than 4 to 5 mm at C3–4, and more than 15 to 20 mm at C6 is suggestive of soft-tissue edema and injury (39,40). A recent study by Herr et al. (40) sought to determine the sensitivity of the soft-tissue measurements at C3 in patients with proven cervical spine fractures or dislocations and to determine if this measurement correlates with the location of injury. Their findings concluded that this measurement was an insensitive marker of cervical spine fractures and did not correlate with the location of injury. Therefore, the finding of prevertebral soft-tissue swelling, when taken alone, is of limited diagnostic value, but may have better predictive value when used in combination with other clinical and radiographic findings.

The examination of the lateral cervical spine film should include visualization of four imaginary lordotic lines, which aid in the evaluation of alignment and the presence of other subtle fractures or dislocations. The first two lines involve the anterior and posterior aspects of the vertebral bodies, essentially tracing the longitudinal ligaments. The third line is the spinolaminar line, which is formed by the joining of the lamina with the anterior cortical margin of the spinous processes. The last line is the spinous process line, which is formed by joining the tips of the spinous processes. If malalignment is noted at a motion segment, then the amount of relative angulation and displacement should be determined as described by White and Panjabi (41). It is generally regarded that angulations greater than 11 degrees as compared to a contiguous level and translations greater than 3.5 mm are unstable.

Localized flexion angulation, or kyphosis, noted on the lateral film is most often the result of wedging of the anterior vertebral body as in compression or burst fractures. One or more of the reference lines may be disrupted as a result of these injuries. A misleading situation may arise when evaluating the lateral cervical spine film in children. It has been shown that laxity of the ligaments in up to 30% of normal children up to 8 years of age can account for mild kyphotic angulation at C2–C3 and C3–C4 (42). This "pseudosubluxation" should not be present at other levels and can be confirmed by examining the spinolaminar line, which remains intact in cases of pseudosubluxation. Another misleading finding in up to 20% of this age group is the greater than 50% incidence of a high riding anterior arch of C1, which may be found cephalad to the tip of the dens. This may initially imply a near or complete C1–C2 dislocation; however, in this clinical population these findings may represent a normal variant. In addition, a persistent synchondrosis of C2 may simulate a hangman's fracture. Finally, it should be remembered that the atlanto–dens interval in normal children might widen in flexion up to 6 mm, while it remains unchanged with flexion in the adult population.

The lateral view of the c-spine may demonstrate a simple wedge fracture of a vertebral body, which occurs as a result of compressive forces to the anterior aspect of the vertebra. This is demonstrated by anterior loss of height, but may be a stable injury without involvement of ligamentous structures. Posterior spinous process widening or intervertebral disk space asymmetry would herald ligamentous injury in the presence of the same fracture pattern. Teardrop-like fractures are caused by significant hyperflexion of the cervical spine and are often associated with severe posterior ligamentous disruption that contributes to retropulsion of bony fragments into the spinal canal.

With flexion of the cervical spine, motion and translation occur through the intervertebral disk and ligamentous complex as the inferior articular facets translate up to 30% over the superior articular facets of the segment below (43). With hyperflexion and disruption of the disk and posterior ligaments, the facets may become perched or may be dislocated unilaterally or bilaterally. A unilateral jumped facet generally occurs with hyperflexion in conjunction with a component of rotation and will demonstrate anterior translation of the affected vertebra of less than 50% relative to the inferior vertebra. Bilateral jumped facets are evidenced by translation of greater than 50% of the vertebra with respect to the subsequent level. In the situation of bilateral jumped facets, neurological involvement is likely secondary to narrowing of the spinal canal unless a fracture of the posterior elements allows for decompression of the cord.

Fractures of the spinous processes are often the result of flexion mechanisms but may be the result of a direct blow or whiplash injury as well. Classically known as "clay shoveler's" fractures, these have been traditionally stable injuries and rarely require intervention (36,44). However, as noted by Matar et al. (45), spinous process fractures with extension into the lamina and canal may demonstrate a breach of the spinolaminar line on the lateral x-ray and warrants further workup to rule out unsuspected instability.

Fractures of the upper cervical spine may also be demonstrated on a lateral plain x-ray. In hyperextension injuries in which the patient's head strikes the windshield forcing hyperextension, fracture of the posterior arch of the atlas may occur as a result of compression between the occiput and spinous process of C2 (Fig. 3).

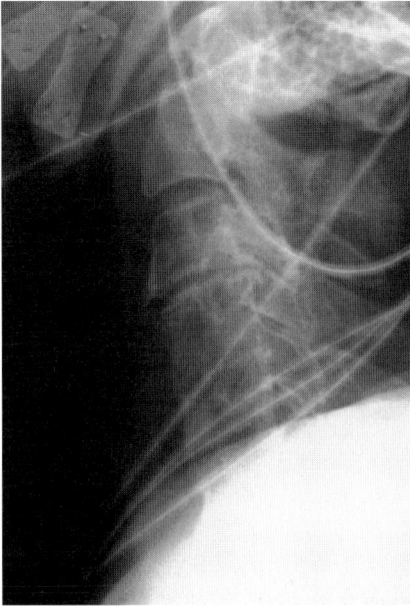

Figure 3 Trauma-bay lateral of a 68-year-old male following blunt head trauma. Despite the poor visualization of the lower subaxial spine and cervicothoracic junction, the presence of a posterior displaced odontoid fracture and C1 ring fracture are evident. Further evaluation with a CT scan is recommended to exclude a noncontiguous injury and evaluate the upper cervical spine fractures.

This may also cause various fracture configurations to the body of C2, such as a hangman's fracture. The historical hangman's fracture consisted of bilateral fractures through the pars interarticularis of C2 and was reproducible through significant cervical hyperextension (46). Neurological injury with these injuries is variable secondary to the relatively wider diameter of the spinal canal at this level. The lateral x-ray may also demonstrate disk space asymmetry with wider spaces anteriorly indicating anterior ligamentous injury. This may signify the presence of significant instability.

A teardrop fracture may also occur with hyperextension injuries. It usually represents an avulsion of the anterior superior aspect of the upper cervical vertebrae caused by pull of the anterior longitudinal ligament with hyperextension. As with other hyperextension injuries, intervertebral disk space asymmetry may be noted with anteriorly widening. This generally does not carry the degree of instability that hyperflexion teardrop fractures can and is differentiated from a flexion injury in that hyperflexion teardrop fractures usually involve the lower cervical levels and the anterior fracture fragment is generally larger and involves the anterior inferior aspect of the vertebral body (23).

Axial compression mechanisms may lead to burst fractures that are apparent on the lateral x-ray. Loss of vertebral body height with or without angulation of the segment may be noted. The main risk of neurological injury with this fracture pattern is the resulting posterior displacement of fracture fragments into the spinal canal and associated spinal cord impingement. This may be visualized on a good-quality lateral x-ray, but is usually difficult to assess with plain radiography, therefore necessitating additional studies (i.e., CT or MRI). Another injury pattern of the upper cervical spine occurs as a result of axial compression across the C1 vertebrae. This fracture, with one variant known as a Jefferson fracture, is best assessed by an open-mouth odontoid view.

The open-mouth odontoid view allows visualization of the atlas, the dens, and the articulation between C1–C2. The central issue with regard to the Jefferson fracture is whether the transverse ligament is intact. This can be assessed on the lateral plain x-ray by evaluating the atlanto–dens interval. In an adult, if this measurement is greater than 4 mm it can be assumed that the ligament is attenuated or ruptured and there is potential instability at this level (47). The open-mouth odontoid view may indirectly demonstrate incompetence of the transverse ligament through the lateral spread of the C1 lateral mass. Spence et al. (48) stated that if the combined overhang of the lateral masses of C1 over the edges of the inferior articulation with C2 was greater than 6.9 mm, it should be assumed that the transverse ligament is ruptured. Heller et al. further clarified the radiographic interpretation of potential instability at this level by taking into account radiographic magnification and amended this value so that if the total overhang is greater than 8 mm, the transverse ligament could be assumed to be incompetent (49). Obviously, more sophisticated imaging modalities such as CT or MRI will allow more precise evaluation and even direct visualization of the transverse ligament.

The open-mouth odontoid view also allows visualization of the odontoid process. Fractures of the odontoid usually occur with high-energy mechanisms in the young adult such as motor vehicle accidents or falls in the elderly. Neurological impairment has been reported to range from 5 to 10% (50). Anderson and D'Alonzo developed a classification of odontoid fractures in 1974 (51). Type I fractures are rare oblique fractures involving the uppermost aspect of the dens and are believed to be a result of avulsion of the apical ligament. Type II fractures involve the base of the dens and are thought to be the result of a lateral or oblique force (52). Type III fractures involve disruption of the cancellous bone of C2. If nondisplaced, fractures of the odontoid, particularly the lower type II and III, may be difficult to visualize and therefore require additional studies for further investigation. In 1984, Harris et al. (53) described the axis ring on the lateral view of the cervical spine which is a ring-shaped cortical density superimposed on the superoposterior body of the axis. The anterior aspect of the ring is formed by the anterior cortex of the axis at the junction of the body and contiguous lateral mass. The superior portion is composed of the upper articulating facets of the axis superimposed on the superior cortex of the body. Finally, the posterior aspect is formed by the posterior cortex of the body of the axis. Disruption of the ring is highly indicative of a low-type dens fracture and can be a useful radiological sign of injury (54).

Some controversy exists over the utility of flexion–extension lateral cervical spine films in the acute setting of trauma. The American College of Radiology Musculoskeletal Task Force concluded that flexion and extension views were highly appropriate for patients who had normal plain films but were symptomatic with persistent cervical pain, thus raising the suspicion of ligamentous injury (55,60–77). It is recommended that these views be obtained in an erect position, as this will better demonstrate instability (56–63). Several authors have demonstrated that flexion–extension radiographs taken 1 to 2 weeks after the acute trauma are valuable in detecting subacute ligamentous instability (57, 58–143, 59–44). Patients at risk for this are generally under 25 years of age and have greater than 1.5 mm of displacement and 5 degrees of angulation on initial radiographs. Wilberger and Maroon (58–143) found that, on follow-up, 8 of 62 patients in their study progressed with horizontal displacement greater than 3.5 mm and angular displacement greater than 11 degrees 2 to 4 weeks following injury. There is some consensus that flexion–extension films should be avoided in acute trauma patients with other distracting injuries or in those who may be obtunded and unable to reliably report the onset of pain or other symptoms and are therefore at risk for iatrogenic neurological injury. However, neurological injury is unlikely in the alert, unsedated patient who is supervised and self-limits the degree of flexion or extension based on elicitation of pain or neurological symptoms.

One of the obvious limitations of plain films of the cervical spine is the lack of sensitive evaluation of soft tissues, including the ligamentous structures and the spinal cord. One particular problem area is at the cervicothoracic junction. This may be due to patient body habitus and overlying shoulders or clavicles. While plain films may indirectly imply ligamentous injury and instability, they cannot definitively demonstrate soft tissue disruption or the presence of an acutely herniated disk or vascular injury. Plain x-rays are also limited in their ability to clearly delineate the position of fragments in upper cervical spine injuries and may be insensitive in detecting traumatic injury to the atlanto-occipital articulation.

Although not part of the standard trauma-screening x-ray series, films of the thoracic and lumbar spine are indicated if the patient's history and physical examination suggest a possible injury involving these spinal regions. As discussed earlier, in the presence of an identified injury at any level of the spine, there is a significant chance of noncontiguous fractures and this mandates, at the minimum, complete spine radiographs including the cervical, thoracic, and lumbar spine (24–27).

In 1983, Denis (60) introduced the concept of the three-column theory of spinal stability in relation to the thoracolumbar spine. This has also been applied subsequently to the cervical spine (60). The Denis classification divides the spine into three columns—anterior, middle, and posterior. The anterior column is composed of three structures—the anterior portion of the vertebral body, the anterior longitudinal ligament, and the anterior aspect of the annulus fibrosis. The middle column is made up of the posterior portion of the vertebral body, the posterior longitudinal ligament, and the posterior annulus fibrosis. The third column is composed of the posterior elements, including the facet joints and their capsules, the ligamentum flavum, the interspinous ligaments, and the posterior aspect of the neural arch. Therefore, it is very important that imaging of a known region of the spine allow evaluation of these structures so that stability can be assessed.

Initial radiographs of the thoracolumbar spine should include AP and cross-table lateral views. Anteroposterior and lateral chest films and abdominal films are not adequate for assessment of the spine. The lateral view should be centered at approximately the L2 level, which will give optimal resolution of the lower thoracic and upper lumbar spine. It has been shown that, in adults, up to 60% of fractures of the thoracolumbar spine occur at the junction between the thoracic and lumbar spine. Several reasons may account for this, including the transition from a relatively rigid thoracic spine, which has supporting rib and muscular structures, to the relatively mobile, unsupported lumbar spine. Additional reasons include the change in sagittal orientation of the kyphotic thoracic spine to the lordotic lumbar spine, as well as the change in spatial orientation of the apophyseal joints. An additional lateral view centered over the lumbosacral junction may be necessary for better evaluation of this area. Adequate lateral views of the upper three or four thoracic vertebrae may be difficult to obtain secondary to superimposed shoulder structures and some authors advocate the swimmer's view or oblique views for better visualization (32,61). Evaluation of posterior column elements of the thoracic spine can also be very difficult secondary to overlying ribs and soft tissue structures (62). AP views may indicate posterior column injuries by showing widening of the interpedicular distance, discontinuity of bony structures, or disruption of the pedicles or neural arch structures. The AP and lateral views should also be evaluated for malalignment, loss of height, and angulation.

In 1983 McAfee et al. (63) proposed a new classification of thoracolumbar injuries based on the mechanism of injury and the involvement of the osteoligamentous columns described by Denis (60). This classification included the (1) wedge compression fracture; (2) stable burst fracture; (3) unstable burst fracture; (4) flexion–distraction injury; (5) chance-type fracture; and (6) translational shear injury. Simple wedge compression fractures involve a hyperflexion injury with failure of the anterior column. This is obvious on a lateral plain x-ray and is generally a stable injury except when the degree of compression exceeds 50%. However, one cannot be certain that what appears to be a simple anterior column injury on plain x-ray does not involve the middle or posterior column, and this is why CT and/or MRI is indicated for more definitive evaluation.

Stable burst fractures demonstrate compression of the anterior and middle column with an intact posterior column. Some degree of kyphosis may be noted on the lateral view, usually less than 15 degrees, but otherwise alignment is maintained (Fig. 4A–D). Bony retropulsion is usually less than 50% and these injuries usually may be treated nonoperatively. In contrast, the unstable burst fracture has complete disruption of the posterior column in either flexion or distraction and may be an extremely unstable injury. Plain films most likely will not be able to appreciate the degree of posterior column involvement or fragment retropulsion with associated canal encroachment, so further advanced imaging studies are indicated.

The chance fracture is a special type of hyperflexion injury, that occurs due to distraction forces of the middle and posterior columns. This is classically a deceleration injury, usually involving a person wearing a seat belt, and is most common in the upper lumbar region. X-rays may demonstrate fracture through bony structures of all three columns; however, this may also be a purely discoligamentous injury or may involve a combination of bony and ligamentous structures. Garrett and Braunstein (64) proposed the term "seat belt syndrome," which consists of the seat belt chance fracture in addition to other associated injuries. These may include injury to the spinal cord or cauda equina, rupture of the spleen, pancreas, or duodenum, and tears of the small bowel or sigmoid colon. Therefore, when this type of injury is suspected, a thorough evaluation of the peritoneum with CT or MRI must be performed to rule out these other associated injuries.

Flexion–distraction injuries involved distraction and failure of the posterior column and compression of the anterior column. This is a highly unstable injury pattern and lateral x-rays may demonstrate only an innocuous-appearing anterior

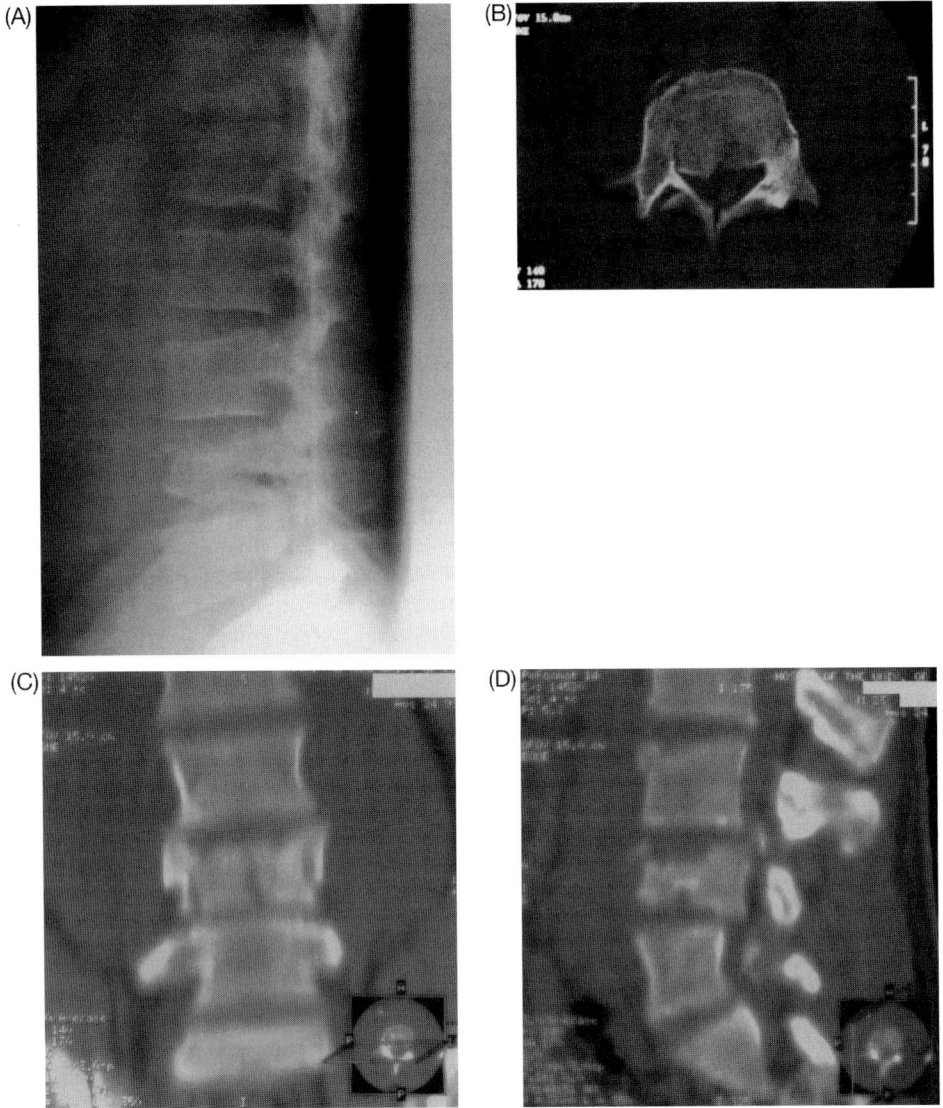

Figure 4 (A) Recumbent lateral plain x-ray of the lumbar spine in a 21-year-old male who sustained a low L4 burst fracture. There is loss of lumbar lordosis and evidence of an incidental L5-bilateral spondylolytic defect of L5. (B) An axial CT scan through the L4 burst. Note the CT scans ability to detect canal encroachment and identify posterior element involvement, which may have gone undetected with plain radiographs or magnetic resonance imaging alone. (C) Coronal and (D) sagittal CT reconstructions of the L4 burst fracture.

wedge fracture, while the AP view may show a wide separation between the spinous processes indicative of these injuries. Translation injuries of the thoracolumbar spine involve a shearing injury with failure of the middle osteoligamentous column. This has also been called a "slice" fracture; it is extremely unstable and has the highest incidence of paraplegia and complete neurological deficit (65). Again, further imaging will be necessary to clearly delineate bony and ligamentous involvement.

Plain films are limited in their visualization and resolution of the posterior spinal elements and posterior vertebral body cortex. Overlying soft tissue and ribs often obscures these structures. Considering that stability of the thoracolumbar spine is significantly influenced by the integrity of the middle and posterior column, more sophisticated imaging modalities are necessary to adequately assess these structures.

III COMPUTED TOMOGRAPHY

In the presence of adequate plain radiographic studies, 5 to 8% of patients with a spinal fracture may still have what appears to be normal radiographs (66,67,71,74–76). In more recent years, computed tomography (CT) has gained wide acceptance as an important adjunct to plain films in evaluating spine injuries. In comparison to plain films, CT imaging provides greater detail and resolution when evaluating the bony elements of the spine and also allows for evaluation of the integrity of the spinal canal. Some authors have even proposed that CT should be the preferred screening modality in the evaluation of spinal trauma (65–72). In general, it is agreed upon that CT scans should be used in the following situations: (1) obtunded or intoxicated patients with high suspicion for cervical spine injury; (2) awake patients with negative plain films but with positive clinical findings; (3) patients in which adequate plain films are not obtained; (4) patients with suspicious findings on plain films; and (5) patients with equivocal fracture patterns on adequate plain film examinations (8,55). CT scans are also useful in evaluating well-defined fracture patterns on plain films in that they may identify occult injuries in adjacent vertebrae and bony elements (Fig. 5A,B).

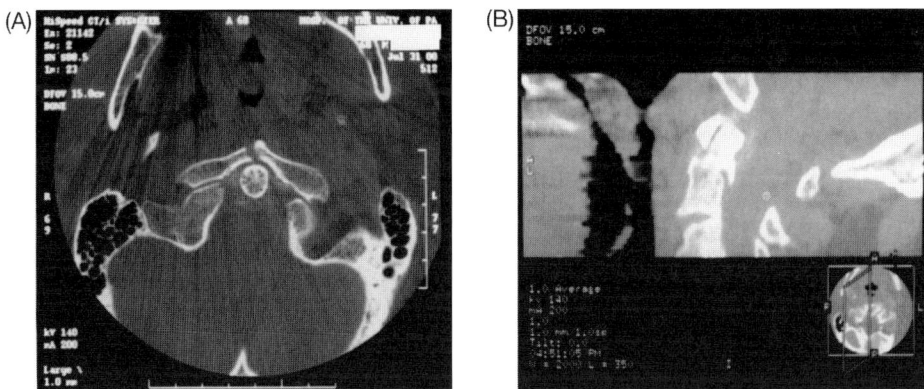

Figure 5   (A) Axial and (B) sagittal CT scans of the upper cervical spine confirming a high type III odontoid fracture with posterior displacement and an associated C1 anterior arch fracture not appreciated on plain radiography.

Other inherent advantages of CT over plain radiography include its independence from technical problems associated with patient positioning and improved visualization of the lower cervical spine in patients with large shoulders or other aspects of body habitus that makes plain film imaging difficult (23). The speed of modern spiral scanners allows a thorough evaluation in an expeditious manner. CT imaging may also be reformatted, allowing reconstruction of the bony architecture in different planes. One must also keep in mind that subtle, nondisplaced fractures in the axial plane may be completely missed on plain films. CT reformats are particularly useful in detecting these subtle injuries in addition to clearly delineating the posterior elements.

Plain films of the upper cervical spine may lack resolution especially in nondisplaced fractures of C1 or C2. CT images with thin slices and sagittal reformats are especially well suited for delineating these injuries. Injuries of the facet joints, pedicles, and lamina are also much better demonstrated by CT (5) (Fig. 6). However, if imaging acquisition is obtained in the plane of the fracture, this injury may be missed on CT reformatted views.

CT imaging is especially well suited for the evaluation of intracanal fragments. Ballock et al. (77) found that of 67 patients with burst or wedge fractures, 20% would have been misdiagnosed based solely on plain film findings. CT scans allow clear demonstration of the posterior vertebral body as well as the degree of canal compromise by retropulsed fragments (78,79) (Fig. 7).

Lumbar burst fractures may also have vertical fractures involving the lamina and associated cauda equina nerve entrapment. This is an uncommon complication in which the roots of the cauda equina herniate through a posterior dural tear and are entrapped in the lamina fracture. It has been shown that CT imaging can dem-

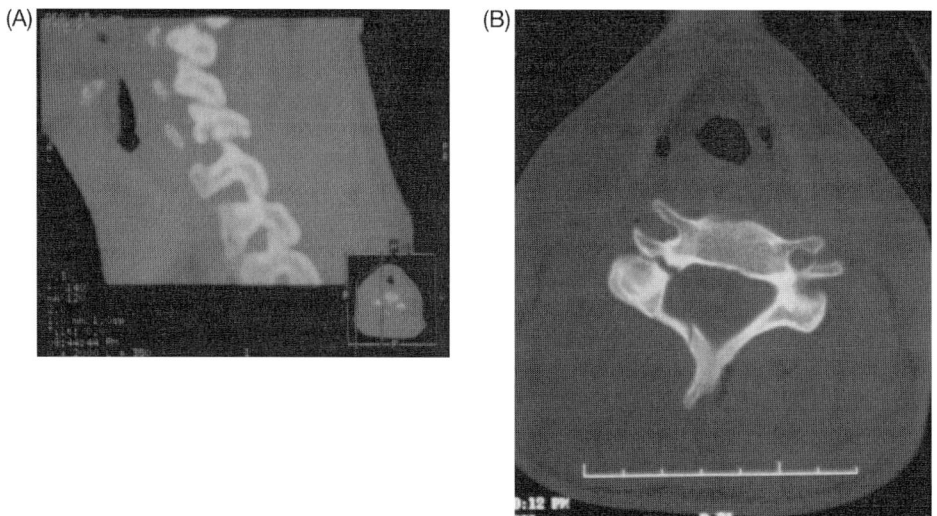

Figure 6   (A) Sagittal reconstruction of the cervical facet complexes. Note the disruption of the C5–C6 facet joint complex with joint diastasis. (B) An axial cervical CT scan of the C5 vertebral body identifying a floating lateral mass with fracture of the lamina–facet junction and base of pedicle.

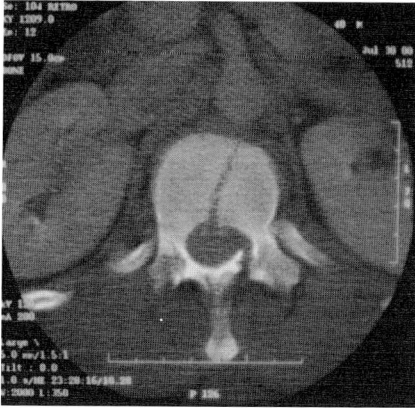

Figure 7 Axial CT scan of T12. Note the sagittal vertebral body fracture and posterior element disruption indicative of an unstable 3-column injury.

onstrate the presence of soft tissue material between the laminar fracture sites. This finding alters surgical management, in that a posterior laminectomy and release of the entrapped roots may be necessary in this setting (80). CT is also invaluable in defining bony spatial relationships and dimensions so that adequate measurements may be made in determining decompression size or the size of surgical implants (Fig. 8A,B).

The new state-of-the-art CT scanners offer unparalleled 2-D and 3-D images of spinal bony architecture and are now much more readily available than in past years. Newer machines are extremely fast, with scan times now often on the scale of minutes. Still, one must keep in mind that reformatted images are somewhat operator-dependent and that the visualized images are reconstructed by smoothing the edges of the rectangular voxels, which has the potential to obscure subtle fracture lines. Another potential pitfall is that patient motion during the examination may result in artificial lines or step-offs, which can mimic fractures. It is very possible that in the not-so-distant future, as CT scanners become even more available and as technology continues to improve, the CT scanner may assume a role as the initial method of screening for suspected spinal injuries.

IV MAGNETIC RESONANCE IMAGING

The advent of magnetic resonance imaging has revolutionized the evaluation of spinal soft tissues and associated pathological processes. Plain films are extremely limited in their ability to assess soft tissue anatomy of the spine, which is critical when evaluating spinal stability. Newer high-quality CT scanners offer some insight into soft tissue injury through identification of spinal hematomas, cord displacement, bulging disks, and cord edema, particularly when used in conjunction with myelography. Still, information regarding the soft tissue detail is limited using these modalities. Although primarily useful in evaluating soft tissue structures such as the ligamentous envelope of the spine, the intervertebral disk, and the spinal cord, recent improvements in MR imaging technology have led to an increasing role in the evaluation of spinal fractures. However, there are several disadvantages to using MRI in

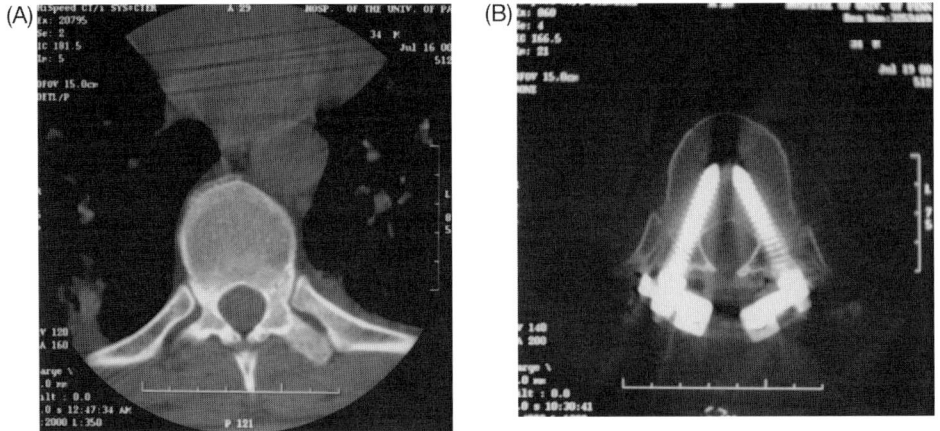

Figure 8 (A) Preoperative and (B) postoperative axial CT scans of T12 following the operative management of an L1 unstable burst fracture. The preoperative study is essential for operative planning when considering transpedicular fixation. In addition, postoperative evaluation of screw placement is best done with computerized tomography.

the evaluation of spinal trauma. These include the expense of the technology, limited availability, logistics, and long-image acquisition time. Patient accessibility is made somewhat difficult while in the magnet, which may be a significant problem in a critically injured spinal trauma patient requiring monitors, ventilators, and other supportive devices that are not compatible with the strong magnetic fields.

Magnetic resonance imaging employs a strong stationary magnetic field, which induces a parallel alignment of the hydrogen proton dipole moments with the tissue being evaluated (18,81). Next, with the application of an external radiofrequency (RF) pulse, the hydrogen protons in the tissue absorb energy and exist in a higher energy state. As the RF pulse dissipates, the protons "relax" to a more stable, unsynchronized energy state with release of the stored energy from the RF pulse. This energy is then gathered and assimilated to result in an electronic image. The efficiency with which different tissue types dissipate the stored energy is what allows the differentiation of different tissue types. Manipulation of the parameters of the RF pulse may modify the contrast and definition of specific soft tissue processes enhancing visualization of pathological disease processes. Certain image acquisition sequences will give maximum resolution of ligamentous structures while others will define and highlight anatomy of the spinal cord, intervertebral disks, nerve roots, vascular structures, or any other tissue in question.

Newer techniques are also allowing improved evaluation of the bony anatomy of the spine, yet at this point the literature continues to support CT as the study of choice for evaluation of bony anatomy. The difficulty in imaging certain bony structures of the spine with MRI, particularly the posterior elements, is related to the low water content present in these structures. The sensitivity of CT imaging for the detection of spinal fractures has ranged from 80 to 100% (82), while studies have shown MR imaging to have a sensitivity ranging from 25 to 70% in the evaluation of spinal fractures (83–85).

Regardless of these limitations, there are certain clinical situations in which MR imaging is indispensable. One such scenario is in the presence of a neurological deficit. MRI findings in the acute trauma setting have been shown to correlate closely with the temporal histopathological findings in spinal cord injury. This implies that MR imaging may be useful in prognosticating long-term functional improvement following a spinal cord injury. A classification to prognosticate neurological recovery following spinal cord injury has been developed based on MR findings of spinal cord parenchymal changes following trauma. Type I spinal cord changes are characterized by severe cord parenchymal damage with physiological or anatomical transection. Patients with these changes have a complete spinal cord deficit and very poor prognosis for motor recovery. Type II injuries are characterized by intramedullary edema. Patients often have incomplete neurological deficit and carry a good prognosis for some functional recovery. Type III injuries represent mixed hemorrhagic and edematous changes. This finding carries a guarded, favorable prognosis for neurological recovery (20,86,87). This information and expected outcome may influence treatment in that an injury with a stable fracture pattern, which would be amenable to conservative treatment, may now benefit from an operative decompression in the setting of cord compression if the potential for recovery exists (88).

In patients with a previous history of spine trauma, MR imaging is useful in distinguishing new, acute injuries from preexisting old trauma and may avoid unnecessary intervention. MRI is extremely useful in the setting of a cervical dislocation. While there is some controversy over the need for a prereduction MRI to rule out the presence of a herniated disk, there is general agreement that following an attempted closed reduction in an alert, awake, and cooperative patient or prior to

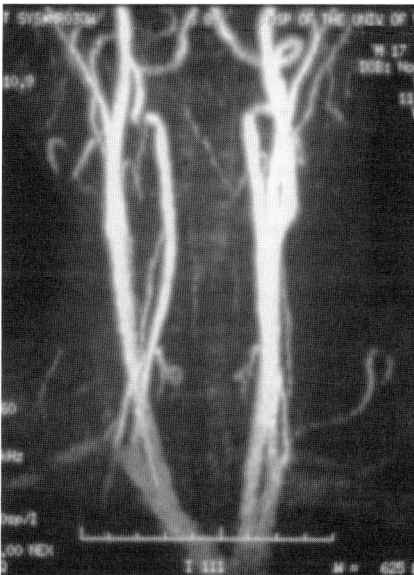

Figure 9 Normal magnetic resonance angiography following a fracture subluxation of the subaxial cervical spine. Excluding a vertebral artery injury is an essential part of the preoperative evaluation of subaxial spine trauma.

a reduction in a cognitively impaired patient, MRI is invaluable in detecting the presence of intracanal pathology that may influence treatment (89–91). The presence of a prereduction intervertebral disk herniation secondary to cervical dislocation has been estimated to be as high as 18% (89). In the patient who is unable to alert the surgeon as to the onset of neurological symptoms, a reduction prior to MR imaging may lead to further spinal cord compression and a worsening neurological deficit. A prereduction MRI in this setting would demonstrate the presence of a disk herniation and allow for an initial anterior diskectomy, followed by an open reduction and stabilization procedure. Alternatively, in a patient who is alert and cooperative, it has been shown that a cervical dislocation can safely be reduced with skeletal traction without the need for a prereduction MRI (89,92,93). The reduction itself may result in an asymptomatic disk herniation, and therefore a postreduction MRI is recommended; a diskectomy in conjunction with stabilization may then be indicated in order to prevent further disk migration and spinal cord or nerve root compression (89).

MRI with magnetic resonance angiography (MRA) is also useful as a screening modality for vascular injury in the setting of cervical spine trauma. Friedman et al. (94) reported abnormal MR angiograms in 24% of a series of cervical spine fractures. In that series, arterial injury was present in 50% of patients with complete neurological deficits, in contrast to 12% of patients with incomplete neurological injuries (94). Another study also found that in approximately 20% of cervical spine injuries there was an injury to the vertebral arteries (95). Certain injury patterns, such as

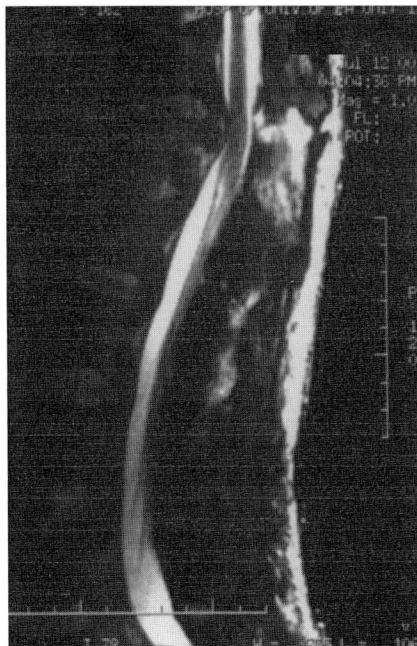

Figure 10   T2 sagittal MRI following a traumatic L1 burst fracture. Despite the mild compression deformity, complete disruption of the posterior ligamentous tension band was identified. Note the increased signal posteriorly at the injury level.

fractures involving the foramen transversarium or cervical dislocations, may have a higher incidence of vertebral artery injury (Fig. 9). In the presence of symptoms and signs of vertebral artery insufficiency such as blurred vision, tinnitus, dizziness, and difficulty swallowing, an MRA is a relatively expeditious and noninvasive method of definitive assessment of the vertebral vasculature (95).

In other areas of the spine, certain fracture patterns may warrant MRI investigation. For example, in thoracolumbar burst fractures, chance fractures, and flexion–distraction injuries, an MRI is valuable in assessing the integrity of the posterior column ligamentous complex (96) (Fig. 10). Plain films and CT imaging will accurately delineate fracture anatomy and spinal canal encroachment by bony fragments, but undetected ligamentous injury could prove catastrophic if not treated and stabilized adequately. MR imaging is especially useful in these situations. MRI is of equal value in assessing cervical spine ligament injuries. Edema demonstrated on MRI may be the only hint of ligamentous injury in the patient with persistent neck pain, but normal plain films. In patients who are obtunded, intoxicated, or with impaired consciousness for other reasons, an MRI is a sensitive tool in evaluating cervical ligamentous structures without the need for dynamic plain films (97) (Fig. 11). MRI is also a useful modality in directly evaluating the integrity of the upper cervical spine ligamentous structures. The ligamentous structures such as the transverse alar ligaments may be visualized directly and, if injured, treated in an expeditious manner without frequent delay as experienced with other, less sensitive, imaging tools (98).

Syrinx formation following a spinal cord injury is a potential cause of late neurological deterioration following trauma. MRI is well suited for evaluation of this pathological process and allows early intervention if necessary (82,99).

In summary, magnetic resonance imaging of the spine offers unparalleled evaluation of the soft tissue anatomy, including the enveloping musculature, ligamentous structures, intervertebral disks, spinal cord, and vascular anatomy. It is most useful in conjunction with plain x-rays and, at times, CT scanning, which together give an

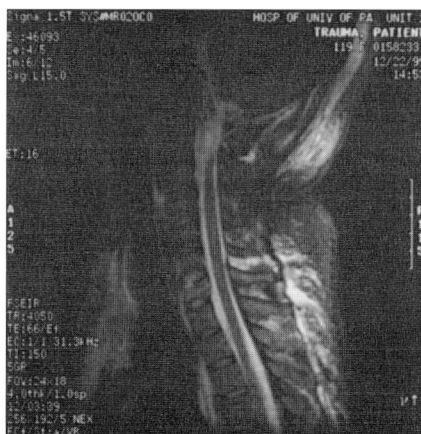

Figure 11 A sagittal T2-weighted MRI of the cervical spine following a flexion-distraction injury to the C6–C7 level. Note the compression deformity of C7 and the posterior C6–C7 ligamentous injury.

optimal assessment of the bony and ligamentous pathology present. Limitations pertaining to MRI utility exist and include its limited availability, at times incompatible monitoring equipment, and contraindications to its use, including cardiac pacemakers or aneurysmal clips. Still, availability is increasing and MRI-compatible ventilators, traction devices, and other monitoring equipment are now being made readily accessible.

REFERENCES

1. Gehweiler JA Jr, Becker RF. The Radiology of Vertebral Trauma. Philadelphia, PA: Saunders, 1980.
2. Freemyer B, Knopp R, Piche J, Wales L, Williams J. Comparison of five-view and three-view cervical spine series in the evaluation of patients with cervical trauma. Ann Emerg Med 1989; 18:818–821.
3. MacDonald RL, Schwartz ML, Mirich D, Sharkey PW, Nelson WR. Diagnosis of cervical spine injury in motor vehicle crash victims: how many x-rays are enough? J Trauma 1990; 30:392–397.
4. Turetsky DB, Vines FS, Clayrnan DA, Northup HM. Technique and use of supine oblique views in acute cervical spine trauma. Ann Emerg Med 1993; 22:685–689.
5. An HS. Cervical spine trauma. Spine 1998; 23:2713–2729.
6. Alexander RH, Proctor HJ. Resource document 5: roentgenographic studies. In: Alexander RH, Proctor JH, eds. Advanced Trauma Life Support Course for Physicians. Chicago, IL: American College of Surgeons, 1993:335–351.
7. Dalinka MK (panel chairman). Musculoskeletal imaging. Topic: cervical spine. In: Cascade PN (chair), American College of Radiology Task Force on Appropriateness Criteria, eds. Appropriateness Criteria for Imaging and Treatment Decisions. Reston, VA: American College of Radiology, 1995:MS-2.2.
8. Katz MA, Beredjiklian PK, Vresilovic EJ, Tahernia AD, Gabriel JP, Chan PS, Heppenstall RB. Computed tomographic scanning of cervical spine fractures: does it influence treatment? J Ortho Trauma 1999; 13:338–343.
9. Cacayorin ED, Kieffer SA. Applications and limitations of computed tomography of the spine. Radiol Clin North Am 1982; 20:185–206.
10. Daffner RH. Imaging of Vertebral Trauma. Rockville, MD: Aspen, 1988.
11. Federle MP, Brant-Zawadski MN, eds. Computed Tomography in the Evaluation of Trauma. Baltimore: Williams & Wilkins, 1983.
12. Keene JS, Goletz TH, Lilleas F. Diagnosis of vertebral fracture: a comparison of conventional radiography. J Bone Joint Surg Am 1982; 64:586–594.
13. Roab IW, Drayer BP. Spinal computed tomography: limitations and applications. Am J Roentgenol 1979; 133:267.
14. Steppe R, Bellemans M, Boven F. The value of computed tomography scanning in elusive fractures of the cervical spine. Skeletal Radiol 1981; 6:175–178.
15. Wojcik WG, Edeiken-Monroe BS, Harris JH Jr. Three-dimensional computed tomography in acute cervical spine trauma: a preliminary report. Skeletal Radiol 1987; 16:261–269.
16. Wojcik WG, Harris JH Jr. Three dimensional CT scanning in the evaluation of acute spinal trauma. Radiology 1985; 157:236.
17. Blam OG, Vaccaro AR. The use of MRI in the evaluation of cervical spine trauma. Lantern 2000; 7:9–12.
18. Slucky, AV, Hollis GP. Use of magnetic resonance imaging in spinal trauma: indications, techniques, and utility. J Am Acad Orthop Surg 1998; 6:134–145.

19. Goldberg AL, Rothfus WE, Deeb ZZ. Impact of magnetic resonance on the diagnostic evaluation of acute cervicothoracic spinal trauma. Skeletal Radiol 1988; 17:89–97.
20. Kulkarni MY, McArdle CB, Kopanicky D. Acute spinal cord injury: MR imaging at 1.5T. Radiology 1987; 164:837–843.
21. Mirvis SE, Geisler FH, Jelinek JJ. Acute cervical spine trauma: evaluation with 1.5T MR imaging. Radiology 1988; 166:807–816.
22. Tarr RW, Drolshagen LF, Kerner TC. MR imaging of recent spinal trauma. J Comput Assist Tomogr 1987; 11:412–419.
23. Young JWR, Cure JK. Radiologic Evaluation of the Spine-Injured Patient.
24. Atlas SW, Regenbogen V, Rogers LF, Kim KS. The radiographic characterization of burst fractures of the spine. Am J Roentgenol 1986; 147:575–582.
25. Vaccaro AR, An HA, Lin S, Sun S, Balderston RA, Cotler JM. Noncontiguous injuries of the spine. J Spinal Disord 1992; 5:320–329.
26. Saifuddin A, Noordeen H, Taylor BA, Bayley I. The role of imaging in the diagnosis and management of thoracolumbar burst fractures: current concepts and a review of the literature. Skel Rad 1996; 25:603–613.
27. Colterjohn NR, Bednar DA. Identifiable risk factors for secondary neurologic deterioration in the cervical spine-injured patient. Spine 1995; 20:2293–2297.
28. An HS, Vaccaro A, Cotler JM. Spinal disorders at the cervicothoracic junction. Spine 1994; 15:2557–2564.
29. Bohlman HH. Acute fractures and dislocations of the cervical spine: an analysis of three hundred hospitalized patients and review of the literature. J Bone Joint Surg (Am) 1979; 61:1119–1142.
30. Chiroff RT, Sachs BL. Discontinuity of the spinous process on standard roentgenographs as an aid in the diagnosis of unstable fractures of the spine. J Trauma 1976; 16:313–318.
31. Cintron E, Gilula LA, Murphy WA, et al. The widened disk space: a sign of cervical hyperextension injury. Radiology 1981; 141:639–644.
32. Daffner RH, Deeb ZL, Rothfus WE. Fingerprints of vertebral trauma—a unifying concept based on mechanisms. Skeletal Radiol 1986; 15:518–525.
33. Edeiken-Monroe B, Wagner LK, Harris JH Jr. Hyperextension dislocation of the cervical spine. AJNR 1986; 7:335–341.
34. Evans DK. Anterior cervical subluxation. J Bone Joint Surg Br 1976; 58:318–325.
35. White AA, Johnson RM, Panjab MD, et al. Biomedical analysis of clinical stability in the cervical spine. Clin Orthop 1975; 109:85–93.
36. Harris JH, Mirvis SE, eds. Hyperflexion Injuries, 3rd ed. Baltimore: Williams & Wilkins, 1995:245–289.
37. Rogers LR. Radiology of Skeletal Trauma. New York: Churchill Livingstone, 1982.
38. Evans DK. Dislocations at the cervicothoracic junction. J Bone Joint Surg Br 1983; 65:124–127.
39. Templeton PA, Young JWR, Mirvis SE, et al. The value of retropharyngeal soft tissue measurement in trauma of the adult cervical spine. Skeletal Radiol 1987; 16:98–104.
40. Herr CH, Ball PA, Sargent SK, Quinton HB. Sensitivity of prevertebral soft tissue measurement at C3 for detection of cervical spine fractures and dislocations. Amer J Emerg Med 1998; 16:346–349.
41. White AA III, Panjabi MM. The problem of clinical instability in the human spine: a systematic approach. In: White AA, Panjabi MM, eds. Clinical Biomechanics of the Spine, 2nd ed. Philadelphia: JB Lippincott, 1990:277–378.
42. Cattell HS, Filtzer DL. Pseudosubluxation and other normal variations of the cervical spine in children. J Bone Joint Surg Am 1965; 47:1295.
43. Scher AT. Anterior cervical subluxation: an unstable position. Am J Roentgenol 1979; 133:275–283.

44. Hirsch LF, Duarte LE, Wolfson EH, Gerhard W. Isolated symptomatic cervical spinous process fracture requiring surgery. J Neurosurg 1991; 75:131–133.

45. Matar LD, Helms CA, Richardson WJ. "Spinolaminar breach": an important sign in cervical spinous process fractures. Skeletal Radiol 2000; 29:75–80.

46. Mirvis SE, Young JWR, Lim C, et al. Hangman's fracture: radiologic assessment in 27 cases. Radiology 1986; 163:713–717.

47. Oda T, Panjabi MM, Crisco JJ, Oxland TR, Latz L, Nolte LP. Experimental study of atlas injuries: II. Relevance to clinical diagnosis and treatment. Spine 1991; 16:S466–S473.

48. Spence KF, Decker S, Sell KW. Bursting atlantal fracture associated with rupture of the transverse ligament. J Bone Joint Surg Am 1970; 52:543–549.

49. Heller JG, Viroslav S, Hudson J. Jefferson fractures: the role of magnification artifact in assessing transverse ligament integrity. J Spinal Disord 1993; 6:392–396.

50. Clark CR, White AA. Fracture of the dens. J Bone Joint Surg Am 1985; 67:1340–1348.

51. Anderson LD, D'Alonzo RT. Fractures of the odontoid process of the axis. J Bone Joint Surg Am 1974; 56:1663–1672.

52. Doherty BJ, Heggeness MH, Esses SI. A biomechanical study of odontoid fractures and fracture fixation. Spine 1993; 18:178–184.

53. Harris Jr JH, Burke JT, Ray RD, Nichols-Hostetter S, Lester RG. Low (type 3) odontoid fracture: a new radiographic sign. Radiology 1984; 153:353–356.

54. Mortelmans LJM, Geusens EAM, Sabbe MB, Delooz HH. Harris or axis ring: an aid in diagnosing low odontoid fractures. Eur J Surg 1999; 165:1138–1141.

55. Kathol MH. Cervical Spine Trauma: what is new? Radiol Clin of North Am 1997; 35:507–528.

56. American College of Radiology. Appropriateness Criteria for Imaging and Treatment Decisions. Reston, VA: American College of Radiology, 1995.

57. Hadley MN, Dickrnan CA, Browner CM, Sonntag VKH. Acute axis fractures: a review of 229 cases. J Neurosurg 1989; 71:642–647.

58. Wilberger JE, Maroon JC. Occult posttraumatic cervical ligamentous instability. J Spinal Disord 1990; 3:156.

59. Fricker R, Gachter A. Lateral flexion/extension radiographs: still recommended following cervical spinal injury. Arch Orthop Trauma Surg 1994; 113:115.

60. Denis F. The three-column spine and its significance in the classification of acute thoracolumbar spinal injuries. Spine 1983; 8:817–831.

61. Angtuaco EJC, Binet EF. Radiology of thoracic and lumbar fractures. Clin Orthop 1984; 189:43–57.

62. Nicoll EA. Fractures of the dorso-lumbar spine. J Bone Joint Surg Br 1949; 31:376–394.

63. McAfee PC, Yuan HA, Fredrickson BE, et al. The value of computed tomography in thoracolumbar fractures: an analysis of one-hundred consecutive cases and a new classification. J Bone Joint Surg Am 1983; 65:461–473.

64. Holdsworth F. Fractures, dislocations, and fracture-dislocations of the spine. J Bone Joint Surg Am 1970; 52:1534–1551.

65. Link TM, Schuierer G, Hufendiek A, Horch C, Peters PE. Substantial head trauma: value of routine CT examination of the cervicocranium. Radiology 1995; 196:741–745.

66. Borock EC, Gabram SGA, Jacobs LM, Murphy MA. A prospective analysis of a two-year experience using computed tomography as an adjunct for cervical spine clearance. J Trauma 1991; 31:1001–1006.

67. Nunez DB, Ahrnad AA, Coin CG, et al. Clearing the cervical spine in multiple trauma victims: a time-effective protocol using helical computed tomography. Emerg Radiol 1994; 1:273–278.

68. Kaye JJ, Nance PE. Cervical spine trauma. Orthop Clin North Am 1990; 21:449–462.

69. Mace SE. Emergency evaluation of cervical spine injuries. CT versus plain radiographs. Ann Emerg Med 1985; 14:973–975.

70. Nunez DB, Zuluaga A, Fuentes-Bernardo DA, Rivas LA, Becerra JL. Cervical spine trauma: how much more do we learn by routinely using helical CT? Radiographics 1996; 16:1307–1318.

71. Woodring JH, Lee C. Limitations of cervical radiography in the evaluation of acute cervical trauma. J Trauma 1993; 34:32–39.

72. Woodring JH, Lee C. The role and limitations of computed tomographic scanning in the evaluation of cervical trauma. J Trauma 1992; 33:698–708.

73. Blackrnore CC, Deyo RA. Specificity of cervical spine radiography: importance of clinical scenario. Emerg Radiol 1997; 4:283–286.

74. Acheson MB, Livingston RR, Richardson ML, Stimac GK. High-resolution CT scanning in the evaluation of cervical spine fractures: comparison with plain film examinations. Am J Roentgenol 1987; 148:1179–1185.

75. Streitwieser DR, Knopp R, Wales LR, Williams JL, Tonnemacher K. Accuracy of standard radiographic views in detecting cervical spine fractures. Ann Emerg Med 1983; 12:538–542.

76. Ringenberg BJ, Fisher AK, Urdaneta LF, Midthun MA. Rational ordering of cervical spine radiographs following trauma. Ann Emerg Med 1988; 17:792–796.

77. Ballock RT, Mackersie R, Abitbol JJ, Cervilla V, Resnick D, Garfin SR. Can burst fractures be predicted from plain radiographs? J Bone Joint Surg Br 1992; 74:147–150.

78. Fontijne WP, De Klerk LWL, Braakman R, Stijnen T, Tanghe HLJ, Steenbeek R, Van Linge B. CT scan prediction of neurological deficit in thoracolumbar burst fractures. J Bone Joint Surg Br 1992; 74:683–685.

79. Hashimoto T, Kaneda K, Abumi K. Relationship between traumatic spinal canal stenosis and neurological deficits in thoracolumbar burst fractures. Spine 1988; 13:1268–1272.

80. Denis F, Burkus JK. Diagnosis and treatment of cauda equina entrapment in the vertical lamina fracture of lumbar burst fractures. Spine 1991; 16:433–439.

81. Yeakley JW, Harris JH Jr. Magnetic resonance imaging of the spine. Instr Course Lect 1992; 44:275–289.

82. Cornelius RS, Leach JL. Imaging evaluation of cervical spine trauma. Neuroimag Clin North Am 1995; 5:451–463.

83. Klein GR, Vaccaro AR, Albert TJ, Schweitzer M, Deely D, Karasick D, Cotler JM. Efficacy of magnetic resonance imaging in the evaluation of posterior cervical spine fractures. Spine 1999; 24:771–774.

84. Levitt MA, Flanders AE. Diagnostic capabilities of magnetic resonance imaging and computed tomography in acute cervical spinal column injury. Am J Emerg Med 1991; 9:131–135.

85. Flanders AE, Schaefer DM, Dban HT, Mishkin MM, Gonzalez CF, Northrup BE. Acute cervical spine trauma: correlation of MR imaging findings with degree of neurologic deficit. Radiology 1990; 177:25–33.

86. Bondurant FJ, Cotler HB, Kulkarni MV, McArdle CB, Harris JH Jr. Acute spinal cord injury: a study using physical examination and magnetic resonance imaging. Spine 1990; 15:161–168.

87. O'Beirne J, Cassidy N, Raza K, Walsh M, Stack J, Murray P. Role of magnetic resonance imaging in the assessment of spinal injuries. Injury 1993; 24:149–154.

88. Vaccaro AR, Kreidl KO, Cotler JM, Schweitzer ME. Usefulness of MRI in isolated upper cervical spine fractures in adults. J Spinal Disord 1998; 11:289–293.

89. Vaccaro AR, Falatyn SP, Flanders AE, Balderston RA, Northrup BE, Cotler JM. Magnetic resonance evaluation of the intervertebral disc, spinal ligaments, and spinal cord before and after closed traction reduction of cervical spine dislocations. Spine 1999; 24: 1210–1217.

90. Eismont FJ, Arena MJ, Green BA. Extrusion of an intervertebral disc associated with traumatic subluxation or dislocation of cervical facets. J Bone Joint Surg Am 1991; 73: 1555–1560.

91. Robertson PA, Ryan MD. Neurologic deterioration after closed reduction of cervical subluxation. J Bone Joint Surg Br 1992; 74:224–227.

92. Cotler JM, Herbison GJ, Nasuti JF, Ditunno JF Jr, An H, Wolff BE. Closed reduction of traumatic cervical spine dislocation using traction weight up to 140 pounds. Spine 1993; 18:386–390.

93. Starr AM, Cotler JM, Balderston RA, Sitiha R. Immediate closed reduction of cervical spine dislocations using traction. Spine 1990; 15:1068–1072.

94. Friedman D, Flanders A, Thomas C, Millar W. Vertebral artery injury after acute cervical spine trauma: rate of occurrence as detected by MR angiography and assessment of clinical consequences. Am J Roentgenol 1995; 164:443–447.

95. Giacobetti FB, Vaccaro AR, Bos-Giacobetti MA, Deely DM, Albert TJ, Farmer JC. Vertebral artery occlusion associated with cervical spine trauma: a prospective analysis. Spine 1997; 22:188–192.

96. Emery SE, Pathria MN, Wilber RG, Masaryk T, Bohlman HH. Magnetic resonance imaging of posttraumatic spinal ligament injury. J Spinal Disord 1989; 2:229–233.

97. Benzel EC, Hart BL, Ball PA, Baldwin NG, Orrison WW, Espinsos MC. Magnetic resonance imaging for the evaluation of patients with occult cervical spine injury. J Neurosurg 1996; 85:824–829.

98. Dickrnan CA, Greene KA, Sonntag VKH. Injuries involving the transverse atlantal ligament: classification and guidelines based on experience with 39 injuries. Neurosurg 1996; 38:44–50.

99. Perrouin-Verbe B, Lenne-Aurier K, Robert R, Auffray-Calvier E, Richard I, Malduyt de la Greve I, Mathe JF. Post-traumatic syringomyelia and post-traumatic spinal cord stenosis: a direct relationship: review of 75 patients with a spinal cord injury. Spinal Cord 1998; 36:137–143.

8

Classification of Cervical Spine Trauma

ANH X. LE

Alpine Orthopaedic Medical Group, Inc., Stockton, and University of California, Davis, Sacramento, California, U.S.A.

RICK B. DELAMARTER

The Spine Institute at St. John's Health Center, Santa Monica, and UCLA School of Medicine, Los Angeles, California, U.S.A.

Classification of cervical spine injuries requires a clear understanding of the anatomy of the cervical spine and the mechanism of injury. Classifications are useful to clinicians when they provide treatment guidelines and have prognostic values. A better understanding of cervical trauma classifications and mechanisms of injury guides proper care of cervical spine injuries and reduces mortality and associated neurological injuries (1–5).

The cervical spine can be divided into two major segments: the occipitocervical articulation and the subaxial spine. The occipitocervical articulation comprises the spinal segment from the occiput to C2. The lower cervical spine from C3 to the cervicothoracic junction forms the subaxial spine. The difference in patterns of injury between the upper and lower cervical spine reflects a difference in bony anatomy and soft tissue support between the two major cervical spinal segments.

I FRACTURES AND DISLOCATIONS OF THE OCCIPITOCERVICAL ARTICULATION

The cervical spine could be compared to a catapult. The anchor point of the catapult arm is the cervicothoracic junction, and at the end of the catapult arm is a heavy projectile, the occiput. The occipitocervical articulation represents a transition between the cranium and the spinal column. It is the transition point of a heavy object on a long moment arm, and thus the biomechanical demands placed on this joint are of considerable significance. The occipitocervical junction supports a wide range of motion, yet its structural foundation is limited. It relies on strong ligaments for support and has little inherent bony stability. The external craniocervical ligaments consist of the ligamentum nuchae and the joint capsules. The internal ligaments are the tectorial membrane, the cruciate ligament, the alar, and the apical ligaments. The main insertion point for these ligaments is the axis, and the atlas acts as a bushing facilitating atlantoaxial rotation (6).

Unlike the subaxial spine, there is not a simple mechanistic way to classify occipitocervical injuries. This is due in part to the complex soft tissue support and in part to the variation in the bony architecture. The atlas does not have a vertebral body, and there is no intervertebral disk between C1 and C2. The odontoid process extends from the upper aspect of the body of the axis to articulate with the atlas. Similar injury force produces different fracture configurations in the bones of the occipitocervical complex because of this anatomical variation. In this chapter, we will attempt to anatomically subdivide occipitocervical injuries into bony fractures and joint instability. The three bones are the occipital condyles, the atlas, and the axis, and the two joints are the occipitoaxial and the atlantoaxial articulations.

A Bony Fractures

1 Occipital Condyle Fracture

The mechanism of injury at this segment involves a direct blow to the head or rapid deceleration. It is usually associated with head trauma, and many patients present with loss of consciousness (6). These fractures are usually picked up on head CT, and three types of occipital condyle fracture are recognized (1,6). Type I is an impacted fracture with comminution of the occipital condyle. There is minimal displacement of fractured fragments into the foramen magnum, and spinal stability is maintained by the intact tectorial membrane and the contralateral alar ligament (1). Type II injury is an occipital condyle fracture that occurs as part of a basilar skull fracture (1). The fracture line traverses the occipital condyle and extends into the foramen magnum. Type III injury is a wedge-shaped avulsion fracture of the attachment of the alar ligament. Types I and II are stable and can be treated with a hard collar; type III fractures are potentially unstable and require rigid immobilization (1).

2 Fracture of the Atlas

The primary mechanism of injury with atlas fractures is hyperextension of the cervical spine coupled with an axial load (7). Neurological injury due to the fracture itself is rare; however, it is associated with other concomitant cervical spine injury (8–13). The most common type of fracture is a bilateral posterior arch fracture (14,15). The second most common fracture is the burst fracture, where both lateral masses of C1 spread and displace laterally (16).

3 Fracture of the Axis

Fractures of the Odontoid Process.   In adults, dens fractures are usually caused by a violent blow to the head such as from a fall from height or high-speed vehicular accident (2,17,18). However, in elderly patients, dens fractures can occur from simple falls (19–21). Patients may complain of suboccipital pain and headaches and have a normal neurological examination (22). However, neurological injuries ranging from occipital neuralgia to quadriparesis have been reported (2).

The classification proposed by Anderson and D'alonzo was selected by the Cervical Spine Research Society for a multicenter study of fractures of the odontoid process (2,23,24). In this classification, three types of fractures were identified based on the anatomical location of the fracture line. Type I fracture occurs through the tip of the dens and represents an avulsion fracture at the insertion of the alar ligaments. It is the least common type of dens fracture (2). Type II fracture occurs at the junction of the base of the dens and the body of the axis (Fig. 1 A and B). A subtype IIa, which defines type II fractures with marked comminution at the base, was recently proposed (25). This fracture is very unstable and poses a challenge to attempt at reduction and maintenance of reduction by external means. In type III fractures, the fracture line extends into the cancellous bone of the axis body.

Traumatic Spondylolisthesis of the Axis.   Several classifications have been proposed to deal with traumatic spondylolisthesis of the axis; however, the currently accepted and widely used classification was initially proposed by Effendi and associates and was later modified by Levine and colleagues (26–29). In type I, the fracture line travels through the neural arch just posterior to the body. It has no angulation and displaces less than 3 mm. Type IA is the atypical hangman's fracture, where the fracture line is oblique with one arm extending into the vertebral body of the axis. On plain radiographs, the fracture lines are not parallel and the C2 body may translate 2 to 3 mm anterior to the C3 body. The mechanism of this fracture is

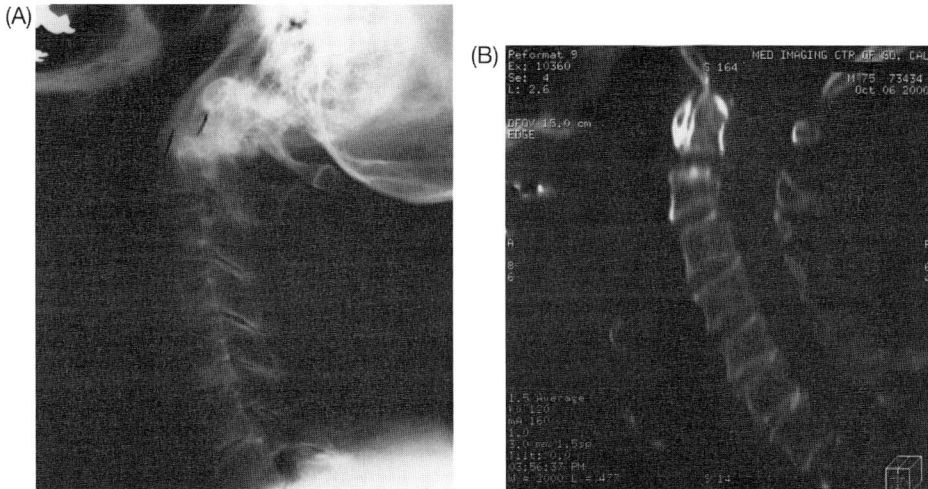

Figure 1   Type II fracture of the odontoid process. (A) Lateral radiograph of the cervical spine of a 75-year-old man who was involved in an automobile accident demonstrates a transverse fracture at the base of the odontoid process. There is a 7-mm anterior subluxation of the C2 vertebral body. (B) Computed tomography sagittal reconstruction of the cervical spine shows a displaced fracture at the base of the odontoid process.

a combination of hyperextension and lateral bending (27). The second group of injuries is separated into two types: type II and type IIA. Type II is caused by a combined mechanism of initial hyperextension followed by hyperflexion with deceleration. Type II fractures involve more than 3 mm of translation and significant angulation across C2–C3 disk space. Type IIA has an oblique fracture line through the pars with significant angulation but little translation across the C2–C3 disk space. The primary mechanism injury of type IIA is flexion distraction. Type III is typically a type I pars fracture with an associated C2–C3 bilateral facet dislocation. The primary deforming force involves an initial flexion injury causing facet dislocation followed by a hyperextension force fracturing the pars (27). Another group of injuries that can produce traumatic spondylolisthesis without pars fracture are bilateral lamina and facet fractures of C2 (27).

B   Occipitocervical Subluxation and Dislocation

1   Atlanto-occipital Subluxation and Dislocation (Occiput-C1)

Atlanto-occipital subluxation of more than 2 mm indicates a loss of integrity of the major occipitocervical stabilizers, the alar ligaments, and the tectorial membrane (6,7). Occipitocervical dislocation is usually associated with a fatal brain-stem injury. However, with improving cardiopulmonary resuscitation in the field, cases of survivors have been reported (30,31). The incidence of atlanto-occipital injury in children (15%) was significantly higher than in the adult population (6%) (9). Occipitocervical subluxations and dislocations are classified according to the direction of occiput displacement (6). Type I is the most common type, where the occipital condyles sublux anterior to the atlantal lateral masses. Type II is a vertical displacement of the occipital condyles greater than 2 mm from their articulation with the superior articular processes of C1. Type IIB is a variant of type II, where there is a vertical displacement between the atlas and the axis. Type III is rare and involves a posterior dislocation of the occipital condyles.

2   Atlantoaxial Instability

Incompetence of both bony and soft tissue can cause instability of the atlantoaxial joint. Pure subluxation without associated bony fractures is caused by transverse atlantal ligament rupture alone or in conjunction with C1–C2 facet joint incompetence (atlantoaxial rotatory subluxation).

II   CLASSIFICATION OF LOWER CERVICAL INJURIES

Clinical instability is an important concept in understanding lower cervical spine injuries. White and Panjabi defined clinical instability as a loss of the ability of the spinal segment to maintain a normal relationship between the vertebral segments under physiological loads (7). In general, low-energy injuries to the cervical spine that do not involve significant disruption of the posterior tensile or anterior load-bearing structures are stable. Injuries that cause substantial disruption of anterior or posterior elements, loss of anterior load-bearing capacity, compromise of the spinal canal, or facet joint subluxation, dislocation, or fracture should be considered unstable (32–34). Instability may lead to damage of the neurological structures and may lead to late deformity and pain. Radiographic and clinical findings are assigned a score of one or two depending on the severity (Table 1). A total point score of five or more suggests an unstable cervical spine. Instability is indicated with vertebral translation of more than 3.5 mm or angulation greater than 11° between adjacent segments (34).

Classification of lower cervical spine injuries requires a clear understanding of the anatomy of the cervical spine and the mechanism of injuries. The bony and ligamentous anatomy of the subaxial spine is more uniform and, therefore, the patterns of injury are consistent with a given deforming force. A commonly used classification of lower cervical spine injuries was proposed by Allen and Ferguson and colleagues (35). Based on a study of 165 cervical spine injuries, they noted that, depending on the position of the neck at the time of injury, a single-vector force could cause different injuries in the cervical spine. They identified six common patterns of indirect injury to the lower cervical spine. Each pattern or phylogeny was named according to the initial, dominant force of injury and the presumed attitude of the cervical spine at the time of failure. The three most commonly occurring injuries were compressive flexion, distractive flexion, and compressive extension. Vertical compression occurred at an intermediate frequency, and distractive extension and lateral flexion were the less common phylogenies. In addition, these phylogenies were also subdivided into stages according to the severity of injury.

A   Neurological Injury

Although neurological injury was not a major component of this classification, the risk of associated neurological injury was observed to rise with increased anatomical disruption. However, the severity of neurological injury and the degree of osteo-ligamentous destruction did not always observe a direct relationship (36). Normal neurological examination was documented in severe cases of compressive extension injuries (CES5), and total cord lesions were observed in cases with less impressive radiographic findings (CES1) (35). Thus, the importance of maintaining adequate cervical spine protection in the initial phase of assessment and of conducting a thorough secondary survey cannot be overemphasized.

Table 1   Checklist for the Diagnosis of Clinical Instability in the Lower Cervical Spine[a]

Element	Point value
Anterior elements destroyed or unable to function	2
Posterior elements destroyed or unable to function	2
Relative sagittal plane translation >3.5 mm	2
Relative sagittal plane rotation >11°	2
Positive stretch test	2
Spinal cord damage	2
Nerve root damage	1
Abnormal disk narrowing	1
Dangerous loading anticipated	1

[a]Total of 5 or more = unstable.
Source: Ref. 34.

B   Compressive Flexion

The injury force in this phylogeny is directed obliquely downward and posterior in the sagittal plane with stress concentration at the anterosuperior margin of the vertebral body. It applies compressive force while flexing the spinal column at the same time. There are five identified stages of increasing severity in this phylogeny. In compression flexion stage 1 (CFS1), the anterosuperior margin of the vertebral body is depressed and reduced to a rounded contour (Fig. 2A). CFS2 consists of CFS1 injury plus loss of anterior vertebral body height and breaking of the anteroinferior margin of the cephalad–vertebral body (Fig. 2A). In both CFS1 and 2, the posterior ligamentous structures are intact maintaining segmental stability. These fractures usually heal by nonoperative means (32,36,37). The fracture line of CFS3 passes through

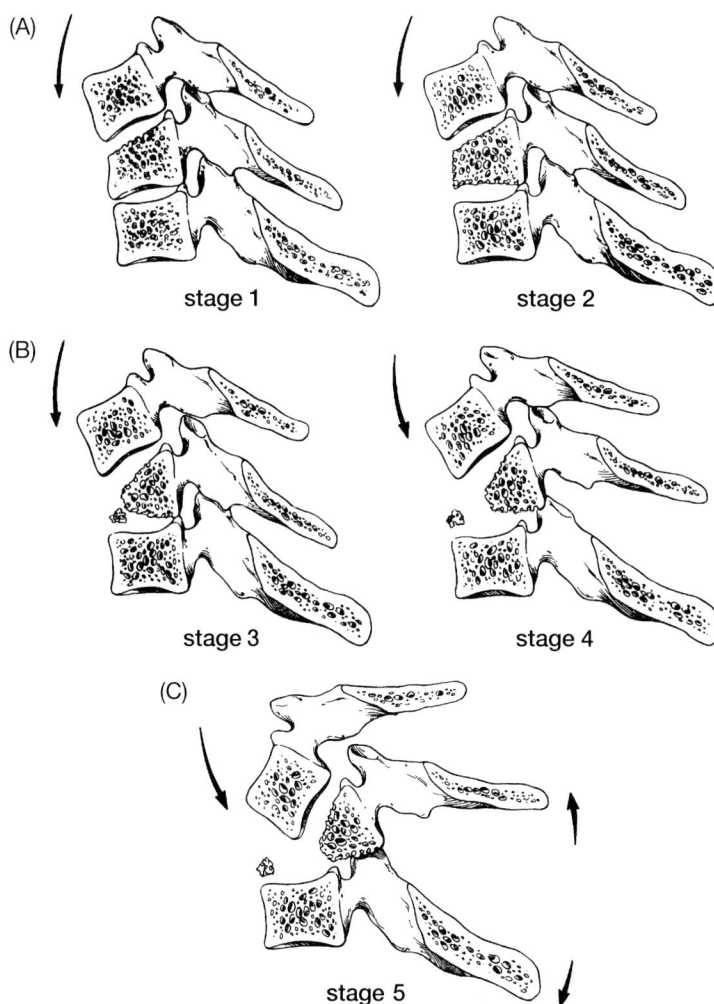

Figure 2   Compressive flexion injury of the subaxial spine. (A) Compressive flexion injury stage 1 and 2. (B) Compressive flexion injury stage 3 and 4. (C) Compressive flexion injury stage 5.

the subchondral plate with moderate collapse and minimal displacement (Fig. 2B). There is moderate comminution of the vertebral body in CFS4, and the inferoposterior margin displaces less than 3 mm into the neural canal (Fig. 2B). CFS5 represents the most severe injury in this phylogeny. There is severe vertebral body comminution and marked displacement of bony fragments into the canal (Fig. 2C). The facet joints are separated, increasing the distance between the spinous processes, and there is complete failure of the posterior longitudinal ligament (PLL) and partial failure of the anterior longitudinal ligament (ALL) (35). In higher stages of compressive flexion injuries, as the fracture propagates through the inferior endplate, the major compressive injury force vector is converted to a shear force, placing the posterior ligaments under tension. Thus, in addition to anterior bony failure, the posterior ligamentous structures are also disrupted, partially in CFS4 and totally in CFS5, rendering the injured segment potentially unstable.

C Distractive Flexion

The major injury force in this phylogeny is directed away from the trunk with the neck in flexion placing the posterior elements in tension and shear (35). There is also a minor compressive force vector causing failure of the inferior vertebral centrum. Significant posterior ligamentous disruption occurs leading to frank dislocation of the facet joints with relative preservation of bony integrity. Head injury can be an associated injury complicating initial neurological assessment (38).

Distractive flexion stage 1 (DFS1), also known as a flexion sprain, represents a disruption of the posterior ligaments with facet subluxation and spinous process divergence in spinal flexion (Fig. 3). This injury can be easily missed because radiographic changes are often minimal. Initial radiographic findings may be limited to just disk space narrowing. Thus, the importance of supervised flexion–extension radiographs cannot be overemphasized (39).

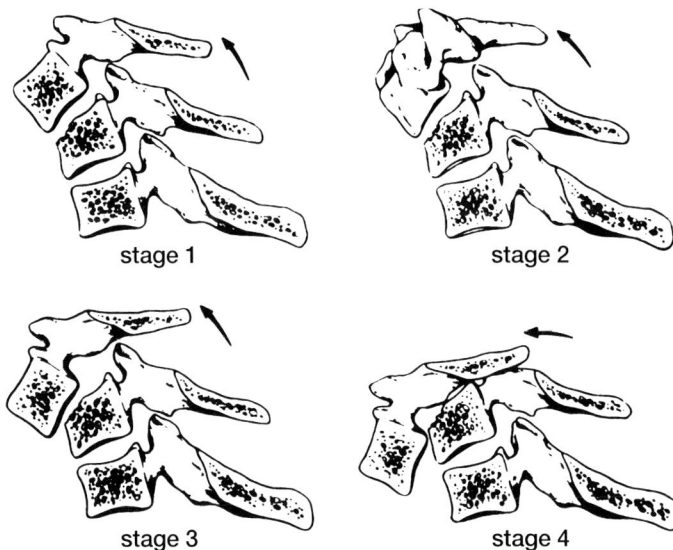

stage 1　　　　　　　　stage 2

stage 3　　　　　　　　stage 4

Figure 3 The four stages of distractive flexion injury.

DFS2 represents a unilateral facet dislocation. The upper vertebral body of the injured segment subluxes less than 50% anterior to the lower vertebral body (Fig. 3) (36,38,40). Anteroposterior radiographs may show tilting of the spine away from the subluxed facet and rotation of the spinous process toward the lesion (38,41). On lateral radiographs, projection of the dislocated facet through the vertebral body gives a "bow-tie" or "bat wing" appearance (38,42). This injury occurs most frequently at C6–C7 (36,38,41).

DFS3 and DFS4 represent bilateral facet dislocation. In DFS3, there is bilateral facet dislocation with approximately 50% anterior vertebral displacement (Fig. 3). The posterior surfaces of the superior facets are pressed against the anterior surfaces of the inferior facet or in a perched position. DFS4 is the most severe injury in this phylogeny, where there is complete vertebral body dislocation and the facet joints show a complete loss of contact giving the appearance of a floating vertebra (Fig. 3).

In early stages of distractive flexion, bony failure of the lowermost vertebral body in the injured segment may occur (36). However, it must be distinguished from a compressive flexion injury. In a unilateral dislocation, root injury is more common than cord injury, and neural recovery may be observed with reduction (37). Bilateral facet dislocation is associated with a higher incidence of complete neurological injury (32,33,42). The healing process of soft tissue is unpredictable, and therefore all distractive flexion injuries should be considered a risk for further displacement.

D Compressive Extension

Compressive extension stage 1 (CES1) consists of unilateral vertebral arch fracture with or without anterorotatory vertebral body displacement. It is further divided into three subcategories based on the location of the fracture lines (Fig. 4A) (43). The

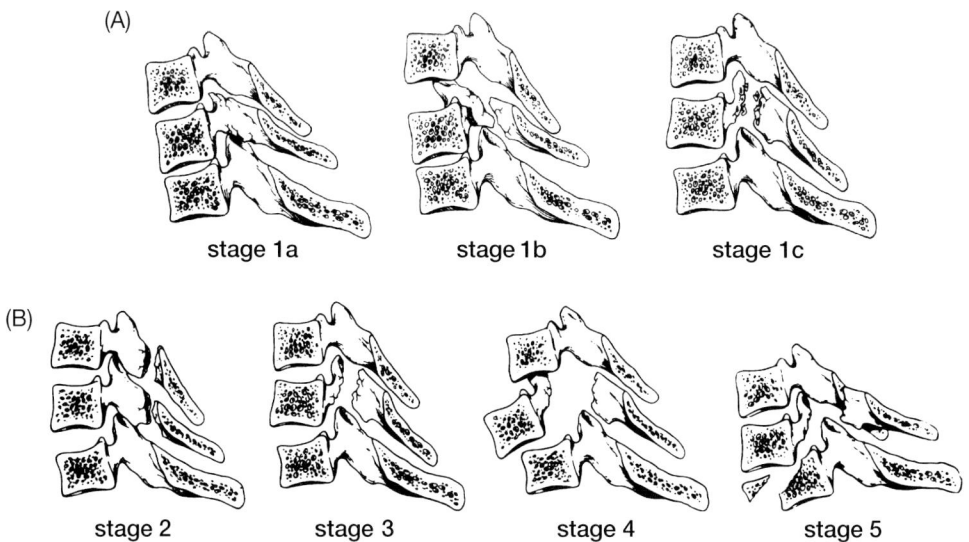

Figure 4 Compressive extension injury of the subaxial spine. (A) Compressive extension injury stage 1 a, b, and c. (B) Compressive extension injury stage 2, 3, 4, and 5.

fracture occurs at the articular process for CES1A, at the pedicle for CES1B, and the lamina for CES1C. This injury often is not evident on the initial lateral radiographs and oblique or pilar views may be necessary to establish the diagnosis (36). CES2 involves bilateral laminar fractures at multiple levels (Fig. 4B). CES3 and CES4 are characterized by fractures of both vertebral arches with increased degree of partial anterior vertebral body displacement (Fig. 4B). These are hypothetical stages because they were not encountered in the study population (35). In CES5, there is a full-width anterior body translation (Fig. 4B). The posterior portion of the vertebral arch does not displace. In this phylogeny, the injured segment consists of three adjacent vertebrae. Ligamentous failure occurs at two places, above and below the fractured vertebra, allowing complete displacement of the vertebral body from its neural arch. The severity of osteoligamentous damage does not correlate well with the severity of the observed spinal cord lesion in compressive extension injury.

E   Vertical Compression

The primary deforming force of this phylogeny is an axial load on the cervical spine. Vertical compression fractures are also known as burst fractures and are associated with severe, incomplete, and, more frequently, complete neurological injury (24). In the first stage (VCS1) of vertical compression injury, there is a central cupping fracture of either the superior or the inferior endplate (Fig. 5). In stage 2, the fractures occur at both endplates, but there is minimal displacement (Fig. 5). VCS3 consists of fragmentation and comminution of the vertebral body with displacement of fractured fragments into the neural canal (Fig. 5).

In late stages of vertical compression injuries, positioning of the neck after the initial application of the deforming force determines associated ligamentous injury (35,36). If the neck is forced into a flexed position, tension will be placed on the posterior ligaments, resulting in disruption (35). On other hand, if the neck is forced into extension, the compressive force may lead to vertebral arch fractures (35).

F   Distractive Extension

The deforming force is directed away from the trunk stressing the anterior elements in tension. These injuries are associated with falling directly onto the face forcing the neck in extension (35). Stage 1 (DES1) consists of anterior ligamentous failure

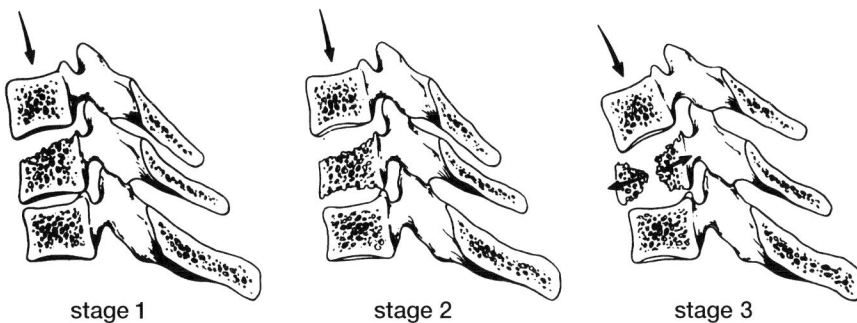

stage 1   stage 2   stage 3

Figure 5   Vertical compression fracture stage 1, 2, and 3.

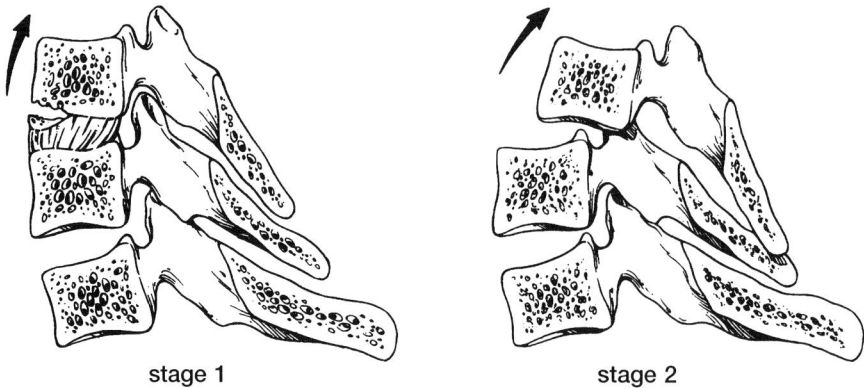

Figure 6   Distractive extension injury stage 1 and 2.

(Fig. 6). There may be widening of the disk space and/or a teardrop fracture of the anteroinferior margin of the vertebral body. In stage 2, the posterior ligaments are also disrupted, allowing the superior vertebra to sublux posteriorly into the canal (Fig. 6).

Distractive extension injuries are often missed because vertebral displacement tends to spontaneously reduce when the head is placed in neutral or flexion position (35). Thus, initial radiographs are usually normal (44). Flexion and extension views and MRIs are usually required to make a diagnosis.

The most common injury associated with distractive extension injuries is central cord syndrome (35). Significant spontaneous recovery is often observed (36). Most of the distractive extension lesions are stable and rarely go on to develop late instability.

G   Lateral Flexion

This is the least common phylogeny of injury. Stage 1 consists of asymmetric compression fracture of the vertebral body with associated ipsilateral vertebral arch fracture (Fig. 7). In stage 2 injuries, the fractured vertebral arch is displaced on anteroposterior radiographs (Fig. 7).

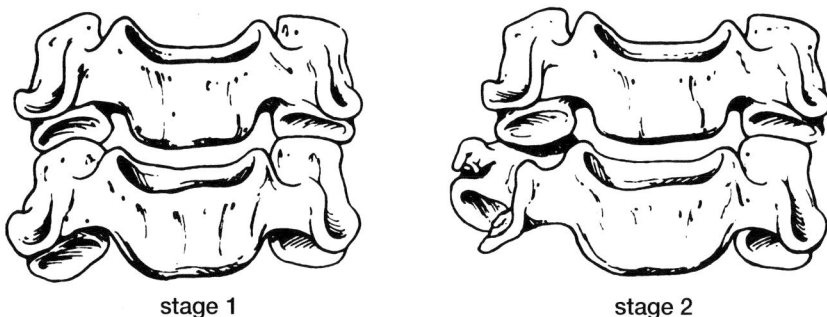

Figure 7   Lateral flexion injury stage 1 and 2.

III SUMMARY

Differences in the bony and ligamentous anatomy between the upper and lower cervical spine result in different injury patterns in these two cervical regions when subjected to similar deforming forces. Multiple noncontiguous fractures may be observed with significant frequency in impact loading of the cervical spine (45). Thus, a clinician must be wary when screening patients with cervical spine injury. Cervical spine fractures resulting from direct injuries such as gunshot wounds and pathological fractures are biomechanically different from those resulting from indirect injuries. Often, the degree of anatomical disruption to the involved segment is much less in direct injury cases, requiring a precise biomechanical understanding prior to instituting fracture management.

REFERENCES

1. Anderson PA, Montesano PX. Morphology and treatment of occipital condyle fractures. Spine 1988;13:731–736.
2. Anderson LD, D'Alonzo RT. Fractures of the odontoid process of the axis. J Bone Joint Surg [Am] 1974;56:1663–1674.
3. Capen DA, Zigler J, Garlan DE. Surgical stabilization of cervical spine trauma. Contemp Orthop 1987;14:25–32.
4. Murphy MJ, Ogden JA, Southwick WO. Spinal stabilization in acute spinal injuries. Surg Clin North Am 1980;60:1035–1047.
5. Garfin SR, Botte MJ, Walters RL, Nickle VL. Complications in the use of halo fixation. J Bone Joint Surg [AM] 1986;68:320–325.
6. Anderson PA. Injuries to the occipital cervical articulation. In: Clark RC, ed. The Cervical Spine, 3rd ed. Philadelphia: Lippincott-Raven, 1998:387–399.
7. White AA, Panjabi MM. Kinematics of the spine. In: White AA, Panjabi MM, eds. Clinical Biomechanics of the Spine, 2nd ed. Philadelphia: JB Lippincott, 1990.
8. Alker GJ, Oh YS, Leslie EV. Postmortem radiology of head and neck injuries in fatal traffic accidents. Radiology 1975;114:611.
9. Bucholz R, Burkhead W. The pathological anatomy of fatal atlanto-occipital dislocations. J Bone Joint Surg [Am] 1979;61:248–250.
10. Esses S, Langer F, Gross A. Fracture of the atlas associated with fracture of the odontoid process. Injury 1981;12:310–312.
11. Levine A. Avulsion of the transverse ligament associated with a fracture of the atlas: a case report. Orthopaedics 1983;6:1467–1471.
12. Levine AM, Edwards CC. Fracture of the atlas. J Bone Joint Surg [Am] 1991;73:680–691.
13. Lipson S. Fracture of the atlas associated with fractures of the odontoid process and transverse ligament ruptures. J Bone Joint Surg [Am] 1977;59:940–943.
14. Baumgarten M, Mouradian W, Boger D, Watkins R. Computed axial tomography in C1-C2 trauma. Spine 1985;10:187–192.
15. Segal L, Grimm J, Stauffer E. Non-union of fractures of the atlas. J Bone Joint Surg [Am] 1987;69:1423–1434.
16. Kurz LT. Fractures of the first cervical vertebra. In: Clark RC, eds. The Cervical Spine, 3rd ed. Philadelphia: Lippincott-Raven, 1998:409–413.
17. Amyes EW, Anderson FM. Fracture of the odontoid process. Arch Surg 1956;72:377–393.
18. Osgood RB, Lund CC. Fractures of the odontoid process. N Engl J Med 1928;198:61–72.

19. Hanigan WC, Powell FC, Elwood PW, Henderson JP. Odontoid fractures in elderly patients. J Neurosurg 1993;78:32–35.

20. Pepin JW, Bourne RB, Hawkins RJ. Odontoid fractures with special preference to the elderly patients. Clin Orthop 1985;193:178–183.

21. Wisoff HS. Fracture of the dens in the aged. Surg Neurol 1984,22:547–555.

22. Stroobants J, Fidlers L, Storms JL, Klaes R, Dua G, Van Hoye M. High cervical pain and impairment of skull mobility as the only symptoms of an occipital condyle fracture: case report. J Neurosurg 1994;81:137–138.

23. Clark CR, White AA III. Fractures of the dens: a multicenter study. J Bone Joint Surg [Am] 1985;67:1340–1348.

24. Ducker TB, Bellegarrigue R, Salzman M, Walleck C. Timing of operative care in cervical spine cord injury. Spine 1984;9:525–531.

25. Hadley Mn, Browner CM, Liu SS, Sonntag VKH. New subtype of acute odontoid fractures (type IIA). Neurosurgery 1988;22:67–71.

26. Effendi B, Roy D, Cornish B, Dussalt RG, Laurin CA. Fractures of the ring of the axis: a classification based on the analysis of 131 cases. J Bone Joint Surg [Br] 1981;63:319–327.

27. Francis WR, Fielding JW, Hawkins RJ, Pepin J, Hensinger R. Traumatic spondylolisthesis of the axis. J Bone Joint Surg [Br] 1981;63:313–318.

28. Levine AM, Rhyne AL. Traumatic spondylolisthesis of the axis. Semin Spine Surg 1991; 3:47–60.

29. Starr JK, Eismont FJ. Atypical hangman's fractures. Spine 1993;18:1954–1957.

30. De Beer JDV, Thomas M, Walters J, Anderson P. Traumatic atlantoaxial subluxation. J Bone Joint Surg [Br] 1988;70:652–655.

31. Eismont FJ, Bohlman HH. Posterior atlanto-occipital dislocation with fractures of the atlas and the odontoid process: report of a case with survival. J Bone Joint Surg [Am] 1978;60:397–399.

32. Stauffer ES. Management of spine fractures C3-C7. Orthop Clin North Am 1986;17: 45–53.

33. Stauffer ES. Subaxial injuries. Clin Orthop 1989;239:30–39.

34. Delamarter RD. Lower cervical spine injuries: Classification and initial management. In: Levine AM, ed. Orthopaedic Knowledge Update, Trauma, 1st ed. Rosemont: American Academy of Orthopaedic Surgeons, 1996:329–334.

35. Allen BL Jr, Ferguson RL, Lehmann TR, O'Brien RP. A mechanistic classification of closed, indirect fractures and dislocations of the lower cervical spine. Spine 1982;7:1–27.

36. Rah AD, Errico TJ. Classification of lower cervical fractures and dislocations. In: Clark RC, ed. The Cervical Spine, 3rd ed. Philadelphia: Lippincott-Raven, 1998:449–456.

37. Stauffer ES, Kelly EG. Fracture dislocation of the cervical spine: Instability and recurrent deformity following treatment by anterior interbody fusion. J Bone Joint Surg [Am] 1977;59:45–48.

38. Robacek CH, Rock MG, Hawkins AJ, Bourne RB. Unilateral facet dislocation of the cervical spine: an analysis of the results of treatment in 26 patients. Spine 1987;12:23–27.

39. Rifkinson-Mann S, Mormino J, Sachdev VP. Subacute cervical spine instability. Surg Neurol 1986;26:413–416.

40. Beatson TR. Fractures and dislocations of the cervical spine. J Bone Joint Surg [Br] 1963;45:21–35.

41. Clark CR, Wessels WE. Unilateral cervical facet fracture-dislocation. Surg Rounds Orthop 1987;45:15–19.

42. Maiman DJ, Barolat G, Larson SJ. Management of bilateral locked facets of the cervical spine. Neurosurgery 1986;18:542–547.

43. Connolly PJ, Abitbol JJ, Martin RJ, Yuan HA. Spine: Trauma. In: Garfin SR, Vaccaro AR, eds. Orthopaedic Knowledge Update, Spine, 1st ed. Rosemont: American Academy of Orthopaedic Surgeons, 1997:197–218.
44. Harris WH, Hamblen DL, Ojemann RG. Traumatic disruption of cervical intervertebral disc from hyperextension injury. Clin Orthop 1968;60:163–167.
45. Nightingale RW, McElhaney JH, Richardson WJ, Best TM, Myers BS. Experimental impact injury to the cervical spine: relating the motion of the head and the mechanism of injury. J Bone Joint Surg [Am] 1996;78:412–421.

9

Traumatic Injuries of the Occipito–Cervical Junction

R. ALDEN MILAM IV

University of Pennsylvania, Philadelphia, Pennsylvania, U.S.A.

JEFF S. SILBER and ALEXANDER R. VACCARO

Thomas Jefferson University Hospital and the Rothman Institute, Philadelphia, Pennsylvania, U.S.A.

I ANATOMY

The occipito-atlanto-axial region of the spine is uniquely complex in both its bony and ligamentous composition. The skull articulates with the cervical spine through congruent articulations of the occipitoatlantal joints, with stability conferred by strong and stout ligamentous structures. The occipitoatlantal joints are composed of the convex occipital condyles, which articulate with the reciprocally concave superior articular facets of the atlas. Because of the long anteroposterior diameter of this articulation and its radius of curvature, this joint provides up to 30° of cervical spine flexion and extension. The anterior occipitoatlantal membrane is the physical continuation of the anterior longitudinal ligament. It connects the anterior rim of the foramen magnum to the anterior arch of the atlas. Homologous to the ligamentum flavum, the posterior occipitoatlantal membrane unites the posterior rim of the foramen magnum to the posterior arch of the atlas. The tectorial membrane, running from the dorsal surface of the odontoid process to the ventral surface of the foramen magnum, is the structural continuation of the posterior longitudinal ligament and is believed to be the prime ligament responsible for stability of the occipitoatlantal articulation (1). Hyperextension is limited by the tectorial membrane and by contact between the posterior arch of the atlas and the occiput (Fig. 1).

The atlas is a bony ring formed by an anterior and posterior bony arch connected together by two lateral masses. The ring of the atlas is quite thin immediately

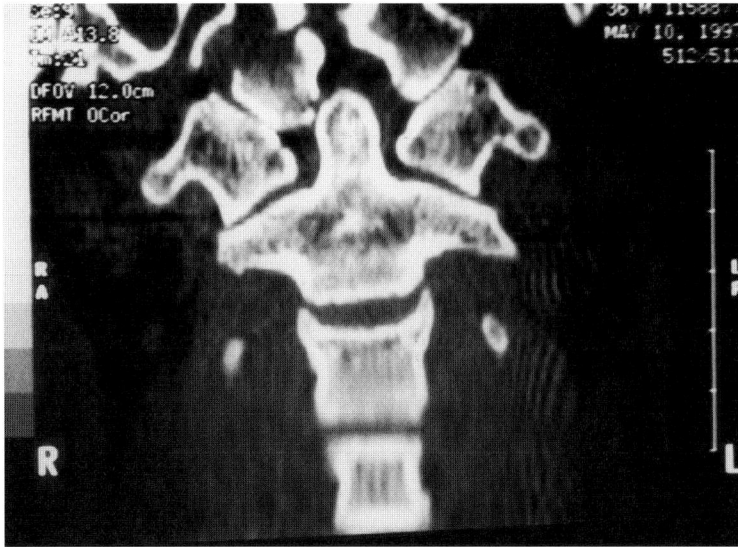

Figure 1   Coronal CT reconstruction demonstrating a right occipital condyle fracture.

posterior to the facet joints due to a depression on its superior aspect bilaterally, which carries the vertebral artery as it passes from the foramen transversarium of the atlas before it enters the foramen magnum. Fractures of the atlas frequently occur in this thin area. The atlantoaxial articulation comprises three joints, the paired lateral atlantoaxial facet joints and the central atlantodental joint. The central atlantodental joint represents the articulation of the odontoid process with the atlas and is stabilized by the transverse atlantodental ligament, which is also part of the cruciform ligamentous complex. This strong ligament can be as thick as 10 mm and takes its origin from two internal or medial tubercles on the posterior aspect of the anterior arch of C1. The function of this ligament is to hold the dens against the anterior arch of the atlas. This allows normal head rotation, which is the primary function of this articulation; however, it also permits limited motion in flexion, extension, and lateral bending.

The atlantoaxial joints provide 40° of rotation to each side, which is half of all cervical rotation. Three additional ligaments, a single apical and paired alar ligaments, attach the odontoid to the occiput stabilizing the occiput–C1–C2 articulations in all ranges of motion especially rotation and lateral bending. The paired alar ligaments are extensions of the cruciform ligamentous complex, and attach to tubercles on the lateral rim of the foramen magnum and serve to provide additional rotational and translational stability to the occipitoatlantal articulation. The apical dental ligament runs from the tip of the odontoid process to the ventral surface of the foramen magnum and is only a minor stabilizer of the craniocervical junction (2,3). Additional ligamentous structures supporting the occipital–C1–C2 junction include the anterior occipitoatlantal membrane, the tectorial membrane, and the capsules of the occipitoatlantal joints.

The second cervical vertebra or axis is designed to provide rotation at its superior articulation with C1 and limited forward flexion, lateral flexion, and rotation at its inferior articulation with C3. The body of C2 is the largest of the cervical vertebrae. The superior projection of the odontoid is stabilized to the C1 ring by the transverse ligament against its posterior surface. The lateral masses of C2 have a foramen that contains the traversing vertebral artery. The pedicles and/or isthmus of C2 are a frequent site of fracture. The C2 pedicles measure approximately 7 to 8 mm in height and width. They project approximately 30° to 35° medially in the axial plane and approximately 20° to 22° superiorly in the sagittal plane. There is no significant difference in dimensions between males and females (4). The vertebral artery begins to angulate laterally at the base of the C2 pedicle as it courses through the foramen transversarium of C2 into the foramen transversarium of C1 and then moves medially and superiorly into the foramen magnum.

II OCCIPITAL CONDYLE FRACTURES

Occipital condyle fractures are most commonly associated with other injuries to the cervical spine, most notably atlas fractures. Because of the location and rarity of these injuries, reformatted computed tomography (CT) scans are invaluable for diagnosis. Patients with occipital condyle fractures often complain of pain at the base of the skull and may have a tilted and rotated position of the head that resembles a C1–C2 rotary subluxation. In addition, occipital condyle fractures should be suspected in patients with associated cranial nerve deficits, as these fractures are commonly associated with cranial nerve injuries (5–7). A CT scan from the occiput to C2 should be obtained in the presence of lower cranial nerve deficits, a basilar skull fracture, or persistent severe neck pain despite normal plain radiographs to rule an occult injury to the occipital condyles (8).

Anderson and Montesano have classified occipital condyle fractures based on the mechanisms of injury (Fig. 2) (5). Type I injuries are impaction fractures of the condyle secondary to an axial load. Type II injuries represent a basilar skull fracture that extends through the condyle and communicates with the foramen magnum, usually the result of a direct blow to the occipital region. Type III injuries are avulsion fractures of the condyle due to tension placed on the alar ligaments secondary to shear, lateral bending, or rotational forces, or a combination of these forces.

Treatment of these injuries is largely based on the degree of associated occipitoatlantal instability. Types I and II fractures are stable injuries and are therefore best treated with a rigid cervical orthosis or halo/vest for 3 months. Due to significant ligamentous instability, type III injuries, in the majority of cases, are more reliably managed with surgical stabilization. Because of the rarity of this fracture, surgical indications are not well defined. Any findings of occipitoatlantal joint instability require halo stabilization and/or an arthrodesis (occipito–atlanto–axial). Contemporary methods of internal fixation utilized for the occiput include unicalvarial or bicalvarial (bicortical) screws attached to a rod or plate device. Use of unicortical screws in areas where the occipital bone is thicker than 7 mm offers comparable pullout strength to bicortical screws at other locations without the potential complications of overpenetrance and neural or vessel (sinus) injury (9,10).

III OCCIPITOATLANTAL DISLOCATIONS

Occipitoatlantal dislocation, also referred to as craniocervical dissociation, has historically been thought of as a nonsurvivable event with only occasional reports of

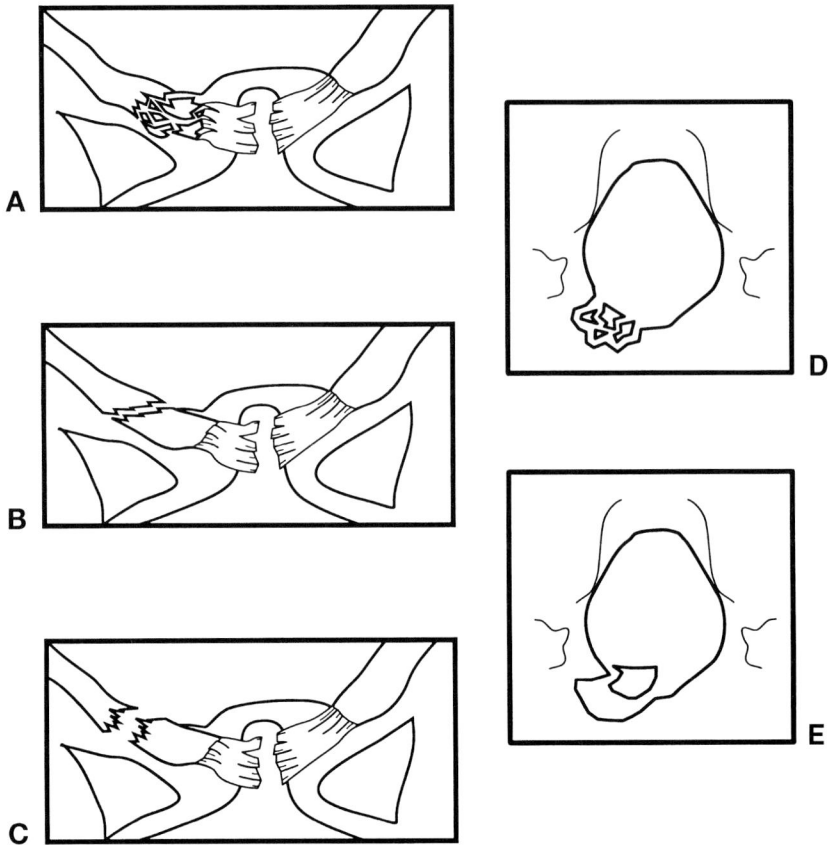

Figure 2   An illustration of the Anderson and Montesano classification of occipital condyle fractures: (A) Type I impacted fracture; (B) type II basilar skull-type fracture; (C) type III avulsion-type fracture; (D) axial view of the type I fracture; (E) axial view of the type III fracture.

survivors. Recently, with improved emergency medical care and immediate resuscitation, survival is more frequently reported (11). This type of injury is thought to represent approximately 0.67 to 1.0% of all acute cervical spine injuries, although the true incidence is unknown due to the often fatal nature of these injuries (12–14). Bucholz and Burkhead noted evidence of occipitoatlantal dissociation in 8% of all victims following a fatal motor vehicle accident (15). Patients sustaining these injuries are typically involved in high-energy motor vehicle accidents resulting in a combination of hyperextension, distraction, and rotational forces to the craniocervical junction. Due to this high-energy trauma, associated injuries are frequently noted in survivors. The most susceptible areas of neurological injury involve the brain stem, the proximal portion of the spinal cord, the upper three cervical nerves, and the ten most caudal pairs of cranial nerves with the abducens nerve (cranial nerve VI) being most frequently injured (2,3,14,16–18). Thus, patients may present with a variety of neurological deficits ranging from complete C1-level flaccid quadriplegia to mixed incomplete spinal cord syndromes such as a Brown–Séquard syndrome. Fatalities

are usually caused by complete transsection at the medulla oblongata or the spino-
medullary junction.

The clinical long-term prognosis of this injury varies from mild disability to
catastrophic neurological deficits, depending on the nature and degree of traumatic
dissociation. Although the prognosis for improvement of incomplete spinal cord lesions is variable; improvement in function of central cranial nerve deficits is rare
(3). Injury to the extracranial vertebral vascular system has also been reported
(19–21).

A popular classification system has described three different types of craniocervical dislocations by the direction of displacement of the occiput in relationship
to the atlas (22–25) (Fig. 3). The first type occurs when the occipital condyles
dislocate anterior to the lateral masses of the atlas. The second type is a pure distraction injury with the condyles separated superiorly from the atlas without translation (Fig. 4). In the third type, the condyles dislocate posterior to the lateral masses
of the atlas. Although anterior, posterior, and longitudinal dislocations have been
reported, by far the most common is the anterior dislocation type, occurring in nearly
all of the reported cases (14,26). Because of anatomical variances and inherent soft
tissue laxity, this injury is thought to be twice as common in children as in adults

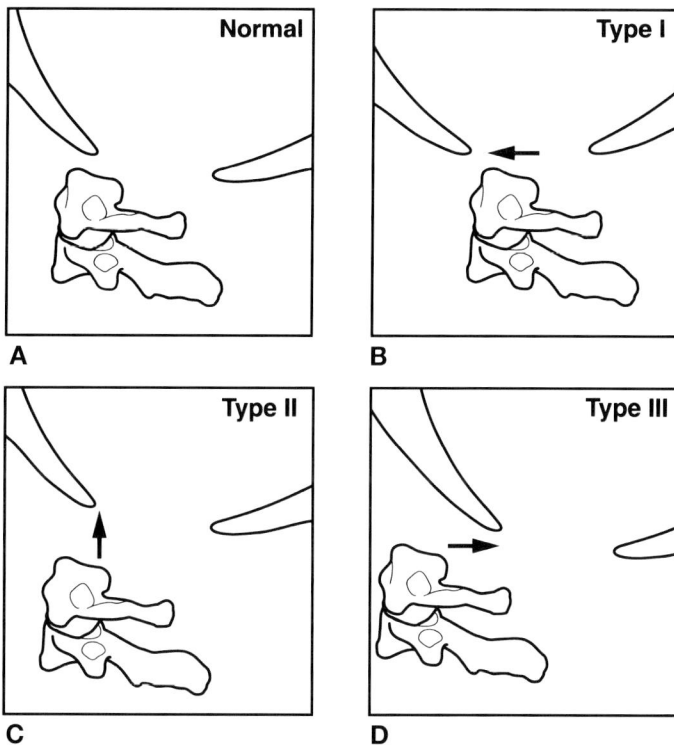

Figure 3 An illustration of the classification of occipital cervical dissociations: (A)
normal; (B) type I anterior displacement of the occiput on the atlas; (C) type II longitudinal displacement of the occiput on the atlas; (D) type III posterior displacement of
the occiput on the atlas.

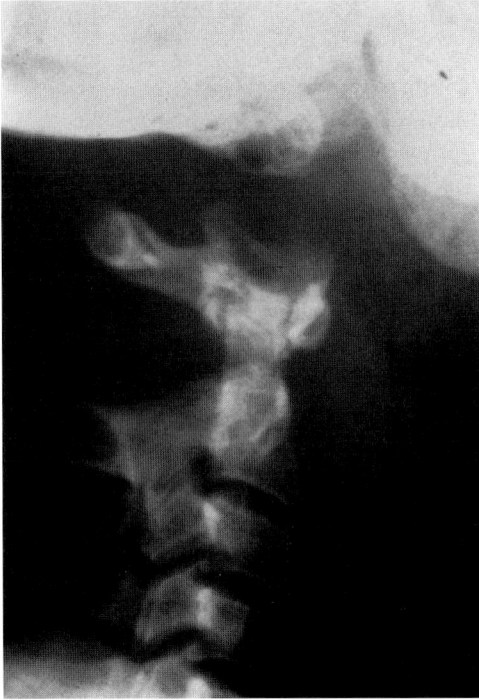

Figure 4 A lateral plain radiograph demonstrating a longitudinal occipito–cervical dissociation.

(2,15). This difference may also result from the smaller occipital condyles and horizontal plane of the occipitoatlantal joints in children as compared to adults (2, 15,27,28).

Anterior occipitoatlantal dislocations are usually the result of high-energy injuries (motor vehicle accidents) following a hyperextension and distraction mechanism. This was demonstrated by Kissinger and Malgaigne and Werne in cadaveric specimens (1,29,30). Their frequent association with submental lacerations, mandibular fractures, and posterior pharyngeal wall disruptions is consistent with this mechanism (2,3,15–18,21,27). Werne demonstrated through cadaveric dissections that certain anatomical constraints limit occipital motion. Flexion of the occiput is limited by bony contact with the odontoid peg and occipital extension is limited by bony contact with the posterior atlas arch and the tectorial membrane. Lateral bending is limited by the paired alar ligaments. By carefully dividing the tectorial membrane and the alar ligaments, Werne was able to demonstrate that these structures were the primary stabilizers of the occipitoatlantal junction, as all specimens demonstrated a forward dislocation of the occiput on the atlas and axis (1).

The radiographic appearance of an occipitoatlantal dislocation is often dramatic, with a marked diastasis at the craniocervical junction. However, some patients present with subtle radiographic findings that often go unrecognized after initial radiographic assessment. Although frequently overlooked, radiographic diagnosis of this injury is usually made from the lateral cervical spine radiograph taken in neutral flexion extension. The dens–basion relationship and Powers' ratio are useful in making the diagnosis. Anatomically, the tip of the odontoid should be in vertical alignment with the occipital basion in neutral cervical flexion extension (2,3,31–33). In the adult patient, the distance between the basion and odontoid peg should be approximately 4 to 5 mm. This distance may be as great as 10 mm in the child (32,33). The maximum amount of translation between the basion and odontoid should be approximately 1 mm (32–34). Any increase in this value may represent instability.

Since these relationships are somewhat dependent on the position of the skull, Powers et al. described a method to aid in the diagnosis of a potential occipitoatlantal dislocation based on radiographic assessment (14) (Fig. 5). Using this technique, two distances are measured between four points: the distance between the basion (B) and the posterior arch of the atlas (C), which is divided by the distance between the opisthion (O) and the anterior arch of the atlas (A). This is expressed as a ratio (BC/OA). If greater than 1, then radiographic evidence of anterior occipitoatlantal dissociation is present. Ratios less than 1 are normal, except in situations involving a posterior occipitoatlantal dislocation, congenital abnormalities of the foramen magnum, and associated fractures of the odontoid process or ring of the atlas with fracture translation (14,27). Normally, this ratio does not vary with occipito–cervical flexion or extension and is not affected by magnification. If difficulties are encountered interpreting the relationships on a lateral plain radiograph, lateral tomography or sagittal computer tomography reconstruction of the region will often suffice.

Definitive treatment is not universally agreed upon. Traction should be avoided and the goal of treatment is stabilization of the skull to the cervical spine. This is

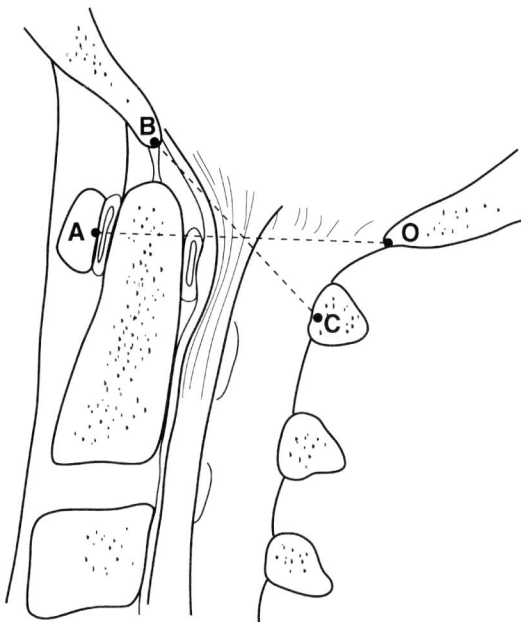

Figure 5 A pictorial measuring Power's ratio (BC/AO). Normal ratio is <1; A = anterior arch of atlas; O = opisthion of occiput; B = basion of occiput; C = posterior arch of atlas.

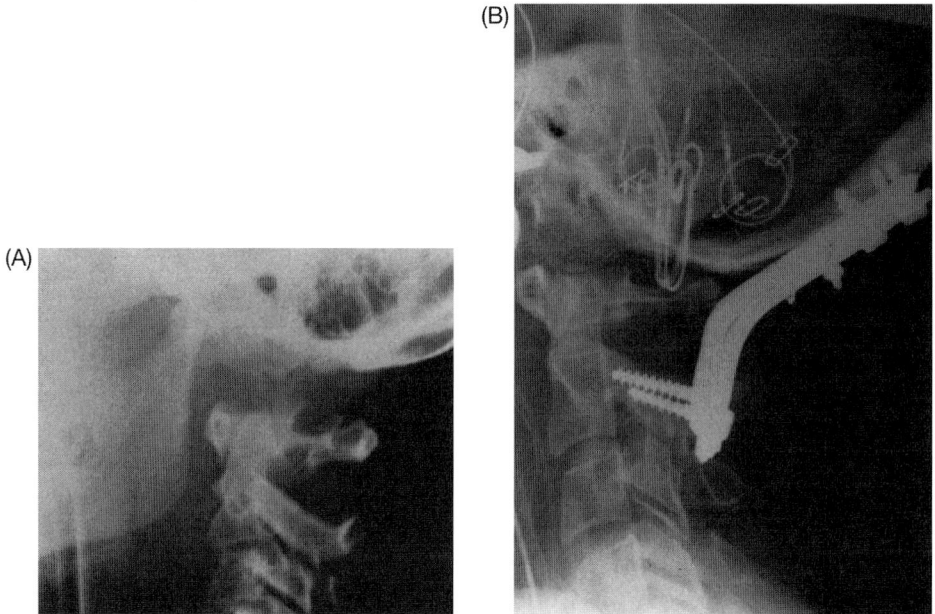

Figure 6   (A) A lateral plain radiograph showing an occipto–cervical dislocation and (B) a postoperative lateral radiograph following an occiput to C2 posterior fusion.

best performed with initial careful application of a halo/vest. Any attempts at reduction should be undertaken with great care and preferably with radiographic (fluoroscopic) guidance. Since this injury results almost entirely from ligamentous failure, an occipito–cervical fusion is required for long-term stability. Most authors advocate surgical stabilization in preference to prolonged halo immobilization because of the potential dangers of persistent instability at the occipitoatlantal junction (2,3, 14,18,20,21). A posterior occipito–cervical stabilization procedure with segmental internal fixation (i.e., occipito–cervical plates or screws and rods with or without wires) is often preferred for long-term stability (Fig. 6A and B). Because of the high risk of potential neurological decline with subtle injury level translation, definitive stabilization should be done relatively early—as soon as the patient's overall medical condition permits.

IV   CONCLUSION

Injuries involving the occipito–cervical junction are frequently associated with significant neurological sequelae. The diagnosis of these injuries requires a heightened index of suspicion and timely use of appropriate imaging modalities. This approach will allow for immediate immobilization and definitive stabilization as determined by the degree of bony and ligamentous instability present.

REFERENCES

1.   Werne S. Studies in spontaneous atlas dislocation. Acta Orthop Scand 1957;23(Suppl): 1–150.

2. Evarts CM. Traumatic occipito-atlantal dislocations. Report of a case with survival. J Bone Joint Surg 1970;52A:1653–1660.
3. Georgopoulos G, Pizzutillo PD, Lee M. Occipito-atlantal instability in children. A report of five cases and review of the literature. J Bone Joint Surg 1987;69A:429–436.
4. Xu R, Nadaud MC, Ebraheim NA, Yeasting RA. Morphology of the second cervical vertebra and the posterior projection of the C2 pedicle axis. Spine 1995;20:259–263.
5. Anderson PA, Montesano PX. Morphology and treatment of occipital condyle fractures. Spine 1988;13:731–736.
6. Levine AM, Edwards CC. Treatment of injuries in the C1-C2 complex. Orthop Clin North 1986;17:31–44.
7. Levine AM, Edwards CC. Traumatic lesions of the occipito-atlanto-axial complex. Clin Orthop 1989;239:53–68.
8. Tuli S, Tator CH, Fehlings MG, Mackay M. Occipital condyle fractures. Neurosurgery 1997;41(2):368–376.
9. Haher TR, Yeung AW, Caruso SA, Merola AA, Shin T, Zipnick RI, Gorup JM, Bono C. Occipital screw pullout strength. A biomechanical investigation of occipital morphology. Spine 1999;24(1):5–9.
10. Roberts DA, Doherty BJ, Heggeness MH. Quantitative anatomy of the occiput and the biomechanics of occipital screw fixation. Spine 1998;23(10):1107–1108.
11. Montane I, Eismont FJ, Green BA. Traumatic occipitoatlantal dislocation. Spine 1991;16:112–116.
12. Blackwood NJ. Atlanto-occipital dislocations. Ann Surg 1908;47:654–658.
13. Bohlman HH. Acute fractures and dislocations of the cervical spine—An analysis of 300 hospitalized patients and review of the literature. J Bone Joint Surg 1979;61A:1119–1142.
14. Powers B, Miller MD, Kramer RS, et al. Traumatic atlanto-occipital dislocation with survival. Neurosurg 1979;4:12–17.
15. Bucholz RW, Burkhead WZ. The pathological anatomy of fatal atlanto-occipital dislocations. J Bone Joint Surg 1979;61A:248–250.
16. Dublin A, Marks WM, Weinstock D, Newton TH. Traumatic dislocation of the atlanto-occipital articulation. J Neurosurg 1980;52:541–546.
17. Furin AH, Pirotte TP. Occipital dislocation. Case report. J Neurosurg 1977;46:663–666.
18. Page CP, Story JL, Wissinger JP, Branch CL. Traumatic atlanto-occipital dislocation. Case report. J Neurosurg 1973;39:394–397.
19. Finney HC, Roberts TS. Atlanto-occipito instability. Case report. J Neurosurg 1978;48:636–638.
20. Gabrielson TO, Maxwell JA. Traumatic atlanto-occipital dislocations with case report of a patient who survived. Am J Roentgenol 1966;97:624–639.
21. Woodring JH, Selke AC, Duff DE. Traumatic atlanto-occipital dislocation with survival. Am J Roentgenol 1981;137:21–44.
22. Banna M, Stevenson GW, Tumiel H, Tumiel A. Unilateral atlanto-occipital dislocations complicating an anomaly of the atlas. J Bone Joint Surg 1983;65A:685–687.
23. Dickman CA, Papadopoulos SM, Sonntag VKH, Spetzler RF, Rekate HL, Drabier J. Traumatic occipitoatlantal dislocations. J Spinal Disord 1993;6:300–313.
24. Eismont FJ, Bohlman HH. Posterior atlanto-occipital dislocation with fracture of the atlas and odontoid process. Report of a case with survival. J Bone Joint Surg 1978;60A:397–399.
25. Kauffman RA, Dunbar JA, McLaurin RL. Traumatic longitudinal atlanto-occipital distraction injuries in children. Am J Neuroradiol 1982;3:415–419.
26. Gehweiler JA, Osborne RL, Jr, Becker RF. The radiology of vertebral trauma. Philadelphia: W.B. Saunders, 1980:132–133.

27. Collato PM, De Muth WW, Schwentker EP, Boal DK. Traumatic atlanto-occipital dislocations. J Bone Joint Surg 1986;67A:1106–1109.

28. Englander O. Nontraumatic occipito-atlanto-axial dislocation. A contribution to the radiology of the atlas. Br J Radiol 1942;15:341–345.

29. Kissinger P. Lexations Fraktur im Atlanto-occipitagelenke. Zentralbl Chir 1900;27:933–934.

30. Malgaigne JF. Traite des Fractures et des Luxations. Paris: J.B. Bailliere, 1850:320–322.

31. Bailey DK. The normal cervical spine in infants and children. Radiology 1952;59:712–719.

32. Wiesel SW, Rothman RH. Occipito-atlantal hypermobility. Spine 1979;4:187.

33. Wholey MH, Browner AJ, Baker HL, Jr. The lateral roentgenogram of the neck (with comments on the atlanto-odontoid-basion relationship). Radiology 1958;71:350–356.

34. Shapiro R, Youngberg AS, Rothman SLG. The differential diagnosis of traumatic lesions of the occipital-atlanto-axial segment. Radiol Clin North Am 1973;11:505–526.

10

Atlantoaxial Rotatory Instability

ALEXANDER R. VACCARO and JEFF S. SILBER

*Thomas Jefferson University Hospital and the Rothman Institute,
Philadelphia, Pennsylvania, U.S.A.*

R. ALDEN MILAM IV

University of Pennsylvania, Philadelphia, Pennsylvania, U.S.A.

HUGH L. BASSEWITZ and HARRY N. HERKOWITZ

William Beaumont Hospital, Royal Oak, Michigan, U.S.A.

JUSTIN P. KUBECK

*Thomas Jefferson University Hospital and the Rothman Institute,
Philadelphia, Pennsylvania, U.S.A.*

I INTRODUCTION

The atlantoaxial region of the spine is a transition zone that helps allow the head to properly function on top of the spine. Specifically, the atlantoaxial joint allows a large degree of head rotation. Its stability is provided by both bony and soft tissue structures. As opposed to the well-fitting, convex–concave design of the occipital–atlantal joints, which provide for weight bearing and some flexion extension, the corresponding facet joints of C1 and C2 are both convex in design. This allows for approximately 50% of the axial rotation of the entire cervical spine. Flexion and extension are approximately 13° to 15° and rotation is 45° to each side at this articulation. This biconvexity also explains the vertical approximation seen with rotation. The low point of each joint surface is at maximal rotation and the highest point is at neutral rotation. Rotation past 63° to 65°at the C1–C2 articulation will start to result in dislocation of the C1–C2 facet joint, with upper cervical canal narrowing down to 7 mm. Rotatory injuries of the atlantoaxial joint thereupon range from a

minor subluxation that preserves normal C1–C2 motion correctable with collar immobilization to frank dislocation with an attendant dense neurological deficit (1–4).

A Anatomy

The cruciate ligament stabilizes the atlantoaxial complex. The horizontal limb of the
cruciate ligament is the thick and sturdy transverse atlantal ligament, which attaches
to the condyles of the axis. The ascending limb of the cruciate ligament attaches to
the anterior margin of the foramen magnum while the descending limb attaches to
the body of the axis. Just posterior to the cruciate ligament is the tectoral membrane.
Anterior to the cruciate ligament are the paired alar ligaments and the single apical
ligament. The alar ligaments attach from each side of the odontoid process to the
medial aspect of each occipital condyle. The apical ligament attaches from the apex
of the odontoid process to the anterior rim of the foramen magnum.

The odontoid process projects upward from the body of the axis, forming a
pivot axis about which head rotation occurs. The odontoid–atlas articulation is a
synovial joint; there is also synovial fluid between the odontoid and the transverse
ligament. Steel's rule of thirds divides the anterior–posterior diameter of C1 into
three equal parts (5). The odontoid occupies the anterior centimeter, the spinal cord
occupies the middle centimeter, and free space occupies the posterior centimeter of
diameter at this level. The free space behind the cord at this level allows for minor
subluxations to avoid neurological damage. However, subluxations that close down
this 10 mm of room will put the spinal cord in danger. Rotary dislocations, odontoid
fractures, os odontoideum, and insufficiency of the transverse ligament can all allow
dangerous narrowing of this free space.

B Biomechanics

Since the bony articulation of C1 and C2 allows such a high degree of motion,
ligaments of the atlantoaxial complex primarily provide stability. Dvorak has shown
that the transverse ligament is nearly twice as strong as the alar ligament and is
considered the primary stabilizer of anterior translation of the atlas (6). The alar
ligaments, the apical ligament, the dens, and the facet joint capsules provide additional stability. Cadaver studies have been done to examine the strength and function
of the transverse ligament. An intact transverse ligament will allow up to 3 mm of
anterior translation of the atlas on the axis and a range of 3 to 5 mm may be
indicative of the potential for sudden transverse ligament failure. The ligament will
fail most commonly as an intrasubstance tear but can fail as an avulsion off its C2
attachment. Although age and ligament strength cannot be correlated, some transverse ligaments will have minimal strength, even without the presence of systemic
illnesses such as rheumatoid arthritis. Current parameters for normal atlantoaxial
motion with flexion extension lateral x-rays are up to 3 mm in adults and up to 5
mm in children. These values have been confirmed by radiographic studies in normal
patients. It was found that in asymptomatic patients, the maximum anterior translation was 2.5 mm in adults and 4 mm in children (7,8).

II ETIOLOGY

Levine and Edwards stated that rotatory subluxations/dislocations at the C1–C2 articulation rarely occur in adults and are significantly different from those in children

(9). Possible mechanisms are thought to be a flexion extension–type of injury with an associated rotatory force. Often there may be an associated fracture of one or both C1 or C2 lateral masses. The force magnitude may be as insignificant as a relatively minor blow to the head. Subluxations in children are often related to a localized inflammatory process and respond well to collar immobilization. Wittek proposed that an effusion of the synovial joint, which produces stretching of the C1–C2 ligaments, may develop in children following an upper respiratory viral illness as a precursor to atlantoaxial rotatory subluxation (10). Furthermore, Coutts suggested that synovial fringes, when inflamed or adherent, might block atlantoaxial reduction if subluxated (2). Persistent malalignment may then lead to capsular and ligamentous contractures with resultant fixation. Multiple authors have proposed other etiologies for rotatory subluxation. Fiorani-Gallotta and Luzzatti postulated the possibility of a rupture of one or both of the alar ligaments and the transverse ligament (11). Watson-Jones hypothesized hyperemic decalcification at specific ligamentous insertion sites with loosening of the ligaments leading to subluxation (4). Finally, Grisel felt that muscle contractions and spasms, often associated with swollen capsules and synovial tissues, may contribute to facet joint subluxation in the early stages (12,13). Additionally, a rotatory facet subluxation is occasionally associated with C1 and C2 lateral mass articular fractures (14).

III DIAGNOSIS

Signs and symptoms of C1–C2 rotatory subluxation may range from complaints of neck pain only to signs of torticollis. The patient may present with the typical "cock-robin" posture with the head tilted toward one side and rotated toward the other. Plagiocephaly, a distortion of the facial geometry, can be seen in the younger patient with late presentation (15). A high index of suspicion is necessary in the adult patient. Suspicion for abnormalities at this level is heightened in patients with complaints of suboccipital or upper cervical neck pain following trauma with radiographic or clinical evidence of angulatory or rotatory deformities of the cervical spine.

Wortzman and Dewar advocated using dynamic radiography in differentiating rotatory fixation from torticolli, and Fielding and coworkers recommended cineradiography and dynamic CT scanning as useful adjuncts to plain radiography to establish an accurate diagnosis (14–16). The evaluation of a patient with C1–C2 rotatory subluxation begins with orthogonal (AP, lateral, and open-mouth odontoid) plain radiographic views. The atlanto–dens interval (ADI) is the measurable space between the posterior edge of the anterior ring of C1 and the anterior margin of the odontoid. This interval in the normal adult should be no more than 3 mm in adults or 5 mm in children. Flexion-extension views are very revealing and can be done if the patient is awake and cooperative and can perform this maneuver on his own. Passive flexion extension of the cervical spine by hospital personnel or physicians should be avoided in the comatose or uncooperative patient. In the acute setting, however, flexion-extension films may not reveal any motion, normal or abnormal, secondary to spasm of the surrounding muscles. In this case, patients may be immobilized in a cervical collar and repeat x-rays can be done in 10 to 14 days, after the spasm has subsided.

The AP open-mouth radiograph is used to assess rotation of the lateral masses. If the space between the lateral masses and the odontoid is asymmetric, there may be atlantoaxial rotary fixation. When the atlas rotates to the right, the distance between the dens and the right lateral mass appears to increase. The same effect appears on the left side, when the atlas rotates to the left. However, one cadaveric study demonstrated that an intact odontoid lateral mass interspace might appear misleadingly asymmetric (18). On the open-mouth odontoid view, the C1 lateral mass on the side of anterior subluxation appears larger and closer to the midline, while the lateral mass rotated posteriorly appears to overlap the C2 lateral mass (the so-called wink sign) and is farther from the midline (19). In the chronic setting, when plain cervical spine radiographs demonstrate evidence of a rotational anomaly at the atlantoaxial joint, additional radiographic investigation is indicated. This workup should consist of open-mouth odontoid views with the patient's head rotated 15° to each side to determine whether true atlantoaxial fixation is present. Persistent (not correctable by rotation) asymmetry of the relationship between the odontoid and C1 and C2 lateral masses forms the basic radiological criterion for the diagnosis of atlantoaxial rotatory fixation (17). Alternatively, a dynamic computed tomography scan through the C1–C2 articulation, with the patient's head rotated to the right and to the left approximately 15°, will aid in documenting the presence of rotatory fixation at the atlantoaxial joint and is considered to be the diagnostic imaging modality of choice Fig. 1A and B).

Both anatomical and CT studies have shown that the transverse ligament is between 2- to 3-mm thick and is thickest at its midportion, posterior to the dens. CT scans can be helpful in differentiating a midsubstance transverse ligament rupture and an avulsion from C2, by revealing a bony fleck at the site of avulsion. CT scans have also shown the presence of a triangular space. This has been described posterior to the transverse ligament and anterior to the dura. It is thought to contain veins and fatty tissue. This periodontoidal venous plexus may be in connection with the hypertrophic peripharyngeal lymphoid tissue shown in children. This has been theorized as the anatomical rationale and cause for Grisel's syndrome. Magnetic resonance imaging (MRI) can also be utilized to see the transverse ligament. The ligament appears like most ligaments, homogeneous with low signal intensity. A tear in the ligament will appear as a high-intensity zone at the site of the rupture or avulsion. Because of their superiority in detecting these injuries, both MRI and thin-cut CT scans may be used in addition to dynamic flexion-extension radiographs for evaluating the ring of C1 for transverse ligament tears (20).

A   Traumatic Rupture of the Transverse Ligament

1   Diagnosis and Treatment

When an acute isolated traumatic rupture of the transverse ligament occurs, the outcome is usually fatal, although survival is possible. Head trauma frequently accompanies this injury. The mechanism is most likely from a shearing force and has clinically been reported to be from a flexion injury. More commonly, this injury is seen in children who appear to have the ability to survive more than adults. The symptoms will vary widely from simple neck stiffness and neck pain to frank transient quadriparesis. Quadriparesis is frequently transient, as significant spinal cord injury of this level is often fatal. However, because of the location of the injury, respiratory functions can be affected due to the proximity of the medulla oblongata. The vertebral arteries are tortuous in the course in C1–C2 articulation and they may

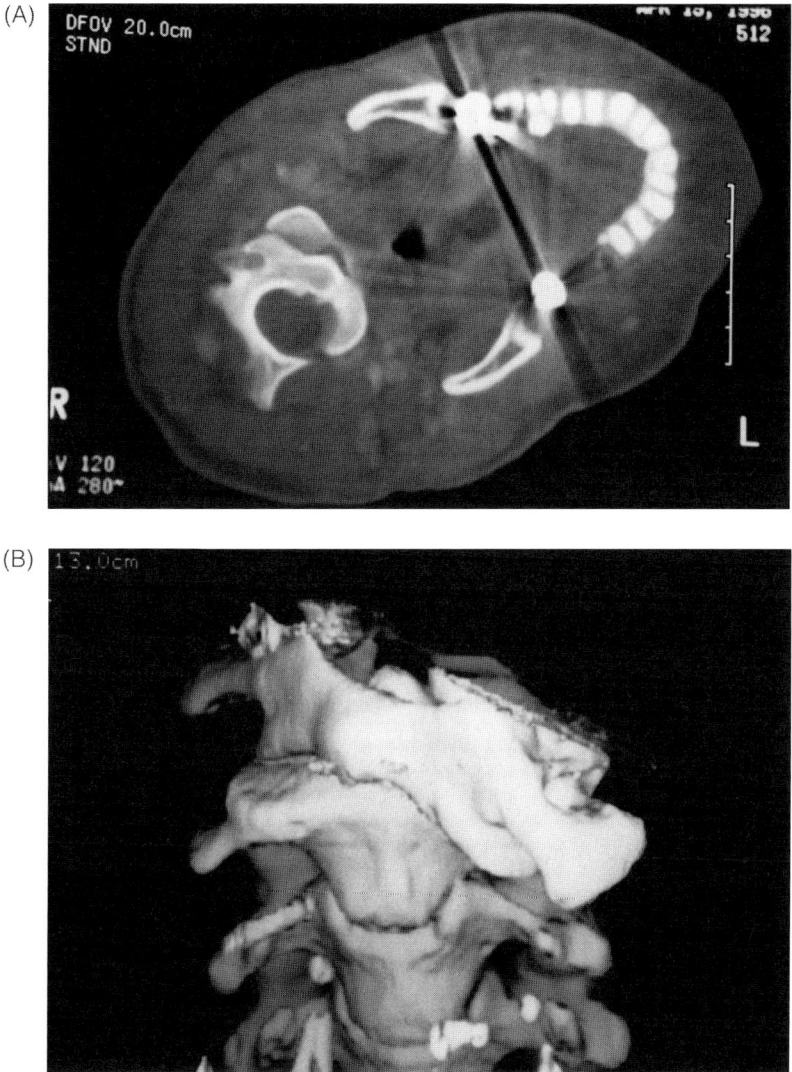

Figure 1   (A) An axial CT view in left rotation demonstrating a fixed subluxation of C1 on C2. (B) A three-dimensional CT reconstruction clearly showing the C1–C2 rotatory subluxation.

be compressed, affecting circulation in the circle of Willis. This may present as syncope or blurred vision. The neurological exam can reveal unilateral or bilateral numbness or weakness in one or more multiple extremities.

Dickman et al. reported on their experience with 39 TAL injuries (20). Using radiographs, CT scans, and MRI, the authors developed a new classification for traumatic TAL ruptures. Type I injuries were classified as intrasubstance tears (IA) or tears at the periosteal insertion (IB). Type II injuries involve a bony fracture that separates the tubercle from the condyle. Type IIA injuries describe a comminuted fracture of the lateral mass, while type IIB injuries describe a tubercle avulsion from an intact lateral mass (Fig. 2).

Reports have described cases in children with ADIs in flexion from 7 to 15 mm. Because of this varied clinical presentation, TAL injuries can be missed initially and present late as chronic atlantoaxial instability. Acute management involves lateral x-rays as well as flexion-extension films initially, if feasible, or in early follow-up.

The treatment of traumatic rupture of the transverse ligament is primarily a C1–C2 arthrodesis as the ligament has a poor propensity to heal, even when the upper cervical spine is immobilized in a halo. Dickman et al. found that type I injuries did not heal primarily, and recommended early surgery (20). Type II TAL injuries, which did actually involve tearing of the ligament, had a 74% chance of healing with treatment with a cervical orthosis. They suggest close monitoring of these patients, with surgical stabilization after 3 to 4 months of observation if there is evidence of nonunion and instability.

When the transverse ligament is ruptured, there is no effective restraint to prevent anterior displacement of the atlas on the axis. If there is any site of neurological injury or compression, a C1–C2 arthrodesis will provide the stability necessary at the atlantoaxial joint and ensure the restoration of the 10 mm of spinal cord free space. In the adult without neurological involvement, a C1–C2 fusion is still the treatment of choice as the ligament has little ability to heal. Children, however, have a better ability to heal the ligament and 2 to 3 months in a brace or halo may be sufficient. If there is still instability after this, a C1–C2 fusion should be performed.

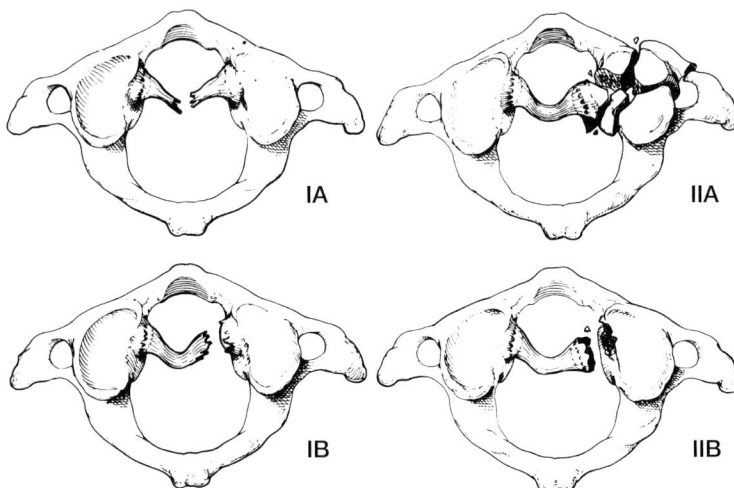

Figure 2 Classification of injuries to the transverse atlantal ligament. Type I injuries disrupt the ligament substance in its midportion (IA) or at its periosteal insertion (IB). Type II injuries disconnect the tubercle for insertion of the transverse ligament from the C1 lateral mass involving a comminuted C1 lateral mass (IIA) or avulsing the tubercle from an intact lateral mass (IIB). (From Ref. 20.)

There are a number of options for posterior cervical fusion at C1–C2 including the Gallic (21), the Brooks (22), and the Magerl (23) techniques. These will be described in detail elsewhere in this book. While the Brooks has a higher fusion rate than the Gallie, the Magerl technique has the best rate of fusion because it employs a transarticular screw through each C1–C2 facet, as well as use of posterior wiring. This technique is obviously more technically demanding, but it is the strongest technique and may eliminate the need for a postoperative halo (24–27). The advantage of the transarticular screws is that they prevent postoperative translation of the C1 on C2 that can occur with posterior wiring alone. This subluxation may possibly be the cause of some C1–C2 posterior wirings developing nonunions.

B Delayed Transverse Ligament Insufficiency

1 Diagnosis and Treatment

Occipitalization of the atlas and the Klippel–Feil syndrome are both congenital ankylosis of the cervical spine. These disorders can impart abnormal forces to the stabilizing ligaments of the atlantoaxial complex and lead to chronic stress and fatigue, and possibly to functional insufficiency and attenuation of the transverse ligament. Developmental disorders, such as Down's syndrome, may have a high incidence of atlantoaxial instability due to laxity of the transverse ligament or odontoid hypoplasia.

With occipitalization of the atlas, most commonly the anterior ring of C1 is fused to the occiput. Thus, the normal 10° to 15° of flexion and extension that usually occurs at the occiput C1 joint is now transferred to the joint below, the C1–C2 joint. This leads to excessive force, which can lead to attenuation of the transverse ligament. Atlantoaxial instability is reported to occur in 39 to 59% of patients with occipitalization of C1. A similar mechanism of abnormal forces happens over time with a congenital fusion of C2 and C3. A combination of this with atlas occipitalization occurs in 47 to 68% of patients with occipitalization. About one-half of these people will develop late, delayed C1–C2 instability. The characteristic feature of this disorder is a prolonged clinical course, with symptoms presenting over a long period of time as the transverse ligament attenuates. Presenting symptoms may be simple neck pain or varied neurological involvement. Patients may present with myelopathy or acute spinal cord injury after trauma.

In the asymptomatic patient, observation is recommended unless the atlanto–dens interval inflection is greater than 7 mm. At that point, a C1–C2 fusion is recommended. If patients have significant pain or any neurological signs or symptoms, a C1–C2 fusion is recommended if the atlanto–dens interval inflection is greater than 5 mm.

C Atlantoaxial Rotational Disorders

This subset of atlantoaxial instability has been termed rotary subluxation or dislocation, rotary fixation, rotary deformity, and spontaneous hyperemic dislocation. The etiology may be either congenital or acquired and may arise spontaneously, secondary from inflammation, or from trauma. Congenital causes related to transverse ligament deficiency or odontoid hypoplasia include Down's syndrome, Morquio's disease, achondroplasia, metaphyseal-epiphyseal dysplasia, and spondyloepiphyseal dysplasia. In these patients, minor trauma can lead to significant atlantoaxial instability. Acquired causes are generally related to an inflammatory process. A recent upper respiratory infection or retropharyngeal inflammation such as tonsillitis or adenoiditis may precede an atlantoaxial malrotation. Grisel first decribed a case of spontaneous rotary subluxation of C1 and C2 after retropharyngeal inflammation (12). It is now thought that the periodontoidal venous plexus may become inflamed due to a connection with the peripharyngeal lymphovenous tissue that becomes inflamed.

Patients present with acute neck pain and torticollis, which is seen primarily in children. With the head rotated approximately 20° in one direction and tilted 20° in the opposite direction, Fielding stated that this position resembled a robin listening for a worm, thus the name cock-robin position was coined (28). When the sternocleidomastoid contracts (shortens), it helps to turn the head to the opposite side (e.g., the right sternocleidomastoid contraction yields a left rotation). In contrast to congenital torticollis, which has a shortened fibrotic sternocleidomastoid on the side toward which the head is rotated, in acquired torticollis the sternocleidomastoid on the side toward which the head is rotated is lengthened. If there were not a fixed rotation of C1 on C2, the sternocleidomastoid would contract to correct the malrotation. When the transverse ligament is intact, C1 will dislocate on C2 at 65° of rotation and narrow the spinal canal to 7 mm. If the transverse ligament is nonfunctional and with 5 mm of anterior–posterior displacement, unilateral facet dislocation can occur at as little as 45° of rotation with narrowing of the spinal canal to 12 mm.

Fielding and Hawkins have identified some key concepts in radiographic imaging of these patients. On the AP open-mouth x-ray, the lateral mass of the atlas that is rotated forward appears wider and closer to the midline, and the contralateral lateral mass appears narrower and farther off the midline. The spinous process of the axis may appear deviated from the midline, opposite to the direction of the lateral tilt. If the spinous process of the axis is tilting in one direction and rotated in the opposite direction, then the chin and spinous process of C2 are usually on the same side, and atlantoaxial rotary fixation is present.

The lateral radiograph is used to measure the atlanto–dens interval. Further abnormalities can be inferred if the two posterior arches of the atlas and axis do not line up and this is usually secondary to tilt. Fielding and Hawkins strongly recommend the use of cineradiography to see if C1 and C2 move together as a unit. CT scans with three-dimensional reconstruction can also show the C1–C2 facet joint complex with a high level of detail.

Fielding and Hawkins have described four types of atlantoaxial rotary fixation (Fig. 3) (28). Type I is rotary fixation without anterior displacement of the atlas. It was the most common in their series and the transverse ligament remained intact with the odontoid acting as the pivot point. In type II, which is the second most common lesion, there is rotary fixation with anterior displacement of the atlas of 3 to 5 mm. The transverse ligament is deficient and the pivot point is now the contralateral nondisplaced C1–C2 facet joint. Type III, seen in three patients, is rotary fixation with anterior displacement of more than 5 mm with both the transverse ligament and secondary structures nonfunctional, both articulations are subluxed anteriorly, one side greater than the other. Type IV, seen in one patient, is rotary fixation with posterior displacement. For this to occur, the odontoid is deficient and C1 translates posterior on C2.

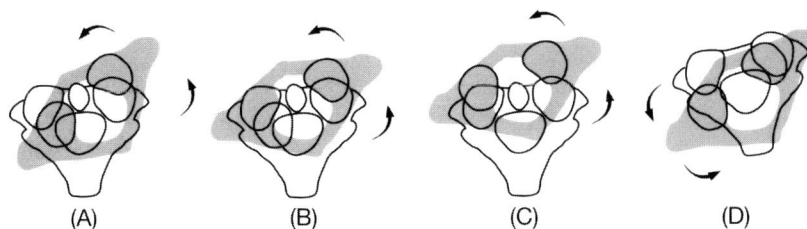

Figure 3 A pictoral demonstrating the classification of rotatory fixation according to Fielding and associates. (A) Type I (ADI < 3 mm); (B) type II (ADI = 3–5 mm); (C) type III (ADI > 5 mm); and (D) type IV (posterior subluxation of C1 on C2). ADI = atlantodental interval.

Most rotary deformities can be treated symptomatically and resolution will occur with time (29). A course of rest, soft collar, and observation will be sufficient for most patients. If significant trauma is present and factors into the history, a more aggressive diagnostic approach may be necessary. If the patient presents with a fixed atlantoaxial rotary deformity, they should initially be treated with head halter traction, sedation, and analgesics. If there is no reduction in the first 1 to 2 weeks, skeletal traction may be instituted. Fielding and Hawkins recommend 3.2 to 3.6 kg in children, with a limit of 6.8 kg increased over time. In adults, they recommend 6.8 kg up to a maximum of 9.1 kg over time. If correction of the deformity occurs in traction, this traction should be maintained for 1 to 2 weeks to ensure correction. The patient is then placed in a halo for 2 to 3 months. A posterior C1–C2 fusion should be considered if the patient has symptomatic instability, presence of a deformity for greater than 3 months, a deformity resistant to nonoperative measures, or recurrence of the deformity after reduction (29). If the transverse ligament is nonfunctional, as in types II and types III, earlier surgery is probably justified. Some authors recommend 1 to 3 weeks of preoperative traction as well as using postoperative traction. A halo vest is probably sufficient for postoperative immobilization. If the Magerl technique is used, a halo is probably not necessary.

IV CONCLUSION

Traumatic atlantoaxial rotatory instability is often the result of an associated bony fracture or significant ligamentous disruption. Due to the potential for chronic long-term instability in the adult patient population, surgical stabilization is often the preferred method of treatment following closed cervical reduction. This spinal disorder is often associated with an inflammatory illness in children and almost universally responds to immobilization with or without halter traction followed by gentle range of motion, flexibility, and strengthening physiotherapy.

REFERENCES

1. Corner ES. Rotary dislocations of the atlas. Ann Surg 1907; 45:9–26.
2. Coutts MB. Rotary dislocations of the atlas. Ann Surg 1934; 29:297–311.

3. Schnieder RC, Schemm GW. Vertebral artery insufficiency in acute and chronic spinal trauma. With special reference to the syndrome of acute central cervical spinal cord injury. J Neurosurg 1961; 18:348–360.

4. Watson-Jones R. Spontaneous hyperaemic dislocation of the atlas. Proc Soc Med 1932; 25:586–590.

5. Steel HH. Anatomical and mechanical consideration of the atlanto-axial articulation. In Proceedings of the American Orthopedic Association. J Bone Joint Surg Am 1968; 56: 1481–1482.

6. Dvorak J, Schneider E, Saldinger P, Rahn B. Biomechanics of the craniocervical region: the alar and transverse ligaments. J Orthop Res 1988; 6:452–461.

7. Jackson H. The diagnosis of minimal atlanto-axial subluxation. Br J Radiol 1950; 23: 672.

8. Werne S. Studies on spontaneous atlas dislocation. Acta Orthop Scand 1957; 23:1–150.

9. Levine AM, Edwards CC. Traumatic lesions of the occipitoatlantoaxial complex. Clin Orthop 1989; 239:530–568.

10. White AA, Panjabi MM. Clinical Biomechanics of the Spine, 2nd ed. Philadelphia: JB Lippincott, 1990.

11. Fiorani-Gallotta G, Luzzatti G. Sublussazione lateral e sublessazione rotatoria dell'ante. Arch di Ortop 1957; 70:467–484.

12. Grisel P. Enucleation de l'atlas et torticollis nasp-pharyngien. Presse Med 1930; 38:50–53.

13. Hess JH, Bronstein IP, Abelson SM. Atlanto-axial dislocations. Unassociated with trauma and secondary to inflammatory foci in the neck. Am J Dis Child 1935; 49:1137–1147.

14. Fielding JW, Hawkins RJ, Hensinger RN, Francis WR. Atlantoaxial rotary deformities. Orthop Clin North Am 1978; 9:955–967.

15. Wortzman G, Dewar FP. Rotatory fixation of the atlantoaxial joint: Rotational atlantoaxial subluxation. Radiology 1968; 90:479–487.

16. Fielding WJ, Stillwell WT, Chynn KY, Spyropoulos EC. Use of computed tomography for the diagnosis of atlanto-axial rotatory fixation. J Bone Joint Surg 1978; 60A:1102–1104.

17. Jones RN. Rotatory dislocation of both atlanto-axial joints. J Bone Joint Surg 1984; 66B:6–7.

18. Sutherland JP, Yaszemski MJ, White AA. Radiographic appearance of the odontoid lateral mass interspace in the occipitoatlantoaxial complex. Spine 1995; 20:2221–2225.

19. Levine AM, Edwards CC. Treatment of injuries in the C1-C2 complex. Orthop Clin North Am 1986; 17:31–44.

20. Dickman CA, Greene KA, Sonntag VKH. Injuries involving the transverse atlantal ligament: classification and treatment guidelines based upon experience with 39 injuries. Neurosurgery 1996; 38:44–50.

21. Gallie WE. Fractures and dislocations of the cervical spine. Am J Surg 1939; 46:495–499.

22. Brooks AL, Jenkins EB. Atlanto-axial arthrodesis by wedge compression method. J Bone Joint Surg Am 1978; 60:279–284.

23. Magerl F, Seeman P. Stable posterior fusion of the atlas and axis by transarticular screw fixation. In: Kehr P, Weidner A, eds. Cervical Spine I. New York: Springer-Verlag, 1987: 322.

24. Grob D, Crisco JJ III, Panjabi MM, Wang P, Dvorak J. Biomechanical evaluation of four different posterior atlantoaxial fixation techniques. Spine 1992; 17:480–490.

25. Grob D, Jeanneret B, Aebi M, Markwalder TM. Atlanto-axial fusion with transarticular screw fixation. J Bone Joint Surg Br 1991; 73B:972–976.

26. Marcotte P, Dickman CA, Sonnatg VKH, Karahaliios DG, Drabier J. Posterior atlantoaxial facet screw fixation. J Neurosurg 1993; 79:234–237.

27. Montesano PX, Juach EC, Anderson PA. Biomechanics of cervical spine internal fixation. Spine 1991; 16:S10–S16.
28. Fielding WJ, Hawkins RJ. Atlanto-axial rotatory fixation (fixed rotatory subluxation of the atlanto-axial joint). J Bone Joint Surg 1977; 59A:37–44.
29. Fielding JW, Hawkins RJ, Ratzan SA. Spine fusion for atlanto-axial instability. J Bone Joint Surg Am 1976; 58-A:400–407.

11

Atlas Fractures

HUGH L. BASSEWITZ and HARRY N. HERKOWITZ

William Beaumont Hospital, Royal Oak, Michigan, U.S.A.

I INTRODUCTION

Fractures of the atlas comprise approximately 2% of all total spinal injuries, 10% of all injuries to the cervical spine, and 25% of all injuries to the atlantoaxial complex (1–4). Whereas most isolated fractures have a favorable prognosis and require only conservative treatment, more aggressive treatment is indicated if there is accompanying atlantoaxial instability. The goals of treatment are achieving bony healing and maintaining atlantoaxial stability. The importance of an anatomical reduction of the lateral masses and the possibility of late-onset C1–C2 arthritis with neck pain is still unclear.

In 1822, Cooper first described a fracture of the atlas in an autopsy specimen (5). The first review of the subject was by Jefferson in 1927. He commented that ''injuries of the first cervical vertebra are, on the one hand, exceedingly rare, and, on the other, extremely fatal. Both of the ideas are wrong . . .'' (6). In 1933, Milward reported a case of atlantoaxial instability due to bilateral posterior arch fractures of the atlas (7). Although there was no sign of radiographic callus at 4 months, the patient had regained stability after 1 month of immobilization. Although there had only been 99 reported cases of atlas fractures from 1822 to 1938, Plaut predicted this number would rise significantly with the increasing use of the automobile (8).

II CLASSIFICATION

Levine and Edwards published a large series of atlas fractures and their treatment (9). The most common type (type I) of atlas fracture was an isolated fracture of the posterior arch, either unilateral or bilateral. These are stable injuries when isolated, as there is no damage to the transverse ligament (Figs. 1 and 2). The mechanism is

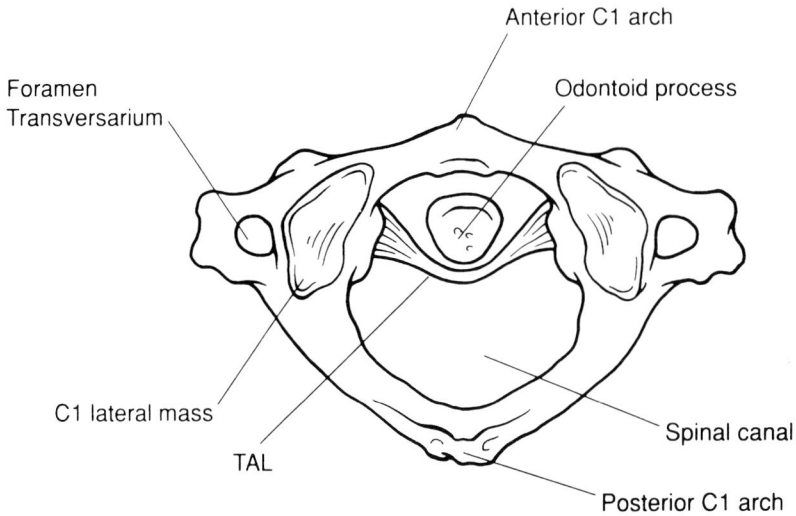

Figure 1 Axial view of the atlas. The transverse atlantal ligament (TAL) attaches to both condyles of C1. (From Ref. 24.)

one of axial loading with hyperextension of the cervical spine. The atlas is compressed between the occiput and the C2 spinous process. The force of the axial compression is translated to the atlas ring through the occiput C1 facets and the ring fails in tension.

Jefferson, or burst, fractures (type III) were the next most common (Fig. 3). When the head is in a neutral position, three or four vertical fractures will occur as the ring fails in tension with axial loading. There will commonly be two bilateral fractures of the anterior ring and one or two fractures of the posterior ring. The least common was a lateral mass fracture (type II) (Fig. 4). When the axial load occurs and there is a lateral bending moment, the ring will fail with the fracture anterior

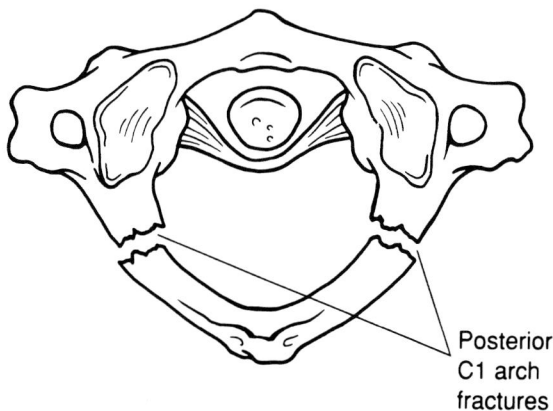

Figure 2 Bilateral posterior arch fractures. The transverse ligament remains intact, maintaining stability, and the lateral mass does not spread. (From Ref. 24.)

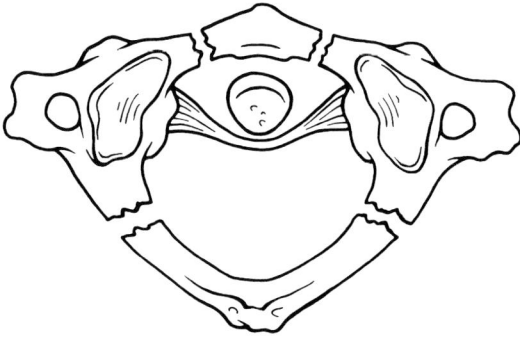

Figure 3 Jefferson (burst) fracture. In this drawing there are bilateral anterior and posterior ring fractures. There will be some spread of the lateral masses, but not more than 6.9 mm, as the transverse ligament remains intact. (From Ref. 24.)

and posterior to the lateral mass, and usually the articular surface will not be affected. Levine and Edwards also reported on the high rate of concomitant fractures with atlas fracture. These include odontoid fractures (Fig. 5), traumatic spondylolisthesis of the axis, occipital condyle fractures, rupture of the transverse ligament, and non-contiguous fracture of the subaxial cervical spine. The most common type of atlas fracture that sustained a concomitant injury was a posterior arch fracture. The most common combination seen with a posterior arch fracture was a type II odontoid fracture followed by a traumatic spondylolisthesis of the axis. Segal et al. noticed an additional type, the comminuted lateral mass fracture, which they suggested carries a worse prognosis, as two of their three nonunions had this fracture type (10).

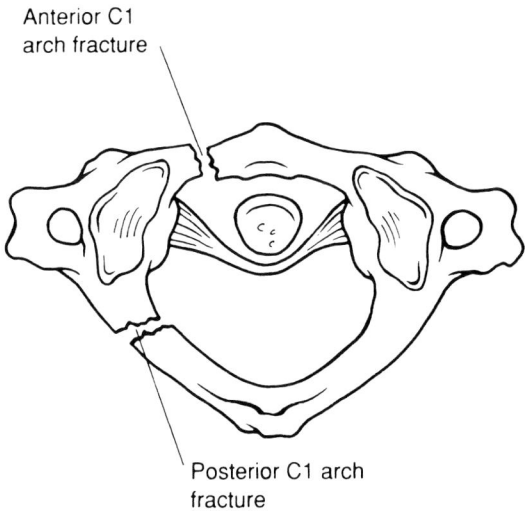

Anterior C1 arch fracture

Posterior C1 arch fracture

Figure 4 Unilateral anterior and posterior ring fractures, resulting in a lateral mass fracture. (From Ref. 24.)

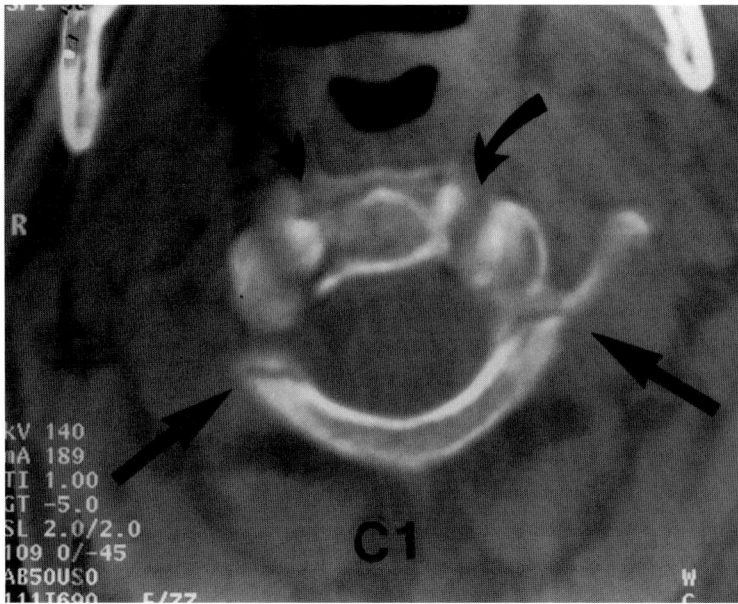

Figure 5 Axial CT scan showing bilateral posterior arch fractures of the atlas (straight arrows) accompanied by an odontoid fracture (curved arrows).

III BIOMECHANICS

The most common force that causes atlas fractures is an axial load to the vertex of the skull. Compression occurs from the occipital condyles onto the facets of the atlas. As the compressive load is transferred to the C1 ring, the ring fails in tension at its weakest point. Additional forces may include rotation, hyperextension, or lateral bending. Experimental work has shown that both the anterior and posterior rings have specific weak points in their bony architecture. As shown in Figure 6, anteriorly the weakest section of the anterior arch is oriented vertically, while the weakest section of the posterior ring is oriented horizontally. Thus, the anterior ring fails under stress while bending horizontally, and the posterior ring is weakest while bending in the sagittal plane (11). Further work has been done that demonstrates that primary instability will be in the flexion-extension plane of motion, while stability is relatively maintained in axial rotation (11,12).

IV CLINICAL PRESENTATION

The majority of patients who present with atlas fractures have been in motor vehicle accidents, but the causes can also include diving, falling from a height, and heavy objects falling on the vertex of the skull (13). Patients who complain of neck pain rarely have neurological injury (10). The lesion is one of canal expansion; thus there is more room for the cord rather than less. The exam may be difficult to assess due to the high incidence of concurrent closed head injury. If there is a neurological deficit, it is usually due to a concomitant fracture of the dens (9). Spreading of the lateral masses can affect cranial nerve function, specifically cranial nerve IX (glos-

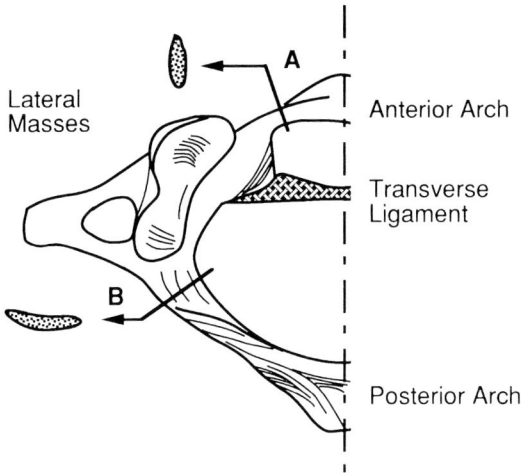

Figure 6 Axial drawing of half of the atlas. Panjabi et al. showed that the weakest section of the anterior arch is oriented vertically, and the weakest section of the posterior ring is oriented horizontally. The anterior ring fails while bending horizontally, and the posterior ring fails while bending in the sagittal plane. (From Ref. 11.)

sopharyngeal), X (vagus), and XII (hypoglossal). Injuries to the vertebral arteries can occur, causing symptoms of posterior fossa vascular insufficiency (3). The majority of patients will complain of high posterior neck pain, and some may have a subjective sense of head-on-neck instability, specifically in flexion and extension (6,11,12,14).

V RADIOGRAPHIC IMAGING

Both the anteroposterior open-mouth x-ray and the lateral x-ray are very helpful in determining the type of fracture, as well as the stability of the atlantoaxial complex. The examiner should assess whether a retropharyngeal soft tissue shadow is present. An isolated posterior arch fracture will have little or no widening of this shadow. However, if a retropharyngeal soft tissue shadow is present, it may be the only indicator that an accompanying anterior ring fracture is present, making the atlas fracture a true burst fracture. The development of this widening is time dependent, however, and may take up to 6 h to be visible. Additionally, in children who are crying, there may be a false shadow present.

The open-mouth AP x-ray is very helpful in determining the state of the transverse ligament. When a burst fracture or lateral mass fracture occurs, there is a tendency of the bony ring to splay open. The anterior ring fractures are medial to the insertion of the transverse ligament. The only structure keeping the lateral masses from spreading apart is the transverse ligament (Fig. 1). Spence has demonstrated that if the lateral masses are displaced by a total of 6.9 mm or more, the transverse ligament is ruptured (Fig. 7a,b,c) (15). Heller redefined that number to 7.9 mm, which accounts for x-ray magnification (16). The mode of failure is usually a midsubstance rupture, but there have been cases of periosteal avulsion. Both conventional tomography as well as computed tomography have been used to better image C1 fractures.

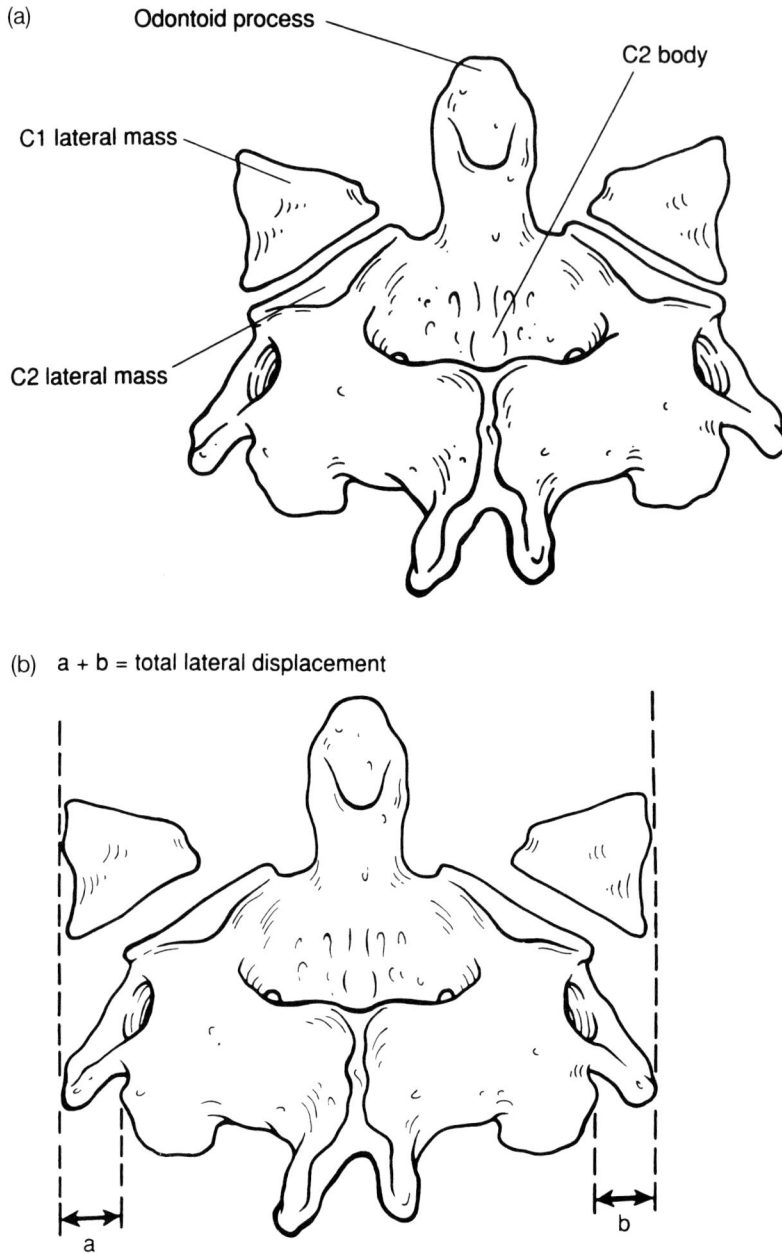

Figure 7 (a) Drawing of what is seen on the AP open-mouth-view radiograph. The lateral edge of the lateral masses of C1 will line up with the lateral edge of the C2 lateral masses. (b) When a burst facture occurs, there will be some spreading of the lateral masses. If a + b is >6.9 mm, the transverse ligament is most likely ruptured. (c) When a lateral mass fracture occurs unilaterally, there may still be a transverse ligament rupture. If b > 6.9 mm, the transverse ligament is most likely ruptured. (From Ref. 24.)

(c)

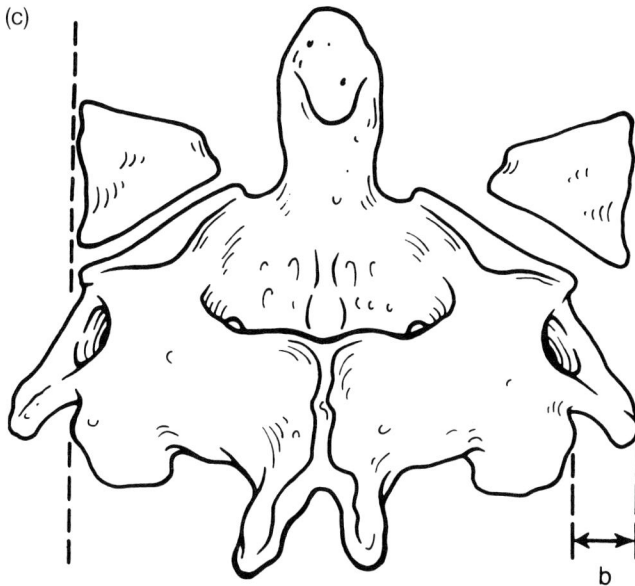

Figure 7 Continued

If the gantry of the CT scan is not in the exact plane of the atlas, fractures of the ring or the dens may be missed. Anteroposterior tomograms are more useful for detecting anterior arch fractures and odontoid fractures, whereas lateral tomograms work best for detecting posterior arch fractures.

VI TREATMENT

Historically a cervical orthosis has been used for isolated posterior arch fractures and an occipitocervical fusion has been used for displaced burst fractures (17). Over time, treatment has evolved with the treatment goals being able to achieve long-term atlantoaxial instability and prevent long-term C1–C2 pain. The most important factor in choosing a treatment for atlas fractures is the associated concomitant injury. For posterior ring fractures that are isolated, a cervical collar for 2 to 3 months is sufficient treatment, as this is a stable injury (2,3,17,18). If there is a concomitant spondylolisthesis of the axis and it is a stable type, a halo vest for 2 to 3 months is recommended, as both injuries are stable. If there was an associated dens fracture, there is some controversy. Options include a halo vest as initial management for 3 months, then checking stability with flexion-extension lateral x-rays. Levine and Edwards treated two patients this way with success. If there is instability, a delayed C1–C2 arthrodesis can now be performed, either with a wiring of the now healed C1 ring to the C2 ring, or with the Magerl technique (9,19,20). Additionally, if the surgeon prefers, an occiput to C2 fusion can be used if the C1 ring is not healed. In the acute setting, odontoid screw fixation followed by a halo vest is another option, provided the transverse ligament is competent (21). A final option is a primary occiput to C2 posterior spinal fusion (Fig. 8). If there is rupture of the transverse ligament with a posterior arch fracture, a halo vest can be tried as initial management

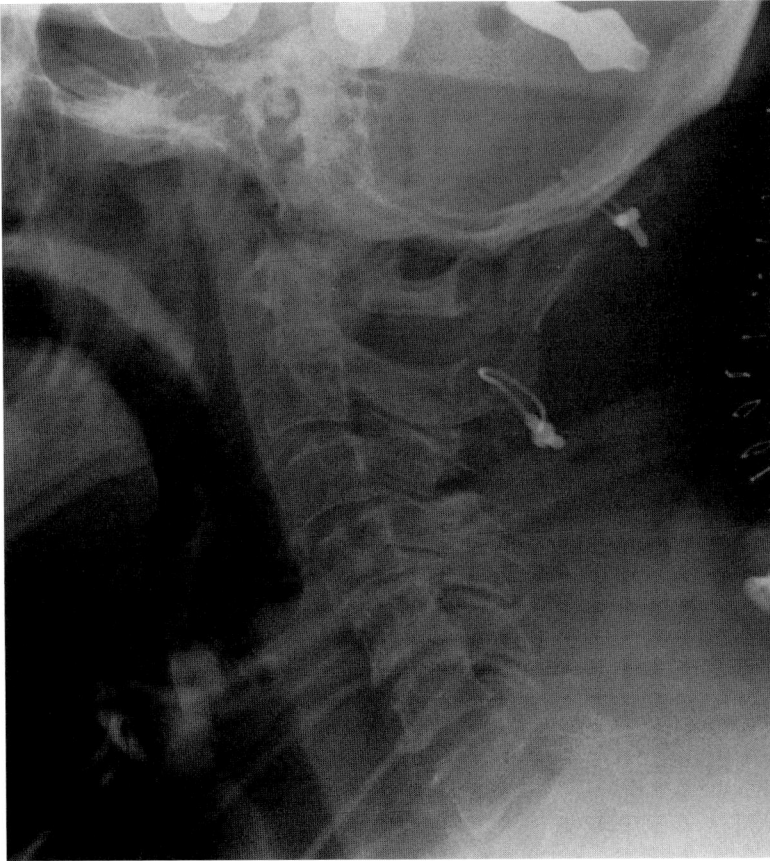

Figure 8   This patient sustained bilateral posterior arch fractures of the atlas with a concomitant displaced type II odontoid fracture. A closed reduction of the odontoid followed by a primary occiput to C2 fusion using wires and iliac crest bone graft was done.

until the C1 ring heals and a late C1–C2 fusion can be performed, if late instability is present.

For lateral mass fractures and burst fractures, the open-mouth AP x-ray should be used to assess the integrity of the transverse ligament. If the lateral masses are displaced by less than 6.9 mm (or perhaps 7.9 mm using Heller's data), the fracture is considered stable, and bracing with either cervical collar, a sternal occipital mandibular immobilization (SOMI), or a halo vest can be used for 3 to 4 months to allow for healing (2–4,22). When the lateral masses are displaced great enough to imply transverse ligament incompetence and instability, treatment recommendations become controversial. Some authors have suggested that although the transverse ligament may be ruptured, the secondary structures (ala ligaments, apical ligament, and tectoral membrane) all afford enough stability to prevent late C1–C2 instability, thus obviating the need for reduction of lateral masses. Others have argued that by leaving the lateral masses displaced, these intact secondary structures will be lax, thus decreasing their functional ability. They suggest that early reduction of the lateral masses is essential, with the option of direct early stabilization with C1–C2 transarticular, transfacet lateral mass screws (23) (Fig. 9). Most authors have suggested that to maintain or obtain reduction of lateral masses is difficult despite the use of prolonged skeletal traction. There appears to be little difference in outcome if the lateral masses are reduced or not, as the majority of patients will complain of some suboccipital pain (9,10). It has been theorized that the reason for this pain is the degenerative change that occurs at the C1–C2 articular facets. This damage may be related to the initial kinetic energy imparted to the cartilage at the time of the initial injury, and not necessarily related to the final joint surface alignment.

If traction is elected, the patient is kept in skeletal traction for 4 to 6 weeks, then x-rays are obtained after a 1-h interval of no traction. If the masses remain reduced, a halo vest is then placed for another 6 weeks. For the lateral masses that have slipped laterally again, traction is reapplied for another week and the process is repeated. Despite the method of treatment selected, the outcome is generally good. Levine and Edwards have had no cases of delayed atlantoaxial instability in their series, although up to 80% of patients complained of some residual neck pain. Hadley, however, found significantly less neck pain at 2½-year follow-up (2). Although

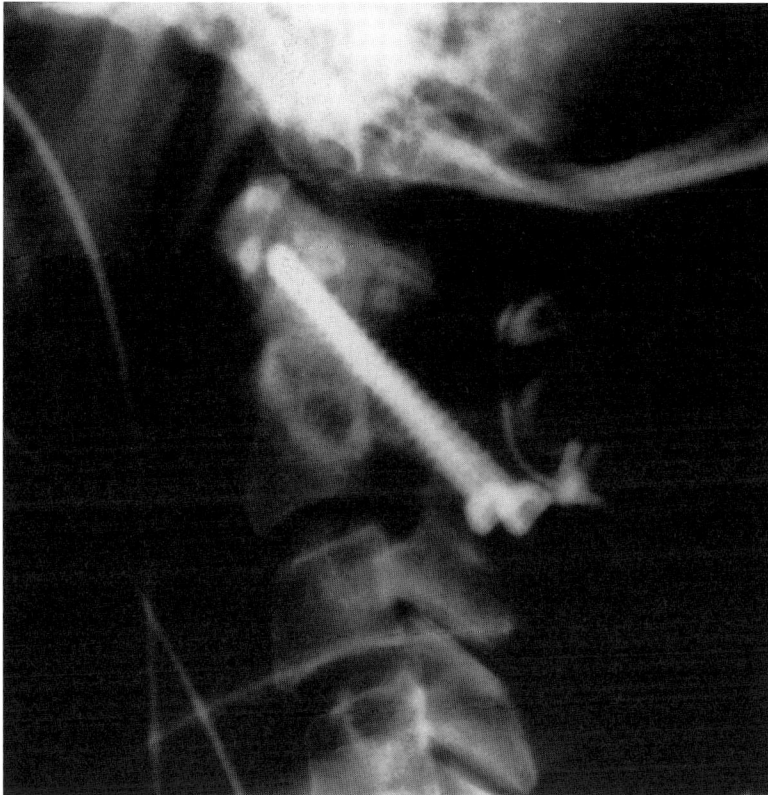

Figure 9   The Magerl technique consists of bilateral C1–C2 transarticular screws and a posterior wiring of C1–C2.

nonunion is infrequent, there is no real statistically significant difference in outcome.

VII SUMMARY

Upper cervical stability in the setting of trauma is based on the integrity of the surrounding bony and soft tissue structures. If the transverse ligament is intact, most fractures of the atlas will respond well to conservative management. When instability is present, there are multiple techniques of stabilization, as well as some controversy in the importance of fracture reduction.

REFERENCES

1. Fowler JL, Sandhu A, Fraser RD. A review of fractures of the atlas vertebra. J Spinal Disord 1990; 3:19–24.
2. Hadley MN, Dickman CA, Browner CM, Sonntag VKH. Acute traumatic atlas fractures: management and long term outcome. Neurosurgery 1988; 23:31–35.
3. Kesterson L, Benzel E, Orrison W, Coleman J. Evaluation and treatment of atlas burst fractures (Jefferson fractures). J Neurosurg 1991; 75:213–220.
4. Landelis CD, Van Peteghem PK. Fractures of the atlas: classification, treatment and morbidity. Spine 1988; 13:450–452.
5. Hatchette S. Isolated fracture of the atlas. Radiology 1941; 36:233–235.
6. Jefferson G. Fractures of the first cervical vertebra. Br Med J 1927; 2:153–157.
7. Milward F. An unusual case of fracture of the atlas. Br Med J 1933; 8:458.
8. Plaut HF. Fractures of the atlas resulting from automobile accidents: survey of the literature and report of six cases. Am J Roentgenol Rad Ther 1938; 40:867–890.
9. Levine AM, Edwards CC. Fractures of the atlas. J Bone Joint Surg 1991; 73A:680–691.
10. Segal LS, Grimm JO, Stauffer ES. Non-union of fractures of the atlas. J Bone Joint Surg 1987; 69A:1423–1434.
11. Panjabi MM, Oda T, Crisco JJ, Oxland TR, Katz L, Nolte LP. Experimental study of atlas injuries I: biomechanical analysis of their mechanisms and fracture patterns. Spine 1991; 16:S460–S465.
12. Oda T, Panjabi MM, Crisco JJ, Oxland TR. Multidirectional instabilities of experimental burst fractures of the atlas. Spine 1992; 17:1285–1290.
13. Dickman CA, Hadley MN, Browner, et al. Neurosurgical management of acute atlasaxis combination fractures. A review of 25 cases. J Neurosurg 1989; 70:45–49.
14. Sherk HH. Lesions of the atlas and axis. Clin Orthop 1975; 109:33–41.
15. Spence KF, Decker MS, Sell KW. Bursting atlantal fracture associated with rupture of the transverse ligament. J Bone Joint Surg 1970; 52A:543–549.
16. Heller JG, Viroslav S, Hudson T. Jefferson fractures: the role of the magnification artifact in assessing transverse ligament integrity. J Spinal Disord 1993; 6:392–396.
17. Bettini N, Bianco T, Di Silvestre M, Ciminari R, Risi M, Savini R. Fracture of the posterior arch of the atlas. Chir Organi Mov 1991; LXXVI:173–178.
18. Sherk HH, Nicholson JT. Fractures of the atlas. J Bone Joint Surg Am 1970; 52A:1017–1024.
19. Zavanone M, Guerra P, Rampini P, Crotti F, Vaccari U. Traumatic fractures of the craniovertebral junction. J Neurosurg Sci 1991; 35:17–22.
20. Stillerman CB, Wilson JA. Atlanto-axial stabilization with posterior transarticular screw fixation: technical description and report of 22 cases. Neurosurgery 1993; 32:948–955.
21. Guiot B, Fessler RG. Complex atlantoaxial fractures. J Neurosur (Spine 2) 1999; 91:139–143.

22. Levine AM, Edwards CC. Treatment of injuries in the C1-C2 complex. Orthop Clin North Am 1986; 17:31–44.
23. McGuire RA, Harkey HL. Primary treatment of unstable Jefferson's fractures. J Spinal Disord 1995; 8:233–236.
24. Kurz LT. Fractures of the first cervical vertebra. In: Clark CC, ed. The Cervical Spine: The Cervical Spine Research Society Editorial Committee. Philadelphia: Lippincott-Raven, 1998:409–413.

12

Odontoid Fractures

DAVID ANDREYCHIK

Geisinger Medical Center, Danville, Pennsylvania, U.S.A.

I INTRODUCTION

Fractures of the odontoid process of the axis comprise 10 to 15% (1) of cervical spine fractures in adults and up to 75% (2) of cervical spine fractures in children. These injuries are common to all age groups. There is a predeliction for upper rather than lower cervical spine injuries in children. In the pediatric population, the atlas and odontoid are secured to the body of the axis and remainder of the lower cervical spine by a thin cartilaginous plate, the basilar sychondrosis. Forces applied to the head tend to disrupt this area more often than other areas (2). Odontoid fractures plague the elderly, often the result of a seemingly trivial fall. High-velocity trauma in the young and middle-aged adult account for upper cervical injuries in this group.

Despite the recent advances in spinal surgery, fractures through the waist of the odontoid remain an enigma. Reports (1–16) of nonoperative treatment have documented nonunion rates ranging from 4.8 (15) to 100% (10). To date, studies have been retrospective, encompassing a variety of treatment methods and patient characteristics. Recent studies (1,9,17–20) using halo–vest immobilization have reported more consistent results with unions ranging from 70 (19) to 90% (18). Certain factors, such as patient age, the degree and direction of fracture displacement, and the adequacy of reduction and immobilization, are known to influence prognosis. Additionally prognosis has often been gauged by union or nonunion. Information concerning the neurological or symptomatic fate of an odontoid nonunion is scant, further clouding the understanding of this fracture subtype.

The last two decades have brought an evolution in the surgical management of odontoid fractures. Direct anterior dens fixation and more reliable, rigid posterior techniques such as transarticular C1–C2 facet screws have greatly enhanced our ability to treat these injuries. With these new techniques, however, come new responsibilities. Identifying those particular fractures with a poor nonoperative prognosis becomes more critical.

II ANATOMY

This axis is unique in that it forms a link between the mobile upper and lower cervical spine. The inferior portion of the axis resembles a lower cervical vertebra having a large bifid spinous process and inferior articular process that slopes downward and backward. The superior facets are slightly convex and face slightly upward and laterally. This configuration is conducive for mobility between the C1 and C2 articulation while compromising stability (Fig. 1). Stability is dependent upon the configuration of the supporting ligaments. The odontoid itself projects upward from just below the C2–C1 facet joints and tends to be truncated at the region of the transverse ligament. The odontoid, transverse ligament, and anterior arch of C1 stabilize the C1–C2 articulation.

The bony architecture of the odontoid has important implications for the surgeon contemplating direct anterior screw fixation. Monu et al. (21), in a radiographic study, determined that 98% of persons have posterior slanting of the dens greater than 6°, with a range of up to 35°. The mean predens angle between the anterior arch of C1 and the odontoid was found to be 5.57° (range 0°–13°) in neutral and 9.27° (range 0°–18°) in flexion. A V-shape predens interval is seen in normal adults and does not necessarily imply Cl–C2 instability or an occult odontoid fracture. This also has important implications, as anatomical reduction is essential prior to direct anterior fixation. Schaffler et al. (22) and Heller et al. (23) described the internal and external morphology of the dens using anatomical specimens and CT measurements (Fig. 2). The dens height was 14.4 mm $\pm$ 1.6 mm with a range of almost 10 mm. Minimum external anteroposterior and transverse diameters were 11.6 (range 8.5–18.6) and 9.3 (range 7.4–12.2) mm, respectively. Using CT scans, Heller et al. (23) were able to quantify the internal, or medullary, diameter. The mean minimal anteroposterior diameter was 6.2 mm (range 2.8–8.7 mm). The mean minimal transverse

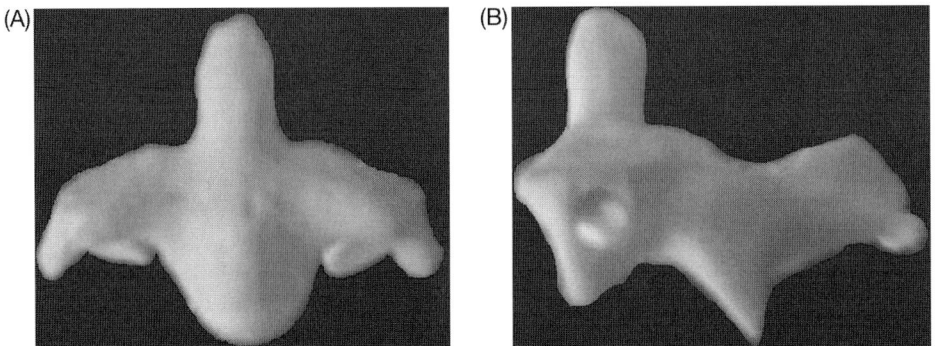

Figure 1 (A) Front and (B) side views of the axis. Note the large bifid spinous process, which serves as origin for the paraspinal muscles, the inferior articular process that project downward and backward, and the relatively flat superior articular processes. The odontoid projects from the body of C2 and is slightly truncated in the region of the transverse ligament.

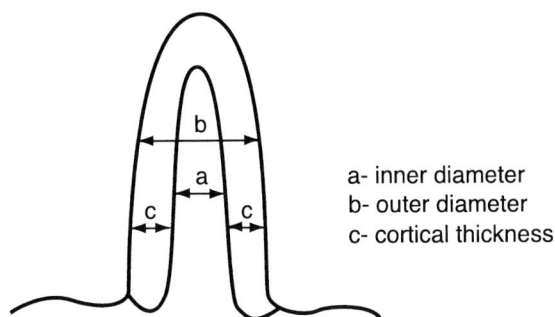

a- inner diameter
b- outer diameter
c- cortical thickness

Figure 2 Morphometric measurements of the dens. (From Refs. 22 and 23.)

diameter was 4.5 mm (range 1.3–8.7 mm) (Fig. 3). Their conclusion was that clearly there are patients whose anatomy will not accommodate two 3.5-mm screws and careful preoperative planning is necessary.

Steel (24) illustrated the transverse anatomy of the Cl–C2 area. He described the rule of thirds in which the odontoid process occupies one-third of the canal, the spinal cord one-third of the canal, with the last one-third being safety zone. This obviously explains the relative infrequency of spinal cord injury with odontoid fractures and provides an estimate of the degree of instability required to produce spinal cord dysfunction. It would also explain why a mild degree of instability (3–5 mm) associated with odontoid nonunions may be reasonably well tolerated.

III LIGAMENTS

The stability of the occipital C1–C2 complex is provided by the odontoid and its supporting ligaments (Fig. 3A and B). The odontoid is tethered to the occiput by the apical and paired alar ligaments. The alar ligaments attach the tip of the odontoid process to the occipital condyles. The transverse ligament is a strong connective tissue band encircling the dens arising from the medial tubercles of the C1 lateral masses. The ligament is separated from the odontoid by a synovial joint (5). Paired accessory ligaments arise with the transverse ligaments and attach to the lateral aspect of the dens at its base (5). The alar ligaments restrain rotation of the upper cervical spine while the transverse ligament resists flexion as well as anterior displacement of the atlas (25). Additional stability is provided by the tectorial membrane (the cranial termination of the posterior longitudinal ligament), the posterior atlanto-occipital membrane, the ligamentous nuchae, and the facet joint capsules.

With a fracture through the base of the dens, upper cervical stability is lost. The relatively flat Cl–C2 facet joints along with its inherent capsular laxity offer little resistance to anteroposterior translation. The skull, atlas, and dens are tethered together by the alar, apical, and accessory ligaments and move as a single unit. Displacement is only restricted by the lax atlantoaxial joint capsules and the cervical musculature (5).

IV VASCULAR ANATOMY

The blood supply to the odontoid was once thought to be scant. Work by Schiff and Parke (26), Althoff and Goldie (27), and Schatzker et al. (5) have elegantly outlined

(A)

apical ligament
alar ligament

transverse
ligament

accessory
ligament

(B)

anterior atlanto-occipital
membrane

transverse ligament

apical ligaments

alar ligaments

tectorial membrane

posterior atlanto-occipital
membrane

ligamentum nuchae

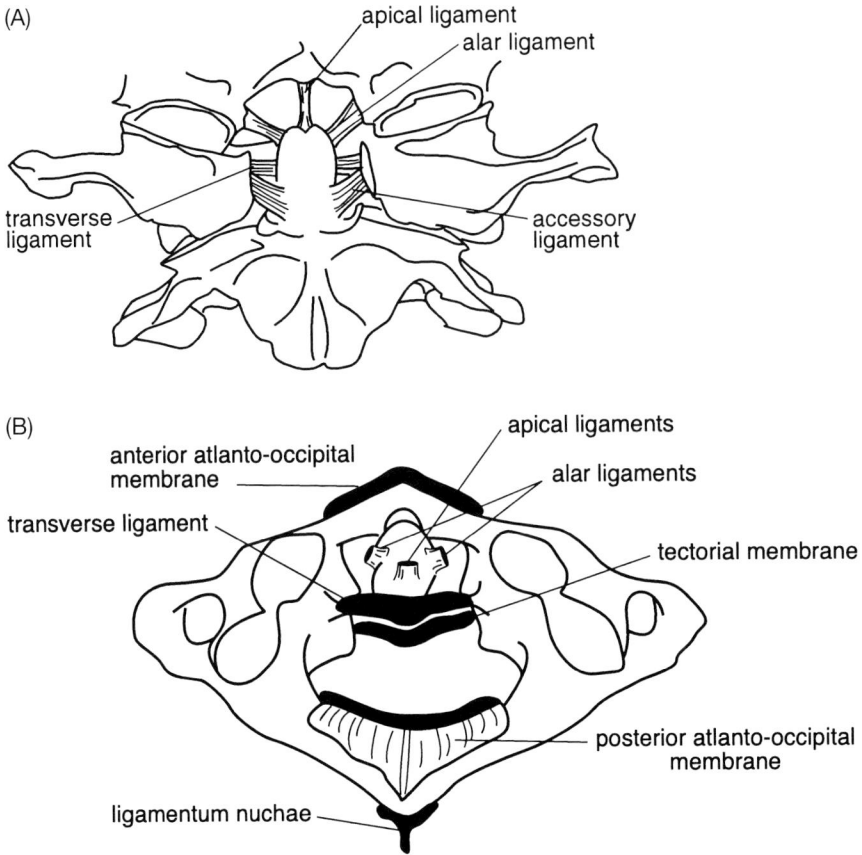

Figure 3 (A) Anterior view of the occiput–C1–C2 complex with a portion of the anterior arch of C1 removed. The apical and paired alar ligaments tether the odontoid to the occiput and lateral masses of the atlas. The transverse and accessory ligaments secure the base of the odontoid to the anterior C1 ring. (B) Transverse section of the odontoid and C1 ring demonstrate additional soft tissue support. The anterior atlanto-occipital membrane and the tectorial membrane represent the cranial termination of the anterior and posterior longitudinal ligaments, respectively. Some additional stability is provided posteriorly with the posterior atlanto-occipital membrane and the ligamentum nuchae.

the rich vascular supply to the dens. The dens receives its blood supply from above and below. Paired anterior and posterior ascending arteries arise from the vertebral artery between the C2 and C3 transverse foramen. They then course rostrally along the anterolateral and posterolateral aspects of the dens sending branches to the base. At the apex of the dens, an arcade is formed with contributions from all four branches. Additional vascularity is supplied by perforators from the internal carotid artery (Fig. 4). Schatzker et al. (5), using microangiography, demonstrated that the dens receives vessels from central and peripheral arteries. Central arteries enter the body anteriorly and course rostrally. Peripheral arteries enter the base through the accessory ligaments and the tip through the alar and apical ligaments.

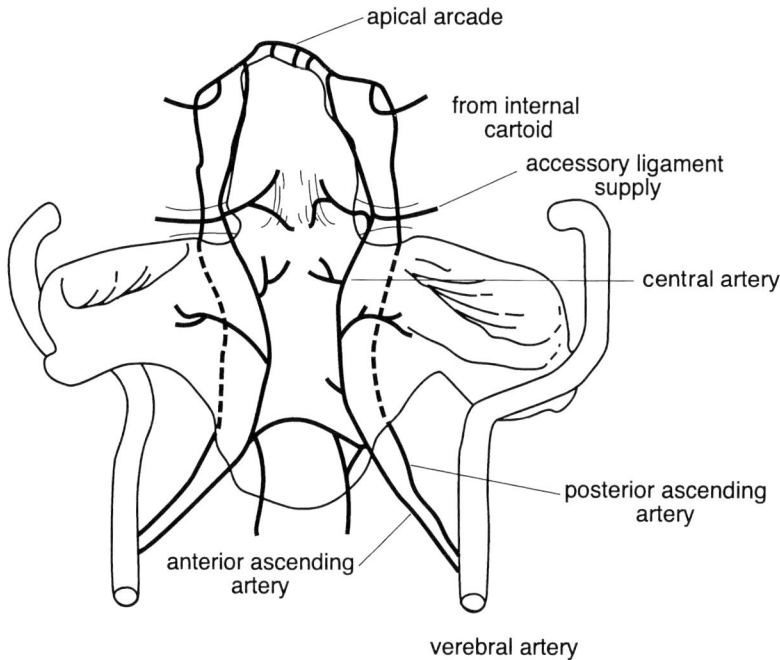

Figure 4 Vascular supply of the odontoid originates from the vertebral and internal carotid arteries. Anterior and posterior ascending arteries, originating from the verte-bral arteries, provide central and peripheral vascularity. Central arteries enter the dens anteriorly and course rostrally to the base of the odontoid. Peripheral vascularity is provided from an apical arcade, which is the termination of the ascending arteries, and from arteries entering the base via the accessory ligaments.

It appears that the odontoid has a rich vascular supply and this may not be the major factor in nonunions. Another plausible mechanism was provided by Bucholz and Burkhead (28). Based upon anatomical studies, they demonstrated that the dens is completely surrounded by synovial cavities—the facet joints laterally and the synovial membranes separating the dens from the anterior arch of C1 and the trans-verse ligament. An injury through the waist of the odontoid, above the accessory ligaments, would essentially leave the fracture surface floating in these synovial cavities (29).

V BIOMECHANICS

The occipito–atlanto–axial joints are the most complex of the various articulations of the spine. The superior facets of C1 are concave and allow 13° of flexion extension and 8° of lateral bending. No axial rotation is possible. Clinically this has signifi-cance. In children, it can be difficult to get a true lateral view of the upper cervical spine. A true lateral view of the skull would accomplish this, sparing pathology at the occipitoatlantal segment. The atlantoaxial joints allow approximately 10° of flex-ion extension and 47° of axial rotation. Obviously fusion of this joint has important kinematic implications as approximately 50% of cervical rotation will be lost. A Cl–

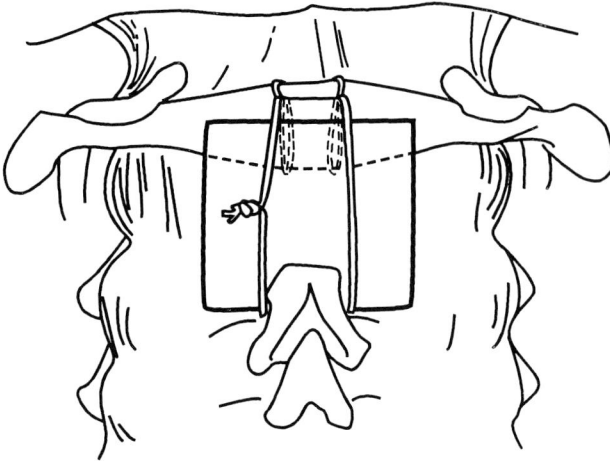

Figure 5   Gallie technique for posterior C1–C2 fusion. A single midline wire loop passed under the C1 arch and around the C2 spinous process secures a single bicortical midline graft.

C2 fusion is therefore less debilitating in an older, less active patient than in a young adult.

A variety of fusion techniques have been described for the C1–C2 complex (Fig. 5). The Gallie technique (single midline graft), Brooks technique (bilateral grafts) (Fig. 6), bilateral posterior clamps (Halifax), and transarticular facet screws (Fig. 7) have all been used successfully. Biomechanically the Gallic and clamp techniques may not be suitable (30,31). Both techniques create a posterior tension band and provide little resistance to extension and axial rotation. This would be particu-

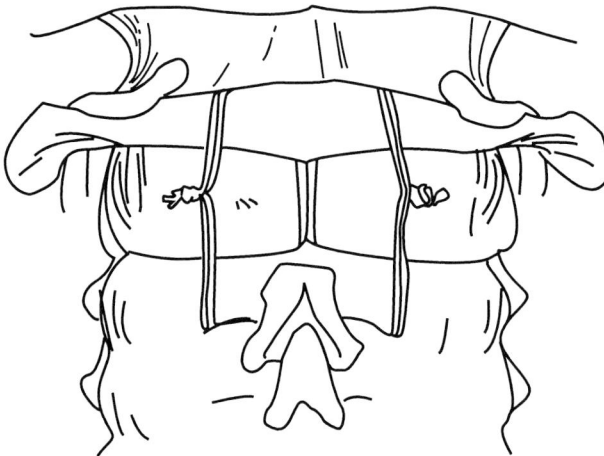

Figure 6   Brooks technique for posterior C1–C2 fusion. Double sublaminar wires secure bilateral, bicortical triangular grafts wedged between the posterior arch of C1 and the lamina of C2.

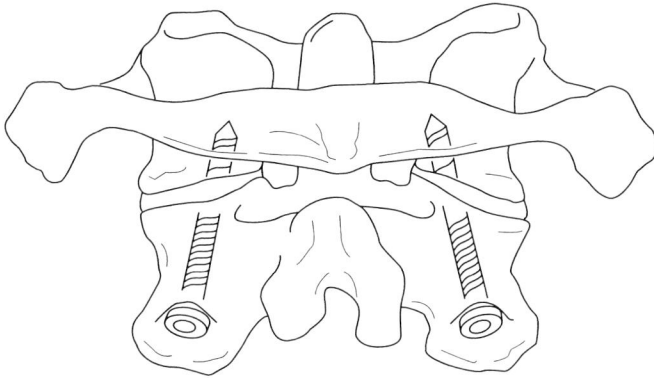

Figure 7 Transarticular facet fixation of the C1–C2 joints.

larly troublesome with posteriorly displaced fractures, as the fixation would tend to displace the dens further into the canal. The Brooks construct provides stability in both flexion and extension. The posterior wires restrict flexion while the bony blocks buttress extension. Some axial stability is thought to occur through friction (30). Transarticular facet screws directly block axial rotation providing the greatest stability.

VI EMBRYOLOGY

The axis, at birth, is composed of four ossification centers (i.e., two neural arches, one body, and the odontoid (32,33). In utero, the odontoid develops as the corpus of the atlas (34). It is initially composed of two lateral ossification centers that coalesce near the fifth month of intrauterine life, although the two centers may persist postnatally.

At birth, the odontoid is separated from the rest of C2 by three cartilaginous plates (Fig. 8). These plates represent synchondroses rather than epiphyses (33,35). The dentocentral synchondrosis, which separates the odontoid from the C2 body, lies well below the articular facets. This area is remote from the typical type II fracture location in adults, but is almost universally associated with dens fractures in children (36). The odontoid typically fuses with the body of the axis between the age of 4 and 7 years, although it may be delayed until young adulthood. As a rule, all synchondroses are fused by the age of 7 to 10 years. At approximately 2 years, an apical ossification appears at the tip of the odontoid. This generally fuses to the remainder of the odontoid by the age of 12. This may cause some diagnostic confusion.

VII CLASSIFICATION

Schatzker et al. (4), in 1971, were the first to classify odontoid fractures. They described fractures as "high" or "low," based upon whether the fracture line traversed above or below the accessory ligaments (5,37). They speculated that fractures above the ligament were inherently less stable as movement of the head would cause motion through the apical and alar ligaments. Additionally, high fractures may be dysvascular as the accessory ligament blood supply is disrupted. Their clinical study,

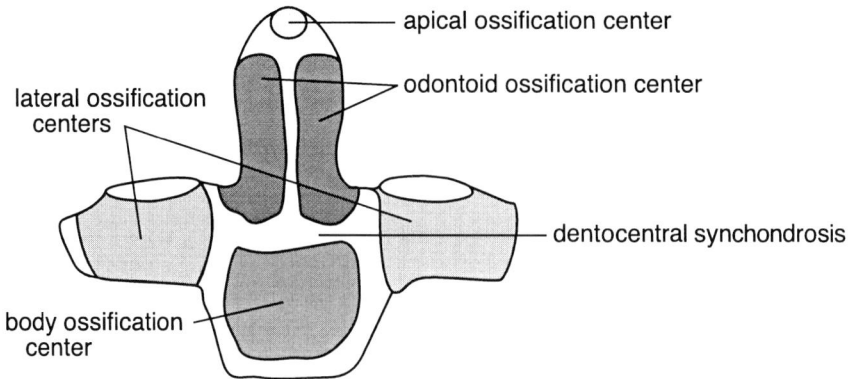

Figure 8   Ossification of C2 and the odontoid. In utero, the odontoid itself is composed of two lateral ossification centers, which generally coalesce prior to birth. At birth, four centers comprise C2—two lateral centers and one each for the body and the corpus. An apical center appears at approximately 2 years.

however, did not bear this out. Comparable union rates were found for high and low fractures.

In 1974, Anderson and D'Alonzo (3) presented a classification based upon an analysis of 60 cases. This classification system has become universally accepted and forms the basis for subsequent reports. The classification is simple, reproducible, and prognostic. Fractures are classified as type I, type II, or type III, based upon the level of the fracture line (Fig. 9).

A type I fracture is an oblique fracture through the upper part of the odontoid and probably represents an alar ligament avulsion. This fracture is rarely of any clinical significance.

A type II fracture occurs at the junction of the dens and the body of the axis. This particular fracture has a guarded prognosis for healing. This has led to current-day controversy in the optimal method of management.

A type III fracture has a fracture line that extends downward into the cancellous C2 body and involves a variable portion of the C2 lateral mass. Prognosis has generally been thought to be good with nonoperative treatment.

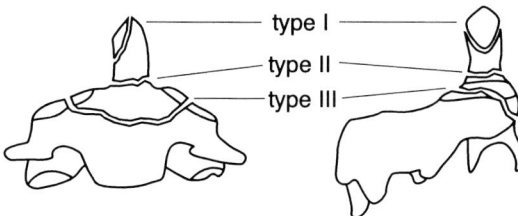

Figure 9   Anderson and D'Alonzo classification of odontoid fractures.

VIII   MECHANISM OF INJURY

Odontoid fractures generally result from blows to the occiput. Falls and motor vehicle accidents account for the majority, with their relative contribution being age-dependent. In young children and older adults, falls account for the majority of injuries. High-velocity trauma predominates in young and middle-aged adults.

Odontoid fractures have been very difficult to reproduce experimentally (5,38). Shear and avulsion vectors have been proposed as possible mechanisms. Fritzsche (39), in 1913, was able to reproduce odontoid fractures in a cadaver by simulating a judicial hanging. Other investigators (40), however, have been unable to reproduce this work. Wastoff felt that odontoid fractures were the result of a shearing force imparted by the transverse ligament. He based this upon the postmortem finding of an intact transverse ligament with fractures of the dens. Other work (41) has subsequently shown the transverse ligament to fail before the odontoid. Mouradian et al. (38) were able to reproduce type III fractures with a flexion force while type II fractures required lateral loading. They suggested that clinically the situation may occur with frontotemporal loading of a rotated upper cervical spine. The ipsilateral lateral mass of C1 would shear the dens from the body. This scenario has questionable clinical significance since laterally displaced fractures are rarely seen.

In reality, some combination of rotation, avulsion, flexion, extension, and shear contributed to these injuries Forces secondary to an occipital blow are transmitted to the odontoid by the surrounding bone and ligaments. Logically some elements of flexion and anterior shear would be necessary to create an anteriorly displaced fracture while extension and posterior shear would be responsible for those posteriorly displaced. Although this may be an oversimplification, this reasoning can be helpful in planning an appropriate reduction.

IX   CLINICAL PRESENTATION

The clinical presentation of odontoid fractures is dependent upon the age, mental status, and level of consciousness of the patient. Children may have minimal complaints but may hold the head fixed and resist any attempt at range of motion (42). The elderly patient with altered mental status may present similarly. An awake, oriented patient will complain of posterior cervical or occipital pain. Physical findings will include cervical tenderness, cervical spasm, and resistance to range of motion.

Neurological deficits are not common but may present as tetraplegia, extremity weakness, subtle myelopathy including exaggerated reflexes and bowel/bladder dysfunction, upper extremity paresthesias, and occipital neuralgia (34,43). The incidence has ranged from 2.5 to 30% (3,5–8,10–13,34,44). Posterior displaced fractures are more frequently associated with neurological impairment (7,13). Incomplete myelopathy and cord syndrome have a favorable prognosis for resolution with appropriate treatment of the fracture (10,13).

Odontoid fractures in the setting of high-velocity trauma and in patients with multisystem injuries present special problems. A severely injured patient may be unable to cooperate with an orthopedic or neurological evaluation. Other, more obvious injuries may divert attention from the upper cervical spine. A high index of suspicion is necessary. Any patient with a closed head injury [40–45% of odontoid fractures may be associated with a closed head injury (8,11)], scalp contusion or laceration, or clinical evidence of facial trauma should be highly suspect of having upper cervical trauma. Odontoid fractures are not uncommonly associated with other cervical spine fractures including C1 ring fractures (44,45).

X   RADIOGRAPHIC EVALUATION

The definitive diagnosis of an odontoid fracture is made with x-ray. Obviously any patient with posttraumatic neck pain, evidence of significant head, facial, or multiple organ system trauma requires a careful radiographic evaluation of the cervical spine. The standard trauma series consists of high-quality AP, lateral, and open-mouth images. Most fractures will be apparent. There will be occasions, however, where the diagnosis may not be readily apparent during the initial evaluation (Fig. 10). Several authors (5,6,8,10,20,46) have described missed diagnoses on initial radiographs. The rate may be as high as 10 to 15% (20). The fracture line may be obscured by overlying facial shadows. Occasionally it may not be possible to obtain an open-mouth view as a result of concomitant facial trauma.

If the diagnosis is in doubt, additional studies are necessary. Tomography can be very helpful especially in subtle, nondisplaced fractures. Anderson and Clark (32) were surprised at the number of fractures identified on tomograms that were not readily apparent on plain radiographs.

At our institution, CT is used to clear a questionable cervical spine. Theoretically the scanner obtains cuts parallel to the typical odontoid fracture line, but with thin slices (1–2 mm), the reconstructions have excellent resolution. CT is routinely used for preoperative planning. The bony dimensions of the dens are ascertained if anterior osteosynthesis is planned. The course of the vertebral arteries is determined if transarticular facet screws are planned. Clearly there is a group of patients, possibly as high as 10%, not suitable for facet screws based on an aberrant vertebral artery. Reconstructions are especially helpful in this regard.

More sophisticated imaging, such as the MRI, has limited use in odontoid evaluation. Any patient with spinal cord injury or neurological deficit, however,

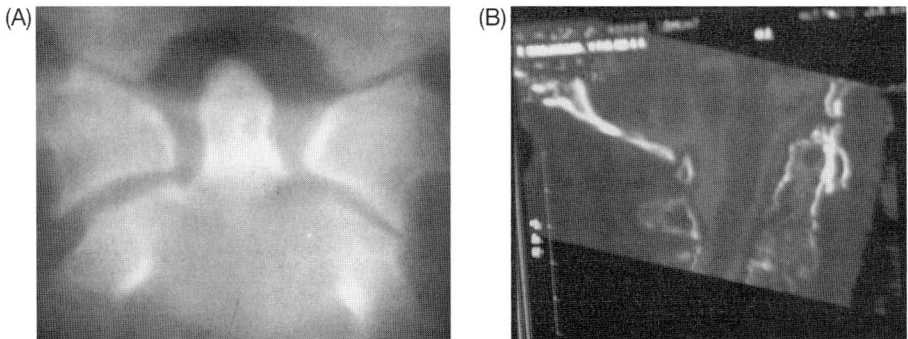

Figure 10   (A) Open-mouth and (B) lateral x-ray of a 55-year-old patient involved in a motor vehicle accident. The patient complained of neck pain but had no neurological dysfunction. Initial x-rays were interpreted as equivocal. Tomograms later demonstrated an obvious fracture through the base of the dens.

should have an MRI. The ability to detect concurrent disk pathology and intrinsic spinal cord abnormalities gives the physician the ability to precisely localize the level and identify additional lesions.

XI   TREATMENT

In general, treatment principles include protection of neurological elements and restoration of spinal stability. For odontoid fracture, the goal has been anatomical reduction and rigid immobilization to promote healing. In selecting an appropriate treatment for a particular patient, the surgeon must rely on personal experience and the literature. Unfortunately, the literature does not supply adequate information that makes it possible to prescribe a standard treatment program for a particular patient with a specific fracture. Treatment options include no treatment, traction, a soft or rigid collar, four-poster bracing, minerva casts, halo braces, anterior osteosynthesis, and posterior cervical fusion. There is no consensus. Staunch advocates of nonoperatives (1,9,13,17–19) and operative (6,10,47–56) treatment persist.

An additional problem in using the literature to guide treatment has to do with the method that outcome is measured. Success and failure of treatment have been classically defined by whether union or stability was obtained. Long-term functional, neurological, and symptomatic outcomes are rarely discussed. In outlining a treatment program, the benefits must outweigh the risks. Certain questions arise:

1.   Is anatomical reduction and solid union a prerequisite for a successful result?
2.   Is a stable nonunion, with minimal motion on flexion extension films, compatible with normal function and minimal neurological risk?
3.   What is the fate of an unstable nonunion and what degree of hypermobility is considered unstable?

Prior to discussing the specifics of fracture treatment, it is helpful to review the symptomatic and neurological outcome of odontoid nonunions. This assures that our treatments are positively altering the natural history of the disease.

XII   NONUNION/LATE MYELOPATHY

This risk of progressive myelopathy or sudden spinal cord injury provides impetus for obtaining a solid union in fractures of the dens. The exact incidence of myelopathy is not known (57). Osgood and Lund (58) reviewed the literature in 1928 and found 55 cases of odontoid fractures. Ten of these patients demonstrated appreciable myelopathy. Anderson and D'Alonzo (3), in their review of the literature, reported 50 cases of delayed myelopathy with variable involvement ranging from occipital neuralgia to quadriplegia. Some deficits were progressive, some were intermittent and static. A delay between the injury and the onset of symptoms was up to 48 years. In their own series, they reported 9 nonunions that were not fused. Five patients had late fusions, three had minor symptoms, and only one developed late myelopathy. Instability was mild, ranging from 2 to 5 mm. Seybold and Bayley (20) reported a patient with type II fracture treated in a collar who developed myelopathy. Pepin et al. (16), on the other hand, described two elderly patients with established nonunions who were alive without neurological complications.

Most information on nonunion outcome have been anecdotal reports as part of larger studies. A few studies (44,57,59,60) have specifically addressed this issue. Crockard et al. (44) presented 16 cases of delayed diagnoses of odontoid fractures with intervals ranging from 4 months to 45 years. Fifteen patients demonstrated second cervical root pain and ten were myelopathic. Ten patients had mobile nonunions, five patients had stable non- or malunions. Patients generally had transoral decompressions followed by posterior stabilizations. Although successful fusion was obtained in all patients, the neurological outcome was not discussed. They concluded that late myelopathy secondary to nonunion or malunion of the odontoid may be more common than previously thought and should be considered in the differential diagnosis of spondylitic myelopathy.

Paradis and Janes (59) presented 29 patients with odontoid nonunions, 22 of which had neurological abnormalities. Interestingly, these patients tended to be younger, with an average age of 29 years. The delay from injury to presentation averaged 13.5 years. These authors recommended stabilization of odontoid nonunions.

Hart et al. (57) identified five elderly patients 77 to 85 years old with established nonunions without myelopathy. Mean excursion on flexion extension was 4.5 mm (range 1–9 mm). No patient deteriorated neurologically nor had more than 1-mm increase in instability. Local symptoms tended to be mild and tolerable.

Information concerning local cervical symptoms in odontoid nonunions is even less available than information concerning neurological sequelae. Several series (3,6,12,16) have addressed nonunions in a cursory manner but did not present the long-term symptomatic and functional outcome. Nachemson (34), in 1960, reported eight pseudarthroses in 26 cases and stated that this group of patients actually had less symptoms than those with healed fractures. His conclusion was that fibrous union was acceptable. One would suspect that instability was minimal. Clark and White (6), on the other hand, found a high rate of symptomatic instability in their patients with odontoid nonunions. Although it is evident that odontoid nonunions can become symptomatic, either through progressive myelopathy or mechanical symptoms, clearly there is a group of patients with nonunions that do not develop symptoms. This is supported by reports (57,60) of nonunions, which were detected during evaluation of unrelated symptoms (Fig. 11).

With the data available it seems imperative to obtain stability, either through fracture union or late stabilization, for younger active patients. Any degree of instability is an absolute indication for surgical stabilization in this group. For elderly, sedentary patients, the risks of treatment need to be carefully assessed, as it appears that a dens nonunion, with mild instability, may be reasonably well tolerated.

XIII TYPE I

Type I fractures represent avulsions of the alar ligament, are rare, and generally can be managed with simple orthotic support. The incidence in selected series has ranged from 0 (9,10,18) to 3.3% (3). Wang et al. (1), Ryan and Taylor (4), and Pepin et al. (16) reported isolated cases that all healed uneventfully. Anderson and D'Alonzo (3) reported two type I of 60 total dens fractures. Both healed with orthotic support.

Although a type I fracture is generally considered benign, its presence should alert the physician to the possibility of more serious occipital–cervical injuries. Eis-

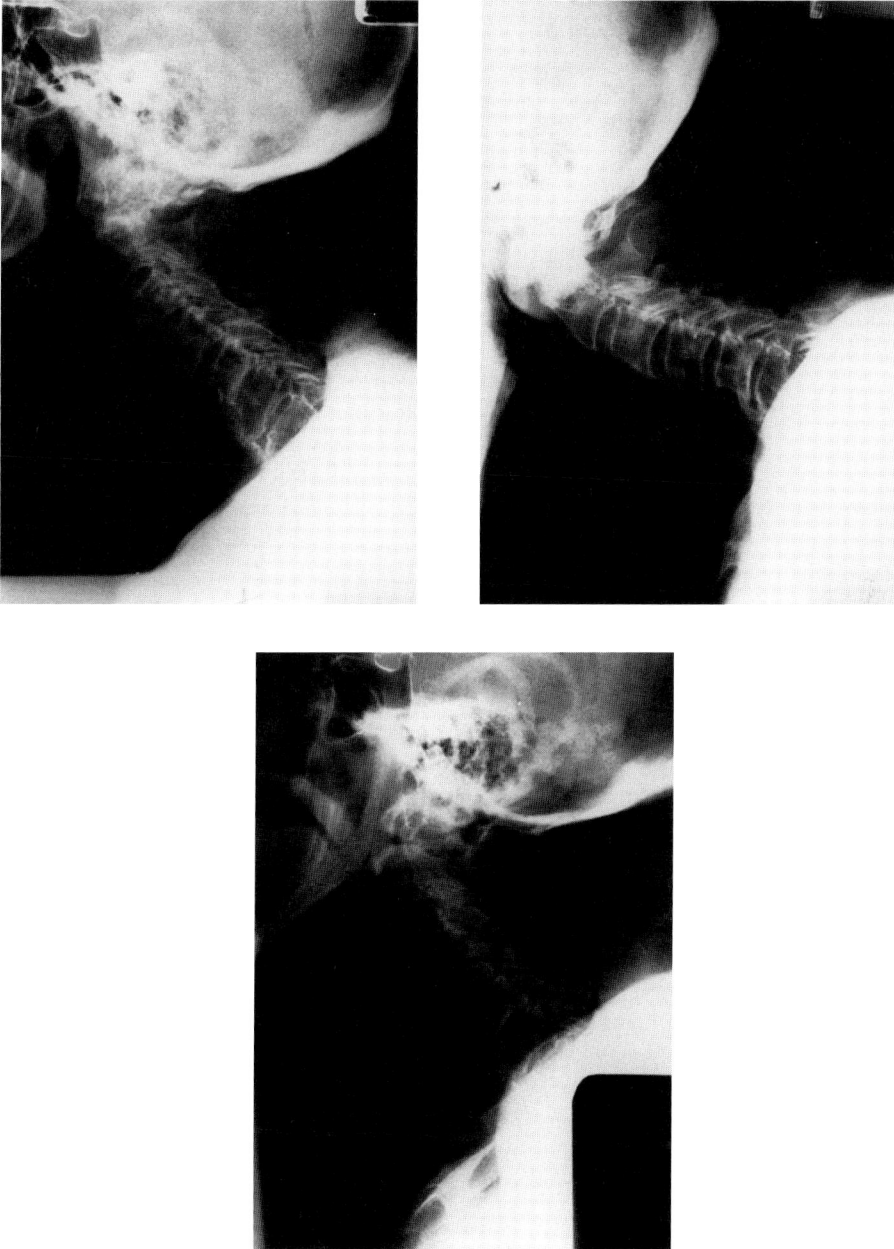

Figure 11 Neutral and lateral flexion extension radiographs of a 76-year-old gentleman seen for the evaluation of atraumatic neck pain. The pain had been present for several years and was nonprogressive. There was no subjective or objective neurological dysfunction. Radiographs demonstrated 7-mm translation. The patient was treated symptomatically.

mont and Bohlman (61) reported a case of a type I odontoid fracture associated with an atlanto-occipital dislocation. Careful attention must be paid to the adjacent cervical spine. Treatment of the concomitant injury takes precedence.

XIV TYPE II

Type II fractures occur at the junction of the dens and the body, or slightly higher, and have a notoriously guarded prognosis. Nonunion rates as high as 100% have been reported with nonoperative treatment (10). Best results appear to occur with anatomical reduction and rigid immobilization. Ryan and Taylor (4) demonstrated that fracture displacements as little as 30% in two planes reduced contact area to less than 50%. They stressed the importance of anatomical reduction. Eleven type II fractures were presented with two nonunions. Both nonunions occurred in unreduced fractures.

Schatzker et al. (37) illustrated the detrimental effect of fracture gap. In an experimental study in dogs, the presence of a gap at the fracture site adversely affected union. Even small amounts of traction may distract fracture fragments. Persistent x-ray evaluation is necessary if this method is to be employed. Prolonged traction may not be indicated.

In addition to the ability to obtain and maintain reduction, various parameters such as patient age, the direction and degree of fracture displacement, fracture comminution, delay in diagnosis, and type of immobilization are thought to influence union rates. Definitive conclusions regarding the importance of these parameters are difficult to glean from the literature. Much of the work has been retrospective, reporting a variety of treatment regimens. As a result, the data have been confusing and often conflicting.

Patient age has been thought to influence nonoperative prognosis. The exact age where prognosis declines in unclear. Apuzzo et al. (12) predicted that patients over the age of 40 with displaced fractures have a nonunion rate approaching 80%. Lennarson et al. (62) felt the patients over the age of 50 have a 21 times higher failure rate with halo immobilization. Elong et al. (13) reported 100% (8 of 8) nonunion in patients over the age of 55. Schatzker et al. (5) noted a trend for increasing nonunion in patients over the age of 60, while Hanssen and Cabanela (8) noted that all nonunions in their services were in patients more than 70 years of age. Several series (6,7,11,18) have not found age to be a significant prognostic indicator and, interestingly, Seybold and Bayley (20) noted higher fusion rates with halo immobilization in those patients over the age of 60 (72.7 vs. 58.3%). Thus, it would appear that age does exert some negative influence on fracture healing but to what degree is unclear. Selecting a surgical approach based upon age alone seems unreasonable.

Magnitude and direction of fracture displacement appear to influence union rates. Displacements ranging from 2 to 6 mm (11) have been found to negatively influence union. Wang et al. (1) noted nonunion rates to climb from 16.7 to 66% with displacements as little as 2 mm. Schatzker et al. (5) had a 100% nonunion rate in those fractures displaced more than 5 mm. Other series have noted displacements of 3 (7), 4 (13), 5 (6), and 6 mm (11) to be detrimental. There are reports (3,16,20), however, that could not correlate degree of displacement with fractures healing.

Most would agree that direction of displacement is related to nonunion. Fractures displaced posteriorly have been consistently shown to have a less favorable prognosis (5,7,8,13). It is difficult to determine, however, if this is more a function of the actual direction of displacement or of the difficulty in obtaining and maintaining reduction.

Other factors that may affect nonoperative outcomes include a delay in diagnosis, fracture comminution, and immobilization method. Ryan and Taylor (4), Seybold and Bayley (20), and Dunn and Seljeskog (7) demonstrated poor results with delays in diagnosis and treatment of as little as 1 week. Surgical stabilization appears warranted for fractures diagnosed late.

Fracture comminution may influence not only the ability to reduce a dens fracture but also its healing potential. Hadley et al. (63) introduced the term type IIA fracture to describe those odontoid fractures with comminution at the base. They spoke of difficulties in maintaining acceptable alignment. This group advocated immediate surgery for comminuted fractures (Fig. 12).

At present, it is not possible to advocate immediate surgery for patients based upon any one parameter. Of all the prognostic indices mentioned probably nothing is more important than the ability to obtain and maintain reduction during healing. The fracture should be aligned in near anatomical position. Choosing the method with the least morbidity is the goal. Treatment must be tailored to the individual patient. It does appear that the method of immobilization is important.

No treatment resulted in very high failure rates. Eighteen of 18 patients in the Clark and White (6) series who were not treated ended up with nonunions and symptomatic instability. Schwiegel (18) found 100% nonunion (6 of 6) in elderly patients not treated. The results of simple collar or brace support are variable, although they may be applicable in a nondisplaced fracture in an elderly, low-demand, patient.

Clearly the halo vest has been shown to provide the most consistent nonoperative results. Overall union rates for halo treatment have been approximately 70% (1,2,9,17–20). The halo vest has been shown to consistently restrict up to 75% of upper cervical motion, compared to 45% with collar orthoses (64). This provides the most rigid external support for this region.

Halo treatment is not benign. Complications, including pin site infections, decubiti, skull perforation, pneumonia, and pulmonary embolism have been reported (20). Several authors (4,16,20,57) have shown that the halo may be poorly tolerated by elderly patients. Seybold and Bayley (20), in comparing halo immobilization to other forms of treatment, noted increased pain scores, a higher complication rate, and less ultimate mobility with this form of treatment. Pepin et al. (16) noted that the halo was poorly tolerated by patients more than 75 years of age and recommended fusion for this group. Complications of the halo included pneumonia, decubiti, pin cellulites, and halo disassembly. Select elderly patients may not be candidates for halo treatment and an alternate treatment may be needed (Fig. 13).

Nonoperative treatment appears most indicated in nondisplaced or easily reducible fractures that demonstrate some intrinsic stability. Patients should be able to tolerate 3 to 4 months of halo immobilization. Fractures that remain reduced in the halo, regardless of patient age and initial displacement, have a union rate of 80 to 90%. Careful, regular, radiographic follow-up is mandatory. Loss of, or inability to maintain, reduction necessitates another option.

Surgical options include anterior osteosynthesis and primary posterior arthrodesis. Absolute indications for surgery include: (1) irreducible or grossly unstable

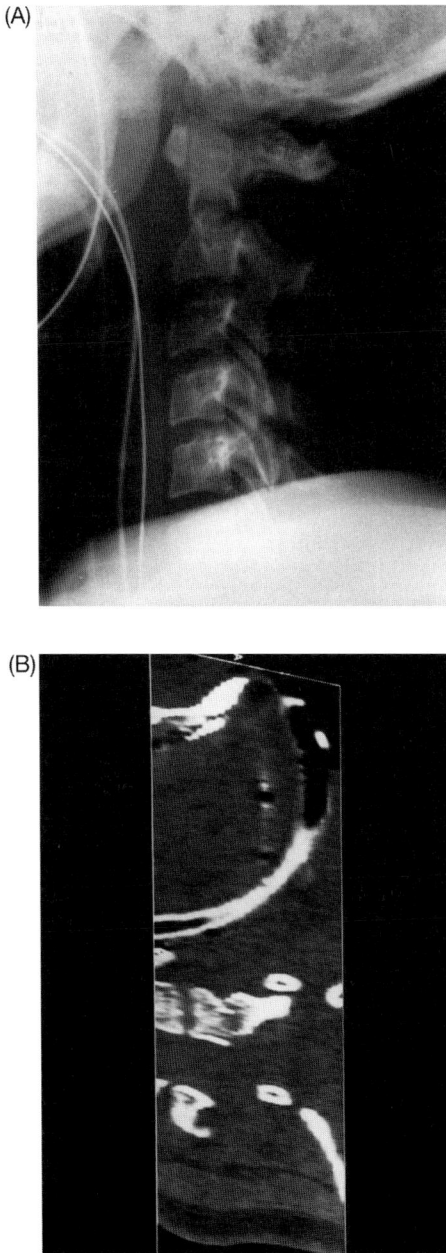

Figure 12 (A) Lateral radiographs and (B) sagittal CT reconstruction of a comminuted type III fracture in a 19-year-old female. (C,D) Reduction was difficult even intraoperatively, but anterior fixation was applied. Despite the slight malreduction, the fracture united uneventfully with simple postoperative collar support.

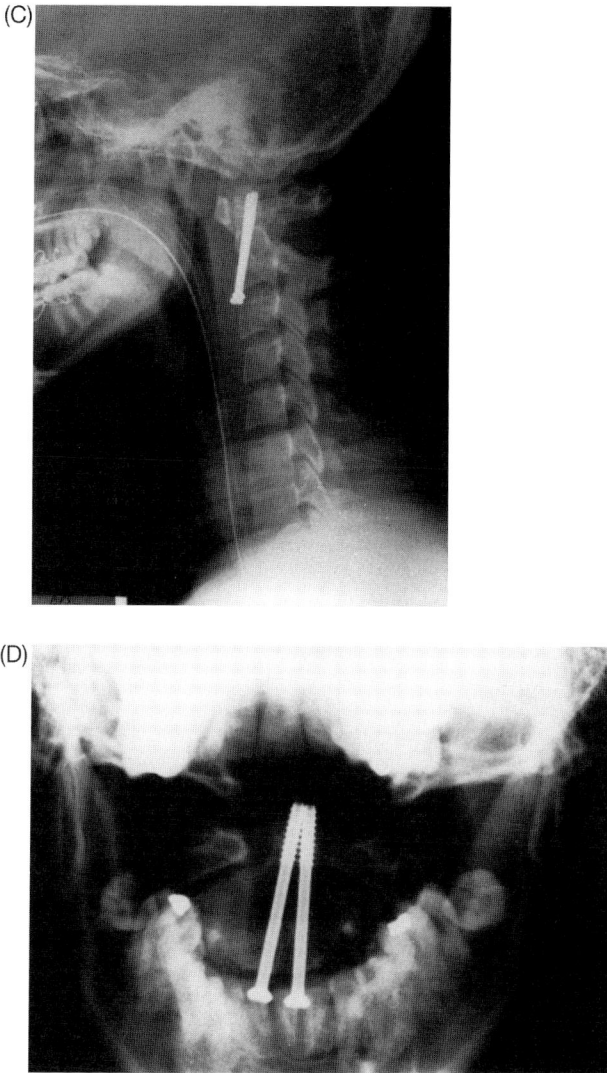

Figure 12 Continued

fractures where reduction is either unobtainable or unmaintainable; (2) associated injuries that preclude halo treatment—skull, facial fractures, chest injuries; and (3) pathological fractures. Relative surgical indications include: (1) significant neurological deficits; (2) comminuted fractures; (3) delay in treatment of more than 1 week; (4) multiple trauma; (5) poor halo candidates—i.e., elderly and debilitated; and (6) patient preference.

Direct anterior osteosynthesis (45,47–52,64,65) appears to be a very appealing method of internal fixation. The procedure uses a standard, generally low morbidity anterior cervical approach. Anterior screw fixation follows the basic principles (interfragmentary compression) of fracture treatment and obviates the need for cum-

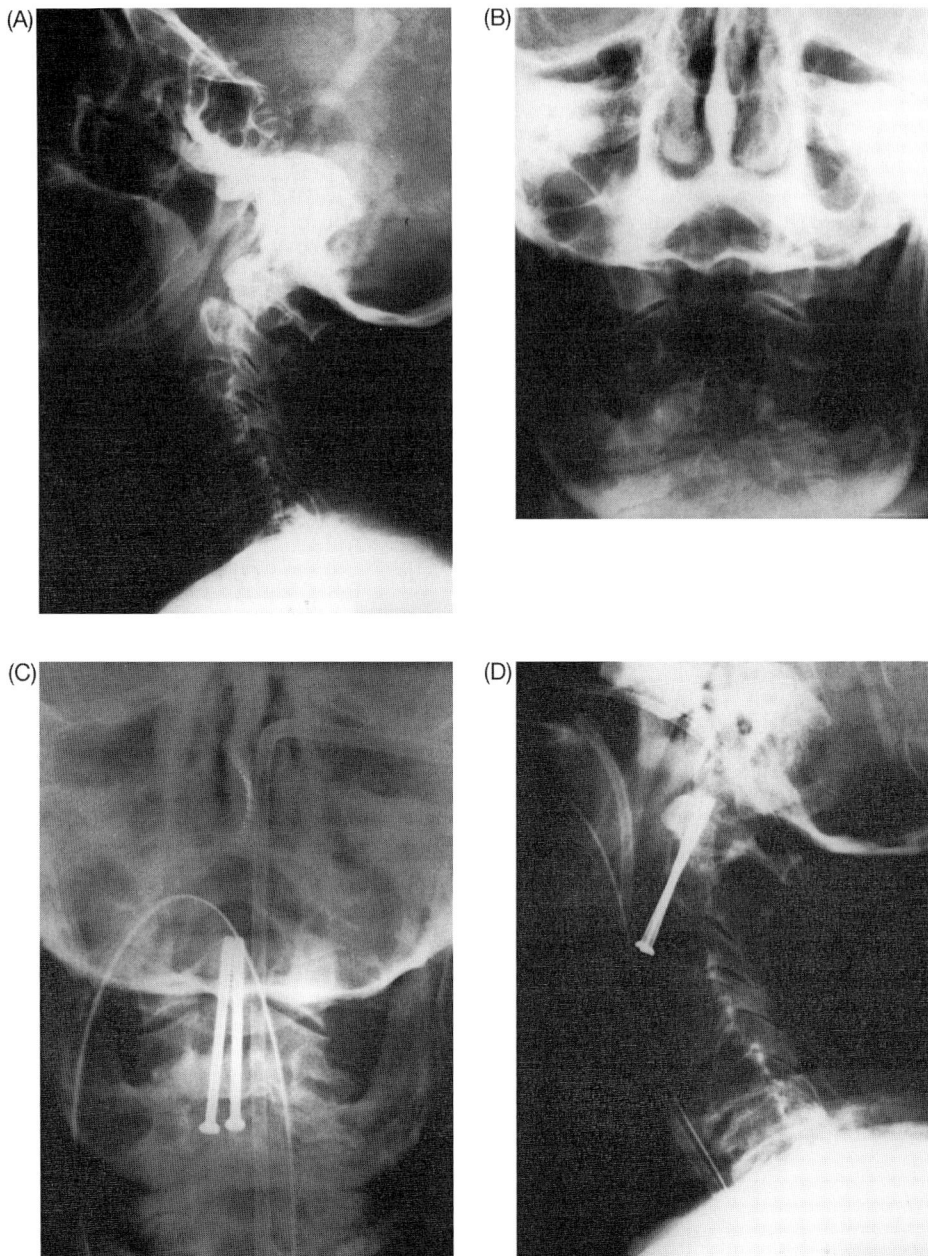

Figure 13 (A) Lateral and (B) open-mouth radiograph of an 80-year-old debilitated patient who sustained a posteriorly displaced type II fracture. The patient was not considered a halo candidate. Because of his age and the direction of displacement, it was assumed that more simple external support would be unsuccessful. (C,D) Anterior fixation was performed. Recovery was uneventful.

bersome postoperative immobilization, and theoretically maintains C1–C2 axial rotation. In actuality, return of C1–C2 mobility has been variable (49,64,65).

The ideal candidates are patients with reducible, transverse, or oblique anterior superior to posterior inferior type II, and shallow type III fractures (Fig. 14). Selected elderly and multitrauma patients who are poor halo candidates would also benefit. Contraindications to the procedure include irreducible fractures, oblique fractures with an anterior inferior to posterior superior configuration (67) (Fig. 15) (an anterior buttress plate is required), pathological bone (osteopenic, atrophic nonunions), and fractures associated with an unstable C1 ring fracture (>7 mm lateral mass offset which implies transverse ligament disruption).

Union rates are very high, ranging from 88 to 100% (45), but this is a technically demanding procedure with potentially catastrophic complications. Aebi et al. (47) in their series of 17 patients reported a major complication rate of 24%, including one early death, one fractured screw, one misplaced screw into the canal, and one fracture redisplacement. Three of these complications occurred late in patients not felt to be appropriate for the procedure—two osteopenic patients and one nonunion. Montesano et al. (51) reported on 14 patients of which three experienced screw cutout, one developed ARDS, and two experienced postoperative dysphagia, both of which resolved.

The procedure is performed with the patient in the supine position with the head supported in tongs or a Mayfield headrest. Patient positioning is critical (Fig. 16). The neck is extended as much as possible. It is helpful to anteriorly translate the lower and hyperextend the upper cervical spine. Simultaneous biplanar fluoroscopy is required for screw insertion (Fig. 17). Anatomical reduction is mandatory. Prior to surgery, the intended path of the screw must be checked with lateral image to verify adequate sternal clearance. A standard Smith Robinson approach is performed, using an incision at the C5–C6 level. The prevertebral fascia is incised and

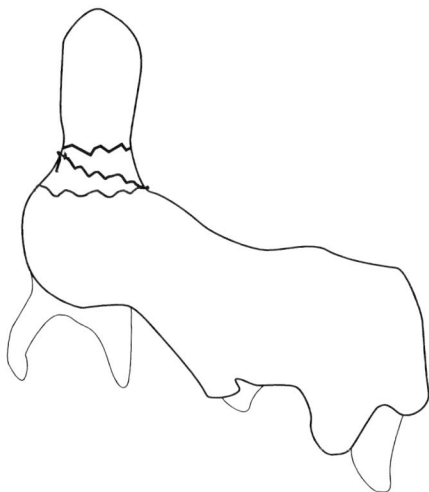

Figure 14 Fractures amenable to anterior osteosynthesis include transverse of oblique fractures that track anterosuperior to posteroinferior. With this configuration, interfragmentary compression is possible.

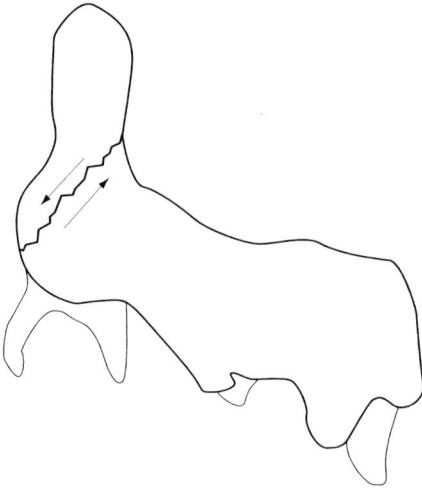

Figure 15 Oblique anteroinferior to posterosuperior fracture configuration not amenable to direct screw fixation. Compression will tend to displace the fracture. An anterior buttress place would be required.

the dissection is carried bluntly up to the C2–C3 disk. Hohman retractors are then inserted around the C2 lateral masses or, alternatively, a single-forked radioluscent retractor can be used (Fig. 18).

The entry point for the screws is actually within the anterior portion of the C2–C3 disk. Generally, the use of a cannulated system and long-threaded guide pins is helpful. Both wires are individually placed with frequent radiographic monitoring. The wires should converge slightly and be angled toward the posterior superior aspect of the dens (Fig. 19). The wires are measured and two self-tapping 3.5-mm screws are placed. The tips of the screws should just exit the posterosuperior portion of the dens. The guidewires are removed and the wound is irrigated and closed in

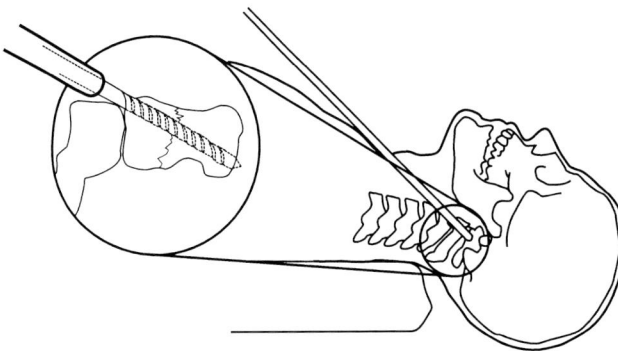

Figure 16 Patient positioning is critical to successful, accurate screw insertion. The neck is extended as much as possible while maintaining reduction. Screw insertion requires a very steep angle. Sternal clearance can sometimes be difficult and even prohibitive.

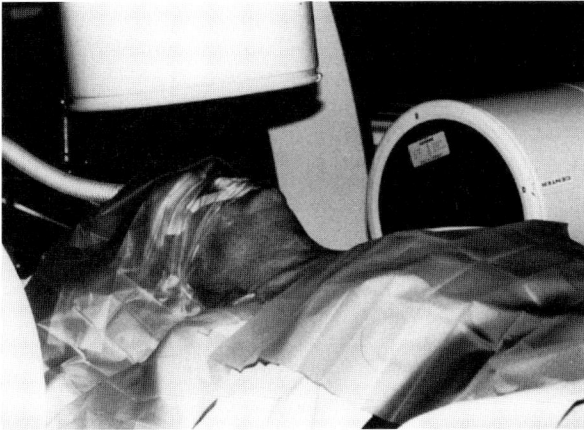

Figure 17 Setup for anterior osteosynthesis. Simultaneous biplanar fluoroscopy is required.

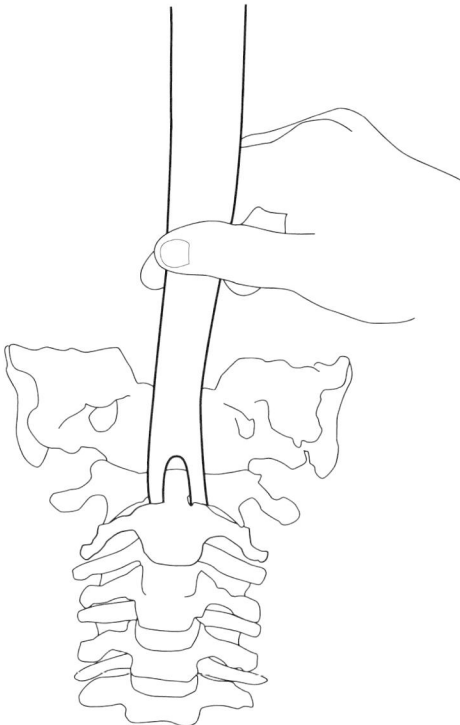

Figure 18 Spiked radioluscent retractor, which is inserted around the base of the odontoid, provides excellent exposure of the upper cervical spine and does not interfere with image acquisition.

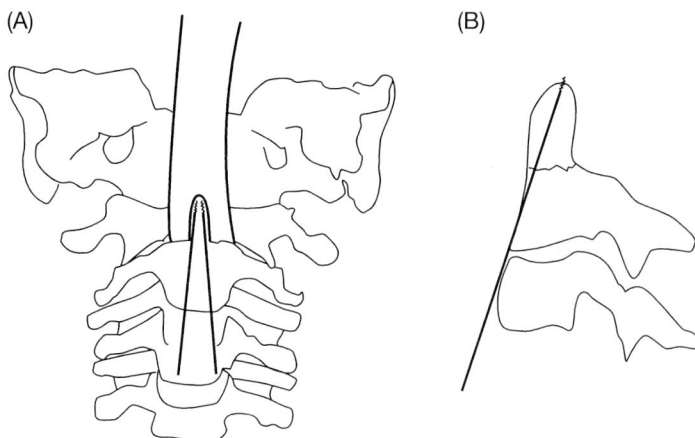

Figure 19 (A) Guidewire inserted prior to placement of cannulated screws. (B) The wires should angled slightly toward the midline (approximately 5–10°) in the coronal plane and be directed toward the posterosuperior portion of the dens in the sagittal plane.

routine fashion. Postoperative immobilization usually consists of a hard collar for 6 to 8 weeks. Theorectically, two screws should improve stability. Occasionally the patient's anatomy or technical problems dictate using only a single screw. This seems to be acceptable biomechanically (65) and clinically (49,51).

Although direct anterior fixation is the treatment of choice for most unstable odontoid fractures, there are situations in which this method may not be possible. Posterior cervical Cl–C2 fusion has proven to be a reliable, time-tested technique for restoring stability (3,6,10,20,53–56,68). Traditional fixation has been achieved using the Gallie (68) or Brooks (53) technique. More recently, transarticular facet screws have been introduced as a method for posterior C1–C2 fixation (31). This technique is not dependent upon an intact C1 arch, making it useful in odontoid fractures associated with Jefferson fractures.

Indications for posterior fusion include irreducible fractures, type II fractures associated with unstable Jefferson fractures, unstable low type III fractures, anterior inferior to posterior superior type II fractures, unstable type II fractures where it is technically impossible to get a working path for anterior instrumentation secondary to patient anatomy, pathological odontoid fractures including severe osteopenia, severely comminuted odontoid fractures, and odontoid nonunions (54) (Fig. 20).

To place transarticular facet screws, the patient is anesthetized and placed prone on the operating table. The Mayfield headrest allows precise positioning of the head, which should be placed in as much flexion as possible while maintaining reduction. Prior to the surgery, it is important to check the intended path of the screw with lateral fluoroscopy. Occasionally, in patients with large, fixed thoracic kyphoses, it will be impossible to get the appropriate trajectory. Intraoperatively pushing the spinous process of C2 superiorly may be helpful.

Exposure of the posterior elements is performed routinely. The upper cervical spine from the occiput to C3 is exposed, with care being taken not to damage the C2–C3 facet joint capsule. Using a small elevator, the superior lamina and isthmus

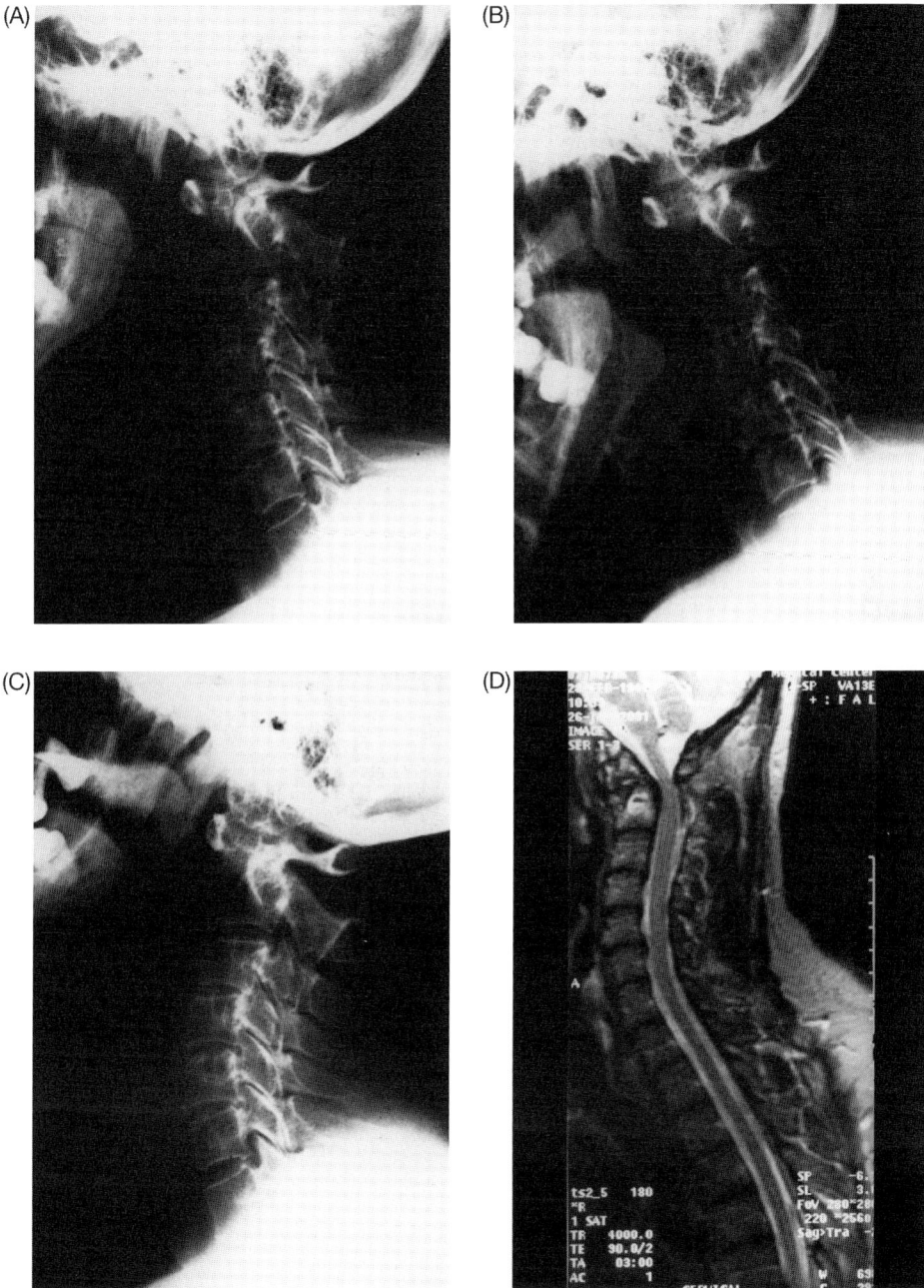

Figure 20 (A) 54-year-old male with odontoid nonunion presenting with neck pain, gait, and upper extremity dysfunction. Initial film demonstrating 100% displacement. (B,C) Flexion and extension films show minimal motion but (D) an MRI scan shows marked spinal canal stenosis. The patient was admitted and placed in Gardner-Wells tong traction. (E) Reasonable reduction was obtained with 10 lbs. (F) The patient subsequently underwent a posterior C1–C2 fusion with slight loss of reduction.

(E)

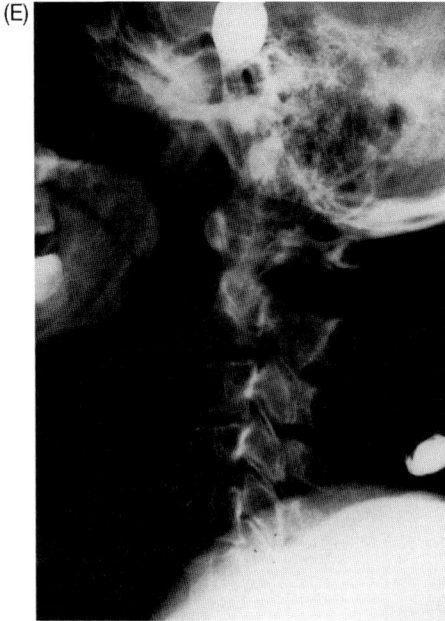

(F)

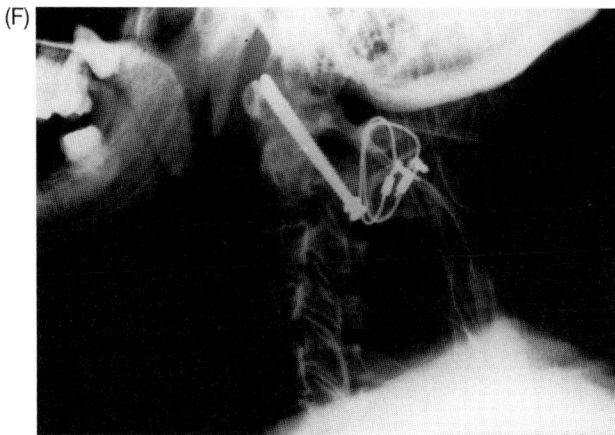

Figure 20   Continued

of C2 is dissected up to the C1–C2 facet joint. Often there is a large venous plexus along the C2 nerve root that can be controlled with bipolar cautery or gelfoam. The medial wall of the C2 pedicle and the posterior aspect of the C1–C2 joints are directly visualized. At this point, a small elevator or a K-wire can be inserted into the joint to retract the C2 root and surrounding venous plexus superiorly. If the Cl lamina is deficient, it is necessary to fuse the C1–C2 joints directly. The K-wire can be drilled into the posterior aspect of the C1 lateral mass and pulled upward. The facet joint capsule is removed and the posterior portion of the joint is decorticated with fine currents. The joints can be packed with bone after screw insertion. A wire loop is then passed around the Cl lamina and may be used to fine tune the reduction.

The screw entry hole is then created with high-speed burr at a point 2 to 3 mm superior and 2 to 3 mm lateral to the medial edge of the C2–C3 facet joint. A cannulated system using a percutaneous approach just distal to the cervicothoracic junction is used (Fig. 21). Two small stab incisions are used. This avoids exposing the entire cervical spine. A trochar and cannula are introduced at the appropriate angle. A 2.5-mm drill bit is used. Drilling is strictly sagittal. When using lateral image intensification, the drill should exit the posterior superior aspect of the C2 facet and be directed toward the anterior arch of C1. During drilling, it is very important to visualize the medial wall of the C2 pedicle to avoid medial or lateral trajectory. The hole is measured, tapped, and the appropriate length 3.5-mm cortical screw is placed. The procedure is repeated on the other side. If the C1–C2 joints are to be grafted, this can be done at this point. A Gallie-type fusion can then be performed to secure the bone graft across the C1–C2 articulation.

As with anterior dens fixation, placement of transarticular facet screws is a technically demanding procedure. Meticulous attention to detail is required. The screw must pass between the vertebral artery laterally and the spinal cord medially. Theoretically, either can be injured with abhorrent screw placement. Direct visualization of the C2 pedicle, the C1–C2 facet joint, and frequent lateral fluoroscopy can minimize the risk. Several series (54–56) have documented that, with careful attention to detail, the screws can be placed with minimal morbidity and high fusion rates. Grob et al. (55) reported 166 cases of transarticular facet screws performed at four centers by 10 different surgeons with varying levels of experience. There were no cases of neurological or vertebral artery injuries and only 5.9% of the complications were screw-related. The pseudarthrosis rate was only 0.6%. Jeanneret and Magerl (54) reported 12 cases with two minor complications. A solid fusion was obtained in all patients. Marcotte et al. (56) similarly reported a 100% fusion rate in 17 patients. One patient developed a wound infection and one patient had malpositioned screws that required replacement. It appears that with careful attention to detail the screws can be safely placed. The procedure provides multidirectional stability to the C1–C2 complex, and is unrivaled by any other form of fixation.

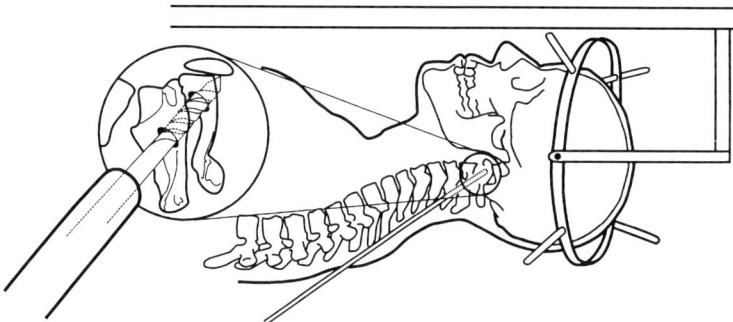

Figure 21 Setup and instrumentation path for posterior transarticular facet fixation. The patient is positioned with the cervical spine flexed as much as possible while maintaining reduction. A very steep angle is required. Exposure of the upper cervical spine and posterior C1–C2 facet joint drilling proceeds. Drilling is strictly sagittal. The trajectory is monitored with lateral fluoroscopy. The screw should cross the posterior portion of the C1–C2 joint and be directed toward the anterior arch of the atlas.

XV   TYPE III

Type III fractures that are technically C2 body fractures generally have a favorable prognosis. Union can be expected in 96% of cases with nonoperative treatment (4,6–8,10,11,13,16,20). Several studies (4,7,8,10,11) have reported 100% union rates with orthotic support, mostly halo vest treatment. Clark and White (6), on the other hand, in a multicenter study conducted by the CSRS, presented a less favorable prognosis. Of 50 type III fractures, they reported a 13% nonunion and a 15% malunion rate with various treatments. Of 10 patients in that series treated with orthosis alone, 50% had a non- or malunion. They recommended the halo vest as the treatment of choice.

Surgical indications of type III fractures would include patients with irreducible fractures, unstable fractures in patients not appropriate for halo application (debilitated, elderly, polytrauma), fractures associated with neurological deficits, pathological fractures, and fractures associated with severe C1–C2 intra-articular comminution. Most type III fractures, because of the location of the fracture line, require C1–C2 posterior fusion. There are, however, certain "shallow" type III fractures that can be stabilized anteriorly.

XVI   PEDIATRICS

Cervical trauma in children predominantly involves the upper cervical spine. Odontoid fractures comprise up to 75% of these injuries (52). From a therapeutic and prognostic perspective, odontoid fractures in children are distinctly different from their adult counterparts. In children, virtually all fractures involve the cartilaginous plate, are displaced or angulated anteriorly, and have a favorable prognosis with nonoperative treatment (25,36,42,69,70). The usual mechanism of injury is a fall or motor vehicle accident. Neurological injury is rare.

In children less then 7 years old, the basilar synchondrosis is generally open and represents a weak area through which the fracture invariably occurs. Sherk et al. (36), in 1978, presented 11 cases of odontoid fractures in children and discussed an additional 24 cases from the literature. In their own series, patients were treated with closed reduction and immobilization with minerva casts or halos. Union occurred in all cases, two of which had residual angulation. In the literature review, treatment methods varied but almost all patients did well. One nonunion was reported in a patient who was not treated.

The diagnosis of odontoid fracture in children requires a high index of suspicion and careful radiographic examination. Clinical examination and x-ray can be difficult. Standard, high-quality x-rays can be difficult to obtain and interpret. A large portion of the upper cervical spine is not yet ossified. Widening the paravertebral soft tissue strip is helpful, but present in less than one half of the cases (36). Seimon (42) reported two cases in which the diagnosis was not made on initial radiographs. Helpful physical findings included an inability to passively or actively extend the neck and a strong resistance to the erect or recumbent position without support of the head. Follow-up x-ray subsequently revealed the fracture.

Treatment involves closed reduction and rigid immobilization. Reduction can be accomplished with traction or with manipulation under anesthesia (Fig. 22). Immobilization is usually with a halo or minerva cast but at times a simple collar may be effective (32,42,69). Anatomical reduction is preferred but may not be necessary for healing. Immobilization is for 2 to 3 months. Subsequent growth disturbances are rare.

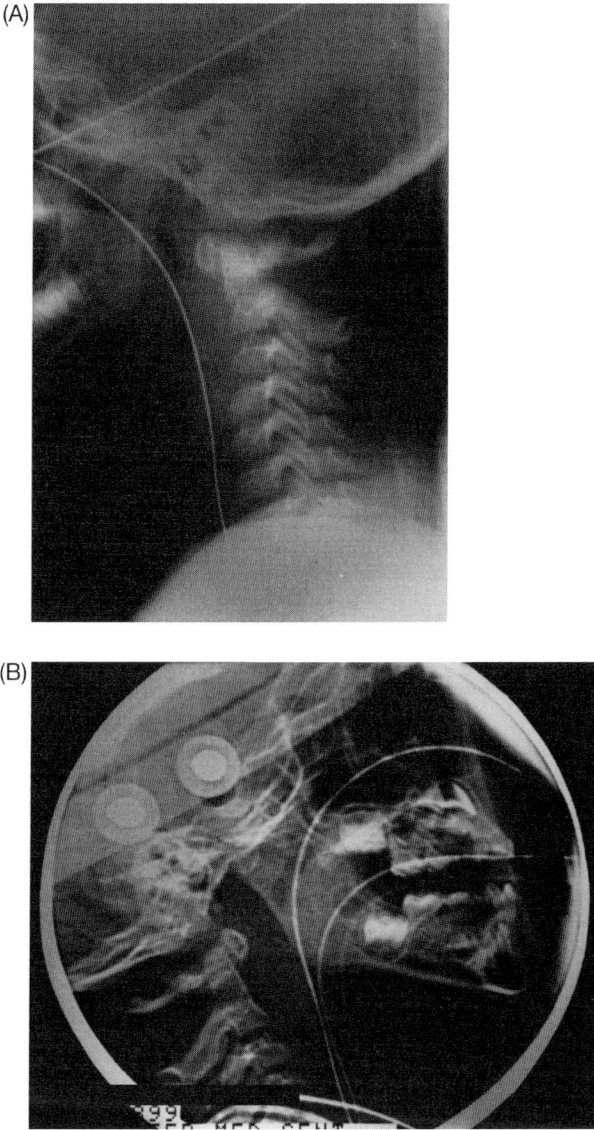

Figure 22 (A) Lateral radiograph of a 5-year-old female involved in a motor vehicle accident demonstrating a displaced odontoid fracture. (B) The patient was taken to the operating room where closed reduction and halo application were performed. (C,D) After 3 months, the halo was disconnected and lateral flexion-extension x-rays demonstrated stable healing. (E) At 6 months, fracture remains in good position. The patient was asymptomatic.

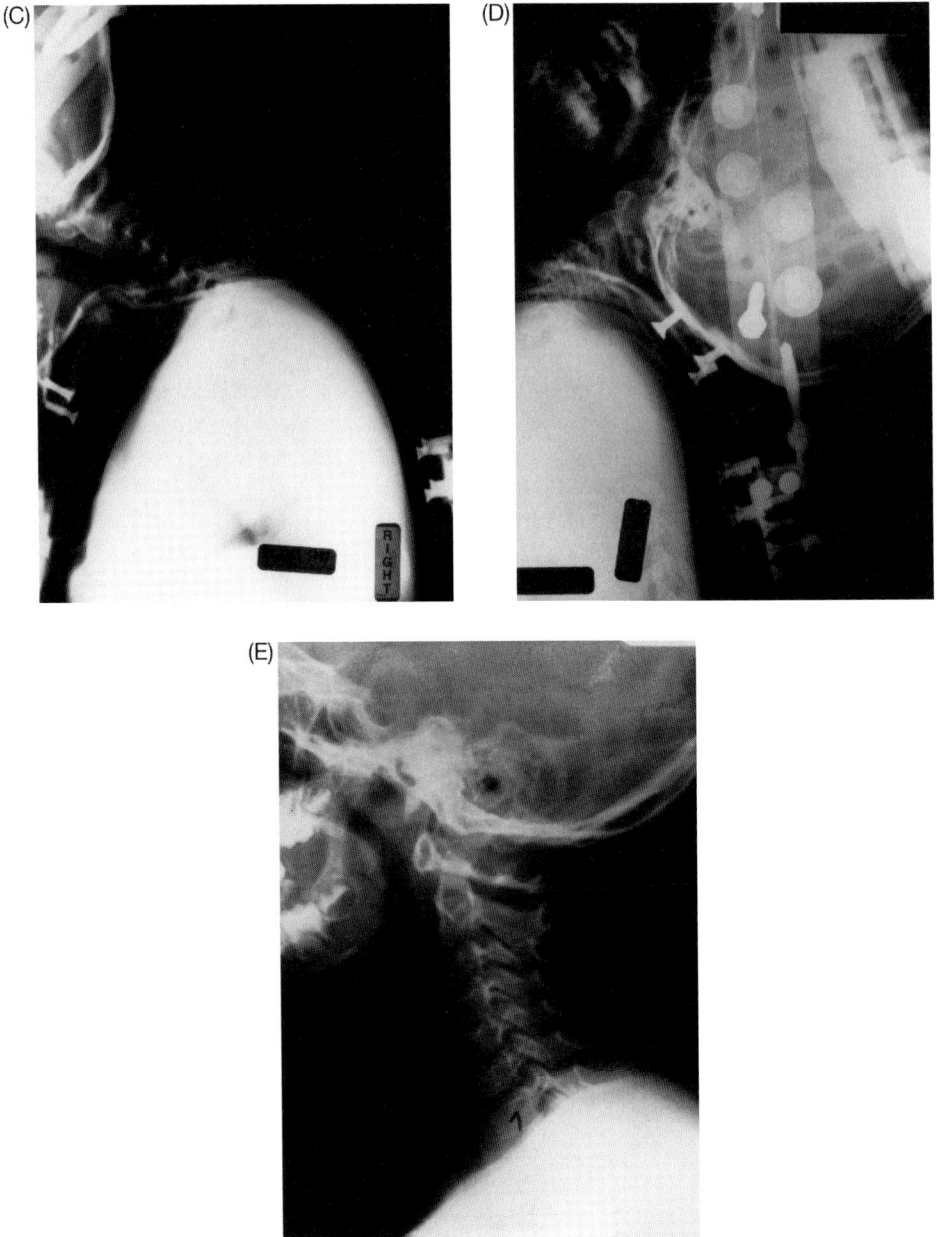

Figure 22 Continued

XVII CONCLUSION

The odontoid process stabilizes the C1–C2 articulation. The complex bone anatomy is designed for mobility. Stability is supplied by the supporting ligaments.

The Anderson and D'Alonzo classification is simple, reproducible, and prognostic. Type I fractures, in the absence of associated upper cervical pathology, can be treated conservatively with good results. Type III fractures have a favorable prognosis with nonoperative treatment. Best results are seen with halo vest immobilization.

There is still no consensus as to the optimal treatment of type II fractures. Treatment must be tailored to the individual patient. Reducible fractures in patients who are halo candidates have an expected union rate approaching 90%. Surgery is indicated for irreducible, or unstable, fractures and for patients who are poor halo candidates.

The choice of approach is dependent upon several factors including the surgeon's experience. Direct anterior osteosynthesis is very appealing but technically demanding. Posterior fusion techniques have stood the test of time. They appear to be most indicated in irreducible fractures. The Brooks or transarticular facet screw techniques are most suitable. Odontoid nonunions may be more prevalent than previously thought. Mild instability in elderly, low-demand patients can be treated with observation in the absence of intolerable symptoms of neurological impairment. Nonunion in the younger patient should be surgically stabilized. High-grade instability (>5–6 mm) should be stabilized regardless of age. Posterior surgery appears to be the procedure of choice, although selected, relatively recent, fractures may be amendable to anterior osteosynthesis.

Fractures in children less than 7 years old invariably occur through the dentocentral synchondrosis. Displacement is generally anterior. Management is with closed reduction and rigid immobilization. Prognosis is excellent.

REFERENCES

1. Wang GWO, Mabie KN, Whitehall R, Stamp WG. The nonsurgical management of odontoid fractures in adults. Spine 1984;9(3):230–231.
2. Sherk HH. Fractures of the atlas and odontoid process. Orthop Clin N Am 1978;9(4): 973–984.
3. Anderson LD, D'Alonzo RT. Fractures of the odontoid process of the atlas. J Bone Joint Surg 1974;56-A(8):1663–1674.
4. Ryan MD, Taylor TKF. Odontoid fractures, a rational approach to treatment. J Bone Joint Surg (Br) 1971;64-B(3):392–405.
5. Schatzker J, Rorabeck CH, Waddell JP. Fractures of the dens (odontoid process). J Bone Joint Surg (Br) 1971;53-B(3):392–405.
6. Clark CR, White AA. Fractures of the dens. J Bone Joint Surg 1985;67-A(9):1340–1348.
7. Dunn ME, Seljeskog EL. Experience in the management of odontoid process injuries: an analysis of 128 cases. Neurosurgery 1986;18(3):306–310.
8. Hanssen AD, Cabanela ME. Fractures of the dens in adult patients. J Trauma 1987; 27(8):928–934.
9. Lind B, Nordwall A, Shilbom H. Odontoid fractures treated with halo-vest. Spine 1987; 12(2):173–177.
10. Maiman DJ, Larson SJ. Management of odontoid fractures. Neurosurgery 1982;11(4): 471–476.
11. Hadley MN, Browner C, Sonntag VKH. Axis fractures: a comprehensive review on 107 cases. Neurosurgery 1985;17(2):281–290.
12. Apuzzo MLJ, Heiden JS, Weiss MH, Ackerson TT, Harvey JP, Kurze T. Acute fractures of the odontoid process: an analysis of 45 cases. J Neurosurgery 1978;48:85–91.

13. Ekong, CEU, Schwartz ML, Tator CH, Rowed DW, Edmonds VE. Odontoid fracture: management with early mobilization using the halo device. Neurosurgery 1981;9(6): 631–637.

14. Benzel EC, Hart BL, Ball PA, Baldwin NG, Orrison WW, Espinosa M. Fractures of the C2 vertebral body. J Neurosurgery 1994;81:206–212.

15. Aymes EW, Anderson FM. Fracture of the odontoid process. Arch Surg 1956;72:377–393.

16. Pepin JW, Bourne RB, Hawkins RJ. Odontoid fracture with special reference to the elderly patient. Clin Orthop Rel Res 1985;193:178–183.

17. Donovan MM. Efficacy of rigid fixation of fractures of the odontoid process—retrospective analysis of fifty-four cases. Orthop Trans 1980;4:46.

18. Schwiegel JF. Management of the fractured odontoid with halo-thoracic bracing. Spine 1987;12:838–839.

19. Traynelis VC. Evidence-based management of type II odontoid fractures. Clin Neurosurg 1997;44:41–49.

20. Seybold EA, Bayley JL. Functional outcome of surgically and conservatively managed dens fractures. Spine 1998;23:1837–1846.

21. Monu J, Bohrer SP, Howard G. Some upper cervical spine norms. Spine 1987;12(6): 515–519.

22. Schaffler MB, Alson MD, Heller JG, Garfin SR. Morphology of the dens: a quantitative study. Spine 1992;17(7):738–742.

23. Heller JG, Alson MD, Schaffer MD, Garfan SR. Quantitative internal dens morphology. Spine 1992;17(8):861–866.

24. Steel HH. Anatomic and mechanical considerations of the atlanto-axial articulations. J Bone Joint Surg 1968;50-A(7):1481.

25. Dvorak J, Schneider E, Saldinger P, Rahn B. Biomechanics of the craniocervical region: the alar and transverse ligaments. J Orthop Res 1988;6(3):452–461.

26. Schiff DCM, Parke WW. The arterial supply of the odontoid process. J Bone Joint Surg 1973;55-A(77):1450–1456.

27. Altloff B, Goldie IF. The arterial supply of the odontoid process of the axis. ACTA Orthop Scand 1977;48(6):622–629.

28. Bucholz RW, Burkhead WZ. The pathological anatomy of fatal atlanto-occipital dislocations. J Bone Joint Surg 1979;61-A:248–250.

29. Southwick WO. Management of fractures of the dens (odontoid process). J Bone Joint Surg 1980;62-A(3):482–486.

30. White AA, Panjabi MM. The clinical biomechanics of the occipitoatlantoaxial complex. Orthop Clin N Am 1978;9(4):867–878.

31. Grob D, Crisco JJ, Panjabi MM, Wang P, Dvorak J. Biomechanical evaluation of four different posterior atlantoaxial fixation techniques. Spine 1992;17(5):480–490.

32. Anderson LD, Clark CR. Fractures of the odontoid process of the axis. In: Sherk HH, et al., eds. The Cervical Spine. 2nd ed. Philadelphia: JB Lippincott, 1989:325–343.

33. Ogden JA. Radiology of postnatal skeletal development XII. The second cervical vertebra. Skeletal Radiol 1984;12:169–177.

34. Nachemson A. Fracture of the odontoid process of the axis. ACTA Orthop Scand 1960; 29(3):185–217.

35. Ewald FC. Fracture of the odontoid process in a seventeen-month old infant treated with a halo. J Bone Joint Surg 1971;53-A(8):1636–1640.

36. Sherk HH, Nicholson JT, Chung SMK. Fractures in young children. J Bone Joint Surg 1978;60-A(7):921–927.

37. Schatzker J, Rorabeck CH, Waddell JP. Non-union of the odontoid process: an experimental investigation. Clin Orthop Rel Res 1975;108:127–137.

38. Mouradian WH, Fiett VG, Cochran GVB, Fielding JW, Young J. Fractures of the odontoid: a laboratory and clinical study of mechanisms. Orthop Clin N Am 1978;9:985–1001.

39. Fritzsche E. Uber die Frakturen des Zahnfortsatzes des Epistropheus Neue Rontgenographische Darstellung des Processus Odontoideus. Deutsche Z Chirurgie 1973;120:7–34.

40. Blockey NJ, Purser DW. Fractures of the odontoid process of the axis. J Bone Joint Surg 1956;38-B:794–816.

41. Fielding JW, Cochran GVB, Lawsing JF III, Hohl M. Tears of the transverse ligament of the atlas. J Bone Joint Surg 1974;56-A:1683–1691.

42. Seimon LF. Fracture of the odontoid process in young children. J Bone Joint Surg 1977; 59-A(7):943–948.

43. Grogono BJS. Injuries of the atlas and axis. J Bone Joint Surg 1954;36-B:397–410.

44. Crockard HA, Heilman AE, Stevens JM. Progressive myelopathy secondary to odontoid fractures, clinical, radiological and surgical features. J Neurosurgery 1993;78:579–586.

45. Geisler FH, Cheng C, Pokra A, Brumback RJ. Anterior screw fixation of posteriorly displaced type II odontoid fractures. Neurosurgery 1989;25(1):30–37.

46. Husby J, Sorensen KH. Fracture of the odontoid process of the axis. Acta Orthop Scand 1974;45(2):182–192.

47. Aebi M, Etter C, Coscia M. Fractures of the odontoid process—treatment with anterior screw fixation. Spine 1989;14(10):1065–1070.

48. Etter C, Coscia M, Aebi M. Direct anterior fixation of dens fractures with a cannulated screw system. Spine 1991;16-(3)S:25–32.

49. Esses SI, Bednar DA. Screw fixation of odontoid fractures and nonunions. Spine 1991; 16-(10)S:483–485.

50. Borne GM, Bedou GL, Pinaudeau M, Cristino G, Hussein A. Odontoid process fracture osteosynthesis with a direct screw fixation technique in nine consecutive cases. J Neurosurg 1988;68:223–226.

51. Montesano PX, Anderson PA, Schlehr F, Thalgott JS, Lowrey G. Odontoid fractures treated by anterior odontoid screw fixation. Spine 1991;16-(3)S:33–37.

52. Bohler J. Anterior stabilization for acute fractures and nonunions of the dens. J Bone Joint Surg 1982;64-A(1):18–27.

53. Brooks AL, Jenkins EB. Atlanto-axial arthrodesis by the wedge compression method. J Bone Joint Surg 1978;60-A(3):279–284.

54. Jeanneret B, Magerl F. Primary posterior fusion of C1/2 in odontoid fractures: indications, techniques and results of transarticular facet screw fixation. J Spinal Disord 1992; 5:464–475.

55. Grob D, Jeanneret B, Markwalder TM. Atlanto-axial fusion with transarticular screw fixation. J Bone Joint Surg 1991;73-B(6):972–976.

56. Marcotte P, Dickman CA, Sonntag VKH, Karahalios DG, Drabier J. Posterior atlantoaxial facet screw fixation. J Neurosurgery 1993;79:234–237.

57. Hart R, Saterbak A, Rapp T, Clark C. Nonoperative management of dens fracture nonunion in elderly patients without myelopathy. Spine 2000;25(11):1339–1343.

58. Osgood RB, Lund CC. Fractures of the odontoid process. N Engl J Med 1928;198:61–72.

59. Paradis G, Janes J. Post-traumatic atlantoaxial instability: the fate of the odontoid process fracture in 46 cases. J Trauma 1973;13:359–366.

60. Blacksin M, Avagliano P. Computed tomography and magnetic resonance imaging of chronic odontoid fractures. Spine 1998;24:158–162.

61. Eismont FJ, Bohlman HH. Posterior atlanto-occipital dislocation with fractures of the atlas and odontoid process. J Bone Joint Surg 1978;60-A(3):397–399.

62. Lennarson PJ, Mostafavi H, Traynelis VC, Walters BC. Management of type II dens fractures: a case-control study. Spine 2000;25(10):1234–1237.

63. Hadley MN, Brown CM, Liu SS, Sonntag VKH. New subtype of acute odontoid fractures (type IIA). Neurosurgery 1988;22(1):67–71.

64. Johnson RM, Hart DL, Simmons EF, Ramsby GR, Southwick WO. Cervical orthoses: a study comparing their effectiveness in restricting cervical motion in normal subjects. J Bone Joint Surg 1977;59-A:332–339.

65. Jeanneret B, Vernet O, Frei S, Magerl F. Atlantoaxial mobility after screw fixation of the odontoid: a CT study. J Spinal Disord 1991;4:203–211.

66. Sasso R, Doherty BJ, Crawford MJ, Heggeness MH. Biomechanics of odontoid fracture fixation. Spine 1993;18(14):1950–1953.

67. Muller ME, Allgower M, Schneider R, Willenegger H, eds. AO Manual of Internal Fixation, 1991:637.

68. Gallie WE. Fractures and dislocations of the upper cervical spine. Am J Surg 1939;46: 495–499.

69. Savader SJ, Martinez C, Murtagh FR. Odontoid fracture in a nine-month-old infant. Surg Neurol 1985;24:529–532.

70. Reis MD, Ray S. Posterior displacement of an odontoid fracture in a child. Spine 1986; 11(10):1043–1044.

13

Axis Fractures

STEPHEN M. HANKINS

*Medical College of Pennsylvania, Hahnemann University Hospital,
Philadelphia, Pennsylvania, U.S.A.*

LOUIS G. QUARTARARO and ALEXANDER R. VACCARO

*Thomas Jefferson University Hospital and the Rothman Institute,
Philadelphia, Pennsylvania, U.S.A.*

Almost 20% of acute cervical spine fractures involve the C2 vertebra (1). Fractures of the axis include three types: odontoid fractures, traumatic spondylolisthesis of the pars interarticularis, or "hangman's fractures," and miscellaneous fractures (Fig. 1).

I ANATOMY

The occipitocervical junction is a complex array of bony and ligamentous structures, and therefore a C2 fracture should not be considered as an isolated bony injury. The body of C2 is the largest of the cervical vertebrae. Its superior articular processes are anterior in the sagittal plane to its inferior articular processes, and articulate with the inferior articular processes of C1. This joint complex provides for approximately 50% of the rotation of the entire cervical spine (2). The inferior articular processes have a similar sagittal orientation as the other subaxial cervical vertebrae and provide limited flexion, tilt, and rotation at its articulation with C3.

Anatomically, the dens or odontoid process has a slight narrowing at its base, where it joins the C2 body. Of clinical importance is the considerable variability in size of the dens. It has been shown that the C2 body size has a poor predictive value in estimating the size of the odontoid (3). This becomes relevant when planning anterior screw fixation of the dens. On the anterior surface of the dens is an oval or nearly circular facet that articulates with the anterior arch of the atlas. On the back of the neck of the dens, and frequently extending to its lateral surfaces, is a shallow

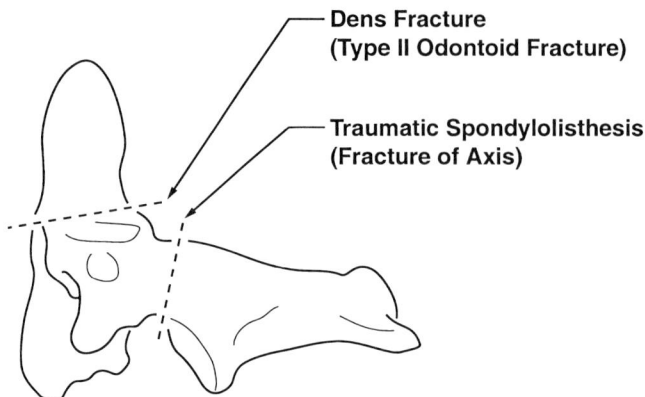

Dens Fracture
(Type II Odontoid Fracture)

Traumatic Spondylolisthesis
(Fracture of Axis)

Figure 1   An illustration of the C2 vertebral body demonstrating common areas of fracture.

groove for the transverse ligament that retains the process in position, preventing anterior displacement of the atlas on the axis. The odontoid tip is pointed and provides attachment to the apical odontoid ligament; below this apex, the odontoid somewhat widens, and, on either side a rough impression exists for the attachment of the paired alar ligaments. These ligaments connect the odontoid process to the occipital bone (Fig. 2). The internal structure of the odontoid process exhibits a bony trabecular density more compact than that of the C2 body. The base of the dens, however, has been shown to have a 55% reduction in the volume of trabecular bone with sparse trabecular interconnection as compared to the remaining odontoid process (4). This finding may account for the predilection for fracture in this region and the high rate of nonunion.

The C2 pedicles are broad and relatively strong compared to the rest of the C2 body, particularly where they join with the C2 body and the odontoid base. They are bordered above by the superior articular processes. The C2 laminae are thick and strong, and the vertebral foramen is large, but smaller than that of the atlas (5). The transverse processes are very small, and each ends in a single tubercle. The transverse processes are perforated by the foramen transversarium, which is directed obliquely lateral and upward. The axis has four ossification centers: the two posterior neural arches, the axis body, and the odontoid process. These centers are joined together by cartilaginous plates or synchondroses and are fused by age 7. The transverse synchondrosis that joins the odontoid to the C2 body lies inferior to the junction of the odontoid and the C2 body and may predispose to a type III fracture before its fusion (6). The anterior longitudinal ligament inserts on the anteroinferior portion of the C2 body. With significant hyperextension, the ligament may avulse a fragment of the anterior, inferior C2 vertebral body at its insertion.

II   TRAUMATIC SPONDYLOLISTHESIS OF THE AXIS

Traumatic spondylolisthesis is the second most common type of axis fracture, behind injuries to the odontoid, accounting for 22% of all C2 fractures (1). These injuries are commonly referred to as "hangman's fractures." This term was coined in 1965

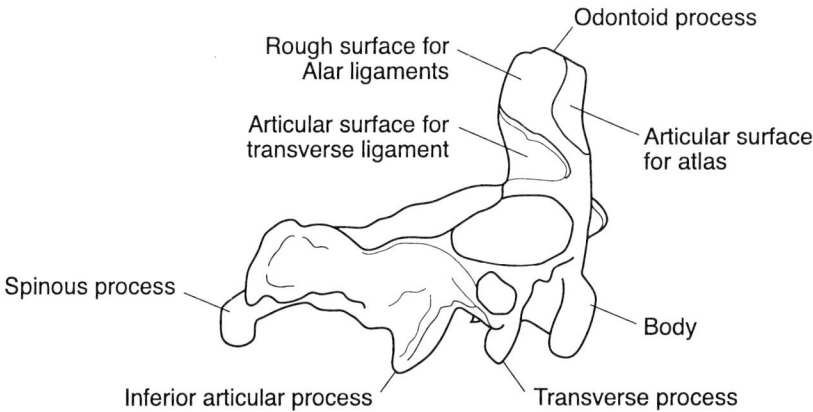

Figure 2   An anatomical illustration of the C2 vertebral body.

by Schneider and associates (7) to describe axis injuries that bear a radiographic resemblance to the injury sustained in a judicial hanging. Despite their radiographic similarity, their mechanism of injury is quite different. The mechanism responsible for traumatic spondylolisthesis is commonly cited as extension combined with axial loading (8,9). As well described by Coric et al. (10), the cervicocranium (base of skull, atlas, odontoid process, and body of the axis) moves in extension as a single unit. As the force magnitude of extension increases, increased stress to the posterior arch of the axis results. The weakest anatomical link (i.e., the pars interarticularis or isthmus of the axis) may eventually fatigue, resulting in displacement of the C2 posterior neural arch and inferior facets. Further loading and hyperextension may lead to rupture of the anterior and posterior longitudinal ligaments. Neurological injury is reported to be present in only 3 to 10% of surviving patients (10–12) due to the "decompressive" nature of these injuries. Associated spinal injuries occur in approximately 31% (1,10) of traumatic spondylolisthesis of the axis. A high incidence of chest, face, and head injuries may also be seen (10).

III   CLASSIFICATION

The most widely accepted system of classification of traumatic spondylolisthesis of the axis is that of Levine and Edwards (13) (Fig. 3), which is a modification of an earlier system by Effendi (11). This system consists of four fracture pattern types as visualized on lateral radiographs. Type I fractures have no fracture angulation and <3 mm of displacement. Type II fractures demonstrate C2–C3 translation >3 mm and fracture angulation. Type IIA fractures have slight or no translation, but severe fracture angulation. Type III fractures show severe fracture angulation and displacement and an associated unilateral or bilateral facet dislocation. Another classification system proposed by Francis (14) (Table 1) describes five fracture types based on the degree of fracture displacement and angulation. In a recent large series, a significant correlation between the Levine and Frances system was noted. The authors also found that both systems were reliable predictors of treatment type and outcome based on fracture classification (1). Types IIa and III are the most infrequent types encountered (1,13) and also the most likely to be unstable.

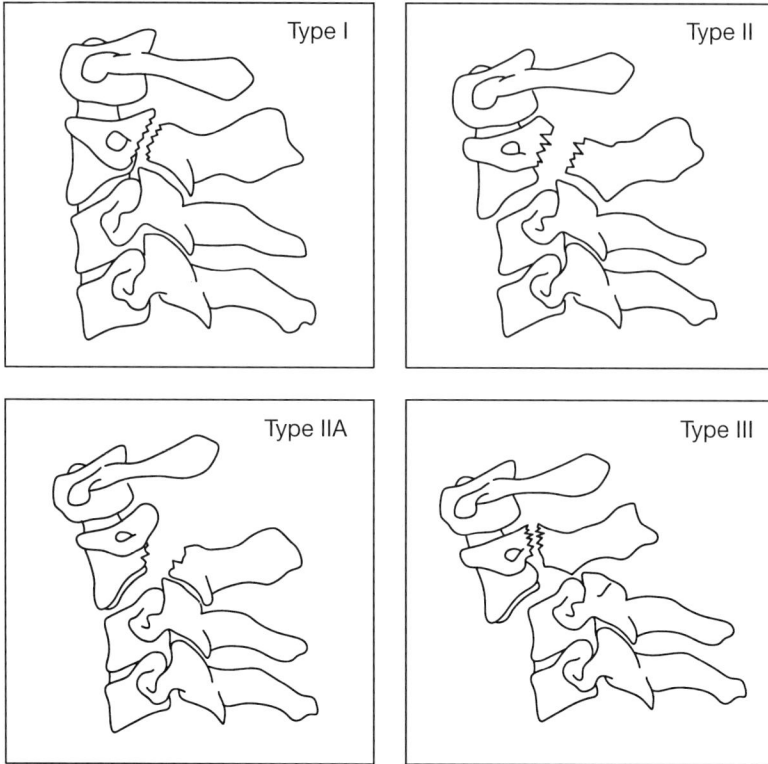

Figure 3 Classification of traumatic spondylolisthesis of the axis: types I, II, IIA, and III. (Reproduced with permission from Ref. 13.)

IV INITIAL MANAGEMENT

All patients with suspected cervical injuries are managed initially with collar immobilization. AP, lateral, and open-mouth radiographs are used to diagnose the presence of a traumatic spondylolisthesis. Careful evaluation of the entire cervical spine

Table 1 Criteria for Classification of Francis Grades

Francis grade	C2–C3 displacement	C2–C3 angulation (degrees)
I	<3.5	<11
II	<3.5	>11
III	>3.5	<11
	<0.5 (vertebral width)	
IV	>3.5	>11
	<0.5 (vertebral width)	
V	Disk disruption	

Source: Reproduced with permission from Ref. 14.

is warranted in light of the significant rate of associated cervical spine injuries with traumatic spondylolisthesis.

V TREATMENT

The authors of large series of patients with traumatic spondylolisthesis of the axis have concluded that conservative management should be the initial treatment approach for almost all of these injuries, except those with a dislocated facet joint (1,10,14,15). The majority of these injuries are stable, and only after disruption of the ligamentous supporting structures and disk space does the fracture become unstable (10). The number of patients undergoing acute surgical intervention in the largest series was 9% (1). Surgical management, excluding Levine and Edward's type III injuries, is reserved only for those patients exhibiting gross instability on dynamic lateral roentgenograms despite extended rigid external immobilization (1).

Type I fractures are stable with an intact C2–C3 disk. There are several commonly encountered subtypes, representing 28 to 72% of all traumatic spondylolisthesis of the axis (1,13). Treatment often involves cervical collar immobilization for 8 to 12 weeks (13,16,17). Some authors recommend flexion/extension radiographs prior to any external immobilization in this fracture subtype; if there is 2 mm or less of motion with flexion and extension and less than a total of 6 mm overall displacement, the patient is immobilized in a Philadelphia collar (10). Type I fractures rarely go on to spontaneous anterior C2–C3 fusion. Levine has shown in long-term follow-up that arthritis is seen in 30% of these patients (13). This may be due to the initial injury sustained at the C2–C3 facet joint, which is then allowed continued mobility and subsequent progressive degeneration. Painful facet arthropathy can be later treated with a C2–C3 fusion.

Type II injuries are treated initially with traction reduction, followed by rigid external immobilization for 8 to 12 weeks. Slight extension of the neck may facilitate reduction. Levine recommended a period of traction for several weeks for displacement >6 mm, followed by halo management for an additional 6 weeks (13,17). This type of treatment has been shown to be unnecessary in two large studies (1,10). It is believed that fractures that heal with some malalignment do not affect functional outcome.

Type IIA injuries, in contrast to type II, should not be reduced with traction. This injury is thought to occur as a result of a unique flexion distraction mechanism (13). Treatment should be with halo immobilization initially, after reduction with compression and extension to counteract the injury mechanism. Surgical management is often reserved for fracture nonunions (1,10).

Type III injuries are the most rarely encountered subtype, the most difficult to treat, and usually require operative intervention. As with type IIA fractures, this type of injury results from a flexion mechanism. A unilateral or bilateral facet dislocation is present along with bilateral posterior element fractures (13,17). This injury pattern is associated with a higher incidence of neurological deficits and a higher mortality rate than all other types of traumatic spondylolisthesis of the axis. Initial closed reduction of the locked facets should be attempted, but is often unsuccessful.

Operative intervention is indicated if closed reduction is unsuccessful, and following a successful closed reduction to stabilize the reduced facet joints (1,10,13). This consists of a posterior C2–C3 instrumented fusion. The hangman's fracture may then be allowed to heal with halo immobilization. A pedicle screw at C2 may be utilized to cross the fracture site in a compressive mode to provide additional fracture stability. Occasionally, C1 may be included in the fusion if the surgeon wishes also to cross the fracture site depending on the amount of comminution to the lateral mass of C2 making screw fixation technically difficult. Additional halo immobilization is recommended following surgical stabilization. An anterior C2–C3 arthrodesis is best suited for treatment of non-healed hangman injuries.

VI MISCELLANEOUS C2 FRACTURES

Other, less common axis fracture patterns exist in addition to odontoid fractures and traumatic spondylolisthesis. These miscellaneous fracture types occur infrequently and no universally accepted classification exists that adequately describes all these subtypes. The vast majority of these fractures are managed nonoperatively, unless associated with instability (1,18). These fractures occur in four basic types: spinous process fractures, lamina fractures, lateral mass fractures, and vertebral body fractures (1). Benzel et al. (16) has described two types of vertical C2 body fractures and a horizontal rostral C2 body fracture, but provides no management recommendations. Fujimura et al. has described four types of body fractures: avulsion, transverse, burst, and sagittal (18). In this series of 31 patients, the authors recommended nonoperative treatment for all patients except those with unstable burst or sagittal fractures. In the largest series of miscellaneous fractures (67 patients), Greene et al. (1) found that only one patient (1.6%) required surgical management for nonunion. All patients were initially managed with external immobilization.

REFERENCES

1. Greene KA, Dickman CA, Marciano FF, Drabier JB, Hadley MN, Sonntag VK. Acute axis fractures: analysis of management and outcomes. Spine 1997; 22:1843–1852.
2. Penning L. Normal movements of the cervical spine. Am J Roentgenol 1979; 130:317–326.
3. Schaffler MB, Alson MD, Heller JG, Garfin SR. Morphology of the dens. A quantitative study. Spine 1992; 17:738–743.
4. Amling M, Hahn M, et al. The microarchitecture of the axis as the predisposing factor for fracture of the base of the odontoid process. J Bone Joint Surg 1994; 76-A:1840–1846.
5. The Cervical Spine Research Society Editorial Committee. The Cervical Spine, 2nd ed. Philadelphia: JB Lippincott, 1989.
6. Anderson LD, D'Alonzo RT. Fractures of the odontoid process of the axis. J Bone Joint Surg 1974; 56A:1663–1674.
7. Schneider RC, Livingston KE, Cave AJ, et al. "Hangman's fracture" of the cervical spine. J Neurosurg 1965; 22:141–154.
8. Garfin SR, Rothman RH. Traumatic spondylolisthesis of the axis (hangman's fracture). In: The Cervical Spine Society Editorial Subcommittee, eds. The Cervical Spine. Philadelphia: JB Lippincott, 1983:223–232.
9. White AA III, Panjabi MM. The clinical biomechanics of the occipitoatlantoaxial complex. Orthop Clin North Am 1978; 9:867–878.
10. Coric D, Wilson JA, Kelly DL Jr. Treatment of traumatic spondylolisthesis of the axis with nonrigid immobilization: A review of 64 cases. J Neurosurg 1996; 85:550–554.

11. Effendi B, Roy D, Cornish B, Dussault RG, Laurin CA. Fractures of the ring of the axis: A classification based on the analysis of 131 cases. J Bone Joint Surg 1981; 63B: 319–327.
12. Francis WR, Fielding JW. Traumatic spondylolisthesis of the axis. Orthop Clin North Am 1978; 9:1011–1027.
13. Levine AM, Edwards CC. The management of traumatic spondylolisthesis of the axis. J Bone Joint Surg 1985; 67A:217–226.
14. Francis WR, Fielding JW, Hawkins RJ, et al. Traumatic spondylolisthesis of the axis. J Bone Joint Surg Br 1981; 63B:313–318.
15. Hadley MN, Dickman CA, Browner CM, Sonntag VK. Acute axis fractures: a review of 229 cases. J Neurosurg 1989; 71:642–647.
16. Benzel EC, Hart BL, Ball PA, Baldwin NG, Orrison WW, Espinosa M. Fractures of the C2 vertebral body. J Neurosurg 1994; 81:206–212.
17. Levine AM, Edwards CC. Treatment of injuries in the C1-C2 complex. Orthop Clin North Am 1986; 17:31–44.
18. Fujimura Y, Nishi Y, Kobayashi K. Classification and treatment of axis body fractures. Orthop Trauma 1996;10:536–540.

14

Distractive Flexion Cervical Spine Injuries: A Clinical Spectrum

MARK DEKUTOSKI and AARON A. COHEN-GADOL

Mayo Clinic and Mayo Foundation, Rochester, Minnesota, U.S.A.

I DEFINITION BY MECHANISM

Distractive flexion (DF) injuries of the cervical spine have long been referred to in the literature as perched, subluxed, or dislocated facet injuries. Formal recognition and distinction of distractive flexion and compression flexion injuries of the cervical spine originated from the mechanistic, clock-face classification first put forth by Drucker et al. in the late 1970s (1). This clock-face representation was further popularized with a subclassification by Allen and Ferguson (2). They describe a continuum of osseous and ligamentous injury that comprises the clinical spectrum of injuries illustrated in their paper as hyperflexion sprains, unilateral facet dislocations, bilateral facet dislocations, and complete-fracture dislocations. The classic article (2) described 165 cervical injuries, including 61 cases of distractive flexion injuries. On the clock-face diagram, these injuries occur with the force vector in the 9:00 to 11:30 direction (Fig. 1). Stages of injury or phylogenes are described. Understanding the pathoanatomical basis of each phylogeny is very helpful in defining the injury and deciding treatment options.

The distractive flexion phylogeny of injuries as described by Allen and Ferguson includes four stages of pathoanatomy. The distractive flexion stage I (DFS I) injury consists of failure of the posterior ligamentous complex as evident by facet subluxation and flexion with abnormally greater divergence of the spinous processes at the injured level. This has been termed a "flexion sprain" in the literature, and may be accompanied by blunting of the anterosuperior vertebral endplate of the caudally involved segment to a rounded contour. It can be confused with a compressive flexion stage I injury. The key difference between the compressive flexion

191

Medical Library Service
College of Physicians & Surgeons of B.C.
1383 W. 8th Ave.
Vancouver, B.C.
V6H 4C4

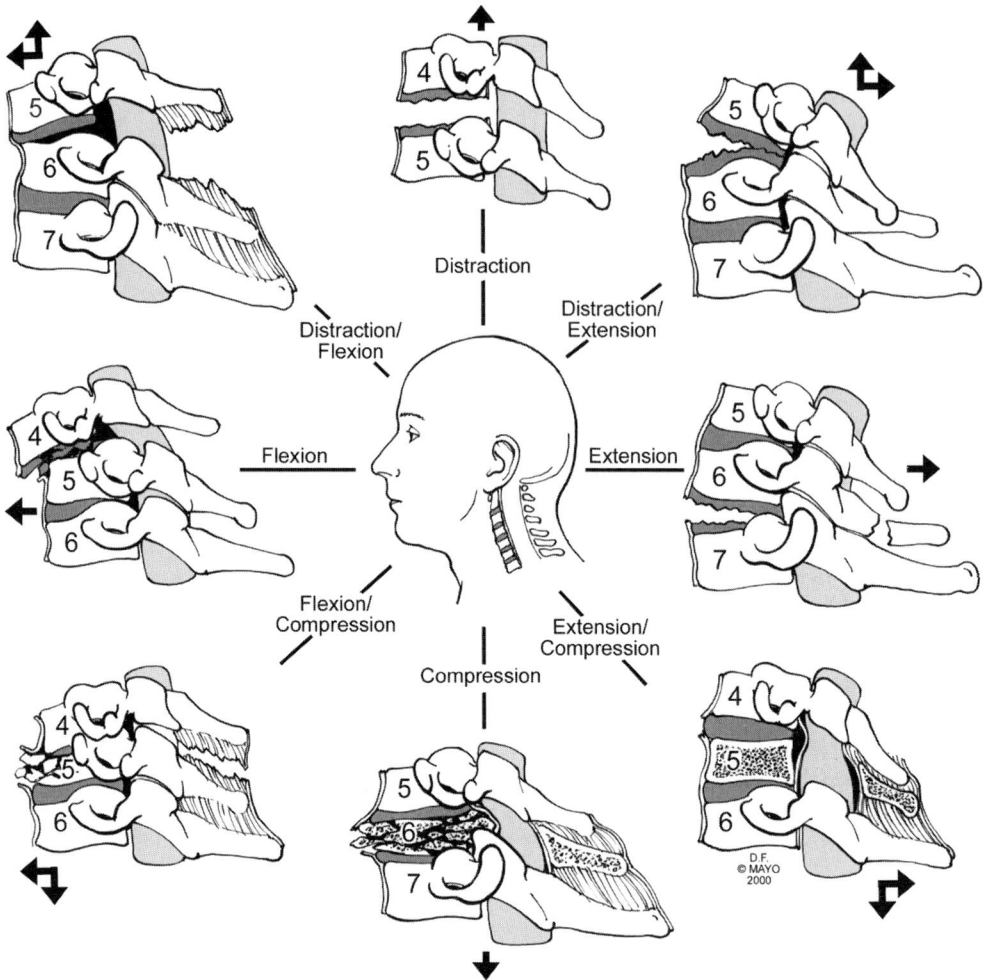

Figure 1 Thomas–Drucker adaptation of the Ferguson and Allen classification.

and the distractive flexion injuries is the widening of the spinous processes on lateral plain radiography (Fig. 2). The distraction injury has interspinous widening and, on clinical exam, posterior midline tenderness. The compressive flexion injury does not characteristically show these findings.

The distractive flexion stage II (DFS II) injury has been described in the literature as a unilateral facet dislocation, interlocked facet, or facet subluxation. The magnitude of the posterior ligamentous injury is greater than what is seen in the flexion sprain injury. In DFS II, the interspinous ligament, ligamentum flavum, and facet capsule disruptions allow for facet displacement. A rotational component has also been recognized in the unilateral distractive flexion injuries. The key element is neck rotation with the center of the moment of force ventral to the vertebral body. There may be bony avulsion of the uncovertebral joint accompanied by tension injuries to the facets. Spinous process distraction and rotation may be noted on the

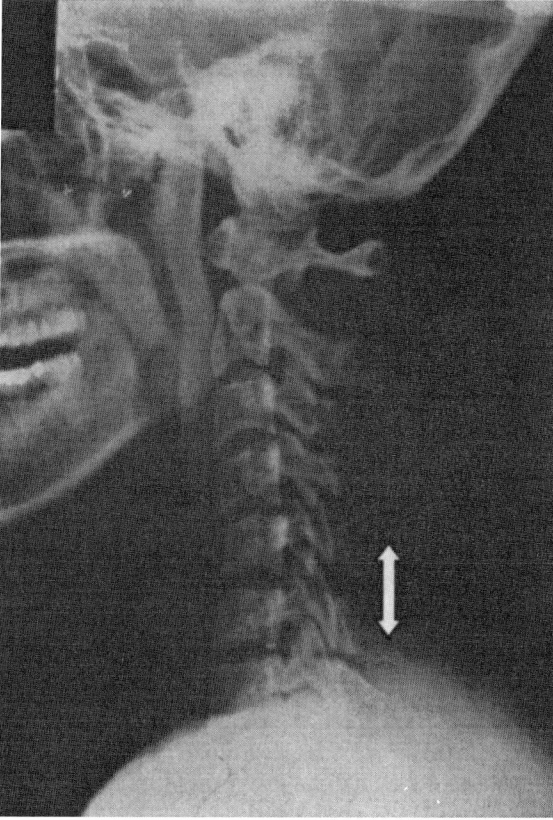

Figure 2   DFSI. Posterior element widening at C5,6 on the lateral C-spine x-ray.

AP radiograph. Lateral pillar injuries are not a common result of distractive flexion injuries, but more characteristic of an extension rotation mechanism of trauma. Translation of less than 25% of the vertebral body width anteriorly on the lateral view is the hallmark of the DFS II injury (Fig. 3).

Distractive flexion stage III (DFS III) injury has been characterized in the literature as a bilateral facet dislocation. Vertebral body translation on the lateral x-ray is typically greater than 25%. The facets are bilaterally subluxated and interspinous widening is noted. The articular facets may be perched with the inferior aspect of the inferior articular process perched ventral to the superior articular processes of the caudal vertebra. There can be blunting of the anterosuperior margin of the inferior vertebra. There is not a significant flexion compression component as seen in compression flexion injuries (Fig. 5).

The distractive flexion stage IV (DFS IV) injuries are characterized by translation and distraction at the motion segment. There is disruption of the anterior and posterior longitudinal ligaments, annulus, and posterior facet capsules. The facets exhibit significant translation associated with distraction at the disk space. This can give the appearance of a "floating or missing vertebra" in the widened disk space (Fig. 6).

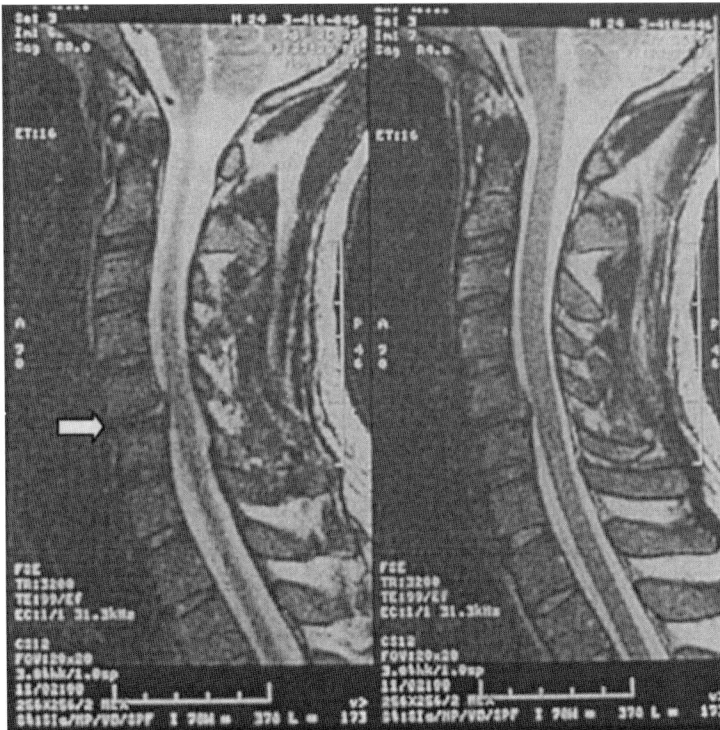

Figure 3 DFSII. Rotation and subluxation with posterior ligamentous failure. The anterior displacement of the vertebral body is less than 25%.

Clinical distinction of unilateral from bilateral facet injuries can be difficult. Many authors have defined these by the extent of vertebral subluxation or position of the facets on axial imaging. The degree of injury displacement may not be typically evident on the postinjury radiographs. The amount of posterior ligamentous disruption found intraoperatively with a radiographic unilateral displaced facet may indeed mimic the complete discoligamentous disruption of a distractive flexion stage III injury (bilateral facet injury). MR imaging can further help define the injury pattern and potential instability.

II EPIDEMIOLOGY

Distractive flexion injuries most commonly occur in motor vehicle trauma. These injuries have also occurred when significant force is applied to the dorsum of the head (Table 1) (2,3).

Cervical distractive flexion injuries frequently present with a neurological deficit. A recent article by Andreshak et al. (4) summarized the literature on unilateral facet injuries. This was inclusive of 308 injuries reported in a series on unilateral facets (5–18). In these series, among the patients with unilateral facet dislocation, 15% were noted to have complete paraplegia and 22% had incomplete cord injuries. In addition, 37% had a root deficit or radiculopathy and only 25% were neurologically intact. The wide variation of neurological severity between series may be due

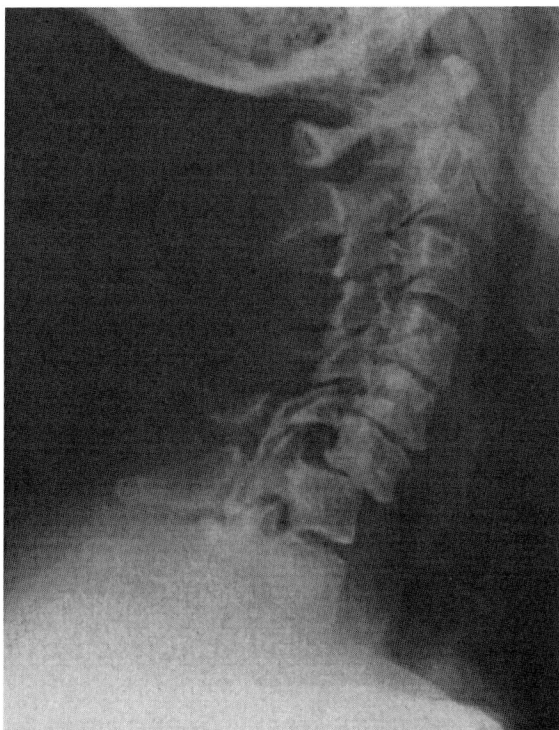

Figure 5   DFSIII. Bilateral facet dislocation as evidenced by about 50% vertebral body translocation on the lateral x-ray.

to the referral bias of tertiary centers and/or the higher proportion of high-energy sporting injuries (19).

In distractive flexion type III injuries, the occurrence of complete cord injury is noted to be between 40 and 90% (21–23). Incomplete lesions are evident in an additional 20%; generally fewer than 25% of these patients will present with an intact neurological status (22,23).

III   INJURY MECHANISM

The biomechanics of unilateral and bilateral facet injuries have been reported in numerous cadaveric studies. In an early biomechanical study by Roaf (24), flexion and rotational moments were applied to the cadaveric spines to reproduce unilateral and bilateral dislocation patterns. This study proved that a rotational moment was necessary while an isolated flexion moment did not replicate the injury. The mechanism studied was a slow manual application of forces in a static mode. However, the sequential static loading does not mimic the dynamic strain patterns induced in high-energy trauma.

Further studies by Holdsworth and Beatson (25) corroborated the component of flexion in combination with rotation causing the unilateral and bilateral facet injuries. The key component to the development of these injuries was the disruption of posterior interspinous and capsular ligaments. Bilateral facet dislocations occurred

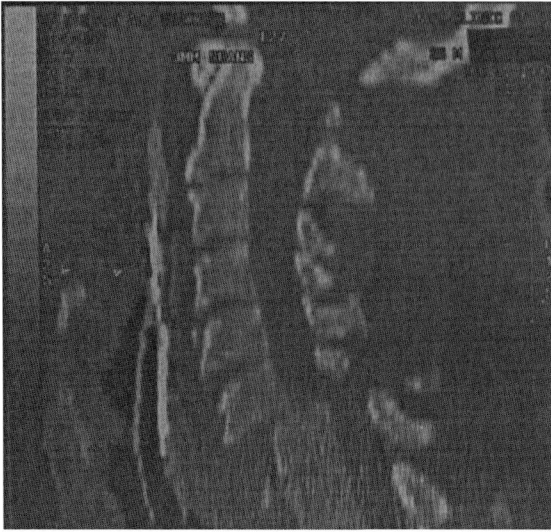

Figure 6 DFSIV. In this severe form of dislocation, an almost full vertebral body width translocation is appreciated on the above sagittal reconstruction CT.

only after the disruption of the posterior annulus and posterior longitudinal ligament. Posterior annular disruption allows for disk herniation in the distractive flexion stage III and IV injuries. Postmortem studies have confirmed these findings.

Cheshire (26) suggested that the spectrum of spine injuries inclusive of unilateral and bilateral facet disruptions was actually a continuum and that spontaneous reduction of bilateral facet injuries could occur causing difficulty with the postinjury classification based upon static x-rays. He also believed flexion and rotation are the major components of force involved. There is a continuum of subluxation and ligamentous disruptions that causes facet injuries. In a pure flexion injury, there is a greater elongation of the spinal cord than seen in a rotational injury, as noted in a cadaveric model (20).

A contemporary cadaveric biomechanical study was conducted by McLain to study distractive flexion injuries (19). The posterior ligamentous complex (inter- and supraspinous ligaments) and facet capsules failed before the posterior longitudinal ligament and annulus in a distractive flexion model. In this study, the changes in spinal cord length were demonstrated. There was a significant lengthening of the cord along its axis concurrent with posterior ligament disruption. The distraction then doubled when the posterior longitudinal ligament and the annulus were disrupted. Spinal cord distraction appears to have the greatest detrimental effect on the neurological recovery in the experimental spinal–cord injury model (26).

Clinically, the instability model, as proposed by White and Panjabi (27), is frequently referenced. In cadaveric models, translation (greater than 3.5 mm) or angulation (greater than 11 degrees) of the vertebral bodies compared to adjacent levels signified instability. The integrity of the facet joint was critical to the development of instability. Sequential resection of the facet capsule in the cadaveric model has demonstrated significant hypermobility in flexion and torsion. This is especially true when the resection is greater than 50%, as noted in the studies by Zdeblick (28,29).

The mechanism of discoligamentous failure in distractive flexion injuries appears to occur along a continuum (29,30).

IV CLINICAL MANAGEMENT

Fortunately, the terminal stage of a distractive flexion injury with complete ligamentous disruption and spinal cord stretching and/or compression is quite rare. The far more common occurrence is the DFS I injury, which can result in a clinical pain syndrome and progressive kyphosis. This has been noted in numerous studies and is frequently the "occult missed fracture" in the emergency room: x-ray findings may be quite subtle except for a mild spinous process widening (31,32). Clinical exam in the alert patient should note midline tenderness.

Distractive flexion stage I injuries are managed initially with cervical collar immobilization. Follow-up flexion and extension lateral radiographs may detect any residual instability. MR imaging with the use of fat suppressed T2-weighted images can help significantly in the detection of posterior ligamentous disruption (33). The discrimination of an annular disruption in flexion stage II and III injuries can also be aided by this technique (34). The sequelae of a missed injury may be neurological injury or development of progressive pain and kyphosis. Axial pain symptoms associated with discoligamentous disruption may be mistaken for whiplash. More critically, missed cervical spine injuries, especially of the distractive flexion stage II to III phylogeny, can result in the development of paraplegia. The characteristic distinction between distractive flexion stage II and III injuries is the disruption of the posterior longitudinal ligament, well defined by MR (35).

Stage IV injuries have complete discoligamentous disruption and are characterized by significant widening of the disk space. This is often associated clinically with a significant spinal cord injury or death. For patients who require infield intubation, in-line cervical immobilization without traction is recommended. The ATLS protocol now designates the preferred neutral cervical position during intubation to avoid exacerbation of this injury (36).

Distractive flexion injuries occur by elongation of the posterior column. The vertebral artery is fixated along its path in the foramina transversaria from C6 to C1. Subluxation of the osseous structures makes it vulnerable to traction injury. When compared to other mechanisms of C-spine trauma, distractive flexion injuries are among the most common associated with vertebral artery injury/occlusion. This vascular injury was evident in 28% of distractive flexion injuries in one series (37). This has gained much notoriety with the current availability of MR angiography imaging and has been the subject of recent studies by Giacobetti et al., Weller et al., and Vaccaro et al., respectively (37–39). Signs of vertebral artery insufficiency include blurred vision, diplopia, dizziness, dysphagia, and/or speech difficulties. In the absence of these findings, routine MRA does not appear necessary. Occlusion of one vertebral artery due to the initial injury should enter into the decision-making process regarding the surgical risk to the contralateral vessel during stabilization.

Stage IV distractive flexion injuries are frequently noticed at autopsy and are associated with high-speed deceleration motor vehicle accidents and fatal pedestrian injuries. The occurrence of complete spinal cord injury is quite common. In certain

Table 1 Vector (Clockface) Representation of the Allen and Fergeson Classification

Time vector	Vector	Phylogeny per Allen	Anterior column injury	Posterior column injury
1:00 to 3:00	30–90 Deg.	Distractive extension		
		DEStg1	Tension injury:ant. long. lig., disk	None
			Widened disk space	
		DEStg2	As above in DES1	Posterior ligaments failure
				Disp. of superior body into canal
4:00 to 5:30	120–165 Deg.	Compressive extension		
		CEStg1	+/− Anterorotatory body subluxation	Unilat. lamina fracture
		CEStg2	As above CES2	Bilaminar fractures often multilevel
		CEStg3-theoretical	Annular avulsions w/out subluxation	As above CES2
		CEStg4-theoretical	Partial body width displacement	As above CES2
		CEStg5	100% vert. displacement	As above CES2
			Shear injury of ant. and post long. lig.	
5:30 to 6:30	165–195 Deg.	Vertical compression		
		VCStg1	Central fracture of sup. or inf. endplate	None
		VCStg2	Fx. of both endplates with resultant	None
			cupping deformity	
		VCStg3	Progression of body comminution	+/− Lamina fractures and ligamentous
			Post. body may retropulse	disruption

6:30 to 8:30	195–255 Deg.	Compressive flexion		
		CFStg1	Blunting of ant. superior endplate	None
		CFStg2	Loss ant. body height with "beaked" appearance	None
		CFStg3	Additional obl. Fx. through body fracture of the "beak"	None
		CFStg4	Add. post. sup. displ. of fracture into canal <3 mm	None
		CFStg5	Add. disp. into canal / Failure of post. long. lig.	Lamina intact w/post. lig. failure
8:30 to 11:00	255–330 Deg.	Distractive flexion		
		DFStg1	Poss. blunting ant. sup body	Post. lig. failure "flexion sprain"
		DFStg2	Rotation and subluxation through disk	Unilateral facet disl. post. lig. failure
		DFStg3	Disp. through disk up to 50% +/− Ant body blunting	Bil. perched or locked facets
		DFStg4	Full body width displacement "Floating vertebra"	Gross widening post. elements
Out of plane		Lateral flexion		
		LFStg1	Asymmetric comp. fx. body or uncovertebral fx.	Ipsilat. arch fx. w/out displ.
		LFStg2	As per LFS1 with separation of contralateral uncovertebral joints	Displ. arch. fx. on AP with contralateral lig. failure

cases, the bilaminar arch fracture may spare the cord from compression. These injuries present with complete posterior longitudinal ligament and annular disruption with or without disk herniation.

V EVALUATION

Patients who are evaluated following an acute (emergency room) or subacute (clinic or hospital) trauma need a thorough review of the mechanism of injury and the symptoms noted at the time of injury. It is important to review the interval changes in the symptoms. These include the changes in neck or arm pain, as well as motor, sensory, and bowel or bladder status since the trauma. Distractive flexion injuries are most common in the high-energy deceleration accidents such as pedestrian versus motor vehicle trauma and, less commonly, from forceful direct blows to the head.

MR imaging is typically conducted in a subacute setting to discern the etiology of a neurological deficit, to detect a disk herniation, or to evaluate the integrity of the dorsal ligamentous structures. While this can be incorporated into the initial trauma management, especially in the comatose patient, it is not typically a part of the routine emergency room evaluation.

Distractive flexion stage I injuries appear as subtle posterior interspinous widening (Fig. 2.) In the stage II injuries, there is interspinous widening, rotation of the spinous processes on the AP view, diastasis of the uncovertebral joint, and displacement of the vertebral body up to 25% of its width anteriorly on the lateral view (Fig. 3). It must be emphasized that the degree of vertebral body displacement alone cannot differentiate a DF type II from III injury. Bilateral facet injuries may have a resting position with significantly less than 50% vertebral body translation.

Distractive flexion stage III injuries or bilateral facet injuries often have greater than 50% translation on lateral plain x-rays (Fig. 5). In facet dislocations, there is a very characteristic appearance of a "naked facet" sign on axial CT or MR imaging (Fig. 4). In DFS IV, an almost full vertebral body width translocation is evident on lateral imaging (Fig. 6).

VI TREATMENT PRINCIPLES

Upon recognition of a distractive flexion stage II or III injury, a decision on the timing and method of reduction is emergently considered.

Closed reduction provides the most expedient means to restore canal diameter and reverse ongoing cord compression. In the patient who has a complete or incomplete spinal cord injury, this should be done most expeditiously in the emergency room with the use of a halo or Gardner-Wells tongs. Initial manual in-line traction supplemented by weights starting at 5 to 10 pounds is performed to provide axial traction in slight flexion without any attempt at rotation. Weights are added incrementally with periodic reexamination of the patient clinically as well as radiographically. Most typically, reduction will occur in the DFS III cases quite early with less than 10 pounds per segment cephalad to the injury. For example, in a C5,6 bilateral facet dislocation, less than 50 pounds of weight is often required. In unilateral facet dislocations, traction weight as high as 120 to 140 pounds has been reported. This higher weight requirement in unilateral facet injuries may be partly caused by the residual intact ligaments that provide the resistance against reduction.

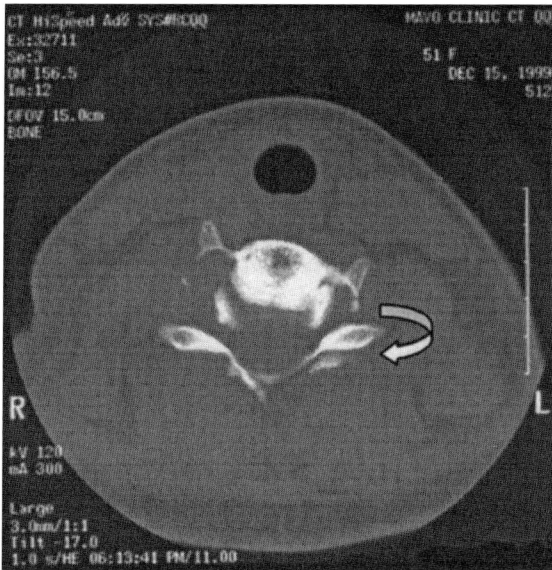

Figure 4 The right "naked facet" often found on axial CT illustrates the facet dislocation.

The neurologically compromised patient who is alert can benefit from expedient axial traction. This method has been quite effective in the centers that routinely manage spine trauma. A review of 131 patients by Rizzolo, et al. (22) proved closed reduction successful in 86% of the cases without any worsening in neurological deficits. The occurrence of a neurological deficit in an awake, alert, and cooperative patient is extremely rare. After reduction of the dislocation and restoration of canal dimensions, the traction weights are reduced and the patient is immobilized by application of a halo vest or Philadelphia collar.

If closed reduction cannot be obtained or the patient has a change in his or her neurological status, an MRI is obtained to discern the status of the posterior longitudinal ligament, annulus, and disk. This is conducted prior to the operative treatment. Some authors have recommended closed or open reduction by manipulation under general anesthesia for neurologically intact patients. This is generally discouraged due to the potential risk for neurological injury as the patient is unable to contribute to the neurological assessment.

There is less urgency to obtain reduction in the case of a neurologically intact patient. In the setting of an alert patient, closed reduction may proceed as mentioned previously. However, many authors will obtain MR imaging to evaluate for disk extrusion. If anterior compression exists, an operative reduction would follow an anterior diskectomy and decompression. The patient's neck must be maintained in neutral alignment during intubation as reduction can occur with pharmacological paralysis and/or manipulation of the neck.

Surgical stabilization after closed reduction proceeds electively, using the posterior cervical fusion techniques. Stabilization with interspinous wiring alone has been reported by Feldborg and Nielsen (40). Most typically, this is conducted by using an oblique wiring method similar to the Roger or Bohlman technique. However, we augment this construct with the posterior lateral mass fixation (Fig. 7).

In neurologically intact patients with a disk herniation who are irreducible, anterior diskectomy with reduction may be performed. Distraction using the Cloward pins in the vertebral bodies will open the disk space. In the anterior reduction maneuver, kyphosis and anterior disk space distraction is required. Most typically, this is conducted with the use of the Cloward pin distraction system. With uncovertebral distraction, a kyphotic moment is used to effect reduction of the dorsal jumped facet.

In the patient without a ventral disk herniation, a posterior approach for open reduction may be performed with a limited resection of the superior articular process. The perched facet will readily reduce, after which time surgical stabilization may follow. It is of paramount importance not to wire the spinous processes during alignment in a manner to drag the cephalad vertebral body dorsally. This overzealous reduction can displace the incarcerated disk material behind the posterior longitudinal ligament into the ventral spinal canal, possibly causing neurological injury. Anecdotally, this has been attributed to the occurrence of neurological deficit following interspinous wiring prior to the recognition of the importance of disk disruption (40).

There are certain controversies among authors regarding the timing of the MRI. Expedient reduction in the patient with a neurological deficit has been shown to

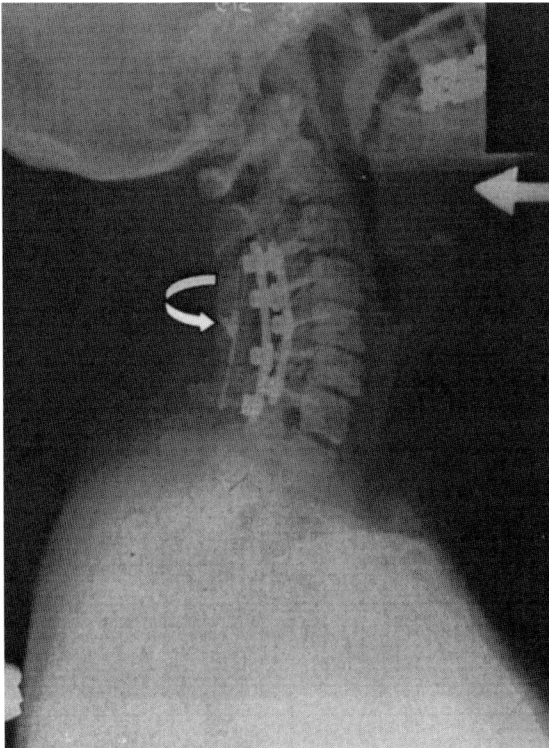

Figure 7   Flexion distraction injuries may be stabilized by recreating the posterior tension band using spinous process wiring (curved arrow) and lateral mass plating, achieving a satisfactory alignment.

improve the neurological outcome. The delay during which imaging is obtained causes ongoing neural tissue compression and potential deterioration. Therefore, patients with a neurological deficit should be immediately reduced prior to MR imaging. In the case of a patient with a focal radiculopathy without evidence of a cord syndrome, some authors believe in performing an elective anterior decompression in the presence of a disk herniation, and therefore closed reduction is not attempted (21). However, many other authors disagree and maintain the need for emergent reduction in all cases of cervical dislocations.

The character of ventral disk herniations has undergone further recognition and definition in the recent literature and is now felt to be overreported in some of the earlier studies. This has been clarified by Vaccaro et al. (22).

VII   OUTCOMES

Deterioration during closed reduction of the awake and neurologically intact patient is extremely uncommon. There have been isolated reports of neurological injury during open reduction under general anesthesia, specifically in those cases with bilateral facet injuries and disk herniation. Furthermore, there have been reported cases of progressive neurological deficit in the perioperative period attributed to disk herniation with permanent paralysis (41). There are two critical issues to consider in these cases. First, these patients underwent closed reduction while being under general anesthesia and, second, interspinous wiring was utilized, which may have dragged the cephalad vertebral body dorsally and may potentially have drawn the disk material into the canal, causing significant cord injury.

Closed reduction has improved the neurological outcome in the patients with facet dislocations significantly. Deterioration has been reported in less than 5 to 6% of these cases (42). In the three large series of unilateral facet dislocations by Rorabeck, Shapiro, and Beyer (10,12,15) significant neurological improvement was noted in approximately 30% of patients with immediate reduction. The success rates with closed reduction and traction alone vary widely. The rate of up to 100% by Vaccaro (22) and others is compared to less than 25% by Cheshire (26) and Sears (43).

Halo immobilization has been utilized without operative stabilization in reduced DFS II injuries, with a failure rate of developing late instability and neurological symptoms in up to 10% of patients, as per Whitehill and Glasser (44). Operative stabilization has been advocated in the series by Rogers (7) and Shapiro (11). Their success is evidenced by the lack of recurrent dislocation in over 95% of their patients. Late kyphosis can develop in spite of an adequate dorsal tension band by wire stabilization due to the mechanical inefficiency of this technique. This has been reported by Hukgle in 5 of 11 patients who developed late kyphosis with DFS II and III injuries. The use of lateral mass plates as reported by Camille (45) and others may augment fusion with the tension band provided by wiring. This technique, without adjuvant use of halo orthosis, provides adequate stabilization with no residual kyphosis in over 90% of patients (45).

REFERENCES

1.   Drucker, McAfee P: Cervical spine trauma. In: Frymoyer WT et al., eds. The Adult Spine. New York: Raven, 1991:1080–1081.

2. Allen BL Jr, Ferguson RL, Lehmann TR, O'Brien RP. A mechanistic classification of closed, indirect fractures and dislocations of the lower cervical spine. Spine 1982;7(1): 1–27.

3. McAfee PC. Cervical Spine Trauma. In: Frymoyer WT, et al., eds. The Adult Spine: Principles and Practice. New York: Raven Press, 1991:1063–1107.

4. Andreshak JL, Dekutoski MB. Management of unilateral facet dislocations: A review of the literature. Orthopedics 1997;20(10):917–926.

5. Burke DC, Berryman D. The place of closed manipulation in the management of flexion-rotation dislocations of the cervical spine. J Bone Joint Surg 1971;53B:165–182.

6. Cotler HB, Miller LS, Delucia FA, Cotler JM, Dayne SH. Closed reduction of cervical spine dislocations. Clin Orthop 1987;214:185–199.

7. Rogers WL. Fractures and dislocations of the cervical spine. An end result study. J Bone Joint Surg 1957;39A:341–376.

8. Evans DK. Reduction of cervical dislocations. J Bone Joint Surg 1961;43:552–555.

9. Rorabeck CH, Rock MG, Hawkins RJ, Bourne RB. Unilateral facet dislocation of the cervical spine. An analysis of the results of treatment in 26 patients. Spine 1987;12(1): 23–27.

10. Webb JK, Broughton RBK, McSweeney T, Park M. Hidden flexion injury of the cervical spine. J Bone Joint Surg 1976:58B:322–327.

11. Shapiro SA. Management of unilateral locked facet of the cervical spine. Rev Neurosurg 1993;33(5):832–837; discussion 837.

12. Hadley MN, Fitzpatrick BC, Sonntag VK, Browner CM. Facet fracture-dislocation injuries of the cervical spine. Neurosurg 1992;30(5):661–666.

13. Beyer CA, Cabanela ME, Berquist TH. Unilateral facet dislocations and fracture-dislocations of the cervical spine. J Bone Joint Surg 1991;73B:977–981.

14. Beyer CA, Cabanela ME. Unilateral facet dislocations and fracture-dislocations of the cervical spine: A review [published erratum appears in Orthopedics 1992 May;15(5): 545]. Rev Orthopedics 1992;15(3):311–315.

15. Argenson C, Lovet J, Sanouiller JL, de Peretti F. Traumatic rotatory displacement of the lower cervical spine. Spine 1988;13(7):767–773.

16. Braakman R, Vinken PJ. Unilateral facet interlocking in the lower cervical spine. J Bone Joint Surg 1967;49B(2):249–257.

17. O'Brien PJ, Schweigel JF, Thompson WJ. Dislocations of the lower cervical spine. J Trauma 1982;22(8):710–714.

18. Goffin J, Plets C, Van den Bergh R. Anterior cervical fusion and osteosynthetic stabilization according to Caspar: A prospective study of 41 patients with fractures and/or dislocations of the cervical spine. Neurosurgery 1989;25(6):865–871.

19. Torg JS, Sennett B, Vegso JJ, Pavlov H. Axial loading injuries to the middle cervical spine segment. An analysis and classification of twenty-five cases. Am J Sports Med 1991;19(1):6–20.

20. McLain RF, Aretakis A, Moseley TA, Ser P, Benson DR. Sub-axial cervical dissociation. Anatomic and biomechanical principles of stabilization. Spine 1994;19:653–659.

21. Vital JM, Gille O, Senegas J, Pointillart V. Reduction technique for uni- and biarticular dislocations of the lower cervical spine. Spine 1998;23(8):949–955.

22. Rizzolo SJ, Vaccaro AR, Cotler JM. Cervical spine trauma. Spine 1994;19(20):2288–2298.

23. Rizzolo SJ, Cotler JM. Unstable cervical spine injuries: specific treatment approaches. J Am Arthrosc Orthop Surg 1993;1(1).

24. Roaf R. A study of the mechanics of spinal injury. J Bone Joint Surg 1960;42B:810–823.

25. Holdsworth FH. Fractures, common dislocations, fractures-dislocations of the spine. J Bone Joint Surg 1963;45(B):6–26.

26. Cheshire DJE. The stability of the cervical spine following the conservative treatment of fracture and fracture-dislocations. Paraplegia 1969;7:193–203.
27. White AA, 3rd, Johnson RM, Panjabi MM, Southwick WO. Biomechanical analysis of clinical stability in the cervical spine. Clin Orthop 1975;(109):85–96.
28. Zdeblick TA, Zou D, Warden KE, McCabe R, Kunz D, Vanderby R. Cervical stability after foraminotomy. A biomechanical in vitro analysis. J Bone Joint Surg 1992;74A(1): 22–27.
29. Zdeblick TA, Abitbol JJ, Kunz DN, McCabe RP, Garfin S. Cervical stability after sequential capsule resection. Spine 1993;18(14):2005–2008.
30. Brooke WS. Complete transverse cervical myelitis caused by traumatic herniation of an ossified nucleus pulposus. J Am Med Assoc 1944;125:117–120.
31. Davis D, Bohlman H, Walker AE, Fisher R, Robinson R. Pathological findings in fatal craniospinal injuries. J Neurosurg 1971;34(5):603–613.
32. Herkowitz HN, Rothman RH. Subacute instability of the cervical spine. Spine 1984; 9(4):348–357.
33. Webb JK, Broughton RB, McSweeney T, Park WM. Hidden flexion injury of the cervical spine. J Bone Joint Surg 1976;58B(3):322–327.
34. Klein GR, Vaccaro AR, Albert TJ, Schweitzer M, Deely D, Karasick D, Cotler JM. Efficacy of magnetic resonance imaging in the evaluation of posterior cervical spine fractures. Spine 1999;24(8):771–774.
35. Halliday AL, Henderson BR, Hart BL, Benzel EC. The management of unilateral mass/ facet fractures of the subaxial spine: The use of magnetic resonance imaging to predict stability. Spine 1997;22(22):2614–2621.
36. Alexander RH, Proctor HJ. Advanced Trauma Life Support (ATLS) Program for Physicians. 1993 Instructor Manual. Chicago: American College of Surgeons, 1993.
37. Giacobetti FB, Vaccaro AR, Bos-Giacobetti MA, Deeley DM, Albert TJ, Farmer JC, Cotler JM. Vertebral artery occlusion associated with cervical spine trauma. A prospective analysis. Spine 1997;22(2):188–192.
38. Weller SJ, Rossitch E Jr, Malek AM. Detection of vertebral injury after cervical spine trauma using magnetic resonance angiography. J Trauma 1999;46(4):660–666.
39. Vaccaro AR, Klein GR, Flanders AE, Albert TJ, Balderston RA, Cotler JM. Long-term evaluation of vertebral artery injuries following cervical spine trauma using magnetic resonance angiography. Spine 1998;23(7):789–794.
40. Feldborg Nielsen C, et al. Fusion or stabilization alone for acute distractive flexion injuries in the mid to lower cervical spine? Eur Spine J 1997;6:197–202.
41. B. Green, personal communication.
42. Eismont FJ, et al. Extrusion of an invertebral disk associated with traumatic subluxation or dislocation of cervical facets. J Bone Joint Surg 1991;73A:1555–1560.
43. Sears W, Fazl M. Prediction of stability of cervical spine fracture managed in the Halo best and indications for surgical intervention. J Neurosurg 1990;72:426–432.
44. Whitehill T, Richman JA, Glasser JA. Failure of immobilization of the cervical spine by the halo vest. J Bone Joint Surg 1986;68A:326–332.
45. Roy-Camille, Saillant G, Laville C, Benazet JP. Treatment of lower cervical spine injuries—C3-C7. Spine 1992;17(10 suppl):S442–446.

15

Compressive Flexion Injuries of the Cervical Spine

MICHAEL J. VIVES

*University of Medicine and Dentistry of New Jersey,
Newark, New Jersey, U.S.A.*

ALEXANDER R. VACCARO

*Thomas Jefferson University Hospital and the Rothman Institute,
Philadelphia, Pennsylvania, U.S.A.*

JEAN-JACQUES ABITBOL

California Spine Group, San Diego, California, U.S.A.

I ANATOMY AND PATHOMECHANICS

While the atlantoaxial joint and subaxial spine contribute equally to rotation, most of the flexion and extension in the cervical spine occurs from C3 to C7. Up to 17 degrees of sagittal plane motion occur at individual motion segments of the subaxial spine. Coronal plane motion ranges from 4 to 11 degrees per motion segment in this region (1). The anterior two-thirds of the vertebral body, in concert with the anterior longitudinal ligament and annulus fibrosis, act as a tension band–limiting extension. Posteriorly, the supraspinous and interspinous ligaments, the ligamentum flavum, and the facet capsules resist flexion (2).

Motor vehicle accidents and shallow dives are the most common scenarios leading to compressive flexion injuries of the cervical spine. Experiments in human cadavers loaded axially posterior to the skull vertex demonstrated cervical motion segment failure in extension, while those loaded anterior to the skull vertex failed in flexion (3). Porcine models have demonstrated great variations in resultant fracture patterns with small variations in distance of load application anteriorly or posteriorly from neutral to the point of axial loading (4–6). The initial head–neck–thorax position and loading conditions determine cervical spine response to impact, as shown in studies of both human cadaveric and calf spines (7–10). When the cervical spine is straight and colinear with an axial force, the spine buckles after a sudden "give" or deformation in structure. In human cadaveric studies, prepositioning the head in a mildly flexed position, eliminating the normal cervical lordosis (straightening the spine), results in the least amount of axial deformation per given axial load. Large amounts of energy are absorbed by the spinal column until it buckles, rapidly dissipating stored energy to the surrounding soft tissues. In theory, the relative straight position of the spine at initial loading may lessen the ability of the surrounding muscles and ligaments to dissipate the applied energy gradually to surrounding structures. Specimens prepositioned in more flexion and axially loaded failed in flexion at substantially lower loads than did the neutrally positioned specimens (3). These studies, along with mathematical models, have suggested that the straightened (rather than the kyphotic) cervical spine will withstand the highest external axial load (11,12).

Even in the absence of an external axial load, excessive flexion or combined flexion rotation may result in injury to the cervical spinal column. Pure flexion injuries generally produce a compression fracture of the vertebral body. More substantial flexion moments can result in associated disruption of the posterior ligaments. The resultant injury is often manifested radiographically as angulation of the compressed anterior vertebral body with widening of the interspinous space. There may be associated perching of the facets with minimal vertebral body translation. Large amounts of translation, however, generally indicate a more substantial rotatory force with facet dislocation (13).

II CLASSIFICATION

While a universally accepted classification system for fractures and dislocation of the lower cervical spine does not exist, those based on mechanism of injury have generally been found useful. Allen et al.'s classification is one of the most widely used today (14). This system is based on a retrospective evaluation of 165 cases of cervical spine trauma. The authors proposed six categories, each named for the presumed position of the cervical spine at the moment of injury and the initial principal mechanism of load to failure. The categories proposed by the authors included vertical compression, compressive flexion, distractive flexion, lateral flexion, compressive extension, and distractive extension (Fig. 1). The authors demonstrated that the probability of related neurological injury could be predicted based on the type and severity of the spinal injury (Fig. 2). The classification discusses a continuum of injury severity related to the force dissipated to the spine at the time of trauma.

A Compressive Flexion Stage I

Compressive flexion stage I (CFS I) lesion manifests as blunting of the anterior–superior margin of the vertebral body, producing a rounded contour. The posterior ligamentous complex remains intact (Fig. 2A).

B Compressive Flexion Stage II

Compressive flexion stage II (CFS II) lesion consists of the changes seen in CFS I, along with obliquity of the anterior vertebral body and loss of some anterior height,

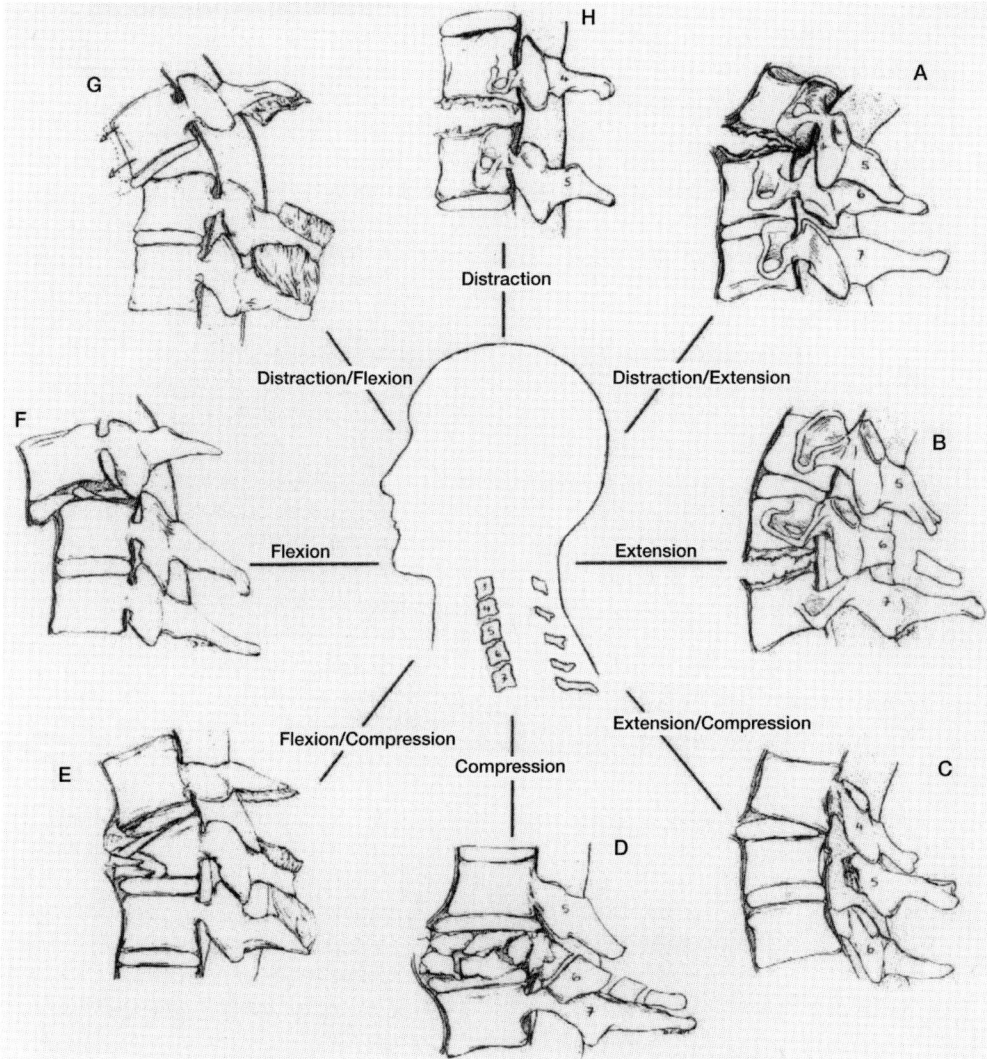

Figure 1 Lower cervical spine injuries. Allen and Ferguson's classification grouped injuries into patterns named for the presumed position of the cervical spine at the moment of injury and the initial principal mechanism of load to failure. (From Ref. 14a.)

resulting in a "beaked" appearance of the anterior–inferior vertebral body. Increased concavity of the inferior endplate may be noted on plain radiographs, but a vertical fracture line through the centrum is often missed (Fig. 2B).

C   Compressive Flexion Stage III

In addition to the features of the CFS II lesion, a compressive flexion stage III (CFS III) lesion also has an oblique fracture extending from the anterior surface

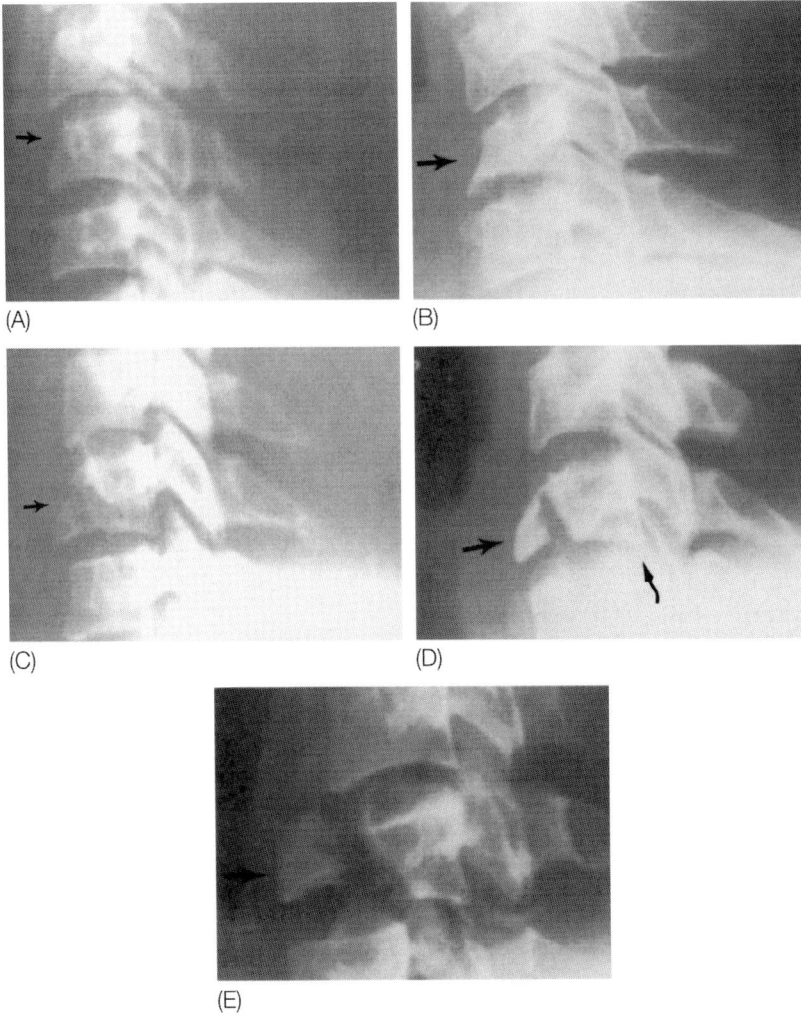

(A)

(B)

(C)

(D)

(E)

Figure 2 (A, upper left) CFS I. (B, upper right) CFS II. (C, middle left) CFS III. (D, middle right) CFS IV. (E, lower right) CFS V. (From Ref. 14.)

of the vertebral body to the inferior subchondral plate with a fracture of the beak (Fig. 2C).

D   Compressive Flexion Stage IV

Along with the findings of a CFS III injury, compressive flexion stage IV (CFS IV) lesions demonstrate mild displacement (less than 3 mm) of the inferior–posterior vertebral margin into the neural canal at the involved motion segment (Fig. 2D).

E   Compressive Flexion Stage V

The compressive flexion stage V (CFS V) lesion has the injury features of a CFS III lesion and more pronounced displacement of the posterior vertebral body fragment into the neural canal. The posteror–inferior margin of the upper vertebrae may approximate the lamina of the subjacent vertebrae. This degree of displacement indicates disruption of the posterior ligamentous complex. The facets are separated or perched, with associated widening of the distance between spinous processes (Fig. 2E).

The authors proposed that the deformation the centrum experiences in CFS I and CFS II indicates a compressive force, oriented obliquely downward and posterior in the sagittal plane, as the predominant injury vector. The oblique fracture of the centrum seen in CFS III patterns was proposed due to shear stress generated by the bending moment across the motion segment. They concluded that the oblique fracture across the centrum resolves the compressive stress since there was no greater deformation of the centrum in CFS IV and CFS V than in CFS III. The ligamentous failure seen with CFS IV and CFS V lesions implies a tension/shear component through the posterior part of the anterior elements and completely through the posterior elements. The transitional axis from compressive to tension/shear failure was inferred as the site where the oblique fracture of the centrum crosses the inferior chondral plate.

In the authors' series of 36 cases with the CF phylogeny, complete spinal cord injury was present in 25% with CFS III, 38% of CFS IV, and 91% of CFS V injuries. Thus, the higher stages of the compressive flexion phylogeny are felt to be caused by greater force and reflect a greater degree of spinal instability.

While radiographic descriptive classifications can be useful for unique injuries, they can often be confusing because of their ambiguity and lack of mechanistic information inferred by their labeling. Two radiographic patterns, however, have been described that are frequently referred to in the neurosurgical and orthopedic literature: the teardrop and quadrangular fractures. The flexion teardrop fracture, described by Harris (15,16), as complete ligamentous and disk disruption at the level of the injury, including disruption of the facet joints. Additionally, a large triangular anterior bone fragment was thought to be "squeezed off" by the vertebral bodies above and below. The spine proximal to the injury level is usually flexed. While Harris felt these injuries were produced by flexion moments, Allen et al. (14) felt these were produced by combined injury mechanisms of compressive flexion and vertical compression. The quadrangular fragment fracture was described by Favero et al. (17) as a variant of a CFS V injury. The four characteristics of this fracture are: (1) an oblique fracture of the vertebral body extending from the anterior–superior margin of the vertebral cortex to the inferior end plate; (2) posterior subluxation of the upper vertebral body on the lower vertebral body; (3) variable degree of angular kyphosis; and (4) disruption of the disk and ligaments anteriorly and posteriorly. The authors felt this pattern implied a greater degree of instability, requiring both anterior and posterior stabilization.

III ASSESSMENT

All patients with head injury, high-energy trauma, complaints of neck pain or neurological deficit should be assumed to have a cervical spine injury. In the field, immediate stabilization and focus on protection of the cervical spine is mandatory. With coordinated movements, the neck should be palpated for tenderness and any evidence of stepoff. A thorough sensorimotor examination should be documented at initial presentation along with documentation of perianal sensory sparing and the presence or absence of a bulbocavernosis reflex.

The initial radiographic evaluation should include an anteroposterior and lateral cervical view (including the cervicothoracic junction), and an open-mouth odontoid view. This radiographic protocol detects the majority of cervical spinal injuries (18–20). Up to 16% of patients will have noncontiguous spine fractures, with fractures at the C1–C2 level along with a remote subaxial fracture as one of the most common patterns (21). The radiographic criteria for spinal stability continue to evolve. Angulation greater than 11 degrees compared to adjacent normal segments or translation greater than 3.5 mm were guidelines developed by serial sectioning studies in cadavers (1).

If plain radiographs reveal osseous abnormalities, computed tomography (CT) may help define the extent of bony damage (Fig. 3). CT is also helpful when the lower cervical spine cannot be adequately visualized on plain radiographs. Magnetic resonance imaging (MR) may be indicated in patients with neurological deficits (to localize and quantify the degree of cord compression); patients with deteriorating neurological status; and cases of suspected posterior ligamentous injury not evident by plain radiographs (22). Controversy exists regarding the timing of these advanced modalities in the acute trauma setting. The authors favor early restoration of cervical alignment and protection, with traction, in the alert and cooperative patient prior to pursuit of an advanced imaging workup, which may require delay or repeated transfers. Flexion extension radiographs are rarely indicated in the acute trauma setting. The patient should be able to position his or her neck voluntarily. These views should not be obtained with physical or radiographic findings of bony, ligamentous, or neurological injury. The information gained in the acute setting is also limited. A negative study does not preclude significant soft-tissue disruption, since muscle spasm can mask instability for up to 2 weeks. Therefore, follow-up films in that timeframe are necessary.

IV   TREATMENT

In CFS I and CFS II injuries, the structural integrity of the anterior column retains partial competence. The posterior annulus and posterior ligamentous structures remain intact. Most patients can be managed with a rigid cervical orthosis, or in cases of questionable compliance a halo-vest, until bony healing. Ten to 12 weeks of immobilization are often necessary. Patients should be monitored for improvement of symptoms and radiographic signs of healing. Flexion extension lateral radiographs should be obtained prior to cessation of immobilization. Abnormal motion in this circumstance may be an indication for a posterior fusion (13).

Stage III injuries (teardrop fragment without subluxation) are potentially unstable. Evaluation by MR imaging should be performed to assess possible injury to the disk and posterior ligamentous complex. In the absence of injury to these soft tissues, the fracture may be managed in a halo brace until healing. For those injuries with associated posterior ligamentous injury, anterior or posterior fusion may be indicated because of the risk of late kyphotic deformity. The authors prefer the anterior approach in the management of this fracture pattern, although a posterior fusion with triple wiring (23) or lateral mass plating is often adequate (22,24). In the setting of a neurological deficit, especially with evidence of significant anterior

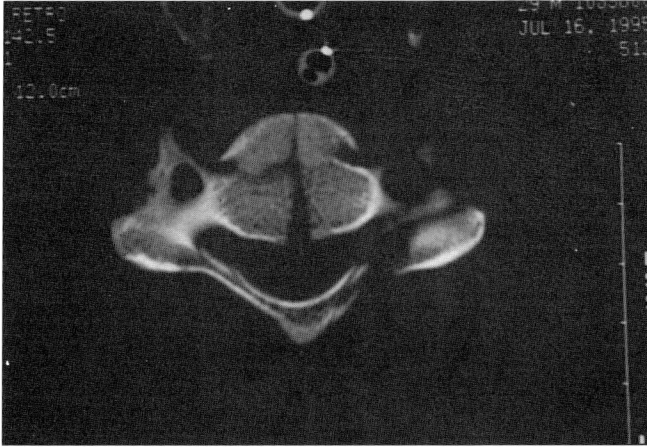

Figure 3   A transaxial CT scan revealing a sagittal plane fracture involving the centrum of the vertebral body.

thecal sac compression from retropulsed bone or an extruded disk fragment, an anterior decompressive and reconstructive procedure is indicated.

Subluxation of the inferior body fragment posteriorly into the neural canal (CFS IV) suggests a more unstable lesion. Traction with Gardner–Wells tongs and an extension roll placed beneath the scapula lengthwise is useful, but often results in incomplete realignment. Definitive halo-vest immobilization without surgical stabilization is often unsuccessful due to progressive loss of cervical alignment over time. In a neurologically intact patient, posterior stabilization may suffice. However, in the presence of an incomplete neurological injury with objective anterior thecal sac compression, anterior decompression, strut graft placement, and plating are often indicated (Fig. 4A, 4B) (25–27). Supplemental posterior fusion may be indicated with extensive posterior ligamentous injury. Fixation posteriorly can be achieved through interspinous wiring or lateral mass plating.

More extensive subluxation (greater than 3 mm) with retropulsion of the postero–inferior vertebral body into the spinal canal defines a CFS V injury. An isolated posterior fusion in this circumstance is inadequate because of the extensive degree of anterior and posterior osteoligamentous instability present. There is disruption of the anterior longitudinal ligament, the entire annulus fibrosus including the disk, the posterior longitudinal ligament, and often the posterior bony elements. Thus all three columns are significantly involved, usually over the course of two motion segments (28). This pattern is more appropriately addressed through an anterior approach. Again, in the presence of a neurological deficit with bony encroachment of the neural canal, this approach facilitates complete decompression of the spinal canal. Strut grafting and anterior plating provide stabilization. More secure stabilization can be achieved through a combined anterior and posterior stabilization approach (Fig. 5A–C). If such a combined approach is necessary, the authors favor performing the anterior procedure first, followed by the posterior procedure under the same anesthesia.

The surgical procedure of choice in these advanced-stage compressive flexion injuries remains controversial. Biomechanical studies in models depicting anterior

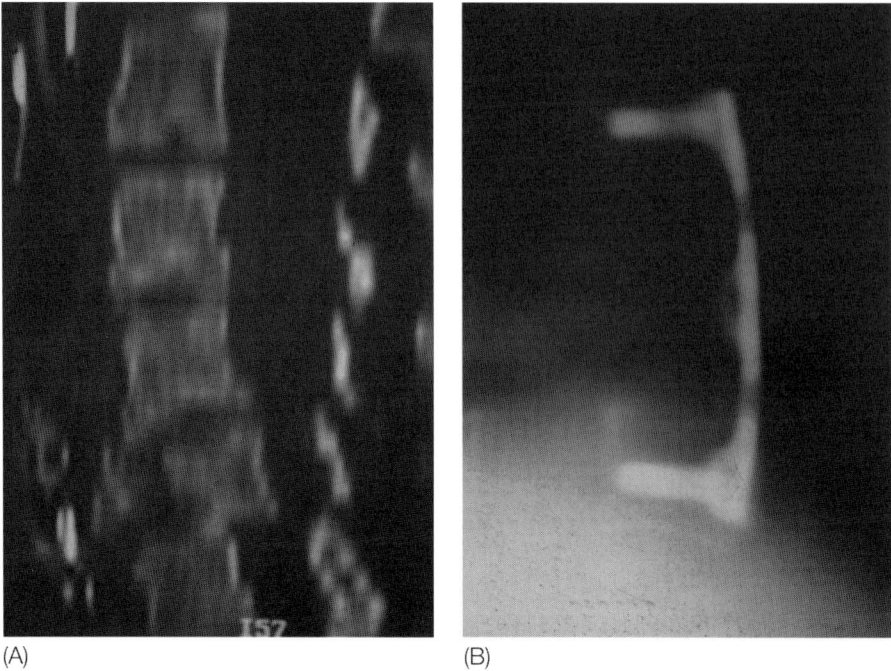

(A)   (B)

Figure 4   (A) A sagittal cervical spine CT reconstruction revealing a compressive flexion stage IV cervical spine injury. Note the retrolisthesis of the C5 vertebral body into the spinal canal. There is no obvious widening of the posterior elements. (B) An anterior-alone approach was used to decompress the cervical canal and stabilize the subaxial cervical spine because of the lack of significant posterior element instability. This is seen on the lateral tomogram following anterior iliac crest strut graft placement and anterior cervical plate instrumentation.

injuries with posterior ligamentous disruption have cited anterior plating techniques as inadequate fixation. In a bovine model, Sutterlin's group found inadequate restoration of flexural or axial stability using anterior Caspar instrumentation. Therefore, they recommended additional posterior stabilization (29). The same group reached similar conclusions in a human cadaver model of distractive flexion injuries treated with anterior plating (but without structural bone graft) (30).

In contrast, clinical reports of anterior plating and structural grafting without supplemental posterior fixation have been more favorable. Several authors have reported success with varied anterior plating systems in lower cervical spine injuries with and without postoperative halo use (25,26,31–33). Garvey and Eismont (34) reported their clinical experience using stand-alone anterior Caspar plating and structural bone grafting. This study focused on a narrow population of 14 patients with mechanically unstable cervical spine injuries (CFS IV or V and distractive flexion stages II or III). At an average follow-up of 30 months, no patient had loss of fixation and all had radiographically solid anterior fusions. Eleven of the 14 patients wore a rigid plastic collar postoperatively, with only three immobilized in halo vests. Based on their results, the authors suggested that the addition of anterior Caspar plating to anterior structural grafting could obviate the need for additional posterior plating.

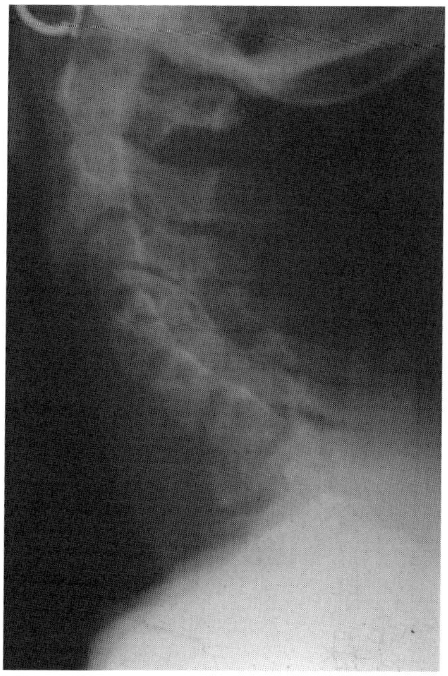

(A)

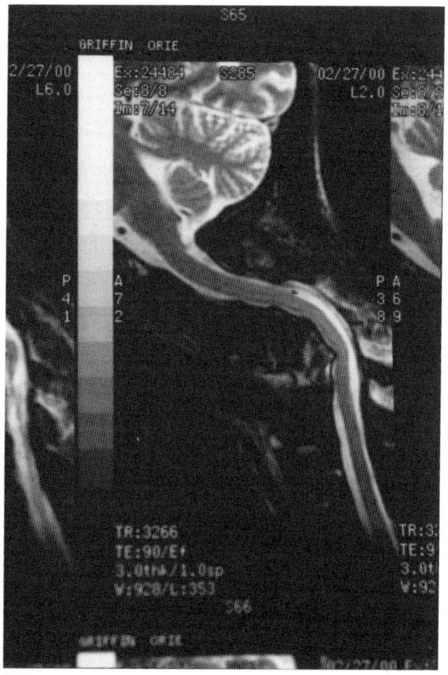

(B)

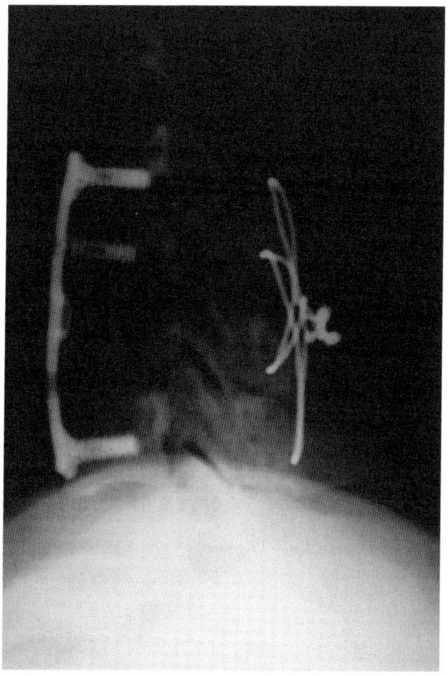

(C)

Figure 5 (A) A lateral plain roentgenograph revealing a compressive flexion stage V injury involving the C7 vertebral body. (B) A sagittal MRI revealing a significant sagittal plane deformity with retropulsion of the C7 body within the spinal canal, causing significant anterior thecal sac compression. (C) An anterior–posterior cervical decompression and stabilization procedure was performed because of the significant amount of anterior and posterior spinal instability present. This is seen on the lateral plain roentgenograph, where an anterior iliac crest strut graft placement and cervical plating were performed followed by a posterior cervical wiring procedure.

In summary, compressive flexion injuries of the lower cervical spine can be mechanistically classified with higher stages representing more unstable lesions. Cervical orthoses may suffice for benign compression fractures with little deformity. Higher grade lesions, however, may require single or combined stabilization procedures. While the classification system presented may help outline treatment recommendations, more unstable injuries may warrant individualized strategies since their specific treatment approaches remain controversial.

REFERENCES

1. White AA III, Southwick WO, Panjabi MM. Clinical instability in the lower cervical spine-a review of past and current concepts. Spine 1976; 1:15–27.
2. White AA III, Panjabi MM, Saha S, Southwick WO. Biomechanics of the axially loaded cervical spine: development of a clinical test for ruptured ligaments. J Bone Joint Surg Am 1975; 57:582.
3. Maiman DJ, Sances A, Myklebust JB, Larson SJ, Houterman C, Chilbert M, El Ghatit AZ. Compression injuries of the cervical spine: a biomechanical analysis. Neurosurgery 1983; 13:254–260.
4. Oxland TR, Panjabi MM, Southern EP, Duranceau JS. An anatomic basis for spinal instability: a porcine trauma model. J Orthop Res 1991; 9:452–462.
5. Panjabi MM, Durancea JS, Oxland TR, Bowen CE. Multidirectional instabilities of traumatic cervical spine injuries in a porcine model. Spine 1989; 14:1111–1115.
6. Southern EP, Oxland TR, Panjabi MM, Duranceau JS. Cervical Spine injury patterns in three modes of high-speed trauma: a biomechanical porcine model. J Spinal Disord 1990; 3:316–328.
7. Alem NM, Nusholtz GS, Melvin JW. Head and neck response to axial impacts. Proceedings of the 28th STAPP Car Crash Conference. Society of Automotive Engineers, Warrendale, PA, 1984.
8. Hodgson VR, Thomas LM. Mechanisms of cervical spine injury during impact to the protected head. Proceedings of the 24th STAPP Car Crash Conference, Society for Automotive Engineers, Warrendale, PA, 1980:17.
9. Nusholtz GS, Huelke DE, Lux P, Alem NM, Montalva F. Cervical spine injury mechanisms. 27th STAPP Car Crash Conference. Society of Automotive Engineers, Warrendale, PA, 1983:179–197.
10. Shono Y, McAffe PC, Cunningham BW. The pathomechanics of compression injuries of the cervical spine. Spine 1993; 18:2009–2019.
11. Helleur C, Gracovetsky S, Farfan H. Tolerance of the human cervical spine to high acceleration: a modeling approach. Aviat Space Environ Med 1984; 55:903–909.
12. Yoganandan N, Sances A, Maiman DJ, Myklebust JB, Pech P, Larson SJ. Experimental spinal injuries with vertical impact. Spine 1986; 11:855–860.
13. Abitbol JJ, Kostuik JP. Flexion injuries to the lower cervical spine. In: Clarke CR, Ducker TB, Dvorak J, Garfin SR, Herkowitz HN, Levine AM, Pizzutillo PD, Sherk HH, Ullrich CG, Zeidman SM, eds. The Cervical Spine, 3rd ed. Philadelphia: Lippincott-Raven, 1998:457–464.
14. Allen BL, Ferguson RL, Lehmann TR, O'Brien RP. A mechanistic classification of closed, indirect fractures and dislocations of the lower cervical spine. Spine 1982; 7:1–27.
14a. Frymoyer JW, ed. The Adult Spine: Principles and Practice. New York: Raven, 1991.
15. Harris JH, Edeiken-Monroe B, Kopaniky DR. A practical classification of acute cervical spine injuries. Orthop Clin North Am 1986; 17:15–30.

16. Harris JH. Radiographic evaluation of spinal trauma. Orthop Clin North Am 1986; 17: 75–86.
17. Favero KJ, Van Petegham PK. The quadrangular fragment fracture: Roentgenographic features and treatment protocol. Clin Orthop 1989; 239:40–46.
18. Streitweiser DR, Knopp R, Wales LR, Williams JL, Tonnemacher K. Accuracy of standard radiographic views in detecting cervical spine fractures. Ann Emerg Med 1983; 12:538–542.
19. Clark CR, Ingram CM, El-Khoury GY, Ehara S. Radiographic evaluation of cervical spine injuries. Spine 1988; 13:742–747.
20. Freemyer B, Knopp R, Piche J, Wales L, Williams J. Comparison of five-view and three-view cervical spine series in the evaluation of patients with cervical trauma. Ann Emerg Med 1989; 18:818–821.
21. Vaccaro AR, An HS, Lin SS, Sun S, Balderston RA, Cotler JM. Noncontiguous injuries of the spine. J Spinal Disord 1992; 5:320–329.
22. Rizzolo SJ, Cotler JM. Unstable cervical spine injuries: Specific treatment approaches. J Am Acad Orthop Surg 1993; 1(1):57–63.
23. Stauffer ES. Wiring techniques of the posterior cervical spine for the treatment of trauma. Orthopedics 1988: 11:1543–1548.
24. Anderson PA, Henley MB, Grady MS, Montesano PX, Winn HR. Posterior cervical arthrodesis with AO reconstruction plates and bone graft. Spine 1991; 16:s72–79.
25. Bohler J, Gaudernak T. Anterior plate stabilization for fracture-dislocations of the lower cervical spine. J Trauma 1980; 20:203–205.
26. Cabenela ME, Ebersold MJ. Anterior plate stabilization for bursting teardrop fractures of the cervical spine. Spine 1988; 13:888–891.
27. Ripa DR, Kowall MG, Meyer PR, Rusin JJ. Series of ninety-two traumatic cervical spine injuries stabilized with anterior ASIF plate fusion technique. Spine 1991; 16:s46–55.
28. Meyer, PR. Cervical spine fractures: Changing management concepts. In: Bridwell KH, DeWald RL, eds. The Textbook of Spinal Surgery. Philadelphia: Lippincott-Raven, 1997:1679–1742.
29. Sutterlin III SE, McAfee PC, Warden KE, Rey RM Jr., Farey ID. A biomechanical evaluation of cervical spine stabilization methods in a bovine model. Static and cyclic loading. Spine 1988; 13:795–802.
30. Coe JD, Warden KE, Sutterlin III SE, McAfee PC. Biomechanical evaluation of cervical spine stabilization methods in a human cadaveric model. Spine 1989; 14:1122–1131.
31. Abei M, Mohler J, Zach GA, Morscher E. Indications, surgical technique, and results of 100 surgically treated fractures and fracture-dislocations of the cervical spine. Clin Orthop 1986:244–256.
32. Caspar W, Barbier DD, Klara PM. Anterior cervical fusion and Caspar plate stabilization for cervical trauma. Neurosurgery 1989; 25:491–502.
33. Suh PB, Kostuik JP, Esses SI. Anterior cervical plate fixation with the titanium hollow screw plate system. A preliminary report. Spine 1990; 15:1079–1080.
34. Garvey TA, Eismont FJ, Roberti LJ. Anterior decompression, structural bone grafting, and Caspar stabilization for unstable cervical spine fractures and/or dislocations. Spine 1992; 17(10 Suppl):S431–435.

16A

Vertical Compression Injuries of the Cervical Spine

ROBERT A. McGUIRE

University of Mississippi Medical Center, Jackson, Mississippi, U.S.A.

I INTRODUCTION

Cervical spine elements can fail by various methods, with the resulting injuries being described in multiple manners (1–4). Most of the injuries that occur do so as a result of a combination of two or more mechanical forces overpowering the stability of the spinal elements leading to failure. Allen et al. published a mechanistic classification to cervical spine injury that allows determination of the injury by the vectorial forces involved (1). This chapter discusses the vertical compression mode of failure.

II VERTICAL COMPRESSION

The failure mechanism for this injury is a loading of the spine in a neutral position with a pure compression force. Due to the positioning of the spine during failure, the transitional axis lies posterior to the anterior column and, as the severity of the injury increases, this mechanical vector causes the injured cephalad vertebral body to retrolisthes, resulting in severe canal compromise. These injuries tend to be located in the lower cervical spine.

These injuries can be divided into three stages, depending on the amount of compressive energy applied. Each has a distinct radiographic appearance determined by the injury severity. Stage 1 consists of a centrally directed fracture of either the superior or inferior endplate leading to a "cupping-type" deformity. There is no injury to either the anterior aspect of the vertebral body, posterior elements, or ligamentous structures in this stage. Stage 2 injury is present when fractures of both superior and inferior endplates occur. The fracture may extend through the vertebral body, but little or no displacement occurs and the ligaments remain intact (Fig. 1). Stage 3 lesions consist of continued progressive damage with fragmentation of the body in multiple directions. The posterior aspect of the body may be displaced into the canal leading to neural compromise. If the posterior arch remains intact, an acute kyphotic angle may occur at the injury site. If the posterior elements fail, posterior translation of the cephalad vertebrae upon the caudal vertebrae can occur. As the severity of vertebral body injury increases, there is a greater likelihood of posterior element involvement and resulting displacement.

III DIAGNOSIS AND TREATMENT

The use of routine cervical radiographs and CT scanning provides excellent evaluation of the bony detail of the injury, but often does not adequately assess the soft-tissue involvement. The use of magnetic resonance imaging provides a method to evaluate the disk, ligaments, and neural elements when determining the extent of these injuries (2).

Treatment of these injuries is determined by severity. Stage 1 and minimally displaced stage 2 fractures are stable injuries and can be adequately managed in a cervical orthosis. For the severely compressed stage 2 with acute kyphosis present, loss of anterior column support has occurred and can be reestablished with corpectomy, vertebral body reconstruction and stabilization with anterior plate fixation. Stage 3 injuries are grossly unstable and treatment begins in the emergency depart-

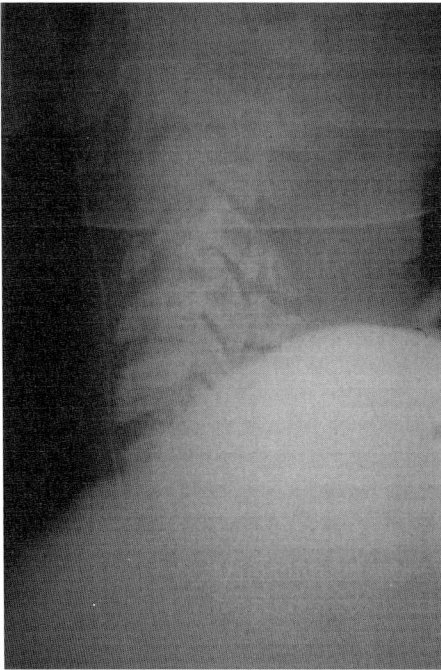

Figure 1   Lateral radiograph depicting a stage 2 vertical compression injury. Note the fracture of both the superior and inferior endplates of the fourth vertebrae with very little angulation or retropulsion of bone into the canal.

ment. Skeletal traction is applied to realign the spine and indirectly decompress the neural elements. Once this has been performed, definitive treatment can be instituted. Since the major destructive force is compression, the injured segment can be distracted, a corpectomy performed with decompression of the neural elements and reconstruction of the vertebral body using autograft, allograft, or cages with anterior plate stabilization. If the posterior elements have been fractured and are causing neural compromise, a posterior approach with decompression and stabilization using lateral mass plate and screw fixation may also be necessary.

IV CONCLUSIONS

A high index of suspicion must be present for vertical compression injuries of the cervical spine. The use of magnetic resonance imaging provides an excellent means for definitive diagnosis, especially in subtle injuries involving the cervicothoracic region. Surgical stabilization of unstable segments may be accomplished by either the anterior or posterior method. The anterior approach is the treatment of choice in cases of symptomatic anterior thecal sac compression.

REFERENCES

1. Allen BL, Fergusion RL, Lehmann TR, O'Brien RP. A mechanistic classification of closed, indirect fractures and dislocations of the lower cervical spine. Spine 1982; 7:1–27.
2. Kerslake RW, Jaspan T, Worthington BS. Magnetic resonance imaging of spinal trauma. Br J Radiol 1991; 64:386–402.
3. Taylor AR, Blackwood W. Paraplegia in hyperextension cervical injuries with normal radiographic appearance. J Bone Joint Surg 1948; 30B:245–248.
4. Klein GR, Vaccaro AR, Albert TJ, Schweitzer M, Deely D, Karasick DJM. Efficacy of magnetic resonance imaging in the evaluation of posterior cervical spine fractures. Spine 1999; 24:771–774.

16B

Distraction Extension Injuries of the Cervical Spine

ROBERT A. McGUIRE

University of Mississippi Medical Center, Jackson, Mississippi, U.S.A.

I INTRODUCTION

Cervical spine elements can fail by various methods, with the resulting injuries being described in multiple manners (1–4). Most injuries occur as a result of a combination of two or more mechanical forces overpowering the stability of the spinal elements, leading to failure. Allen et al. published a mechanistic classification to cervical spine injury that allows determination of the injury by the vectorial forces involved (1). This chapter discusses the distraction extension mode of failure.

II DISTRACTION EXTENSION INJURY

The failure mechanism for this injury is one of tension disruption of the anterior structures of the cervical spine as the force is directed away from the trunk and subsequently transmitted to the posterior elements as the force continues. These injuries can involve both bone and soft tissue structures, although the predominant component is the ligament and disk injury. A high index of suspicion must be present, as these injuries can be more severe than indicated on routine radiographs. Taylor and Blackwood described cases in which significant neurological deficit occurred in patients in whom the radiographs appeared innocuous (3).

There have been two stages described by Allen et al. of this injury. Stage 1 consists of either failure of the anterior longitudential ligament and disk or a transverse nondeforming fracture of the vertebral body without translation. Stage 2 occurs when the force is continued posteriorly, causing disruption of the posterior column, allowing retrolisthesis of the cephalad vertebrae upon the caudal vertebra resulting in potential canal compromise (Fig. 1).

III DIAGNOSIS AND TREATMENT

A high index of suspicion is needed to detect this injury, as radiographs often reveal only subtle abnormalities. Often a subtle widening of the disk space is all that will be evident on the initial radiographs. A small avulsion of the anterior margin of either the cephalad or caudal vertebral body with widening of the prevertebral soft tissue space may be present. Evidence of trauma to the face and forehead will give a hint of the possible mechanism to produce this injury. The use of magnetic resonance imaging is an excellent method to detect this injury, as it is predominantly soft tissue in origin. This technique has been shown to have some problems in detecting and evaluating body posterior column injury in some cases (4).

Once the injury is diagnosed, spinal realignment is performed with the preservation of neural function of paramount importance. Great care must be used in the application of traction in this type of injury, as even the addition of small amounts of force can result in over-distraction through the injured segment (Fig. 2).

If the injury has not destroyed all soft tissue restraints and no neurological deficits exist, then the cervical spine can be immobilized with halo stabilization. The

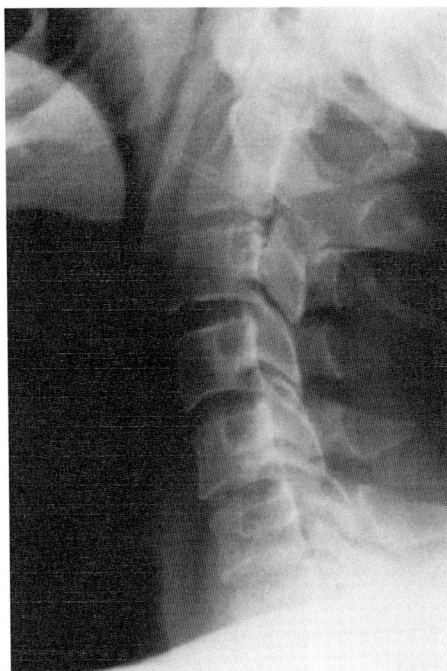

Figure 1   Lateral radiograph revealing failure of the inferior endplate attachment of the anterior longitudinal ligament, widening of the disk space, and retrolisthesis of C3 on C4. This translation classifies this injury as a stage 2 distraction extension failure mode.

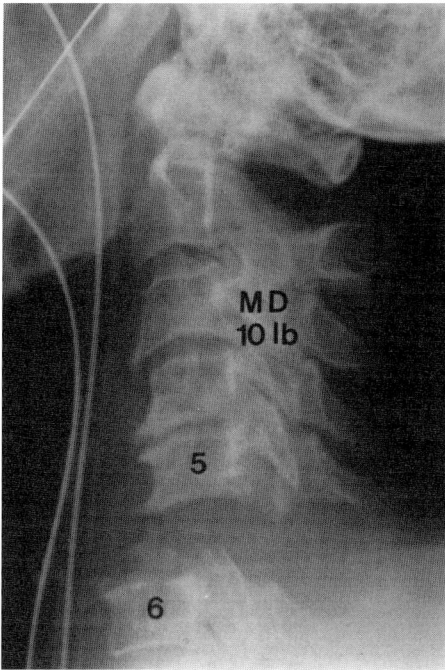

Figure 2   Potentially unstable distraction extension injury. Great care must be used to diagnose the injury correctly prior to adding skeletal traction. As can be seen from this radiograph, the addition of only a small amount of weight led to overdistraction through the injured segment.

bony injury will heal and often the injury through the disk space will ossify reestablishing stability.

Definitive surgical treatment can be provided by either the anterior or posterior route. The use of anterior plate fixation following diskectomy and bone grafting or posterior lateral mass plate fixation following bone grafting reestablishes spinal stability and protects neurological function.

IV   CONCLUSION

Close periodic radiographic follow-up is necessary in patients managed nonoperatively with distraction extension cervical injuries.

Gradual retrolithesis of the cephalad on caudal vertebral segments may result in symptomatic neurological decline, if not detected early. A low threshold for surgical intervention is often recommended with this injury subtype.

REFERENCES

1. Allen BL, Fergusion RL, Lehmann TR, O'Brien RP. A mechanistic classification of closed, indirect fractures and dislocations of the lower cervical spine. Spine 1982; 7:1–27.

2. Kerslake RW, Jaspan T, Worthington BS. Magnetic resonance imaging of spinal trauma. Br J Radiol 1991; 64:386–402.
3. Taylor AR, Blackwood W. Paraplegia in hyperextension cervical injuries with normal radiographic appearance. J Bone Joint Surg 1948; 30B:245–248.
4. Klein GR, Vaccaro AR, Albert TJ, Schweitzer M, Deely D, Karasick DJM. Efficacy of magnetic resonance imaging in the evaluation of posterior cervical spine fractures. Spine 1999; 24:771–774.

17A

Compression Extension Injuries

FEDERICO P. GIRARDI and FRANK P. CAMMISA, Jr.

Hospital for Special Surgery, Weill Medical College of Cornell University, New York, New York, U.S.A.

I INTRODUCTION

This type of cervical injury, originally described by Forsyth (1), is characterized by a fracture of the posterior elements.

The concept of compression extension injuries was readvocated by Allen and coworkers (2), who classified this mechanism into stages; however, the classification was thought to be somewhat hypothetical, at least for the advanced stages.

Stage 1 consists of a unilateral, vertebral arch fracture with or without vertebral body displacement. Stage 2 consists of a bilaminar fracture without evidence of other injuries. Stage 3 consists of bilateral vertebral arch fractures-articular processes, pedicles, lamina, or some bilateral combination without vertebral body displacement. Stage 4 consists of bilateral vertebral arch fractures with partial vertebral body width displacement anteriorly. Stage 5 involves bilateral vertebral arch fracture with full vertebral body width displacement anteriorly. This lesion generally involves a rotational component as well results in rotational instability. This mechanism however, could account for articular mass separation or facet fractures.

Extension of the initial injury to the lamina or pedicle is not unusual. Anterior column involvement with either bony or disk disruption is also possible (3). As a result, rotatory spondylolisthesis can occur by rotation of the superior vertebral body around the intact contralateral lateral mass.

It is important to realize that the injury pattern in cervical spine injuries is a result of a combination of force (energy) impact as well as the direction of the force vector. A high level of impact could produce either a three-column injury or just an isolated facet fracture (Fig. 1) (posterior column injury) (4). Furthermore, there may be a combination of vector forces, including those resulting in hyperextension. Ex-

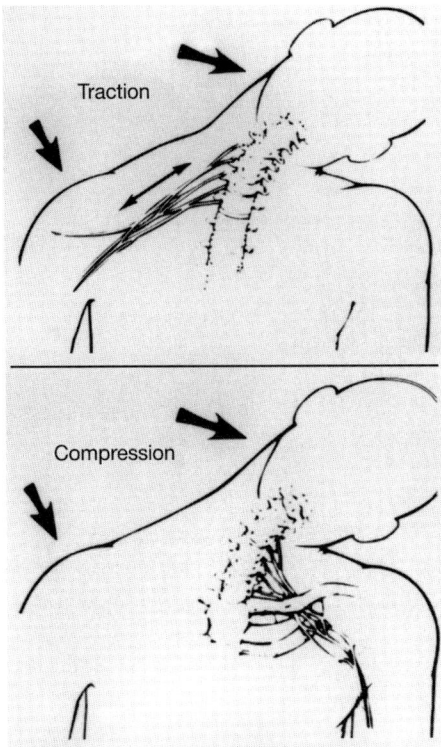

Figure 1   Diagram showing that a lateral flexion–type injury may produce traction and compression on opposite sides.

perimentally, it has been found that injuries to the spine are more severe in extension trauma (3). Extension trauma results in more severe pedicle injuries, often manifesting in rotational instability. Panjabi et al. (5) reported their findings on a porcine model. They ascertained that the extension-compression mechanism produced the greatest instabilities in axial rotation and lateral bending compared with other mechanisms.

The extension-compression mechanism may cause minimal or no bony lesion; however, it may cause the occurrence of "stingers" or transient cord neuropraxia in patients with cervical spine stenosis following a traumatic event (6–9). Patients with a compression-extension fracture mechanism often have facial or anterior scalp trauma, indicating that the mechanism was primarily extension and rotation (10).

Its characteristic pattern involves a fracture through the pedicle and a longitudinal fracture through the lamina, parallel to the articular process on the same side. It occurs most commonly as a unilateral injury; however, bilateral lesions can occur.

The rotationally unstable fracture pattern may either appear innocuous both radiographically and clinically or present as an unstable fracture configuration with neurological injury.

Ligamentous injuries above or below the involved area may also be present. This type of lesion generally creates two levels of instability. Therefore, this rotational unstable condition often requires stabilization of more than one level. Furthermore, any of these fractures can occur in multiple combinations.

It has been reported that 25% of patients with unilateral vertebral arch fractures have a radiculopathy, and 12.5% a central cord lesion in one original series (2). These rates may increase if this injury occurs in patients with a narrow spinal canal or previous spondylotic pathology.

Radiographic findings in this type of injury are very similar to those seen in other unilateral facet injuries. It may be difficult to detect this fracture by routine plain radiographs (11,12). The lateral radiograph may show a "horizontalization" of the lateral mass as it rotates after the injury. This fracture pattern may be radiologically confused with a unilateral facet dislocation, in that both may show evidence of anterior subluxation. The unilateral facet dislocation is a result of a very different mechanism, which involves a flexion-distraction injury (2). The AP radiograph may help to visualize an associated lamina fracture. The injury is best visualized on CT scan (Fig. 2), which may show the extent of the bony lesion and possible extension into the pedicle or through the vertebral artery foramen (13). Associated ligamentous injury and disk herniation are best demonstrated by magnetic resonance imaging (MR) (11–15). Halliday et al. (16) found that plain radiographs lack sensitivity to detect the presence of lateral mass/facet fractures. Furthermore, they concluded that the appearance of the fracture on computed tomography does not indicate instability. The amount of soft tissue disruption demonstrated on MRI correlated with the instability found in these series of patients.

II TREATMENT

Reports in the literature regarding the treatment of this type of cervical injury are rare. Some injuries of the subaxial cervical spine are treated appropriately by nonoperative means. Nonoperative treatment with external immobilization may also play a role in pediatric injuries where there is an exceptional healing potential. On the

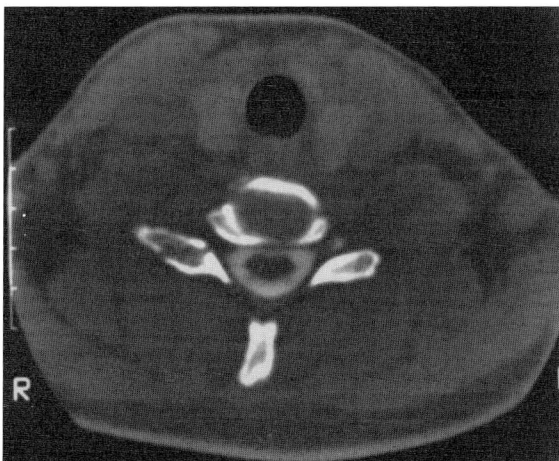

Figure 2 Myelogram followed by axial CT scan demonstrating a fracture of the right C6 lateral mass.

other hand, in the presence of cervical instability, compression of the neural elements, or both, surgical management is often necessary. Many have found that brace or halo vest immobilization proved unreliable in maintaining rotational stability (17–20). Bucholz and Cheung (21) documented a 17% failure rate of halo-vest immobilization for a fractured facet. As a result of this failure rate, they recommended primary fusion for facet injuries with subluxation.

Operative stabilization may be indicated for unilateral lateral mass fractures that present with subluxation or that have injured the facet capsule, intraspinous ligaments, anterior longitudinal ligament, or posterior longitudinal ligament.

The cervical injury may be classified as "major" when there is either radiographically or CT evidence of instability with or without neurological findings and/ or has the potential to produce them at a later stage. These injuries may present with displacement of more than 2 mm in any plane, wide vertebral body in any plane, a widened interspinous/interlaminar space, subluxated facet joints, a vertebral burst fracture, or locked or perched facets (unilateral or bilateral) on CT scan examination (22).

If surgery is indicated, a posterior approach is usually preferred for the majority of unilateral or bilateral facet injuries, unless there is significant anterior column disruption (17). The surgical stabilization used for the facet fractures should take into consideration any deforming forces and instabilities caused by the trauma.

The goals of surgery should be to obtain and maintain satisfactory alignment, promote fusion, and allow safe and early mobilization.

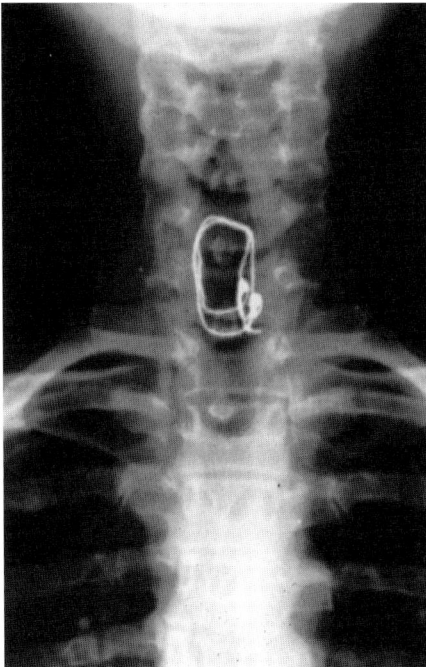

Figure 3 Postoperative AP radiograph showing a C6–C7 posterior fusion with interspinous wiring fixation.

Biomechanical data showed (23) that anterior plate fixation alone is not enough for stabilization in cadaveric cervical spines with bilateral facetectomies. Posterior alone or combined anterior and posterior procedures may be necessary.

Choosing a method of posterior cervical stabilization is dependent on the surgeon's experience and preference (24). Coe et al. (25) have suggested that there is no significant biomechanical difference between any of the posterior stabilization methods. Ebraheim et al. (26) reported their results with posterior plating of 22 patients with traumatic instability with very good results and no major complications. Unfortunately, wiring is not always ideal because of the high association of laminar and lateral mass fractures in this pattern.

The authors generally treat these injuries with posterior methods such as posterior lateral mass plate fixation (26–29). However, we still use the Bohlman triple-wire and other wiring techniques, depending on the type of injury and levels involved (Figs. 3 and 4). There may be a role for pedicle screw fixation at C7 and T1, especially in the face of deficient posterior elements or bilateral laminar fractures. This technique is more demanding and may be done more safely under computerized frameless stereotactic image guidance (30).

Posterior techniques alone are usually sufficient unless there is also anterior cord or nerve root compression or the lack of anterior column support. Posterior plating techniques (31,32) are able to control rotational instability, but if anterior column deficiencies exist, a residual kyphosis might develop (17). In these rare situations, an anterior procedure (decompression, reduction, and stabilization) is performed.

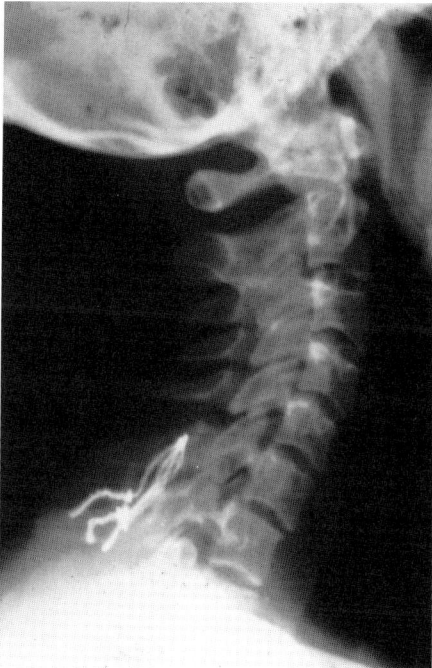

Figure 4   Postoperative lateral radiograph showing a C6–C7 posterior fusion with interspinous wiring fixation.

Some authors recommend anterior surgery for all of these injuries to avoid posterior muscle injury, facet disruption, and possible development of a late deformity (17,30,31).

Final recommendations regarding the best treatment for each particular clinical scenario will only be available after completion of prospective randomized treatment trials and respective outcome assessments.

REFERENCES

1. Forsyth HF. Extension injuries of the cervical spine. J Bone Joint Surg 1964;46A:1792–1797.
2. Allen BL, Ferguson RL, Lehmann TR, O'Brien RP. A mechanistic classification of closed, indirect fractures of closed, indirect fractures and dislocations of the lower cervical spine. Spine 1982;7:1–27.
3. Southern EP, Oxland TR, Panjabi MM, Duranceau JS. Cervical spine injury in three modes of high-speed trauma: A biomechanical porcine model. J Spinal Disord 1990; 3(4):316–328.
4. Zhu Q, Ouyang J, Lu W, Li Z, Guo X, Zhong S. Traumatic instabilities of the cervical spine caused by high-speed axial compression in a human model. An in vitro biomechanical study. Spine 1999;24:440–444.
5. Panjabi MM, Duranceau JS, Oxland TR, Bowen CE. Multidirectional instabilities of traumatic cervical spine injuries in a porcine model. Spine 1989;14(10):1111–1115.
6. Meyer SA, Schultse KR, Callaghan JJ, Albright JP, Powell JW, Crowley ET, el-Khoury GY. Cervical spinal stenosis and stingers in collegiate football players. Am J Sports Med 1994;22(2):158–166.
7. Torg JS, Pavlov H, Genuario SE, Sennett B, Wisneski RJ, Robie BH, Jahre C. Neurapraxia of the cervical spinal cord with transient quadriplegia. J Bone Joint Surg 1986; 68A:1354–1370.
8. Torg JS, Corcoran TA, Thibault LE, Pavlov H, Sennett B, Naranja RJ, Priano S. Cervical cord neurapraxia: classification, pathomechanics, morbidity, and management guidelines. J Neurosurg 1997;87:843–850
9. Levitz CI, Reilly PJ, Torg JS. The pathomechanics of chronic, recurrent cervical nerve root neurapraxia. The chronic burner syndrome. Am J Sports Med 1997;25:73–76.
10. Taylor JR, Twomey LT. Acute injuries to cervical joints: An autopsy study of neck sprain. Spine 1993;18:1115–1122.
11. Harris JH, Mirvis SE. The Radiology of Acute Cervical Spine Trauma, 3rd ed. Baltimore: Williams & Wilkins, 1996:320–339.
12. Woodring JH, Lee C. limitations of cervical radiography in the evaluation of acute cervical trauma. J Trauma 1993;34:32–39.
13. Schaefer DM, Flanders AM Northup BE, Doan HT, Osterholm JL. Magnetic resonance imaging of acute cervical spine trauma: correlation with severity of neurologic injury. Spine 1989;14:1090–1095.
14. Silberstein M, Tress BM, Hennessy O. Prevertebral swelling in cervical spine injury: identification of ligamentous injury with magnetic resonance imaging. Clin Radiol 1992; 46:318–323.
15. Katzberg RW, Benedetti PF, Drake CM, Ivanovic M, Levine RA, Beatty CS, Nemzek WR, McFall RA, Ontell FK, Bishop DM, Poirier VC, Chong BW. Acute cervical spine injuries: prospective MR imaging assessment at a level 1 trauma center. Radiology 1999; 213:203–212.
16. Halliday AL, Henderson BR, Hart BL, Benzel EC. The management of unilateral mass/facet fractures of the subaxial cervical spine. Spine 1997;22:2614–2621.

17. Lifeso RM, Colucci MA. Anterior fusion for rotationally unstable cervical spine fractures. Spine 2000;25:2028–2034.
18. Anderson PA, Budorick, Easton KB, Henley MB, Salciccioli GG. Failure of halo vest to prevent in vivo motion in patients with injured cervical spines. Spine 1991;16:S501–S505.
19. Sears W, Fazl M. Prediction of stability of cervical spine fractures managed in the halo vest and indications for surgical interventions. J Neurosurg 1990;72:426–432.
20. Whitehill R, Richman JA, Glaser JA. Failure of immobilization of the cervical spine by the halo vest: a report of five cases. J Bone Joint Surg 1986;68A:326–332.
21. Bucholz RD, Cheung KC. Halo vest versus spinal fusion for cervical injury: evidence from an outcome study. J Neurosurg 1989;70:884–892.
22. Daffner RH, Brown RR, Glodberg AL. A new classification for cervical vertebral injuries: influence of CT. Skeletal Radiol 2000;29:125–132.
23. Spivak JM, Bharam S, Chen D, Kummer FJ. Internal fixation of cervical trauma following corpectomy and reconstruction. The effects of posterior element injury. Bull Hosp Joint Dis 2000;59(1):47–51.
24. Davis J. Injuries to the subaxial cervical spine: Posterior approach options. Orthopedics 1997;20:929–933.
25. Coe JD, Warden KE, Sutterlin CE 3rd, McAfee PC. Biomechanical evaluation of cervical spine stabilization methods in a human cadaveric model. Spine 1989;14:1122–1131.
26. Ebraheim NA, Rupp RE, Savolaine ER, Brown JA. Posterior plating of the cervical spine. J Spinal Disord 1995;8(2):111–115.
27. Roy-Camille R, Mazel G, Saillant G. Les fractures-separation du massif articulatire. In: Roy-Camille R, ed. Rachis Cervical Inferieur: Sixiemes Journees D'Orthopedie de la Pitie. Paris: Masson, 1988:94–103.
28. Anderson PA, Henley MB, Grady MS, Montesano PX, Winn HR. Posterior cervical arthrodesis with AO reconstruction plates and bone graft. Spine 1991;16:S72–79
29. Nazarian SM, Louis RP. Posterior internal fixation with screw plates in traumatic lesions of the cervical spine. Spine 1991;16:S64–S71.
30. Cammisa FP, Parvataneni KH, Girardi FP, Khan SN, Sandhu HS. Computerized frameless stereotactic image-guided spinal surgery. Bull Hosp Joint Dis 2000;59:17–26.
31. Bohler J, Gaudernack T. Anterior plate stabilization for fracture dislocations of the lower cervical spine. J Trauma 1980;20:203–205.
32. deOliveira JC. Anterior plate fixation of traumatic lesions of the cervical spine. Spine 1987;12:324–329.

17B

Lateral Flexion Injuries

FEDERICO P. GIRARDI and FRANK P. CAMMISA, Jr.

Hospital for Special Surgery, Weill Medical College of Cornell University, New York, New York, U.S.A.

I INTRODUCTION

This lesion consists of anasymmetric compression fracture of the vertebral body, disk, and posterior arch on the ipsilateral side. Similar patterns of anterior (bone and disk) and posterior compression may occur with different degrees of axial rotation superimposed on the initial lateral flexion–injury vector (1,2).

The stage 1 lesion consists of asymmetric compression fracture of the vertebral centrum plus a vertebral arch fracture on the ipsilateral side without displacement of the arch on the anterior–posterior (AP) view.

The lateral flexion stage 2 lesion has both asymmetric compression of the centrum and either an ipsilateral vertebral arch fracture with displacement on the AP view or ligamentous failure on the contralateral side with separation of the articular processes (1).

Lateral flexion of the cervical spine may cause a sagittally oriented fracture of the lateral mass with shearing of all or part of the lateral mass off the vertebral body.

This type of injury may be seen more commonly in patients with disk degeneration and associated cervical lateral flexion instability (3).

No neurological injury is usually associated with this type of trauma. However, brachial plexus and spinal cord injury have been reported (1,4). It is conceivable that compressive lateral flexion and distractive lateral flexion mechanisms may coexist (Fig. 1). Traumatic dissection of the extracranial carotid artery caused by severe stretching of the artery over a cervical vertebral transverse process has been reported (5). The mechanism of injury was thought to be a sudden hyperextension and lateral flexion of the spine causing a spinal fracture and vascular injury.

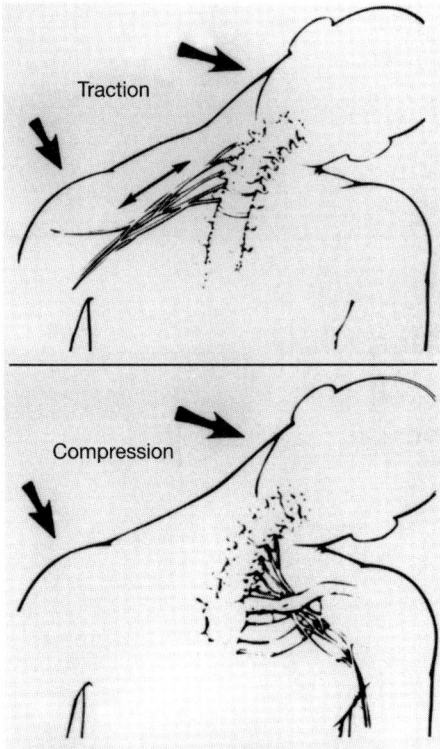

Figure 1   Diagram showing that a lateral flexion–type injury may produce traction and compression on opposite sides.

Cervical lateral flexion injuries may result from motor vehicle accidents or sports-related trauma such as football. Special orthoses have been developed to prophylactically limit motion and prevent the nerve injury known as "burners." These devices try to limit both hyperextension and lateral bending of the cervical spine (6). There has been an increase in these injuries by the sudden lateral air-bag deployment in car collisions (7).

Lateral cervical spine radiographs may demonstrate the presence of a sagittal lateral mass fracture with malalignment or widening of the facet joints. Displaced fracture fragments of the articular pillars, vertebral body, and the transverse and uncinate processes may be discernible. Vertebral subluxation or rotation and displacement of the spine above the level of injury may be evident as well. The anterior–posterior radiograph may show an asymmetric compression fracture of the vertebral body. However, it is very important to understand that radiographs could have a normal appearance as well. Oblique radiographs might be helpful in some cases, although, CT scan with sagittal reformatting will better outline the fracture pattern, while an MRI will illustrate associated soft tissue injuries (Fig. 2). As with other spinal fractures, it is not uncommon to have concomitant spinal lesions caused by different mechanisms. Therefore, it is imperative to examine fully the patient clinically and radiographically for other noncontiguous injuries.

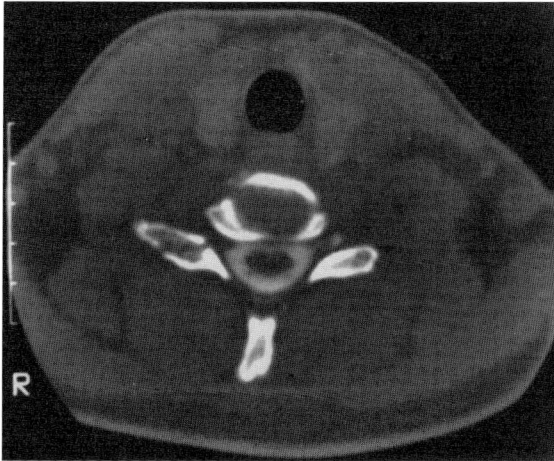

Figure 2 Myelogram followed by axial CT scan demonstrating a fracture of the right C6 lateral mass.

Lateral flexion injuries may be unstable, and neurological compromise, including paraplegia, hemiplegia, and radiculopathy has been reported (1,4). There is a wide range of bony and soft-tissue disruption patterns that may result with associated neurological compromise depending on the principal force vector and the energy dissipated at impact.

II TREATMENT

Many of these injuries can be treated by nonoperative means. However, in the presence of cervical instability, compression of the neural elements, or both, surgical management is often necessary.

Cervical lesions caused by lateral flexion mechanisms are treated with the same surgical principles of extension-compression injuries. A posterior approach and fusion with internal fixation is usually required for the treatment of unstable injuries. We prefer the use of screws and lateral mass plate fixation; however, the use of wiring techniques has shown satisfactory results (8).

Posterior techniques alone are usually sufficient, unless there is also anterior cord or nerve root compression or lack of anterior column support. Severe lateral compression fractures with significant anterior and middle column collapse may need anterior column reconstruction. In these rare situations, an anterior procedure (decompression, reduction, and stabilization) is necessary.

REFERENCES

1. Allen BL, Ferguson, RL, Lehmann TR, O'Brien RP. A mechanistic classification of closed, indirect fractures and dislocations of the lower cervical spine. Spine 1982; 7:1–27.
2. Crowell RR, Shea M, Edwards WT, Clothiaux PL, White AA 3rd, Hayes WC. Cervical injuries under flexion and compression loading. J Spinal Discord 1993;6(2):175–181.

3. Dai L. Disc degeneration and cervical instability. Correlation of magnetic resonance imaging with radiography. Spine 1998;23:1734–1738.
4. Lee C, Woodring JH. Sagittally oriented fractures of the lateral masses of the cervical vertebrae. Trauma-Injury Infec Crit Care 1991;31:1638–1643.
5. Stringer WL, Kelly DL, Jr. Traumatic dissection of the extracranial internal carotid artery. Neurosurgery 1980;6:123–130.
6. Hovis WD, Limbird TJ. An evaluation of cervical orthosis in limiting hyperextension and lateral flexion in football. Med Sci Sports Exerc 1994;26(7):872–876.
7. Martin PG, Crandall JR, Pilkey WD. Injury trends of passenger car drivers in frontal crashed in the USA. Accid Anal Prev 2000;32:541–557
8. Roy-Camille R, Mazel G, Saillant G. Les fractures-separation du massif articulatire. In: Roy-Camille R, ed. Rachis Cervical Inferieur: Sixiemes Journees D'Orthopedie de la Pitie. Paris: Masson, 1988:94–103.

18

Lateral Mass Fractures of the Cervical Spine: Diagnosis and Surgical Management

AARON A. COHEN-GADOL, PAULINO YANEZ, W. R. MARSH, and MARK DEKUTOSKI

Mayo Clinic and Mayo Foundation, Rochester, Minnesota, U.S.A.

I EPIDEMIOLOGY

Lateral mass fractures of the cervical spine are most commonly caused by extension or flexion injuries of the neck that force the facets into distraction or compression. Facet injuries can elude the inexperienced reviewer on the survey lateral cervical spine x-rays. Their recognition has been enhanced by the advent of computerized tomography (CT) using reconstruction views. Radiographic imaging, however, needs to be combined with clinical evaluation of the patient. Specifically, the posterior column needs to be assessed to avoid missed injuries. Facet injuries include a wide spectrum of ligamentous and/or osseous findings. Their varied descriptions have created confusion regarding their diagnostic and therapeutic recommendations.

The true incidence of facet injuries is not well defined. While it is assumed that a thorough evaluation is performed in an acute trauma setting, a number of facet injuries are initially missed. This may explain their presentation in a delayed setting with neck pain and no previous evaluation. Facet injuries represented 6.7% of all the cervical spine fractures treated at one institution over a 12-year interval (1). Unilateral and bilateral facet injuries were most common at the C6–C7 level. Bilateral facet injuries are commonly associated with neurological deficits. These deficits include either root and/or cord syndromes. The presenting patients may have associated head injuries or impaired consciousness due to drug or alcohol intoxication. These factors can limit the clinical examination.

A   Presentation

The cervical spine controls the position of the head relative to the thorax. Direct trauma, acceleration, or deceleration moments may displace the cervical spine outside its "normal" range. Neurological injury may occur from the initial cord deformation or later instability. The initial force to the spine and resulting translation of bony elements into the canal and neural foramen may determine the presenting neurological features. Trauma can also result in ligamentous disruption and instability, leading to progressive deformity. The premorbid canal dimensions play an important role in the degree of neural injury incurred by the trauma. Patients with congenital narrow canals are at a greater risk of developing radiculopathy, myelopathy, or their combinations as a result of "limited" trauma.

The initial spine trauma evaluation requires a detailed neurological exam and palpation for interspinous tenderness or step off. Unilateral facet injuries may present only as persistent neck pain without any obvious radiographic findings. Subsequent CT or MRI imaging can add to the diagnostic yield. Delayed diagnosis of an asymptomatic unilateral facet subluxation has occurred in up to 40% of the patients (2).

Unilateral facet fractures and dislocations commonly cause radiculopathy. Midline cord compression from a disk can present with a myelopathy or asymmetrically with a Brown–Sequard pattern of injury. Rorabeck reported 26 patients with unilateral facet fractures: three had cord and 11 had root injuries (2). In another study, 29% of the patients with unilateral facet dislocations had neurological involvement. In this study, 68% had radicular symptoms and 24% had mixed evidence of cord injury (3).

Bilateral facet injuries have a greater incidence of causing cord injury and myelopathy. Vertebral translation can lead to the deformity of the spinal cord secondary to elongation and compression. In the acute setting, evidence of cord trauma should merit initiation of the methylprednisolone protocol. This is given as a bolus of 30 mg/kg body weight over 15 min followed by a drip at 5.4 mg/kg/h for the subsequent 23 h. Rizzolo reported 40 and 80% rates of disk injury in unilateral and bilateral facet dislocations, respectively (4). This high rate of disk injury becomes an important factor in the closed reduction of these injuries. The displaced disk may cause further narrowing of the canal during reduction under anesthesia. This will be discussed later.

B   Radiographic Evaluation

According to ATLS guidelines, the detailed neurological and spine evaluation should be deferred until the secondary survey. Attention to the primary survey and avoidance of hypotension is critical to avoid secondary ischemic insult to the compromised cord. A three-view cervical spine x-ray series (PA, lateral, odontoid views) should be reviewed prior to obtaining axial imaging, obliques, or flexion extension films. Oblique radiographs may add to the specificity of diagnosis but generally not to its sensitivity. Inspection of the cervical films for rotational malalignment on the PA and lateral views as well as offsets in the anterior body, dorsal body, or spinal laminar line are all critical (Fig. 1). Facet fractures may be evident on lateral C-spine x-rays (Fig. 2). The review of facet congruity on an oblique view is shown in Figure 3.

Widening of the spinous processes may be evident in unilateral and bilateral facet injuries. The "bow-tie" sign seen in the lateral film is caused by visualization

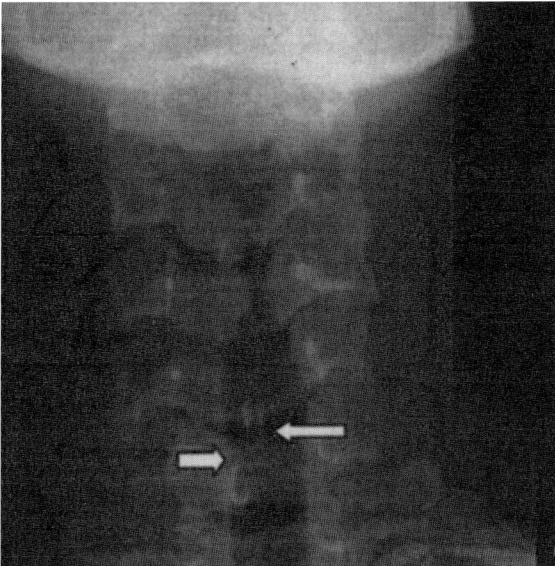

Figure 1 Malalignment of the spinous processes as illustrated in this lateral mass fracture.

of both subluxed facets at the level of the injury (5) (Fig. 4). Anterior subluxation of 3 to 5 mm (about 25% of vertebral body width) on lateral imaging is generally associated with unilateral facet dislocation. A displacement greater than 5 to 7 mm (about 50%) suggests bilateral facet dislocation. Facet fractures can be mobile and may reduce spontaneously in the supine position. Attention to the significant degree of soft tissue injury associated with these radiographic findings is critical.

Computerized tomography (CT) is the study of choice for visualization of lateral pillar injuries. Axial cuts alone may at times be parallel to the plane of fracture. This imaging modality will miss the fracture site. Therefore, spiral imaging algorithms with 2D or 3D reconstructions are invaluable in disclosing these fracture patterns. The "empty" or "naked" facet sign on axial CT is almost pathognomonic of a facet dislocation. The "floating" facet signifies a fracture through the pedicle with a second parallel fracture in the ipsilateral lamina (Fig. 5).

The application of prereduction MRI in the setting of facet fractures has been controversial. Even though up to 60% of patients (see above) may have disk injuries, neurological deterioration during closed reduction of the awake patient is extremely rare. Only a minority of the patients with a large disk herniation require open diskectomy prior to reduction. Performing MRI in a neurologically compromised patient will further delay the reduction of dislocation and neural decompression. The indications for MRI are as follows:

1. Evidence of a neurological deficit not accounted for by the findings on x-rays and CT.
2. Deterioration during awake closed reduction using traction.
3. Planned reduction under general anesthesia.
4. Failure of closed reduction methods.

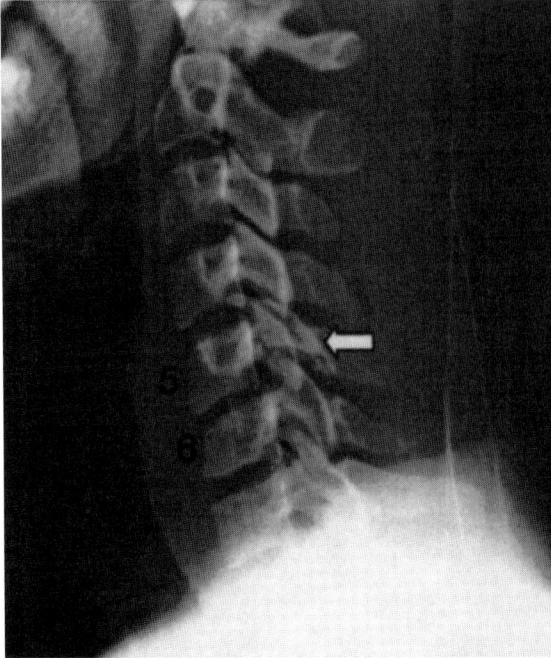

Figure 2   Lateral spine x-ray demonstrating the facet fracture at C5. This fracture in its milder forms may be easily overlooked by the inexperienced reviewer.

C Mechanisms of Injury

A mechanistic classification of cervical spine injuries was described by Thomas Ducker, Robert Bellegarrigue, and Mark Carol in the late 1970s. These categories have been based upon the clockface head position and dominant moment of force and were popularized by Ferguson and Allen (6). This illustration of vectors of force is presented in the chapter dealing with distractive flexion injuries of the cervical spine. The Ferguson and Allen classification is a description of the spectrum of osseous and ligamentous injuries involved in cervical spine trauma. Facet fractures most commonly occur during three major vectors of force: distraction, compression, and/or lateral bending. The other various mechanisms can be subclassified under these three.

Injury to facets and posterior ligaments occur most commonly in compression and tension mechanisms. The laminae, facets, facet capsules, ligamentum flavum, and interspinous ligaments are most commonly disrupted in tension. Compressive injuries to the posterior elements do occur and can manifest occult instability. Compression injuries to the cervical vertebra have been globally referred to as "teardrop" or "burst" fractures. These two terms lack sufficient specificity to warrant their continued use.

1 Distraction

The major classifications follow by prevalence. Distractive flexion (DFS1–4) injuries occur with forces in the 8:00 to 11:00 direction (see Chap. 14). These comprise 37%

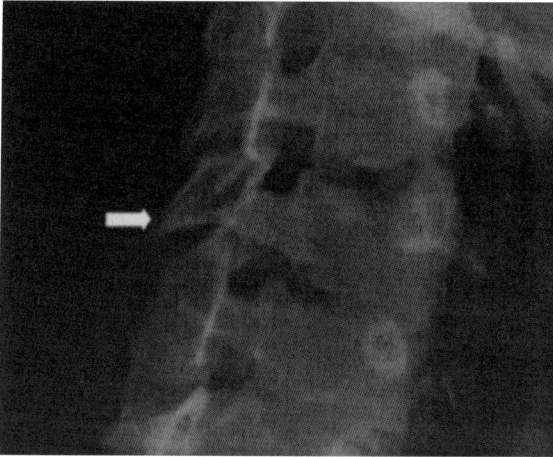

Figure 3 Oblique view of the lateral mass fracture depicted in Figure 2. This view of the spine allows improved visualization of the facets.

of the injuries in Allen's series. DFS1–4 injuries occur with flexion or deceleration trauma and include all unilateral and bilateral facet dislocations. They cause different degrees of injury to the posterior ligaments and therefore result in the loss of the posterior tension band. In this mechanism, the shearing component of injury may cause avulsion fracture of the superior facets, with the fracture possibly extending into the lamina. If the shearing force is significant, the posterior longitudinal ligament and the disk may be disrupted enough to cause noted instability.

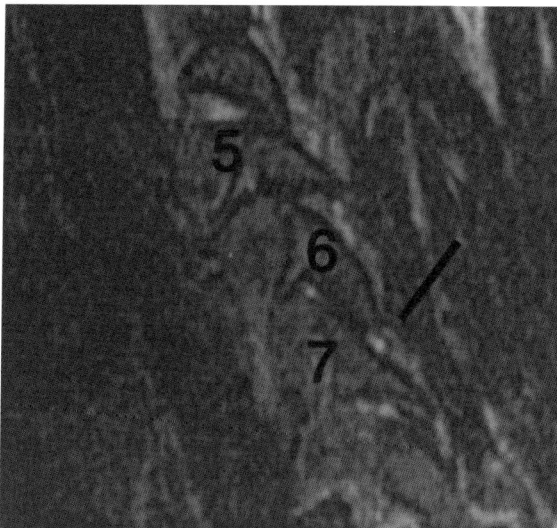

Figure 4 Sagittal MRI of the spine illustrating the facet dislocation (C5,C6.) Please note the "bow-tie" sign at C5.

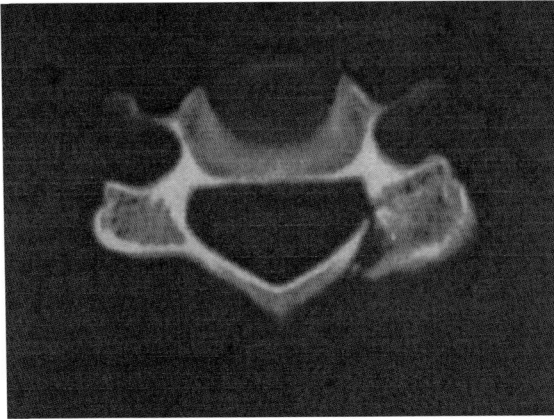

Figure 5 Axial CT of the spine showing the left laminar and facet fractures. This creates a "floating" lateral mass.

Flexion and shearing vectors may also cause bilateral inferior articular process fractures, even though the shearing component may be less prominent in this pattern of fracture (7). The unilateral facet injuries, unlike their bilateral counterparts, are often associated with additional rotational moments. This rotation contributes to the malalignment of the spinous processes on the PA x-rays (Fig. 1). Unilateral facet fracture with contralateral facet dislocation is rare and is caused by lateral bending/flexion/rotation injury mechanisms.

Distractive extension injuries (DES1–2) occur with neck hyperextension or sudden acceleration from rear impact and are represented on the clockface in the 1:00 to 3:00 direction. Though rare in Allen's series (5%), these injuries in their milder form (stage 1) can manifest as a central cord syndrome, commonly after falls in the older patients with a spondylitic cervical spine. In higher stages, there is significant anterior ligamentous injury with subsequent transmission of the vector force to the posterior elements, causing ligamentous tears and compression facet fractures.

Neurological injury is most commonly associated with pure flexion injuries. This greater degree of neurological injury is felt to be due to both cord traction with the flexion moment as well as compression between the subluxating cephalad lamina, which narrows the spinal canal over the cephalad aspect of the residual inferior disk and body.

2 Compression

Compression flexion injuries are divided into several subtypes. In stages 4 and 5 of flexion compression mechanism, posterior elements may lose their integrity. In stage 5, the articular facets are separated. Displacement of the adjacent segments indicates significant anterior and posterior longitudinal ligament injuries. Compressive flexion (CFS1–5) injuries result from falls or impacts on the top or back of the head with axial loading. This is a common injury seen in football "spearing" tackles/accidents, and comprises 22% of Allen's series.

Flexion compression phylogeny may cause significant facet capsule and disk disruption. This may lead to anterior translation with superior and inferior articular fractures, as discussed above. Vertical compression (VCS1–3) injuries are less common (8%) and occur with direct axial loading. The presence of posterior element disruption predisposes these injuries to significant instability.

3 Lateral Bending

Lateral flexion (LFS1–2) injuries occur by a lateral head impact with asymmetric loading. These injuries may manifest solely as neck pain and are often associated with radicular findings. Asymmetric lateral body or uncovertebral joint fractures with contralateral ligamentous injuries may cause angulation and coronal displacement. A lateral mass fracture associated with a pedicle fracture is actually a dual motion segment injury. These are characterized by instability of the articulation above and below the pedicle. They can cause a rotational subluxation and/or flexion/extension instability. Their myelopathic or radiculopathic signs and symptoms can originate from the level above and/or below the injured pedicle.

D Treatment

Early detection of symptomatic canal compromise and reduction of the dislocation expediently with early axial traction is critical. Reduction of the step-off associated with fracture dislocation of the cervical spine restores spinal canal volume. In the canine cord compression model, the duration of cord compression was inversely related to neurological recovery. Patients with preoperative neurological deficits need to maintain cervical alignment during examination, transport, and imaging procedures. Anatomical alignment will aid in restoration of the space available for the cord and will aid in the definitive stabilization or immobilization options chosen.

1 Ligamentous Injuries

The principal ligaments injured in cervical trauma are interspinous/supraspinous ligaments, facet capsules, and occasionally the ligamentum flavum. These injuries are especially common in distractive flexion mechanisms of trauma. Posterior spine pain or tenderness is suggestive of this ligamentous disruption. Flexion x-rays may show evidence of spinous process divergence or vertebral body malalignment. These injuries tend to reduce spontaneously in extension.

A partial ligamentous disruption may be present when there is widening of the spinous processes on flexion/extension views and limited vertebral body translation of less than 3 to 5 mm. In these cases, a course of nonoperative immobilization with a hard collar may initially be attempted. The patient should be reevaluated later with flexion extension films at a minimum of 8 to 12 weeks. If further instability or malalignment is noted, posterior fusion to reestablish the posterior tension band is warranted. These methods of fusion are briefly mentioned in the section dealing with the treatment for bilateral facet dislocations.

More severe ligamentous disruptions may result in unilateral or bilateral subluxed ("perched") facets. In the more common mechanism of distractive flexion, up to two-thirds of patients will present with neurological deficits (3). Detailed baseline neurological evaluation, followed by infusion of the methylprednisolone protocol, in the setting of cord injury, is now the standard of care. Expeditious use of Gardner-Wells tongs for early closed reduction is also warranted (see below).

When compared to bilateral facet dislocations, unilateral dislocations are less likely to undergo closed reduction successfully. The rate of complete reduction in unilateral injuries has been as low as 25% (2). On the other hand, bilateral facet injuries have been successfully reduced in up to 50 to 75% of cases (8). This difference may be explained by several factors. Unilateral facet injuries tend to be diagnosed in a more delayed fashion than their bilateral counterparts, making closed reduction more problematic. Bilateral facet subluxations are associated with greater ligamentous disruptions, decreasing the resistance against which traction works to cause reduction. The experience of different centers may also contribute significantly to the rate of success.

Major ligamentous injuries tend not to heal well even with adequate immobilization. However, isolated osseus fractures do. Unilateral and bilateral facet subluxations are primarily ligamentous injuries. The inter/supraspinous ligaments and facet capsules are markedly disrupted in these cases. Attempts to maintain reduction in a halo has not been associated with an adequate success rate. Operative stabilization after closed reduction is strongly recommended.

2 Lamina Fractures

Lamina fractures are frequently associated with other ligamentous and osseous injuries. Lamina fractures seen in extension injury patterns are accompanied by anterior injury to the disk or vertebral body, causing instability. Lamina fractures associated with lateral bending or rotation can also be associated with contralateral ligamentous or osseous injuries. Associated neurological findings at the level of the cord, root, or brachial plexus often accompany this pattern.

Treatment of lamina fractures should be based on neurological status. Posterior tenderness is expected. Dysphagia or anterior neck symptoms should raise concern regarding significant anterior injury and instability. Lack of posterior tenderness may also assist in evaluating the posterior interspinous ligament. When there is no midline tenderness, no neurological deficit, and no sagittal or coronal translation evident, the isolated lamina or lateral mass fracture may be observed closely in a hard collar. More extensive lateral collapse, any translation, or neurological deficit should warrant greater caution and consideration of halo immobilization or operative stabilization.

3 Unilateral Facet Injuries

Treatment of unilateral facet dislocations should commence with an expedient exam and reduction using skull traction (either via halo ring or Gardner-Wells tongs.) Placement of Gardner-Wells tongs dorsal to the sagittal axis of external auditory canal will assist with reduction of dislocation. General guidelines recommend an initial traction of less than 10 pounds to balance the head. The patient is then re-examined clinically and radiographically so as to detect any neurological change or distraction of an undetected occipitocervical or subaxial injury.

Closed reduction mandates the participation of an awake, cooperative, and alert patient. The use of mild sedation and muscle relaxants may aid in reduction. These have to be tempered so as not to interfere with an adequate exam. General traction guidelines utilize additional weights to a maximum of 5 lb for each level below C2

(9). Traction is typically applied until the facets are distracted or perched. With adequate muscle relaxation, reduction occurs and traction is then reduced. Reduction may be further assisted by slight flexion and is maintained by positioning the head in slight extension.

As a guideline, an increase of greater than 10 mm in the height of disk space indicates overdistraction and warrants caution. Neurological deterioration mandates reduction in traction and follow-up axial imaging. In these situations, the lack of reduction with reasonable weights would make operative open reduction and fusion the safer and preferred management plan. For the reasons mentioned previously, unilateral facet dislocations may require more weight to achieve reduction than bilateral facet injuries. There is also less ligamentous resistance to closed reduction involved in fractures compared with pure dislocations. Therefore, facet fracture dislocations may require less weight to reduce than the facet dislocations with no associated osseous injuries.

It is exceptionally rare for neurological deterioration to occur during closed reduction in an awake and alert patient. This deterioration has been attributed to disk herniation within the canal during reduction. The incidence of radiographic disk injury with facet injuries has been reported to be as high as 47% (4). However, numerous large series have reported safe reduction of these injuries without MRI (7). Although there was a significantly higher disk herniation incidence in the Rizzolo study, all patients were reduced with progressive traction without neurological deterioration. Further examination of the reductions reported to be associated with neurological deficits revealed that, in each case, the reduction was carried out under general anesthesia (10).

The use of manual manipulation to achieve reduction is controversial. Slight flexion associated with rotation away from the perched facet will aid in unlocking the facets. The use of manipulation under anesthesia is a less accepted treatment option. The awake patient provides a safe means of neurological evaluation. Neurological risk is greatest for the anesthetized patient undergoing closed reduction. Therefore, an awake and alert patient in the preoperative setting has the optimal environment for reduction of injury. Some authors advocate anterior diskectomy and intraoperative reduction for all neurologically intact patients with MR evidence of disk herniation (11) (Fig. 6). However, in these cases, concern exists regarding fracture displacement and cord function during intubation, induction of anesthesia, and positioning of the patient. Inability to effectively reduce the subluxed facet from the anterior approach has required posterior reduction and stabilization.

In the awake patient with unilateral facet fracture/dislocation and cord symptoms, expedient reduction, prior to obtaining axial imaging studies, is most reasonable. Acquisition of axial imaging may further delay reduction. Immediate reduction has the potential to reduce ongoing cord compression and allow for enhanced recovery. Should closed reduction fail or neurological symptoms appear, then MR imaging should be conducted.

If closed reduction has failed, MR imaging should be conducted prior to operative reduction under anesthesia. Reduction of the jumped facet should be conducted by resection of the cephalad aspect of superior articular process, local limited distraction, and dorsal rotation of the interior articular process. Using spinous process wiring to lever the reduction has the potential to increase ventral canal compromise by dragging the disk fragment dorsally into the canal. Operative stabilization of the

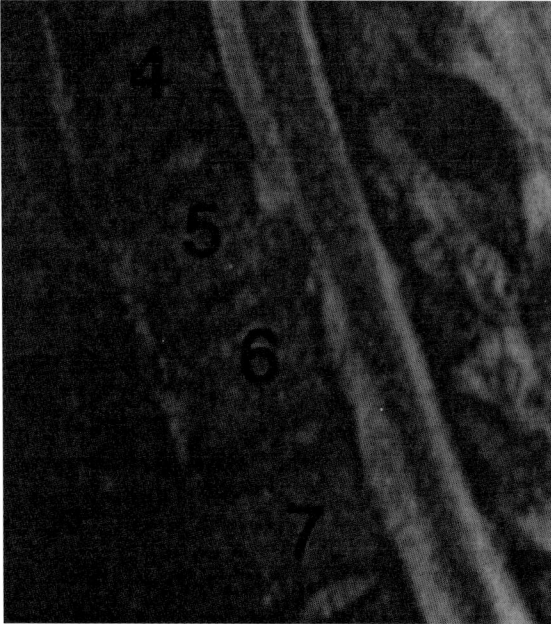

Figure 6   Sagittal MRI showing the disk injury.

reduced facet dislocation requires consideration of the rotational component of the injury. It is not uncommon to discover significant contralateral facet and capsular injury during surgical stabilization of a reduced "unilateral facet dislocation." Oblique wiring and fusion with use of a halo has been advocated. However, local arthrodesis with lateral mass plate fixation and postoperative hard collar has enhanced perioperative mobility and comfort.

4   Bilateral Facet Injuries

Both facet capsules, disk annulus, posterior, and commonly anterior longitudinal ligaments are disrupted in bilateral facet dislocations. These injuries are frequently associated with neurological compromise. Methylprednisolone protocol (see Sec. I.A) should be initiated in the setting of cord injury and closed reduction attempted prior to axial imaging. The role of open versus closed reduction in treatment of the neurologically intact patient with bilateral facet subluxations is controversial. MR imaging may assist in this decision as discussed previously.

If a neurological deficit occurs during reduction, then axial imaging followed by decompression, reduction, and stabilization should promptly be conducted. For the irreducible injury, anterior decompression of the retropulsed disk fragment is indicated prior to reduction to avoid additional cord compromise. Operative treatment of bilateral facet injuries is dependent upon the nature of the anterior vertebral body injury. In pure flexion distraction injuries, restoration of the posterior tension band via interspinous wiring and lateral mass plates can expedite functional recovery and rehabilitation of the injured patient.

Anterior fusion in the patient with bilateral facet dislocation has a significant risk of nonunion or hardware failure due to deficiency of the posterior tension band.

A simple interspinous wiring as an adjunct to the anterior buttress may reduce this risk. The cases involving both facet and anterior vertebral body injuries such as the compressive flexion injuries CFS3, 4, and 5 often require combined anterior and posterior procedures for stabilization. Most successful treatments have involved the use of anterior decompression followed by restoration of the posterior tension band with interspinous wiring or lateral mass plates.

5 Facet Avulsions

Facet avulsions most commonly occur at the base of the superior facet (7). These fractures are predominantly osseous. The remainder of the superior facet is attached through at least a partially intact capsule to the inferior facet. Patients may present with a radiculopathy due to the displacement of the fracture fragment into the foramen. Plain x-rays note rotational deformity. As mentioned previously, the plane of the fracture can be parallel to that of the CT cuts and therefore may be missed on the initial imaging. Two-dimensional CT reconstructions are invaluable in revealing these fracture patterns. There is often an associated disk injury due to the rotational components of the trauma.

Inferior facet avulsions also occur in flexion rotational injuries and are typically accompanied by more facet capsule disruption. The fracture line may extend into the lamina. There appears to be no difference in the mechanisms by which superior or inferior facet avulsions occur. Both patterns of fracture are best managed through closed reduction followed by posterior decompression and single-level fusion.

6 "Floating" Lateral Mass Fracture

This uncommon group of fractures includes pedicle fractures and concurrent lamina fractures parallel to the ipsilateral articular mass. These injuries dissociate the facets from the remaining anterior and posterior bony elements, thus creating a "floating" lateral mass. The mechanism of this injury is extension with rotation and/or lateral bending. Patients may present with radicular symptoms due to traumatic narrowing of the foramen. There is often rotation across the fractured segment, accounting for malalignment of the vertebral bodies on x-rays.

These fractures cause instability at the segments above and below the fractured pedicle. The predominant component of the instability exists at the level of or below the pedicle fracture. Less than one-quarter of these patients present with instability at the level above. This injury is considered to be more osseous than ligamentous. Three level posterior fusion techniques have the greatest likelihood of restoring stability and avoiding further deformity. In select patients, MR imaging may assist in the isolation of the motion segment injury. In some cases, anterior fusion of this motion segment may restore enough stability to allow for the pedicle or lateral mass fracture to heal (Fig. 7). However, these patients must be followed for the potential instability above the fused level. Malalignment of the residual lateral mass also remains a concern.

E Vascular Injuries

The vertebral artery is particularly prone to injury in cervical spine trauma. It is confined along its second segment in the foramen transversaria from C6–C1. The extracranial portion of the artery is tethered to its bony confines and is therefore

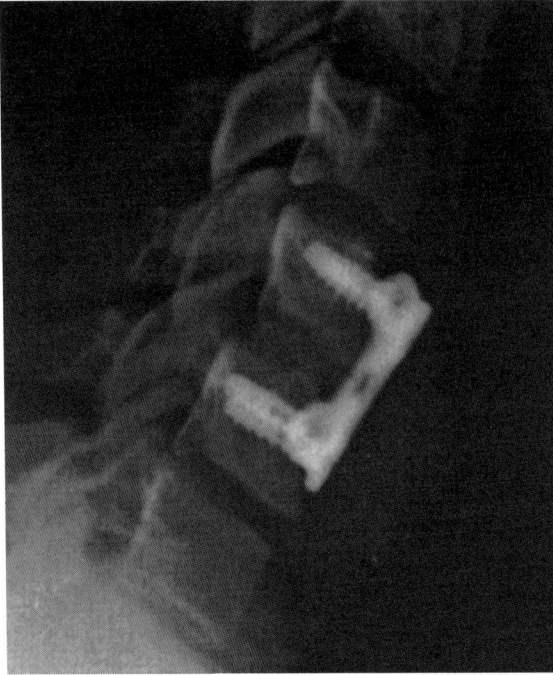

Figure 7   Anterior diskectomy with bone graft instrumented fusion.

prone to various traction injuries. Further direct injuries can be caused by the fractures of lateral masses and foramina.

1   Incidence

The incidence of vertebral artery insufficiency is difficult to determine since a number of the patients with traumatic vertebral artery occlusion may remain asymptomatic. This is due to the adequate collateral circulation unless embolization from the site of occlusion occurs. These patients may undergo treatment of their cervical fractures without further imaging. Patients with CT evidence of foramen transversarium fracture are at high risk for vertebral artery injury and therefore require further evaluation.

Benzel and associates evaluated prospectively the incidence of vertebral artery injury after acute fracture or dislocation of the mid-cervical spine by angiography (12). They found evidence of arterial injury in 46% and total occlusion in 35% of these patients. The spectrum of these vascular injuries included arterial dissection, formation of an intimal flap, arteriovenous fistula, or pseudoaneurysm. In another study (13), complete disruption of flow was demonstrated on MRI/A in 19.7% of the patients with significant cervical injuries. Flexion distraction was the most common mechanism involved (28%), followed by flexion compression (18%). The rotational component of the initial insult plays an important role in causing arterial occlusion.

2   Signs and Symptoms

Vertebrobasilar ischemic symptoms can be associated with violent neck movements during trauma, chiropractic manipulations, endotracheal intubation, or fractures and dislocations of the spine (14). The most common mechanism of injury is distractive flexion with the resultant fracture located at C5–C6 (15). Vertebral artery insufficiency may present itself after an acute cervical trauma by any symptoms of brainstem dysfunction such as altered level of consciousness, dysarthria, blurred vision, nystagmus, ataxia, or dysphagia. A high clinical index of suspicion is paramount in revealing the diagnosis (16).

Unilateral vertebral artery injury remains occult in the majority of cases because of the collateral supply through the contralateral vertebral artery and posterior inferior cerebellar arteries (PICA) (16). Preexisting conditions such as underdevelopment of these collaterals (vertebral artery ending as PICA) or atherosclerosis may, however, cause a unilateral vertebral artery occlusion to become symptomatic. In addition, embolism from the site of partial occlusion remains a possibility. Heros et al. (17) documented a case of unilateral vertebral occlusion resulting in cerebellar infarction by extension of the proximal thrombosis distally into the corresponding PICA.

3 Imaging

Since the treatment of post-traumatic vertebral artery injury is most commonly conservative, cerebral angiogram is generally not necessary. MR angiography can evaluate the vessels as well as any area of ischemic changes in the distribution of the vertebral arteries. This technology is noninvasive and may be more practical for the critically ill patient. Studies confirm the ability of MRI to detect arterial occlusion and dissection in about 80% of the cases (18).

MRI findings of dissection include an "enlarged" vessel with intramural hematoma. These can present as an eccentric signal void with a surrounding semilunar-shaped signal intensity representing the dissecting clot. The age of the hematoma will produce different signal changes. An MRI/A is also very helpful in the follow-up evaluation of these patients with vertebral artery dissection (19). On angiogram, a dissecting aneurysm appears as elongated, ovoid collections extending beyond the lumen of the vessel wall (9).

4 Treatment

The treatment for nonpenetrating vertebral artery injuries is rather controversial; the treatment for the asymptomatic completely occluded unilateral vertebral artery is conservative. Propagation of the thrombus in an occluded artery to the distal intracranial circulation is rare. However, if the occluded vertebral artery has no collaterals, it may cause brain-stem infarction and subsequent neurological deficits. In the latter case, the nonreversible neurological disabilities have to be addressed individually.

The more controversial case involves the treatment of partially occluded vertebral artery. Dissecting injuries and pseudoaneurysms can act as the sources of emboli. These emboli may be distributed to the end arteries distally, resulting in ischemia. Care of these lesions has to be evaluated on a case-by-case basis. Anticoagulation may be rather risky in trauma patients with possible closed head injuries. Treatment with aspirin may remain as one option, since anticoagulation may be contraindicated in patients with multiple systemic injuries. In at least one study, there was no difference in the final outcome with or without anticoagulation (4).

Endovascular obliteration of a partially thrombosed vessel may be feasible if balloon occlusion studies confer (20). Thromboembolectomy using open surgical techniques has significant risks. More up-to-date thrombolytic agents such as intra-arterial recombinant tissue plasminogen activator are in early stages of evaluation and therefore not yet available.

5 Follow-Up

Patients with arterial injury on initial hospitalization may be followed by MRI/A for possible restoration of flow in the vertebral arteries. However, Vaccaro reports on a lack of reconstitution of flow in the majority of these patients (83%) with an average follow-up of 25.8 months studied with MRA (21). Restoration of flow was seen only with the patient with presumed arterial spasm. The lack of reconstitution of the vessel lumen after thrombus formation may point to the significant initial intimal injury.

REFERENCES

1. Hadley MN, Fitzpatrick BC, Sonntag VKH, et al. Facet fracture-dislocation injuries of the cervical spine. Neurosurgery 1992;30:661–666.
2. Rorabeck CH, Rock MG, Hawkins RJ, et al. Unilateral facet dislocation of the cervical spine: an analysis of the results of treatment in 26 Patients. Spine 1987;12:23–27.
3. Roy-Camille R, Mazel G, Edourard B. Luxations et luxations-fractures. In: Roy Camille R, ed. Rachis Cervical Inferieur; Sixiemes Journees D'Orthopedie de Pitie. Paris: Masson, 1988:94–103.
4. Rizzolo SJ, Piazza MR, Colter JM, et al. Intervertebral disk injury complicating cervical spine trauma. Spine 1991;16:187–189.
5. Andreshak JL, Dekutoski MB. Management of unilateral facet dislocations: A review of the literature. Orthopedics 1997;20(10):917–926.
6. Allen BL Jr, Ferguson RL, Lehman TR, O'Brien RP. A mechanistic classification of closed, indirect fractures and dislocations of the lower cervical spine. Spine 1982;7(1): 1–27.
7. Levine AM. Facet fractures and dislocations. In: Levine A, Garfin SR, Eismont F, Zigler JE, eds. Spine Trauma. Philadelphia: W.B. Saunders, 1998:331–366.
8. Sonntag VK. Management of bilateral locked facets of the cervical spine. Neurosurgery 1981;8:150–152.
9. Colter HB, Miller LS, De Lucia FA, et al. Closed reduction of cervical spine dislocations. Clin Orthop 1987;214:185–199.
10. Rizzolo SJ, Vaccaro AR, Colter JM. Cervical spine trauma. Spine 1994;19(20):2288–2298.
11. Eismont FJ, et al. Extrusion of an invertebral disk associated with traumatic subluxation or dislocation of cervical facets. J Bone Joint Surg 1991;73-A(10):1555–1560.
12. Willis BK, Greiner F, Orrison WO, Benzel EC. The incidence of vertebral artery injury after midcervical spine fracture or subluxation. Neurosurgery 1994;34(3):435–442.
13. Willis BK, Greiner F, Orrison WO, Benzel EC. The incidence of vertebral artery injury after midcervical spine fracture or subluxation. Neurosurgery 1994;34(3):435–442.
14. Bose B, Northrup BE, Osterholm JL. Delayed vertebrobasilar insufficiency following cervical spine injury. Spine 1985;18:108–110.
15. Alexander JJ, Glagov S, Zarins CK. Repair of a vertebral artery dissection. J Neurosurg 1986;64:662–666.
16. Veras LM, Pedraza-Gutierrez S, Castellanos J, Capellades J, Casamitjana J, Rovira-Canellas A. Vertebral artery occlusion after acute cervical spine trauma. Spine 2000; 25(9):1171–1177.
17. Heros RC. Cerebellar infarction resulting from traumatic occlusion of a vertebral artery. J Neurosurg 1979;51:111–113.

18. Quint DJ, Spickler EM. Magnetic resonance demonstration of vertebral artery dissection. J Neurosurg 1990;72:964–967.

19. Atlas SW. Magnetic resonance imaging of the brain and spine. Philadelphia: Lippincott-Raven, 1996:1571–1573.

20. Aymard A, Gobin YP, Hodes JE, Bien S, Rufenacht D, Reizine D, George B, Merland JJ. Endovascular occlusion of vertebral arteries in the treatment of unclippable vertebrobasilar aneurysms. J Neurosurg 1991;74:393–398.

21. Vaccaro AR, Klein GR, Flanders AE, Albert TJ, Balderston RA, Colter JM. Long term evaluation of vertebral artery injuries following cervical spine trauma using magnetic resonance angiography. Spine 1998;23(7):789–795.

19

Cervical Whiplash Injuries

KANWALDEEP S. SIDHU

St. Clair Orthopaedics and Sports Medicine, Detroit, Michigan, U.S.A.

JEFFREY S. FISCHGRUND

Private practice, Southfield, Michigan, U.S.A.

Whiplash injury or cervical sprain syndrome is often the end result of rear-end vehicle collisions. The term whiplash lacks exact definition, and may present with a variety of symptoms—the only common factor being neck pain. When defined as a syndrome, the term whiplash has been typically used to describe the initial injury and subsequent sequelae associated with the acceleration extension of the head and neck during a rear-impact collision.

Whiplash injuries are a common source of disability and litigation after motor vehicle accidents. It is estimated that over 250,000 cervical whiplash injuries occur every year in the United States (1). For most patients, symptoms associated with whiplash injuries will resolve spontaneously by 4 to 6 weeks. However, up to 25% of patients may go on to develop chronic neck pain, and 10 to 15% may have severely disabling symptoms (1). These injuries account for 85% of compensated claims from litigation associated with motor vehicle accidents (2).

I SYMPTOMS

Initial presentation is that of a musculoligamentous sprain of the cervical region. Neck pain or limitation of range of motion may not be severe immediately; however, within 48 to 72 h these symptoms may intensify. Other symptoms may include fatigue, headache, dizziness, vertigo, loss of concentration, irritability, and loss of memory (3) (Table 1). Spitzer and colleagues reported on the relative predominance of various symptoms associated with whiplash (4).

255

Table 1 Symptoms Associated
with Whiplash

Symptom	Frequency
Neck pain	88–100%
Headache	54–66%
Shoulder pain	40–42%
Dizziness	17–25%
Paresthesias	13–62%
Visual disturbance	8–21%
Auditory disturbances	4–18%

Contusion to the brain may occur in association with whiplash injuries. Skull movement associated with sudden acceleration may cause contrecoup-type injury to the cerebral cortex and cerebellum (5). This may be responsible for some of the cognitive disorders seen in association with whiplash injuries.

The Quebec Task Force on Whiplash-Associated Disorders has recommended a classification for whiplash injuries based on clinical presentation (4) (Table 2).

According to the above classification, Norris and Watt concluded that 43% of the whiplash patients in their study corresponded to Quebec grade I, 29% to grade II, 12% to grade III, and 6% to grade IV (6). In their series, Burke and colleagues reported a 41% correlation with grade I, 56% in grade II, and only 3% in grade III (7).

II BIOMECHANICS

Useful information regarding the intensity of forces experienced by the cervical spine during rear impact collision includes speed at impact, presence or absence of head rests, and whether the patient was wearing a seat belt. Seat belts have saved countless

Table 2 Proposed Clinical Classification of
Whiplash-Associated Disorders

Grade	Clinical presentation[a]
0	No complaint about the neck/no physical sign(s)
I	Neck complaint of pain, stiffness; tenderness only No physical sign(s)
II	Neck complaint **and** musculoskeletal sign(s)[b]
III	Neck complaint **and** neurological sign(s)[c]
IV	Neck complaint **and** fracture/dislocation

[a]Symptoms and disorders that can be manifest in all grades, including deafness, dizziness, tinnitus, headache, memory loss, dysphagia, and temporomandibular joint pain.
[b]Musculoskeletal signs include decreased range of motion and point tenderness.
[c]Neurological signs include decreased or absent deep tendon reflexes, weakness, and sensory deficits.

lives by preventing life-threatening injury; however, since their use has become widespread, the incidence of whiplash injuries has increased (8). A 3-year study in Scotland found that the number of cervical strains associated with automobile accidents doubled since the introduction of mandatory seat-belt laws (9). The U.S. National Highway Transportation Safety Administration found that the rate of whiplash injuries in drivers of vehicles with headrests was 10% lower than in drivers of vehicles without headrest restraints (10). Headrests limit the amount of extension that is allowed in the case of rear-end collisions. They should be ear level, which approximates the center of gravity of the skull (5).

McNab simulated whiplash injuries in animals by subjecting monkeys to sudden deceleration forces (11). The most frequent and reproducible injuries were ruptures of the anterior longitudinal ligament and fibers of the annulus fibrosus. Head motion following a collision involves initial flexion followed by hyperextension within 0.2 s (5).

III RADIOLOGICAL SIGNS

Most patients with whiplash symptoms have normal cervical radiographs. Loss of physiological cervical lordosis often seen on radiographs after whiplash injuries may denote underlying spasm. Widening of the prevertebral soft tissue shadow may indicate underlying hematoma secondary to injury of the anterior longitudinal ligament and other soft tissues (12). Miles and colleagues reported on a 2-year radiographic and clinical follow-up of 73 patients with soft tissue cervical spine injuries (13). They concluded that patients with angular deformity have good prognosis and special treatment is not necessary if there is no spinal cord injury. In addition, degenerative changes signal a poor outcome. If there is no spinal cord injury or spinal fracture, the presence of soft tissue swelling does not appear to affect patient outcomes significantly. If ligamentous injury is suspected, then flexion extension radiographs or MRI may be the study of choice.

Magnetic resonance imaging is an ideal tool to assess soft tissue neck injuries. Tears of the supraspinous and interspinous ligaments and cord contusions are best seen on MRI. In the absence of neurological signs, the role of computed tomography or MRI in the acute setting is minimal (14). Bone scan in addition to CT scan may be utilized occasionally in the chronic setting to identify occult injuries to the bony structures.

IV TREATMENT

Most patients with whiplash injuries will do well with nonoperative management. Surgical treatment may be indicated only in patients with proven ligamentous/bony instability or fractures as seen on CT, MRI, or flexion extension studies.

The natural history studies of whiplash injuries indicate that 75% of patients will improve spontaneously (1). However, 25% may suffer from persistent pain at 1 year following the injury. Treatment during the acute phase may involve a soft cervical collar to provide support to the neck during the phases of muscular spasm and stiffness. Depending on the severity of injury and symptoms, a prescribed treatment regimen may include rest, immobilization, local modalities (ice/heat), anti-inflammatory medication, and muscle relaxers. Immobilization should be limited so as to avoid dependence and muscle atrophy. Long-term use of narcotics should be discouraged.

After the initial pain and spasms have subsided, patients should be weaned off the medication and started into a mobilization and exercise program. An initial program of isometric exercises may be better tolerated than aggressive physical therapy and traction. Formal physical therapy for eight to twelve sessions may be beneficial for certain patients who need a structured treatment protocol for compliance. Mealy and colleagues compared two treatment modalities in 61 patients with whiplash: collar immobilization and active exercises (16). They reported a superior outcome at 8 weeks in the active exercise group. Pennie and Agambar compared rest in a soft collar/unsupervised mobilization to early traction/physiotherapy in 135 patients with whiplash (17). At 5-month follow-up, there was no difference in outcome between the two groups. McKinney reported on 126 patients treated in one of three ways: mobilization, physiotherapy, and no treatment (18). He concluded that mobilization treatment was superior to physical therapy or no treatment. Borchgrevink and colleagues reported a single-blind, randomized trial for treatment of acute whiplash (19). Patients were treated within 2 weeks of injury by either (1) resumption of normal activities or (2) soft collar immobilization and time off from work. At 6-month follow-up, patients who were allowed to resume normal activities of daily living had better outcomes.

Injection therapy either with saline, lidocaine, or steroids has no role in acute treatment. Select studies have hinted toward the cervical zygapophyseal joints as being a source of chronic pain in whiplash syndrome (20). Lord and colleagues reported a double-blind study of 68 chronic whiplash patients treated with either saline (placebo) or local anesthetic blocks (20). The authors concluded that the overall prevalence of cervical facet pain in this group was 60%. In addition, they postulated that headaches in this group of patients may originate from dysfunction of the C2–C3 facet joint. Such injections should be used sparingly due to the discomfort associated with the procedure and lack of proven efficacy over the natural history of the disease.

The role of steroids in the treatment of spinal cord injury is well established (21). However, use of corticosteroids for the treatment of musculoligamentous strains/sprains is more controversial. Peterson and colleagues reported on a prospective, randomized, double-blind study comparing high-dose methylprednisolone with placebo (22). At 6-month follow-up, the steroid group had better outcome regarding number of sick days and sick leave profile. The sample size in this study was quite small and, at this time, there is no definitive evidence to support the use of high-dose steroids in acute whiplash injuries.

Intra-articular facet injection with corticosteroids has not been proven to affect outcomes for patients with chronic pain due to whiplash (23). Barnsley et al. reported a controlled double-blind study of 41 patients with chronic zygapophyseal pain after motor vehicle accidents (23). Patients were randomized to injections with either bupivacaine or betamethasone. There was no statistically significant difference in outcome between the two groups.

Pulsed electromagnetic therapy has been shown to have anti-inflammatory effects and promote healing. Foley-Nolan and colleagues reported a double-blind study on the effect of pulsed electromagnetic therapy (PEMT) on 40 patients with whiplash (24). At 2- and 4-week follow-up, the PEMT group had statistically significant im-

Table 3 Clinical Factors Associated with Prognosis Following
Soft-Tissue Injury of the Neck

Numbness, paresthesias, or pain in the upper extremity
Reversal of cervical lordosis on x-rays
Restricted motion on flexion extension x-rays at one level
Need for >3 months of immobilization with a cervical collar
Use of home traction
Resumption of physical therapy more than once for symptom exacerbation

provement over the placebo group. The improved outcome continued at 12-week follow-up. The authors concluded that PEMT has a beneficial effect in the treatment of acute whiplash.

V PROGNOSTIC FACTORS

Identification of risk factors for poor prognosis following whiplash injury is important. Hohl retrospectively reported on 146 patients with whiplash injuries (25). Clinical factors associated with poor prognosis following soft tissue injuries of the neck are noted on Table 3.

Norris and Watt analyzed 61 patients with whiplash injuries to develop indicators of prognosis (6). They concluded that preexisting cervical spondylosis, neck stiffness, muscle spasms, and neurological deficit were objective signs that indicated a poor prognosis. A 10-year follow-up was reported by Gargan and Bannister on 43 patients with whiplash injuries (26). Older patients had a worse prognosis, and symptom recovery plateaued at 2 years. At 10.8-year follow-up, 12% of patients had continued severe symptoms.

VI SUMMARY

Whiplash injuries are a leading cause of disability and litigation after rear-impact collisions. Whereas most patients will have self-limiting symptoms, up to 25% may go on to chronic pain. Most patients will respond well to an initial treatment protocol that includes rest, immobilization, medications, and physiotherapy. Surgical treatment is indicated only when neurological deficit or spinal instability is present. Patients with persistent disabling symptoms are a difficult subgroup to treat. This small subset of patients may undergo treatment with injections, traction, steroids, pulsed electromagnetic fields, and nontraditional therapies. However, the efficacy of such treatment protocols is not proven, and good outcomes are marginal at best.

REFERENCES

1. Barnsley L, Lord S, Bogduk N. Whiplash injury—a clinical review. Pain 1994; 58:283–307.
2. Gunzburg R, Szpalski M. Whiplash injuries: Current Concepts in Prevention, Diagnosis and Treatment of the Cervical Whiplash Syndrome. Philadelphia: Lippincott-Raven Publishers, 1998.

3. Radanov BP, Dvorak J, Valach L. Cognitive defects in patients after soft tissue injury of the cervical spine. Spine 1992; 17:127–131.
4. Spitzer WO, Skovron ML, Salmi LR, et al. Scientific monograph of the Quebec Task Force on whiplash-associated disorders: redefining "whiplash" and its management. Spine 1995; 20:1S–73S.
5. White AA, Panjabi MM. Practical biomechanics of spine trauma. In: White AA, Panjabi MM, eds. Clinical Biomechanics of the Spine. Philadelphia: Lippincott, 1990:169–275
6. Norris SH, Watt I. The prognosis of neck injuries resulting from rear end vehicle collisions. J Bone Joint Surg (Br) 1983; 605:608–611.
7. Burke JP, Orton HP, West J, et al. Whiplash and its effect on the visual system. Graefes Arch Clin Exp Ophthalmol 1992; 230:335–339.
8. Barancik JL, Kramer CF, Thode HC. Epidemiology of motor vehicle injuries in Suffolk County, New York before enactment of the New York Senate seatbelt use law. Washington, DC: U.S. Department of Transportation, National Highway Safety Administration, June 1989; DOT HS 807 638.
9. Turbridge RJ. The long term effect of seat belt legislation on road user injury patterns. Crowthorne, UK: Transport and Road Research laboratory, 1989. Research report #239.
10. Stewart JR. Statistical evaluation of the effectiveness of FMVSS 202: head restraints. Chapel Hill, NC: Highway Research Center, University of North Carolina, 1980. Task 3 report 2:1-1-A-10, DOT HS 8 02014.
11. McNab I. Acceleration injuries of the cervical spine. J. Bone Joint Surg 1964; 46A:1797.
12. Pennie L. Prevertebral hematoma in cervical spine injuries. Am J Roentgenol 1981; 136:553–561.
13. Miles KA, Maimaris C, Finlay D, et al. The incidence and prognostic significance of radiologic abnormalities in soft tissue injuries to the cervical spine. Skeletal Radiol 1988; 17:493–496.
14. Borchgrevink GE, Smevik O, Nordby A, et al. MR imaging and radiography of patients with cervical hyperextension-flexion injuries after car accidents. Acta Radiol 1995; 36:425–428.
15. Deans GT, Magalliard JN, Kerr M, et al. Neck sprain—a major cause of disability following car accidents. Injury 1987; 18:10–12.
16. Mealy K, Brennan H, Fenelon GC. Early mobilization of acute whiplash injuries. Br Med J 1986; 292:656–657.
17. Pennie BH, Agambar LJ. Whiplash injuries: a trial of early management. J Bone Joint Surg (Br) 1990; 72:277–279.
18. McKinney LA. Early mobilization and outcome in acute sprains of the neck. Br Med J 1989; 299:106–108.
19. Borchgrevink GE, Kaasa A, McDonagh D, et al. Acute treatment of whiplash neck sprain injuries. A randomized trial of treatment during the first 14 days after a car accident. Spine 1998; 23:25–31.
20. Lord SM, Barnsley L, Wallis BJ, et al. Chronic cervical azygapophysial joint pain after whiplash. A placebo controlled prevalence study. Spine 1996; 21(15):1737–1745.
21. Bracken MD, Shepard MJ, Collins WF, et al. A randomized controlled trial of methylprednisolone or naloxone in the treatment of acute spinal cord injury. N Engl J Med 1990; 332:1405–1411.
22. Pettersson K, Toolanen G. High dose methylprednisolone prevents excessive sick leave after whiplash injury. A prospective, randomized, double blind study. Spine 1998; 23(9):984–989.
23. Barnsley L, Lord SM, Wallis BJ, et al. Lack of effect of intraarticular corticosteroids for chronic pain in the cervical zygapophyseal joints. N Engl J Med 1994; 330:1047–1050.

24. Foley-Nolan D, Moore K, Codd M, et al. Low energy high frequency pulsed electromagnetic therapy for acute whiplash injuries. A double blind randomized controlled study. Scand J Rehabil Med 1992; 24(1):51–59.
25. Hohl M. Soft tissue injuries of the neck in automobile accidents-factors influencing prognosis. J Bone Joint Surg 1974; 56A:1675–1682.
26. Gargan MF, Bannister GC. Long term prognosis of soft tissue injuries of the neck. J Bone Joint Surg 1990; 72B:901–903.

20

Cervical Traction and Reduction Techniques

JEFFREY M. SPIVAK

Hospital for Joint Diseases Spine Center and New York University–
Hospital for Joint Diseases, New York, New York, U.S.A.

AFSHIN E. RAZI

New York University–Hospital for Joint Diseases, New York, New York, U.S.A.

I HISTORICAL PERSPECTIVE

The general population has had a healthy fear of spinal injuries for many centuries, as they are so often associated with paralysis and death. In 2500 BC, a medical author described a clinical finding in the Edwin Smith papyrus: "One having a crushed vertebra of his neck he is unconscious of his two arms and legs and he is speechless—an ailment not to be treated" (1). This phrase is quoted many times in the literature dealing with fracture dislocation of the cervical spine. This condition presents many difficulties in its treatment. In his treatise *On Joint* (2,3), Hippocrates described methods for the management of spinal diseases including fractures. The early methods were primitive, the patient being tied upside down to a ladder, which was violently shaken in order to reduce a dislocation. He later used a more rational form of treatment and applied traction to the neck of a supine patient, but these cases were rarely treated successfully until the beginning of this century.

The management of spinal injuries, particularly those involving the cervical spine, has always been challenging. Differences of opinion regarding the closed management of cervical spine fractures and dislocations have been well documented. The mechanism of injury in cervical dislocations has been evaluated by Bauze and Ardran (4). Distractive flexion injury is the most common injury pattern and is most often caused by motor vehicle accidents and falls from a height. Compressive force applied along the axis of the semiflexed neck causes posterior tension and ruptures the posterior ligaments, causing the posterior facets to slide apart and dislocate. The anterior shift of the superior vertebra completes the rupture of the capsule of the apophyseal joint and the annulus of the disk. The amount of anterior displacement is dependent on the degree of posterior element failure. In general, less than 25% subluxation is indicative of a facet subluxation, between 25 to 50% subluxation is indicative of a facet dislocation, and more than 50% is indicative of bilateral facet dislocations. About 1890, Walton appears to have been the first to use manipulation for the treatment of dislocations in the modern era (5). His reduction maneuver consisted of full rotation to disengage the facets, followed by a full lateral flexion to lift the anteriorly displaced inferior articular process above the posteriorly displaced superior articular process. Rotation in the opposite direction was then done to replace the facets in their normal relationship and the manipulation was completed by hyperextending the neck into a more stable position.

In 1924, Taylor advocated less violent methods (6). He used traction employing his own body weight through a head sling so as to leave both hands free to manipulate the dislocation. By using the head sling, he was able to pull out the locked processes. Brookes described 36 successful manipulations (such as Taylor's) in 40 patients, with no mortalities (7). In 1935, Bohler used heavy traction with manipulation, after infiltration of muscles with a local analgesic (8). Roberts advocated the use of general anesthesia for manipulation of a complete dislocation (9). He stated, "When the dislocation is complete, reduction must be attempted only under anesthesia." Crooks and Birkett introduced the use of Pentothal anesthesia in 1946 (10). They recommended that the simplest and safest way to obtain reduction is by traction of the neck, using a halter, and counter-traction on the legs by assistants, while Pentothal was given. However, they reported a high mortality rate (23%). Ellis used increasing weight and then proceeded with manipulation if traction was not successful; this was then followed by a posterior fusion (11).

Over time, as a consequence of some catastrophic results from forceful manipulations under anesthesia, there developed a growing opinion that manipulation under anesthesia was dangerous and should not be done. This went on until the 1960s, when Evans reviewed his series of dislocations (12). He reported on 17 patients; 6 with complete quadriplegias and most of the others with isolated nerve root lesions only. He reported the use of relaxant anesthesia, such as Scoline, and he followed his closed reduction with posterior wiring and spinal fusion 2 to 3 weeks later. No patient with an incomplete paralysis was made worse and no new neurological deficits were seen postreduction; two of the patients had significant neurological recovery. Burke used manipulation under both anesthesia and muscle relaxation in 21 cases of bilateral and 20 cases of unilateral facet dislocations (13). There were four failures of reduction. No patients suffered neurological deterioration. Holdsworth waited 6 weeks after manipulation and closed reduction for anterior fusion if no bony bar was seen (14). Sonntag reported 15 cases of bilateral dislocations, 6 of which were reduced by traction and manipulation (15). There were no cases of neurological worsening. Recently, Lu presented a small series of six cases of bilateral facet dislocations in which manual closed reduction under general anesthesia and muscle relaxation was used (16). Three had complete (Frankel A) and three incomplete (Frankel B, C, D) neurological deficits. No neurological deterioration was seen and all patients improved to a Frankel C or better. Cotler et al. reported his series with traction and/or manipulation on awake patients with good clinical results (17). There were 13 bilateral and 11 unilateral facet dislocations with 10 patients having incomplete neurological deficits. Approximately 71% of these patients were reduced successfully using traction (up to 140 pounds) and/or manipulation. Ninety percent of patients with neurological deficits improved by one Frankel grade. Twenty-nine percent of patients could not be reduced by closed means. Vital reviewed 168 cases where reduction was performed using gradual traction without manipulation, traction and manipulation under general anesthesia, or open reduction (18). Of the 91 bilateral facet dislocations, reduction was achieved by simple traction in 43%, by manipulation under anesthesia (MUA) in 30%, and by open reduction in 27%. Of the 77 cases of unilateral dislocation, reduction was obtained by traction in 23%, by manipulation in 36%, and by open reduction in 34%. All patients underwent anterior fusion, whether reduced closed or open. No neurological deterioration was observed with this protocol. The authors recommended attempting reduction within 2 h of the patient's arrival. In a series reported by Lee, reduction was attempted by closed traction with serial weight applications in 119 awake patients and by manipulation under anesthesia (MUA) in 91 patients (19). Of the traction group, 88% were successfully reduced. Of the MUA group, 73% had satisfactory reduction. Sixteen patients in the MUA group and four patients in the traction group died within 3 months of their injury. Three of those dying in the MUA group had respiratory failure with neurological deterioration.

Many surgeons have cautioned about the potential complications related to closed manipulation of the cervical spine. Gallie felt that closed reduction of cervical injuries were associated often with poor clinical outcomes (20). Durbin argued that manipulation under anesthesia could potentially increase the level of paralysis (21). Four percent of patients in Durbin's series (53 dislocations and fracture dislocations) required an open reduction. In 1961, Bailey considered closed reduction to be a hazardous maneuver. He stated "Under no circumstances must the grave error be made of trying to reduce any cervical dislocation by closed manipulation" (22). Even Guttmann and Munro, two advocates of conservative treatment of spinal injuries, disapproved of manipulative closed reduction (23–25). Mahale reported on 16 patients with cervical dislocations who worsened neurologically after or during the closed reduction procedure (26). However, the vast majority of authors believe that closed reduction is a safe procedure if it is performed on an awake and cooperative patient.

There is still considerable controversy on the subject of neurological recovery and its relationship to the timing of cervical reduction (27). Early reduction has been advocated by many. The likely mechanism by which reduction may facilitate recovery is by relief of spinal cord compression and minimization of direct and secondary ischemic damage. This may prevent further damage to the spinal cord and may promote neuronal recovery (27).

The common causes of failure of closed reduction of cervical spine dislocations and fracture dislocations include severe pain or spasm, deterioration of neurological function during reduction, fracture fragments physically preventing reduction, and delay in the time to reduction with partial soft tissue and bony healing. When closed reduction is not successful, an MRI should be obtained and an open reduction and spinal stabilization procedure is generally considered the treatment of choice. The success rate reported in the literature of closed reduction in reducing bilateral facet dislocations ranges from 25 to 90%.

II CERVICAL TRACTION DEVICES

Many devices have been used for closed traction reduction of the cervical spine. Depending on the level of injury and the type and degree of tissue damage, variable amounts of traction weight are required to realign the cervical spine. Head halters, cranial tongs, and halo rings are three potential methods of applying traction to the cervical spine. The head-halter apparatus is noninvasive and easily applied. It attaches to the head around the occiput and chin (mandible), and is attached to traction weight via a crossbar (Fig. 1). In general, only small amounts of weight can be tolerated in most patients, and usually for a short period of time. This makes halter traction suitable only for temporarily stabilizing the position of the head and neck but not suitable for use to reduce fracture deformities and dislocations. Prolonged use of cervical halter traction has been associated with transient temporomandibular joint pain and dysfunction.

Cranial tongs allow for the application of large forces on the skull, allowing significant longitudinal traction forces to be applied to the cervical spine. This allows them to be used effectively for reduction of cervical spine fractures and fracture dislocations. Cranial-tong application is not considered rigid immobilization of the spine, and its use restricts patients to bed rest, which makes mobilizing the patient for additional testing, such as CT and MRI, difficult. Crutchfield first used tongs in 1933 in the management of cervical spine trauma (28). His original patient had a mandibular fracture that prevented the use of head-halter traction. His device was modified from a femoral traction rig and was placed using burr holes in the parietal skull region above the widest diameter of the cranium. This location of pin placement near the vertex of the skull above the skull equator unfortunately resulted in a higher chance of pin migration, although it now allowed patients to be turned over more easily in bed. An early complication of this device was inner table blunt pin-tip penetration with repeat tightening. Crutchfield tongs remained popular up until early 1970s (28,29).

Many other tong devices were used and reported on over the ensuing years. In 1935, McKenzie reported on the use of a modified ice tong (30). This tong had a

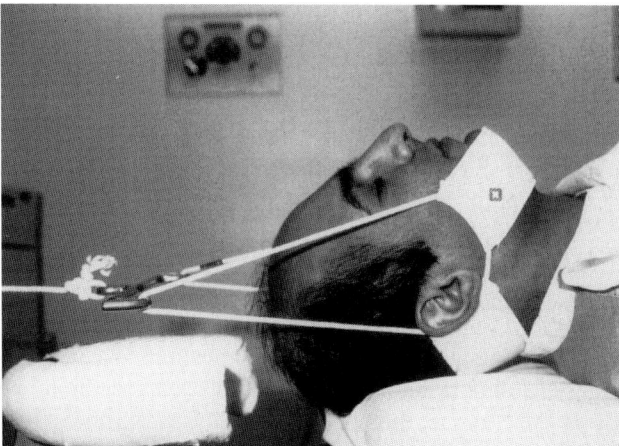

Figure 1 Cervical halter traction.

mechanism for locking the pins into position by having a depth stop about one-eighth inch from the tong points. Barton described a device that was similar to McKenzie's but safer because its points were drilled in place (31). Around the same time, Blackburn introduced a tong with points requiring burr holes into the parietal region of the skull (32). This tong, however, made it difficult for patients to move. Hoen also described another method where wire loops were used through two burr holes on each side of the skull (33). However, a high rate of wire pullout from the skull was seen. In 1948, Vincke introduced another change by placing burr holes in the parietal region using eccentric cutters (34).

Gardner-Wells tongs are currently the most commonly used tong for patients with cervical spine injuries, mainly because of their ease of application, low complication rate, and ability to apply large traction forces to the skull and cervical spine. Gardner first published a description of his tongs in 1973 (35). It consists of a one-piece bow with threaded pins on each side (Fig. 2). One of the pins is spring loaded with an indicator that shows the amount of compressive force exerted by the pin (about 30–35 pounds). The tapered pin tips do not require shaving, incising the

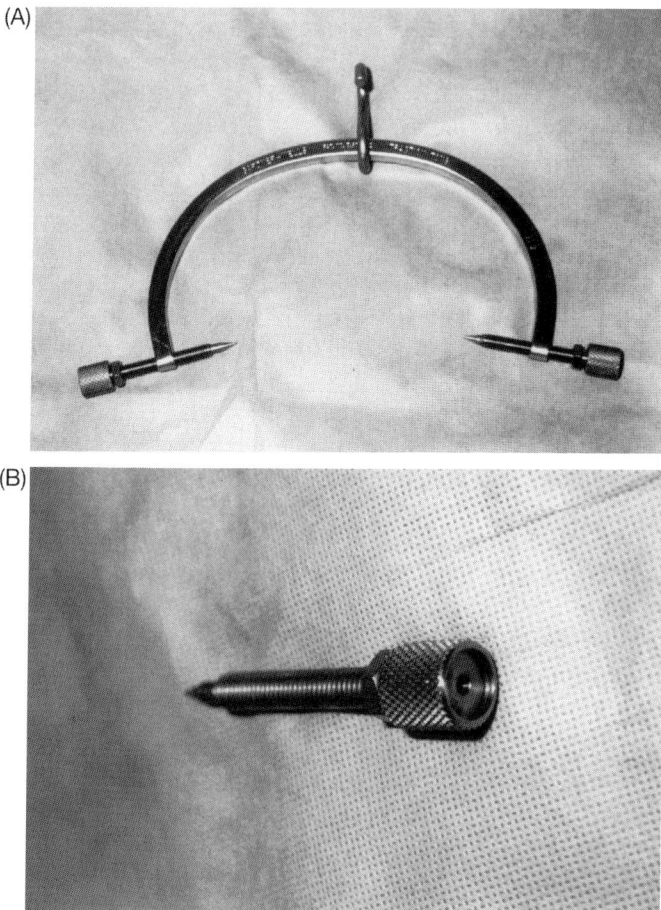

Figure 2 (A) Gardner-Wells tongs; (B) close-up of spring-loaded pin.

scalp, or predrilling into the skull, thus allowing easy and rapid application. The pins are intended to be placed below the temporal ridges, below the maximum biparietal diameter, to obtain maximum pull-off resistance. The pins are inclined or angled toward the vertex of the skull in order to improve the biomechanical advantage of the pin–bone interface and lower the tendency for pin migration with longitudinal traction. Disadvantages of Gardner-Wells tongs are: (1) the lateral protrusion of the pin shafts and the width of the tong itself make it impossible for the patient to turn to the side; (2) pins placed under the temporal ridge are in proximity to certain thin areas of the calvarium; and (3) the fixed size of the hoop can make it difficult to fit extremely small and extremely large heads.

There are several complications related to Gardner-Wells tong application. These include perforation of the inner table of the skull, pin migration or pullout, and infection. Early pin migration is most likely due to inadequate pin tightening and torque. This can be seen with an initial pin setting with less than 0.75-mm shaft protrusion of the spring-loaded mechanism. Late failure may occur due to bone resorption as a response to infection or bone necrosis from pressure (36–38). The earlier version of Gardner-Wells tongs was made of stainless steel. An MRI-compatible graphite tong and titanium pin system is also available and frequently used. A cadaver study compared the failure rates of titanium pins to the standard stainless steel tongs and found that the titanium pins failed because of plastic deformation of the pin tips with subsequent disengagement of the tongs (39). The stainless steel tongs failed only as a result of fractures of the skull. Actual failure loads for the MRI-compatible tongs averaged 75 pounds. Failure loads for the stainless pins averaged 225 pounds. Based on this, the authors recommend that MRI-compatible tongs should be used with caution when more than 50 pounds of traction is considered.

Gardner-Wells tongs are applied under local anesthesia. The skin is prepped in a sterile fashion and infiltrated with an anesthetic down to the skull periosteum. The pins are applied below the equator of the skull, about 1 cm superior to the pinna of the outer ear (Fig. 3). Direct axial traction is applied with the tongs placed longitudinally in line with the external auditory meatus. Placement of the tongs more anteriorly will apply an extension moment to the cervical spine with longitudinal traction; placement of the tongs more posteriorly will result in a flexion moment. With more anterior placement, care must be taken to avoid injury to the temporalis muscle and the superficial temporal artery and vein. Care should be taken to avoid positioning the tong asymmetrically, as this would result in asymmetric forces applied to the left and right sides of the cervical spine. The pins are tightened by hand until the indicator on the spring-loaded side protrudes about 1 mm. At the manufacturer's recommendation of 1-mm stem protrusion, the mean pull-off strength is approximately 137 pounds (36). The tongs need to be retightened 24 h after their application, until the indicator along the protruding stem is again flush with the flat surface of the pin. They should not be retightened after this.

The halo ring can be used for skeletal traction in certain cervical injuries. It is not useful with traction weight as used with Gardner-Wells tongs because the pins are applied directly perpendicular to the skull and have less holding power against longitudinal traction. The four-pin fixation of the halo ring allows for optimum head control and application of specific force vectors for reduction of certain deformities. Use of the halo ring with two traction vectors (bivector) has been described to reduce certain spinal fractures, such as posteriorly displaced odontoid fractures and fractures

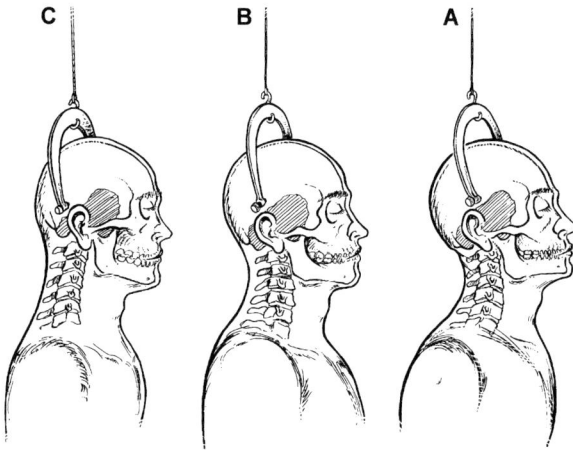

Figure 3 Proper fixation points for Gardner-Wells tong application. (A) Anterior placement of tongs to produce hyperextension of head; (B) normal placement of tongs to produce straight traction; (C) posterior placement of tongs to produce flexion of head.

in the setting of ankylosing spondylitis (40,41). When used with a prefabricated rigid vest or applied body cast, the halo can provide adequate stabilization of the cervical spine to allow early patient mobilization and rehabilitation.

III INDICATIONS FOR CERVICAL TRACTION

The goals of cervical traction are to restore and maintain normal spinal alignment, providing temporary stabilization and indirect decompression of the spinal canal. This potentially allows for improved neurological recovery and prevention of further neurological injury. Traction is often a temporary measure, until more definitive management (usually surgical stabilization) is performed. In the setting of a dislocation, serial traction weights are often required to obtain a reduction of the malaligned spinal elements. Lower weight traction is frequently used in the setting of displaced odontoid fractures, traumatic spondylolisthesis of the axis, rotatory atlantoaxial subluxation, basilar invagination, and cranial settling. Traction may also be used effectively in other nontraumatic cervical spine conditions that result in instability or deformity such as tumors, infections, rheumatoid arthritis and late posttraumatic kyphotic deformity or instability.

Cervical traction is a common means of intraoperative head and cervical spine immobilization, allowing controlled axial distraction and interspace widening for bone graft insertion during anterior cervical reconstructions.

IV TECHNIQUE OF REDUCTION

Physicians involved in the treatment of cervical spine injuries must be aware of the possibility of multiple noncontiguous levels of spinal injury before attempting reduction of any cervical fracture or dislocation. This requires a thorough history and physical examination, as well as complete imaging of the spine in an orthogonal manner in order to identify all levels of anatomical and neurological injury. Good-quality x-rays (including a Swimmer's view, if needed) are necessary in order to visualize the lower cervical spine to the level of T1. If a focal rotational deformity indicative of a unilateral facet joint dislocation is found on the lateral radiograph, it is useful prior to traction application to discern which facet is dislocated. This can be done clinically, by examining head rotation, or radiographically (Fig. 4). On the anteroposterior plain x-ray, the more cephalad spinous process is rotated toward the side of the dislocated facet joint (Fig. 5). However, if there is fracture of the posterior elements, the spinous process direction might be deceptive. In this case, oblique x-rays should be obtained without moving the neck.

Axial traction without general anesthesia using incremental increases in traction weight has been well established by Crutchfield and Gardner (35,42). Several formulas have been offered for determining the weight necessary for a closed reduction of the cervical spine, depending on the level of injury. Crutchfield believed that the force of traction depends on the level of the dislocated vertebra (42). Yashon stated that the maximum weight should never exceed more than 30 kg (43). White and Panjabi advocated using no more than one-third of the patient's body weight or approximately 32 kg (44). Newton advocated a maximum weight of 45 kg, and Venter recommended 5 kg per vertebral level requiring traction down to the site of injury (45,46). Cotler et al. have used up to 140 pounds of weight with successful reductions in 91% of cervical dislocations (47,48). Vital et al. proposed traction equal to 3 to 4 kg plus 2 kg/vertebral level, gradually applied with radiographic monitoring

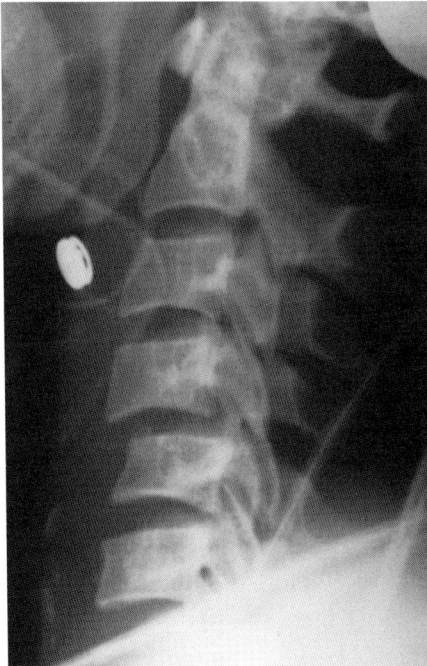

Figure 4   A lateral plain x-ray of a unilateral facet dislocation. Note the subluxation at the C4–C5 level of approximately 25%.

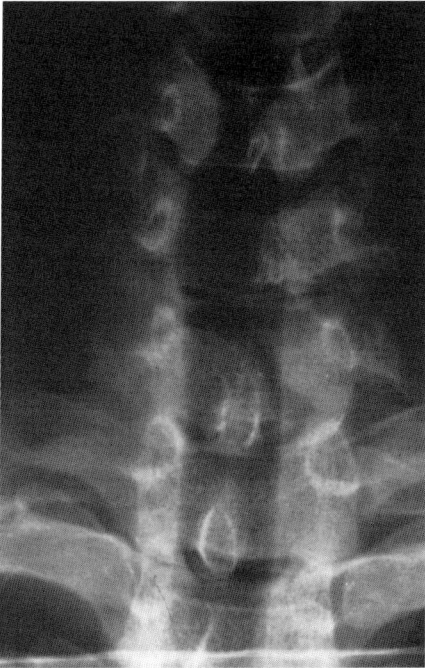

Figure 5   An A-P x-ray of a unilateral facet dislocation. Note the asymmetry of the spinous processes at the C6–C7 level.

(18). Interestingly, Breig demonstrated that traction of only 5 kg stretched the spinal cord approximately 10 mm (49). Cotler et al. also documented that excessive flexion was potentially dangerous because of cord compression by the posterior aspect of the vertebral body (48).

In order to reduce a unilateral or bilateral facet dislocation, the patient is placed on a Stryker frame or a radiolucent table in the supine position. A Gardner-Wells tong is then applied, as previously described, in the neutral position. Tong placement should be more posterior to the neutral axis so that longitudinal traction will cause a flexion moment to the spine and "unlock" the dislocated facet(s). A more anterior tong placement will result in an extension moment on the spine and a more difficult time reducing the facet(s) (see Fig. 3). Such a scenario will likely require additional traction weight to achieve a reduction.

A traction weight of 5 to 10 pounds is initially applied and a lateral x-ray is obtained to make sure that no occult instability, especially at the occipital–cervical junction, is present. Weights are then added in 5- to 10-pound increments. The weights are applied at 10- to 20-min intervals to allow for muscle relaxation and to obtain a soft tissue creep effect. A thorough neurological examination and lateral cervical roentgenogram are performed after *each* weight increase. The use of smaller weight increments (i.e., 5 pounds) is favored initially to avoid any over distraction. If overdistraction or a significant change in the neurological exam occurs, the weights should be quickly removed. Intravenous diazepam in small doses can be used during axial traction to aid in muscular relaxation. The patient should be awake and alert prior to administration of medication, and must remain so during the reduction procedure in order to obtain meaningful interval neurological exams. Infrequently, the patient's lower extremities are either held by an assistant or secured to the frame with ankle weights. A reverse Trendelenburg position can use the patient's body weight to counteract the pull of the traction weights.

In general, significantly more weight is needed to provide enough distraction to reduce a unilateral facet dislocation than a bilateral dislocation. The reason for this is that the intact, nondislocated facet of the unilateral injury provides a significantly greater resistance to distraction with longitudinal traction than the bilateral injury without any intact facet capsule and support ligaments. Reduction weights of 75 pounds and over are fairly common in reduction of a unilateral facet dislocation and fairly uncommon in reduction of a bilateral dislocation.

If reduction cannot be achieved and there is no change in position of the dislocated vertebrae with progressive weight application, a decision must be made whether to pursue further closed reduction. Additional time under traction is often helpful to allow tissue relaxation and may allow reduction to occur. The dislocated facet joint(s) may be locked and unresponsive to axial traction alone. In these cases, it is often helpful to modify the direction of the traction vector. If a patient is on a Stryker frame, in order to increase cervical flexion to approximately 30 degrees, two to three springs of the Stryker frame are removed under the shoulder. This usually tends to unlock the facet joints. A careful neurological exam is then performed. Care should be taken not to produce excessive flexion. Incremental weights can then be added. As soon as cervical distraction has progressed to the point where the articular facets are perched, a slight extension movement can be applied to the cervical spine by replacing the springs on the frame and/or placing a small roll between the shoulder blades to gain some cervical extension. The traction weight is then reduced and x-rays are obtained.

A closed manipulative procedure may assist in the final stages of cervical reduction but should only be performed by an experienced surgeon. The procedure should be discussed with patient, and he or she should be educated to assist in alerting the patient to any symptoms of parasthesias. Before any closed manipulative procedure is performed, the facets must be at a minimum perched. If a reduction maneuver is performed without the facets in this distracted position, the reduction will often be unsuccessful and may potentially result in unnecessary spinal cord compression.

For manipulation of a unilateral facet dislocation, the tongs are grasped by the physician with both hands while standing above the head of the patient. The physician then applies axial compression to the reduced side, as distraction and slight rotation away from the dislocated side are performed. The neck is then gradually turned toward the dislocated facet to about 30 to 40 degrees past the midline. If any resistance is felt, the manipulation should be stopped. A forced manipulation may result in neurological embarassment or a facet fracture. Usually, with a successful reduction, a pop or click is heard or felt. It is important to note that if there is a facet fracture present, neurological injury or loss of reduction may occur with this manipulation. A lateral x-ray should then be obtained and, if adequate reduction is achieved, a small roll is placed under the shoulder to maintain slight cervical extension. The traction weight is then reduced to about 10 to 20 pounds.

For a bilateral facet dislocation, the manipulation maneuver is somewhat different. The facet must be perched or further distracted as in the case of a unilateral facet dislocation. The spinous processes are carefully palpated, and a gap can usually be felt at the level of the dislocation. The physician can apply slight anterior pressure just caudal to the gap, as slight distraction is applied to the tongs. Cotler et al. recommend that the head and the neck be rotated toward one side slowly, about 30 to 40 degrees beyond the midline, then toward the midline, and finally 30 to 40 degrees beyond the midline in the opposite direction to aid in achieving reduction (17). The head and neck are then gently extended. If a closed reduction fails to reduce the dislocation, then an open reduction is performed after the appropriate imaging studies are obtained. Prior to an open reduction procedure under general anesthesia, MRI evaluation for disk herniation should be done, and an anterior diskectomy performed first in cases where a true disk herniation is found.

V MAGNETIC RESONANCE EVALUATION PRIOR TO TRACTION REDUCTION OF DISLOCATIONS

A true disk herniation reduces the space in the spinal canal available for the spinal cord. Disk herniations in cervical spine dislocations before and after reduction have been defined as a displacement of disk material posterior to a vertical line drawn along the posterior vertebral body of the *inferior* vertebra at the level of dislocated level (50) (Fig. 6A,B). The presence of an intervertebral disk herniation seen on MRI

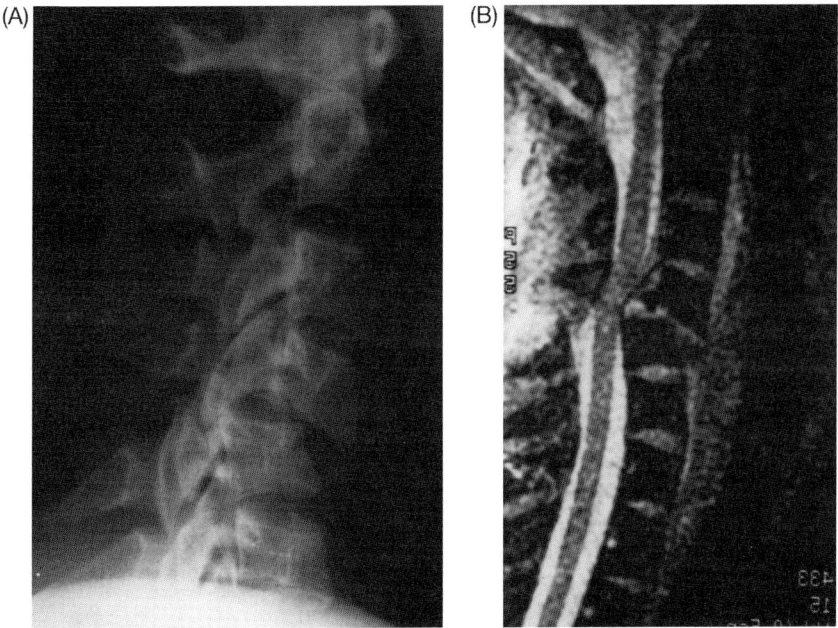

Figure 6 (A) A lateral x-ray of a bilateral facet dislocation. Note the degree of subluxation at the injury site (50%). (B) An MRI of the same patient revealing significant canal narrowing at the dislocation site with a possible large disk fragment cephalad to the C5 vertebral body.

following a cervical spine dislocation has been implicated as the cause of neurological worsening in some patients. Vaccaro et al. reported the incidence of true disk herniation as high as 18% before and 56% after reduction in a series of 11 patients (50). However, no patient had neurological worsening after attempted awake closed reduction, which was successful in 9 of the 11 patients. It has been recognized that about 54 to 80% of patients with dislocations have an associated acute disk herniation at the level of injury. The incidence of disk herniation after closed reduction of cervical spine dislocations has been reported from 9 to 77% (47,51–54). A closed reduction may theoretically result in further disk disruption and displacement of disk material, or it may simply allow the displaced disk material to move more posteriorly along with the cephalad vertebral body. To date, however, no sustained neurological worsening has been reported in an alert, awake, and cooperative patient while undergoing a closed traction reduction.

Eismont and Robertson both advocated that narrowing of the disk space on plain films might suggest the presence of a herniated disk (51,52). However, MRI imaging was not used before reduction to correlate with this finding. There are a number of recent case reports that present acute neurological deterioration after cervical reduction in patients with herniated disks. This has altered the treatment protocols for many centers. These reports, however, involve open or closed reduction under anesthesia rather than closed reduction in an awake, alert patient. As stated previously, there has been no report of a patient with permanent neurological deterioration after closed reduction in the presence of a disk herniation imaged before reduction. Many centers have reported large series of patients treated with awake, closed reduction without prereduction imaging with minimal neurological consequences. At present, there is consensus on the need for MRI evaluation following a successful or failed closed reduction prior to an open surgical reduction in order to evaluate the amount of potential cord compression present, which may worsen during the surgical procedure.

VI NURSING CARE

Any patient maintained in cervical skeletal traction requires skilled nursing care. Assessment of neurological function, maintenance of airway, traction, nutrition, and muscle tone, and persistent reassurance and support are all important nursing duties. A patient who is completely restricted to a supine position by traction must be assessed frequently to ensure that there is sufficient ventilation. Neurological assessment is critical for any patient in traction, and should be performed every hour during the traction period when the patient is awake. Often these patients are placed in a monitored room (ICU or stepdown ICU) while in traction. A patient in traction requires sufficient nutrition for healing and future rehabilitation. Assistance during meals is needed to encourage oral intake and to prevent aspiration. If a patient has difficulty swallowing and is a high risk for aspiration, oral intake should be stopped and a nasogastric tube should be used. Early physical therapy should be initiated to preserve muscle tone and endurance. These patients need constant emotional and physical support by all staff members even for the simplest things, such as positioning to watch television.

Daily pin cleaning is important to prevent future infection. The general recommended procedure involves cleansing the pin sites on a daily basis with hydrogen peroxide with a sterile cotton swab.

REFERENCES

1. Power, Sir D'Arcy. The Edwin Smith Papyrus. Br J of Surg 1934; 21:385.
2. Hippocrates. On Joints. In: Capps E, Page TE, Rouse WHD, eds. Withingtin ET, trans. Hippocrates: The Loeb Classical Library. Vol. III. London: W. Heinemann, 1927:200–397.
3. Marketos SG, Skinadas P. Hippocrates. Spine 1999; 24(13):1381–1387.
4. Bauze RJ, Ardran GM. Experimental production of forward dislocation in the human cervical spine. J Bone Joint Surg (Br) 1978; 60:239–245.
5. Walton GL. A new method of reducing dislocation of cervical vertebrae. J Nervous Mental Dis 1893; 20:609.
6. Taylor AS. Fracture-dislocation of the neck. A method of treatment. Archiv Neurol Psychol 1924; 12:625.
7. Brookes TP. Dislocations of the cervical spine. Surg Gyn Obstet 1933; 57:772.
8. Bohler L. The treatment of fractures, 4th Eng ed. Bristol: John Wright. 1935:110.
9. Roberts SM. Fractures and dislocations of the cervical spine. J Bone Joint Surg 1937; 19:477.
10. Crooks F, Birkett AN. Fractures and dislocations of the cervical spine. J Bone Joint Surg (Br) 1944; 31:252.
11. Ellis VH. Injuries of cervical vertebrae. Proc R Soc Med 1946; 40:19.
12. Evans DK. Reduction of cervical dislocations. J Bone Joint Surg (Br) 1961; 43:552.
13. Burke DC, Berryman D. The place of closed manipulation in the management of flexion-rotation dislocations of the cervical spine. J Bone Joint Surg (Br) 1971; 53:165–182.
14. Holdsworth FW. Fractures, dislocations and fracture-dislocations of the spine. J Bone Joint Surg (Br) 1963; 45:6.
15. Sonntag VKH. Management of bilateral locked facets of the cervical spine. Neurosurgery 1981; 8:150–152.
16. Lu K, Lee TC, Chen HJ. Closed reduction of bilateral locked facets of the cervical spine under general anesthesia. Acta Neurochir 1998; 140:1055–1061.
17. Cotler HB, Miller LS, Delucia FA, Cotler JM, Davne SH. Closed reduction of cervical spine dislocations. Clin Orthoped 1987; 214:185–199.
18. Vital JM, Giulle O, Senegas J, Pointillart V. Reduction technique for uni and bilateral dislocations of the lower cervical spine. Spine 1998; 23:949–955.
19. Lee AS, MacLean JC, Newton DA. Rapid reduction of cervical spine dislocations. J Bone Joint Surg (Br) 1994; 76:352–356.
20. Gallie WE. Fractures and dislocations of the cervical spine. Am J Surg 1939; 46:495.
21. Durbin FC. Fracture-dislocation of the cervical spine. J Bone Joint Surg (Br) 1957; 39:23.
22. Bailey RW. Fractures and dislocations of the cervical spine. Surg Clin North Am 1961; 41:1357.
23. Guttmann L. Surgical aspects of the treatment of traumatic paraplegia. J Bone Joint Surg (Br) 1949; 31:399.
24. Guttmann L. Surgical aspects of the treatment of traumatic paraplegia. J Bone Joint Surg (Br) 1949; 31:399.
25. Munro D. The role of fusion or wiring in the treatment of acute traumatic instability of the spine. Paraplegia 1965; 3:97.
26. Mahale YJ, Silver JR. Neurological complications of the reduction of the cervical dislocations. J Bone Joint Surg (Br) 1993; 75:403–409.

27. Maiman DJ, Barolat G, Larson SJ. Management of bilateral locked facets of the cervical spine. Neurosurgery 1986; 18:542–547.
28. Crutchfield WG. Skeletal traction for dislocation of cervical spine: report of a case. South Surg 1933; 2:156–159.
29. Grundy DJ. Skull traction and its complications. Injury 1983; 15:173–177.
30. McKenzie KG. Fracture, dislocation, and fracture-dislocation of the spine. Can Med Assoc J 1935; 32:263–269.
31. Barton LG. Reduction of fracture dislocations of the cervical vertebra by skeletal traction. Surg Gyn Obstet 1938; 67:94–96.
32. Blackburn JD. A new skull traction appliance. South Surg 1938; 7:16–18.
33. Hoen TI. A method of cervical traction for treatment of fracture dislocations of the cervical spine. Arch Neurol Psychiatr 1936; 36:158–161.
34. Vincke TH. A skull traction apparatus. J Bone Joint Surg (Am) 1948; 30: 522–524.
35. Gardner WJ. The principle of spring-loaded points for cervical traction. J Neurosurg 1973; 39:543–544.
36. Krag MH, Byrt W, Pope M. Pull-off strength of Gardner-Wells tongs from cadaveric crania. Spine 1989; 14:247–250.
37. Krag MH, Monsey RD, Fenwick JW. Cranial morphometry related to placement of tongs in the temporo-parietal area for cervical traction. J Spinal Dis 1988; 1(4):301–305.
38. Feldman R, Kayyat G. Perforation of the skull by a Gardner-Wells tongs. J Neurosurg 1976; 44:119–120.
39. Blumberg KD, Catalano JB, Cotler JM, Balderston RA. The pullout strength of titanium alloy MRI-compatible and stainless steel MRI-incompatible Gardner-Wells tongs. Spine 1993; 18(13):1895–1896.
40. Rowed DW. Management of cervical spinal cord injury in ankylosing spondylitis: the intervertebral disc as a cause of cord compression. J Neurosurgery 1992; 77:241–246.
41. Graham B, Van Peteghem PK. Fractures of the spine in ankylosing spondylitis. Spine 1989; 14(8):803–807.
42. Crutchfield WG. Skeletal traction in the treatment of injuries of the cervical spine. J Am Med Assoc 1954; 155:29–32.
43. Yashon D, Tyson G, Isew M. Rapid closed reduction of cervical fracture dislocation. Surg Neurol 1975; 4:513–514.
44. White AA, Panjabi MM. Clinical biomechanics of the spine. Philadelphia: JB Lippincott, 1978:443–444.
45. Newton DA. Closed reduction of cervical dislocations by traction. J Bone Joint Surg (Br) 1990; 72:744.
46. Venter PJ. Unilateral facet joint dislocation C3-T1. J Bone Joint Surg (Br) 1990; 72: 741.
47. Rizzolo SJ, Vaccaro AR, Cotler JM. Cervical spine trauma. Spine 1994; 19:2288–2298.
48. Cotler JM, Herbison GJ, Nasuti JF, Ditunno JF, Howard A, Wolf BE. Closed reduction of traumatic cervical spine dislocation using traction weights up to 140 pounds. Spine 1993; 18:386–390.
49. Breig A. In: Almquist and Wiksell, ed. Adverse Mechanical Tension in the Cervical Nervous System. Uppsala: J Wiley and Sons, 1978:86–87.
50. Vaccaro AR, Falatyn SP, Flanders AE, Balderston RA, Northrup BE, Cotler JM. Magnetic resonance evaluation of the intervertebral disc, spinal ligaments, and spinal cord before and after closed traction reduction of cervical spine dislocations. Spine 1999; 24(12):1210–1217.
51. Eismont FJ, Arena MJ, Green BA. Extrusion of an intervertebral disc associated with traumatic subluxations or dislocation of cervical facets; case report. J Bone Joint Surg (Am) 1991; 73:1555–1560.

52. Robertson PA, Ryan MD. Neurologic deterioration after reduction of cervical subluxations. J Bone Joint Surg (Br) 1992; 74:224–227.
53. Harrington JF, Likavec MJ, Smith AS. Disc herniation in cervical fracture subluxations. Neurosurgery 1991; 29:374–379.
54. Rizzolo SJ, Piazza MR, Cotler JM, Balderston RA, Schaefer D, Flanders A. Intervertebral disc injury complicating cervical spine trauma. Spine 1991; 16(suppl):187–189.

21

Cervical Orthoses and Halo-Vest Management

DOUGLAS C. BURTON and JOHN NOACK

University of Kansas Medical Center, Kansas City, Kansas, U.S.A.

ALEXANDER R. VACCARO

Thomas Jefferson University Hospital and the Rothman Institute, Philadelphia, Pennsylvania, U.S.A.

D. GREG ANDERSON

University of Virginia School of Medicine, Charlottesville, Virginia, U.S.A.

I   INTRODUCTION

The American Academy of Orthopedic Surgeons has defined an orthosis as an external device applied to the body to restrict motion in that particular segment (1). Cervical orthoses are employed in a wide variety of situations in clinical practice; they can be used for symptomatic treatment of neck pain, postoperative immobilization after cervical surgery, definitive treatment after cervical trauma, and stabilization and extrication in the prehospital setting after injury. Their objective is to provide immobilization to the cervical spine.

The purpose of this chapter is to expose the reader to the various broad categories of cervical orthoses available and to their documented characteristics. Not all orthoses that are commercially available have been scientifically tested in peer-reviewed literature; however, we have attempted to discuss those that have documentation.

II   HISTORY

The use of braces dates back to the Fifth Egyptian Dynasty (2750–2625 B.C.) (2). Galen later used dynamic bracing for scoliosis, and developed a body jacket for this purpose (3). In the sixteenth century, Ambrose Pare developed a metal jacket, lined with leather, called a cuirasse for the treatment of scoliosis (4). Nicolas Andry, an eighteenth-century physician, developed a cervical brace resembling an iron cross attached to a metal ring (5).

The advances in bracing have come as our knowledge of the deforming forces and, more importantly, the materials used in their manufacture have improved. Initially braces were made of wood, metal, and leather. The recent addition of thermoplastics has considerably expanded our ability to produce comfortable, lightweight, yet effective, cervical orthoses.

III BIOMECHANICS OF CERVICAL ORTHOSES

Biomechanical modeling of the spine shows it to be a series of semirigid bodies with intervening viscoelastic linkages (disks) (6). Surrounding the spine is a multitude of structures with varying stiffness, including the rib cage at the level of the thoracic spine and the pelvis at the base of the lumbar spine. Surrounding the cervical spine, however, are vital structures that cannot be subjected to direct pressure (carotid artery, jugular vein, trachea, etc.). Because of this, a cervical orthosis must obtain its seating on stiff structures on either end of the cervical spine, namely, the skull and thorax.

Even when seated on a stiff bony structure, there always exist intervening soft tissues. This becomes important as potential complications such as pressure ulcers are examined. The anatomical orientation of the brace, as well as its material properties, play an important role in determining the risk of skin ulceration with prolonged wear. This is primarily important in patients who remain supine while wearing the orthosis, particularly patients with impaired sensation or with altered sensorium (7).

The effectiveness of the immobilization is directly determined by the mechanical properties of the intervening structures. That is, stiffer materials can apply forces more effectively. This includes the stiffness of the bracing material, as well as the stiffness of the biological structure upon which it is seated.

Normal spine kinematics allows for motion in all six degrees of freedom (6). This includes translation along the three coordinates and rotation along the three axes. Nearly all of the testing of cervical orthoses has been performed on normal subjects, and the evaluation of their effectiveness in limiting motion has been performed in the three clinically relevant motions, namely, sagittal plane flexion and extension, coronal plane lateral bending, and axial plane rotation. These planes of motion will be the focus of this chapter.

IV CLASSIFICATION OF CERVICAL ORTHOSES

Cervical orthoses can be categorized based on type of fixation, such as skin contact versus skeletal, or by the anatomical regions where fixation is obtained. This would include cervical, head–cervical, head–cervical–thoracic, halo–pelvic, or halo–femoral (Table 1). For the purposes of this chapter, we will divide them as follows:

1. Cervical and head-cervical orthoses (cervical collars).
2. Head–cervical–thoracic orthoses.
3. Halo fixation.

Table 1 Recommended Orthoses for Immobilization of the Cervical Spine

	Total flexion extension	Flexion	Extension
Occipital-C1	Halo	Halo	Halo
C1–C2	Halo/CTO	Halo/SOMI	Halo/CTO
C2–C3	Halo	Halo/CTO	Halo/CTO
C3–C7	Halo/CTO/CO	Halo/CTO/CO	Halo/CTO/CO
C7–T12	Halo/CTO	CTO	CTO

A Cervical Collars

Cervical and head–cervical orthoses (cervical collars) have been used for centuries. While the early devices were made of wood, leather, and iron, the cervical collars currently in use are made of foam rubber, polyethylene, and/or plastizote. The varying material properties of these substances define the rigidity of the orthosis. Unfortunately, the more rigid materials tend to be less comfortable for the patient.

There are many different cervical collars commercially available today. These include the soft collar, the hard collar, the Aspen/Newport collar, the Miami J collar, the Philadelphia collar, the NecLoc collar, the Stifneck collar, the Thomas brace, the Camp orthosis, the Mayo collar, the Nebraska collar, the Canadian collar, and the Malibu brace (Fig. 1A–F) (8–10). The differences between these orthoses include price, fabrication material, efficacy, risk of potential complications, and indications for use.

The scientific evaluation of the efficacy of an orthosis in limiting cervical motion is a relatively new phenomenon. This can be accomplished through cineradiography, standard radiography, or by goniometric means. Cineradiography uses fluoroscopy with movie film, while goniometry uses an external device attached to the patient to measure the cervical motion. The advantage of the goniometric method is there is no radiation exposure to the subjects of the study. Fisher et al. found the goniometric method to be a reliable clinical tool, with fair-to-good statistical correlation with radiographic methods (11). However, they noted that the goniometric method was not as accurate as radiography, and it gave no information on the amount of motion at any one particular level.

Jones was the first to study motion in cervical collars (12). He used cineradiography to evaluate cervical motion in 11 patients with various types of cervical orthoses. Hartman et al. used cineradiography to study the ability of five commonly used orthoses to limit motion in normal subjects (13). They studied rotation, flexion extension and lateral bending and found the soft collar to provide little immobilization, with the Thomas collar providing 75% restriction and the Guilford two-poster cervico-thoracic orthosis providing 90 to 95% restriction in all three planes. Unfortunately, they did not detail how the restriction of motion was measured with either the motion picture or cineradiographic techniques.

Colachis et al. studied the effect of the soft collar, the chin–piece collar, and the Queen Anne collar on normal female subjects using radiography (14). They found that the soft collar produced little change in overall motion, the chin-piece collar was more effective in restricting flexion, and the Queen Anne collar was better at

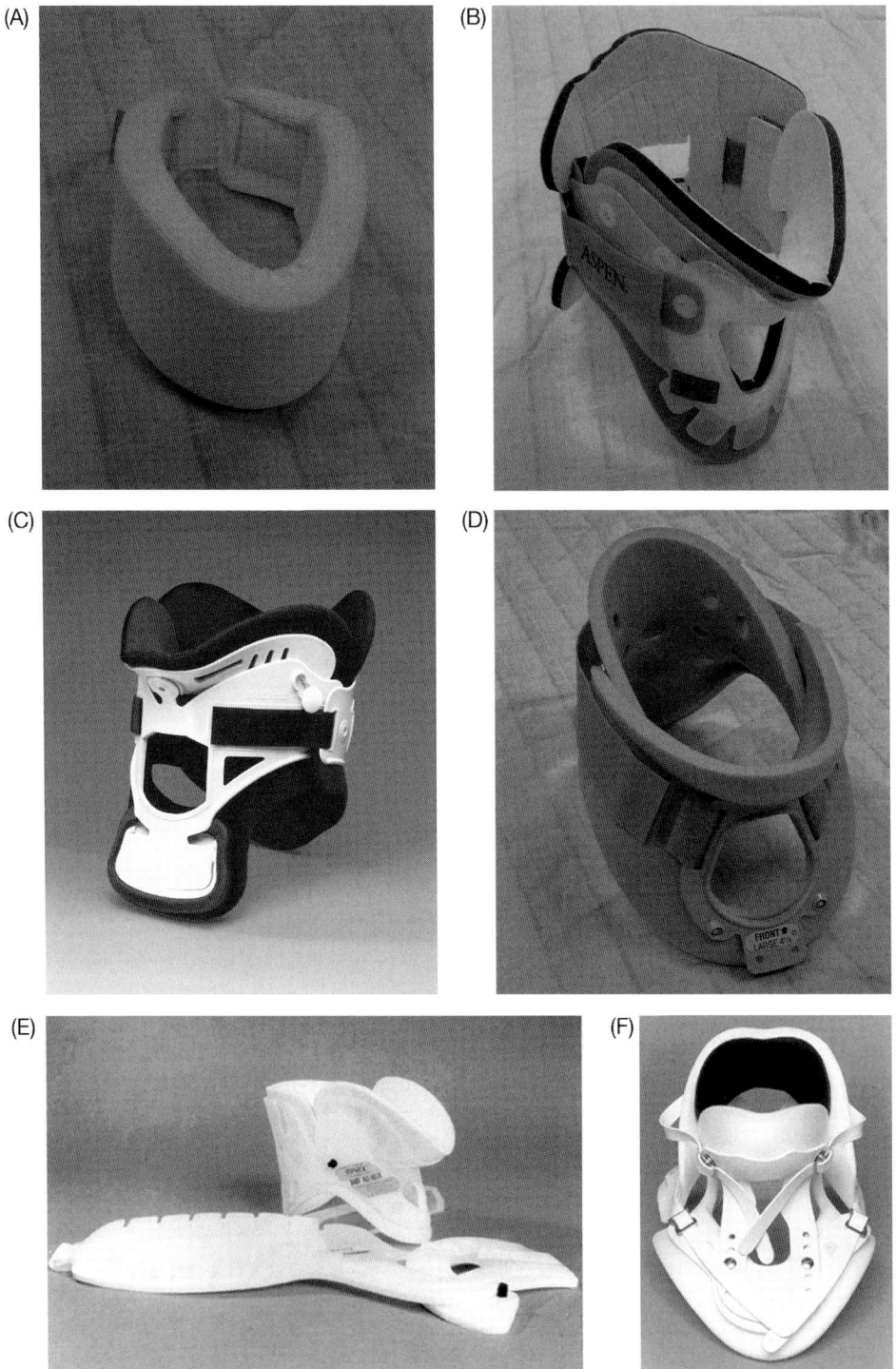

Figure 1 Some types of commercially available cervical collars: (A) soft collar; (B) Aspen collar; (C) Miami J collar; (D) Philadelphia collar; (E) Stifneck collar; and (F) Malibu collar.

restricting extension. They provided quantitative data of motion at each level of the cervical spine, but did not perform statistical analyses of their results.

As noted, Fisher et al. studied motion in collars with both radiographs and goniometry (11). Skin pressure of the various orthoses was also recorded at the chin and the occiput. The collars evaluated included the Camp, Philadelphia, four-poster, and sterno-occipital-mandibular-immobilizer (SOMI) orthoses. They found that the Camp was more effective than the Philadelphia, but poorly tolerated. The SOMI provided the best restriction of flexion, and the four-poster was best at restricting extension. Skin pressures were highest with the SOMI at the occiput and the chin.

In 1977, Johnson et al. published their study evaluating the effectiveness of cervical orthoses in limiting motion of the spine (15). This was a very carefully designed study and its methods have been emulated in many subsequent studies by various authors. The authors studied the soft collar, the Philadelphia collar, the four-poster orthosis, the SOMI, and a cervico-thoracic orthosis in flexion extension, lateral bending, and rotation. They quantified motion for each brace at every level of the cervical spine. Similar to other studies, they found the soft collar to be relatively ineffective in limiting motion in any plane. The Philadelphia collar was better than the soft collar, but not as good in limiting motion as the thoracic extension orthoses. All of the orthoses were best in limiting flexion extension, and performed poorly in limiting lateral bending and rotation. One of the interesting observations from this study was the paradoxical motion seen with halo immobilization. One vertebral level would flex, while the next would extend. This phenomenon has been termed "snaking," and has been noted in other studies (13,16).

Many authors have examined the efficacy of immobilization in the prehospital setting (17–27). Typically, this involves a cervical collar, a short board or sand-bag technique, or a combination of short board and collar. Podolsky et al. compared soft collars, hard collars, the Philadelphia collar, extrication collars, and sand-bag techniques using goniometric methods (25). They found the sand-bag technique to be superior to the others in limiting neck motion, and the addition of a Philadelphia collar to the sand bags was significantly better than sand bags alone. Cline et al. performed a similar study using a short-board technique instead of sand bags, and analyzed the motion radiographically (18). They found the short board to be superior to Philadelphia, Hare extrication, and rigid plastic collars alone. They also found the addition of a collar to the short board provided no benefit. These findings have been supported by other studies (24,28). Graziano et. al. studied the effect of simulated vehicle motion on cervical spine immobilization (20). They found that while the head could be adequately secured to the board during simulated driving, as would occur in ambulance transport, motion between the thorax and the board contributed to motion across the neck.

Askins and Eismont recently published a study comparing the restriction in motion of five different cervical orthoses (29). They studied the Philadelphia collar, the Aspen/Newport collar, the Miami J collar, the Stifneck collar, and the NecLoc collar, which represent 80% of the cervical collars in use today (29). The authors found the NecLoc to be statistically significantly superior to the other collars studied in all planes of motion. The Miami J collar was the next most effective, but statistically superior to the other three collars only in extension and combined flexion/extension.

As with most treatments, use of cervical collars is not without potential complications. The most frequently seen complication is skin ulceration (30). This typically occurs in a supine patient, particularly one with altered sensorium. Chendrasekhar published a 38% rate of collar-related decubitus ulcer formation in patients with severe, closed head injuries (31). Other potential complications include nerve palsy or increased intracranial pressure due to improper tightness of the collar (32,33).

A prospective analysis was performed comparing the skin pressure reached with the Philadelphia, the Miami J, the Aspen/Newport, and the Stifneck collars (34). This study found that the Miami J and the Aspen collar produced the lowest occipital and chin pressures in supine patients, with these pressures being below capillary closing pressure.

B   Cervicothoracic Orthoses (CTOs)

Cervicothoracic orthoses vary greatly in design, but all consist of occipital and mandibular supports rigidly attached to anterior and/or posterior thoracic plates (Fig. 2A–F). Examples include the rigid cervicothoracic brace, SOMI, Yale cervical orthosis, and several forms of the Minerva brace. Johnson and associates distinguished poster braces from cervicothoracic orthoses by their lack of extensive thoracic components and by their flexible rather than rigid connections on each side of the head and over both shoulders (15,35). However, the four-poster brace, the Dennison two-poster brace, and the Guilford brace are considered cervicothoracic orthoses rather than cervical orthoses, based on the more recently standardized classification system (3). Finally, several standard cervical orthoses, including the Philadelphia collar and the Malibu brace, can be fitted with thoracic extensions, converting them to cervicothoracic orthoses. In general, all of the cervicothoracic orthoses allow less flexion extension, particularly at the mid and low cervical spine, when compared to the conventional cervical orthoses. Control of rotation and lateral bending is improved to a lesser extent. These improvements in immobilization typically, but not always, come at the price of decreased patient comfort.

No orthosis, including the halo, restricts all motion. Increasing length and rigidity of cervical orthoses correlates with improvement in ability to restrict motion. In addition, none of the conventional cervicothoracic orthoses effectively limits lateral bending, axial rotation, or flexion extension at the upper levels of the cervical spine.

The traditional four-poster brace consists of padded mandibular and occipital supports attached to anterior and posterior high thoracic plates by four adjustable, rigid, metal uprights. Two flexible leather straps travel over the shoulders to connect the anterior and posterior plates, with the chin and occiput rests connected by straps on either side of the head. The four-poster brace limits 79% of overall cervical flexion extension and is comparable to the rigid cervicothoracic orthoses in limiting flexion over the middle portion of the cervical spine (15,35). Like other conventional orthoses, this brace is not effective in restricting lateral bending, rotation, or sagittal plane motion at the upper portion of the cervical spine (15,35). Although the four-poster brace has been reported to be comfortable and well tolerated by most subjects, these braces are relatively heavy and are infrequently used today (11,15,36). Additionally, Fisher found the four-poster to have average resting pressures at the chin

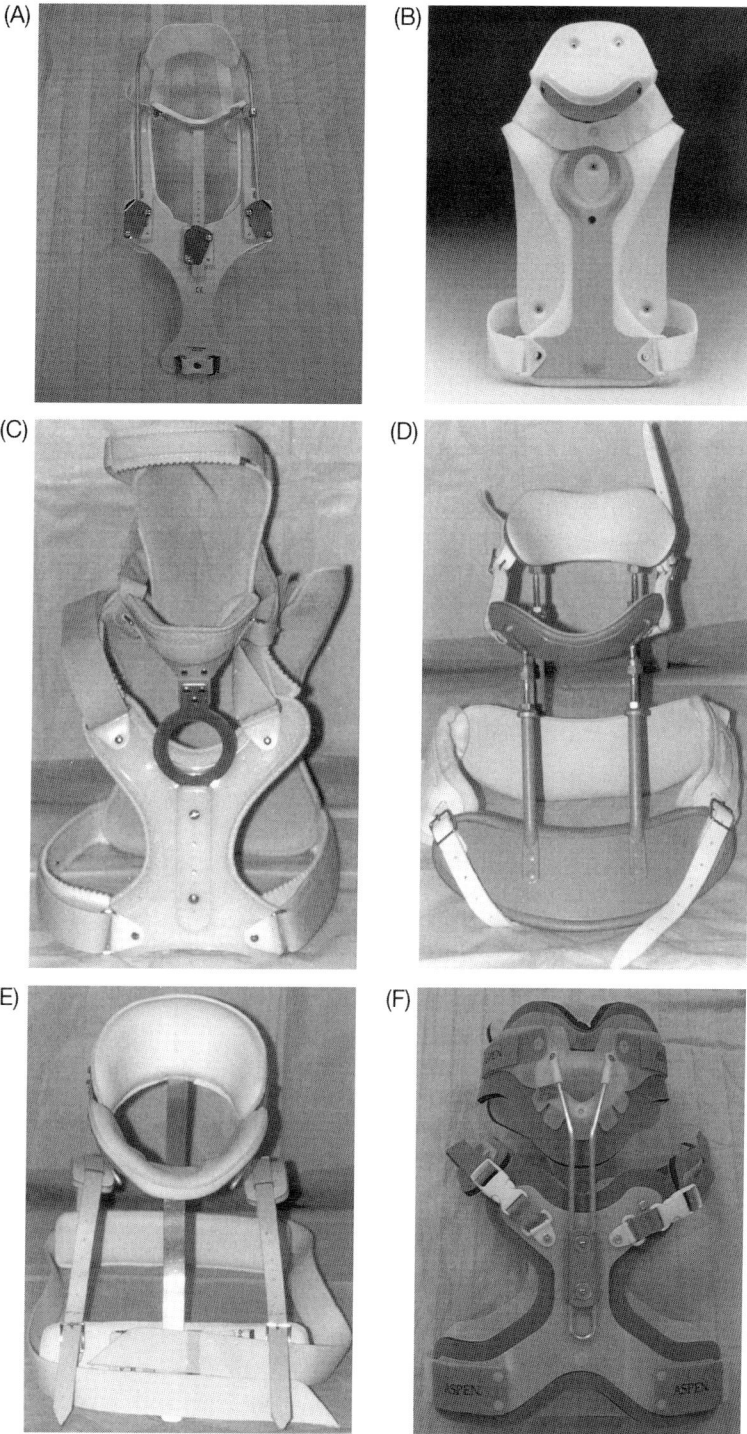

Figure 2   Some types of commercially available cervicothoracic orthoses: (A) SOMI;
(B) Yale orthosis; (C) Minerva brace; (D) four-poster brace; (E) two-poster brace; and
(F) modified Aspen CTO.

and occiput of 65 and 83 mmHg, respectively, which exceed the maximum capillary pressures of human skin (11).

The rigid cervicothoracic orthosis that Johnson tested in his initial studies is essentially a four-poster brace with a lower, more extensive anterior thoracic plate and rigid metal connections over each shoulder and on either side of the head (15,35). In addition, this brace is fixed to the trunk by a circumferential chest strap. The cervicothoracic orthosis in this form was the most effective of the six conventional braces that Johnson and his group studied (15,35). It limits sagittal plane motion by 89%, axial rotation by 82%, but lateral bending by only 50%. This brace is most effective at limiting flexion at the mid-to-low cervical spine and extension at the mid-cervical spine. It was the least effective of the other cervicothoracic orthoses at limiting atlanto-axial flexion, and is also poor at limiting overall lateral bending. Unfortunately, this orthosis is uncomfortable, particularly for long-term use, and is also difficult to fit and adjust (15,35,36). This particular cervicothoracic orthosis has largely been replaced by modern-day versions that incorporate its key features, such as an extensive thoracic attachment and rigid materials of construction.

The SOMI, as its name implies, consists of occipital and mandibular rests connected by rigid metal uprights to an anterior sternal plate. Padded metal straps hook over each shoulder and suspend the sternal plate, which is secured to the thorax by circumferential straps that cross in back. However, there is no true posterior thoracic plate, and supports for the occipital rest originate from the anterior thoracic plate. This construct allows for effective control of the upper cervical spine in flexion, but these posterior supports are flexible enough to allow considerable distortion of this brace during active neck extension (15). Consequently, the SOMI is particularly effective in controlling flexion at the upper cervical spine but is inadequate for control of extension at all cervical levels (15,35). The SOMI restricts 72% of overall flexion extension, 66% of axial rotation, and only 34% of lateral bending (35). It was significantly better at controlling flexion at C1–C2 and C2–C3 than any of the other conventional orthoses tested by Johnson. Advantages include its ease of application, adjustment, and relatively high comfort level (11,15,35,36). However, the SOMI recorded the highest average resting pressures at the chin and occiput (100 and 107 mmHg) in Fisher's study (11).

The Yale cervical orthosis was introduced in 1978 and was designed to be easily fabricated, comfortable for long-term use, and equivalent to the standard cervicothoracic orthosis in limiting cervical spine mobility (37). The original Yale braces consisted of molded anterior and posterior polypropylene extension bibs secured to a standard Philadelphia collar (38). While the original Yale braces were fabricated by physical therapists, modern-day versions are prefabricated. The Yale brace restricts 87% of overall flexion extension, 75% of axial rotation, and 61% of lateral bending (35,37). Of the conventional orthoses tested by Johnson, the Yale brace ranked a close second to the standard cervicothoracic orthosis in limiting flexion extension at most cervical levels (35). The Yale brace effectively controls flexion at each level from C2–C7 and extension at C2–C3, C3–C4, and C7–T1. It is partially ineffective at controlling flexion at C1–C2. The Yale brace compares favorably to the standard cervicothoracic orthosis in terms of effectiveness and is considerably more comfortable (37).

The Minerva brace, in its original form, was a cumbersome plaster jacket that had to be applied in the sitting position. This apparatus was relatively heavy, posed significant obstacles to patient hygiene, and made obtaining adequate radiographs difficult (39). Perry and Nickel introduced the halo in 1959 and overcame most of these problems with their new form of external immobilization (40). With increasing use of the halo came a new set of complications that have been well documented in the literature and are discussed elsewhere in this chapter. The thermoplastic Minerva body jacket (TMBJ) was first described in 1987 and was developed to address the problems of both the halo and the plaster Minerva body jacket (41). The TMBJ consists of a bivalved Polyform shell that encompasses the cervical spine and thorax and is molded to provide support of the occiput and mandible. A circumferential chest strap, combined with nylon screws at the level of the neck and a rigid Polyform headband, holds the anterior and posterior sections together.

Using a study design similar to Johnson's, Maiman et al. quantitatively measured the effects of the TMBJ on cervical spine motion in 20 normal male subjects (42). When compared with previously published results (Johnson et al. and Wang et al.), the TMBJ was found to be more effective at reducing overall flexion extension than the halo (42). Likewise, it was as effective or more effective in restricting flexion extension at each individual cervical vertebral level. Benzel and associates directly compared the TMBJ and the halo in 10 patients with unstable cervical spine injuries (16). Each patient was initially treated in a halo for 6 to 8 weeks and standard radiographic evaluation was performed. Patients were then switched to a TMBJ and were reevaluated radiographically. The TMBJ allowed less movement at every vertebral segment except C1–C2 where the difference in movement was not significant. The average overall cervical flexion extension was 5.2° for both the TMBJ and halo, but the halo produced significantly more of a snaking phenomenon. The sums of the movements at each segmental level were 14.8° for the TMBJ compared with 23.4° for the halo in this study. They followed this study with a retrospective analysis of 155 cases of unstable cervical spine fractures in which they compared clinical results of Minerva immobilization with other methods of external stabilization (39). Based on their results, they concluded that unstable hangman's fractures should be stabilized with a halo, but all other upper cervical spine fractures, in addition to unstable mid-to-low cervical spine fractures, may be safely treated with a Minerva (39).

Obvious advantages of the TMBJ include its noninvasive application, relatively lightweight construct, and low cost. Additionally, the TMBJ is conducive to radiographs and interferes less with rolling and other aspects of rehabilitation (41). Its bivalved nature allows for easy access to the patient's body for hygiene or emergency procedures. In Benzel's initial questionnaire study, 8 out of 10 patients preferred the TMBJ to halo (16). Disadvantages of the TMBJ include less rotational instability than the halo as well as decreasing the potential for skin breakdown (41,42). One of the major disadvantages of the TMBJ is that its proper application is complex and highly dependent upon an experienced orthotist.

The Minerva CTO is a recently developed, prefabricated version of the Minerva body jacket. It is a cervicothoracic brace with a large occipital flare and a flexible forehead strap. It limits overall sagittal plane motion by 79%, axial rotation by 88%, and lateral bending by 51% (43). When compared to the cervicothoracic orthosis tested by Johnson, the Minerva CTO offers significant improvement in immobilization of C1–C2 and in controlling rotation. However, the addition of the occipital flare and forehead strap does not improve immobilization at the occiput to C1 level.

C   Halo-Vest Management

Halo immobilization was developed by Vernon Nickel and Jacquelin Perry in the 1950s at Rancho Los Amigos Hospital in Downey, CA. The polio epidemic of the 1940s and 1950s had left a number of patients with paralysis of the cervical musculature. Rigid immobilization of the head was needed to carry out the occipital–cervical fusions these patients needed and the halo was their response to this need (40,44).

The inspiration for the halo was Frank Bloom. Dr. Bloom developed a similar device to treat the inwardly displaced facial fractures with overlying burns of pilots in World War II (45). Bloom's device consisted of a three-pin tiara open in the back. It was through personal communication with Dr. Bloom that Perry and Nickel saw the application of Bloom's device to their problem of cervical immobilization (40).

The initial halo was a circumferential ring made of stainless steel with four pins fixing the ring to the skull. The ring was then attached to the torso via a body cast and upright posts. The original ring was curved up in the back to allow better access to the cervical spine. Current halo designs have been modified since the initial use nearly five decades ago. Most rings are open in the back. This allows easier placement in a supine patient. In addition, most halos are made of nonferromagnetic materials to allow for MRI compatibility (Fig. 3). Aluminum or graphite–carbon composite materials with plastic spacers that interrupt electrical loops seem to be the most successful components for MR compatibility (46). Multiple pin sites are still recommended, as this allows for optimal pin placement into the skull.

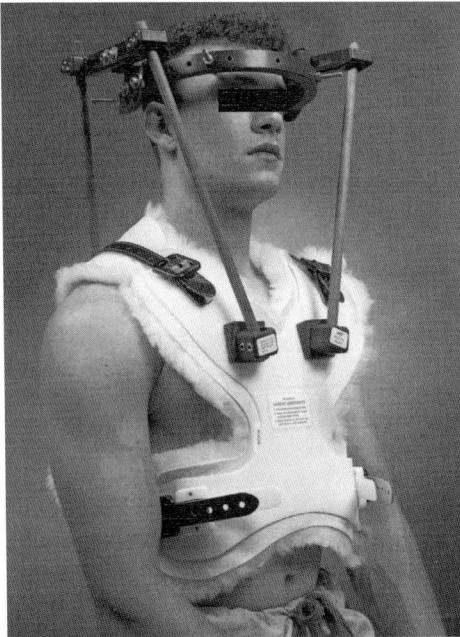

Figure 3   A halo device applied to supplement a posterior cervical fusion following a traumatic spinal injury. Note the graphite composition of the halo device, allowing for MRI compatibility.

Considerable study has been performed on nearly every aspect of halo design. The current pins used are not substantially different from the original ones. Most pins, however, are MRI compatible. A bullet-tipped pin has been studied and found to have advantages over the currently available design (47). This pin is not commercially available.

The precise placement and angle of insertion of the pins has been studied as well. It has been found that perpendicular placement of the pins is biomechanically superior to angled insertion (48). A 90° insertion angle improved both the ultimate load and the amount of deformation prior to failure when compared with 75° and 60° insertion angles.

The optimal sites for pin placement have been determined by studies of the osteology of the skull and biomechanical studies of the pin–bone interface (49–51). Studies of the skull show it to be thickest in the anterolateral and posterolateral positions. Directly anterior, over the underlying frontal sinus, the bone is relatively thin, as it is the temporal region. In addition, the masseter muscle overlies the temporal bone, and placement of pins into this muscle can cause pain with mastication. Some have advocated placement of the anterior pins behind the hairline for cosmetic reasons; however, cosmesis does not seem to be a major concern among most patients (51). The placement of skin incisions prior to pin insertion does not affect the rate of complications, nor does it change the cosmetic outcome, and the use of incisions is not currently recommended (52).

There are at least 3 cm of thick parietal bone from the lateral edge of the frontal sinus to the temporal bone (50). A lateral placement of the pin within this region is recommended to avoid the superior orbital nerve. Based on these data, Garfin et al. concluded that the initial recommendation of pin placement antero- and posterolaterally was appropriate (40,53) (Fig. 4).

It has been suggested that placement of the halo below the equator of the calvarium and above the orbital ridge provides an optimal biomechanical position. Ballock et al. studied nine different pin positions within the anterolateral safe zone (49) and found that the rigidity of the pin–bone interface decreased as the pins were inserted more superiorly on the calvarium in an in vitro model. Based on this information, the authors recommend placing the pins as close to the supraorbital ridge as possible.

Perry et al. recommended an insertion torque of 6 inch-pounds (40). This empirical observation was used routinely until the 1980s. In vitro studies showed that an insertion torque of 8 inch-pounds performed better under cyclic loading (49). In 1987, Botte et al. reported on a prospective study examining the complications associated with an insertion torque of 8 inch-pounds (54). In 42 patients, they found a loosening rate of 7% and an infection rate of 2%. They compared this to their own retrospective study in which they found a loosening rate of 36% (55). Based on biomechanical data, as well as their own clinical experience, Botte et al. recommended changing to an 8 inch-pound insertion torque.

Rizzolo et al. performed a prospective randomized study evaluating the differences between the 6 and 8 inch-pound insertion torques (56). They found no statistically significant differences between the two groups. Their randomization process produced similar groups, although there were slightly more neurologically intact patients in the 8 inch-pound group. They found a trend toward more loosening and more infection in the 8 inch-pound group, but this was not statistically significant.

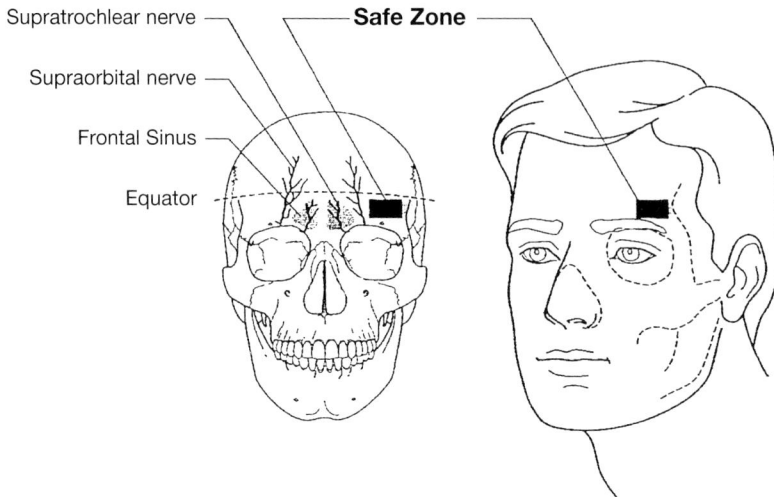

Figure 4 Drawing depicting the "safe zone" for anterior halo-pin placement. Laterally the pin should be placed anterior to the temporalis muscle and fossa to avoid possible painful mastication or penetration through thin cranial bone. Medially, the pin should be kept lateral to the middle portion of the superior orbital rim to avoid the supraorbital and supratrochlear nerves or the frontal sinus. Superiorly, the pin should be kept below the level of the greatest skull circumference (skull equator) to avoid cephalad migration of the pin. Inferiorly, the pin should be kept above the supraorbital ridge to prevent displacement or penetration into the orbit. (Adapted with permission from Ref. 51.)

Because of this trend, they recommended continuing to utilize a 6 inch-pound insertion torque. However, they did not perform multivariate analysis to correct for the differences between the two groups in the number of neurologically intact patients.

A number of studies have been performed on the vest portion of the halo vest apparatus (57–60). Initially, a body cast was used to stabilize the halo ring to the thorax (40,53). Currently, plastic vests with a sheepskin lining are available for thoracic fixation. A vest length that extends to the level of the xiphoid has been found to be adequate for stability throughout the cervical spine (59). Wang et al. found that half-length vests were adequate to control motion above C4, but a full-length vest was needed to improve control below C4 (60). Mirza et al. found that increasing vest tightness, decreasing the deformability of the vest, and ensuring a good fit can decrease motion (58). They also found that most commercially available vests provide similar immobilization (58).

Complications associated with halo use have been well documented (51,61–66). The most common complication is pin loosening (51,56). Pin tract infections have also been noted in most large series (51,62,63). Cerebrospinal fluid leakage or subdural abscess is also a possible, though much less frequent, complication (61,63). Pressure sores under the vest, particularly over the scapula can be problematic, particularly in patients with compromised sensation (Fig. 5) (40,51,67).

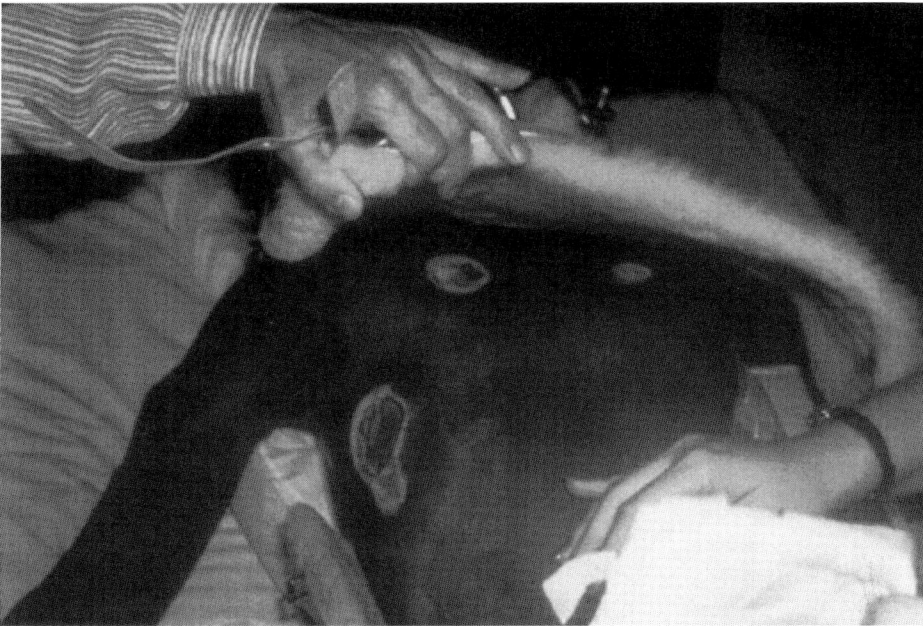

Figure 5 Pressure ulceration underneath the posterior halo-vest in a patient with an unstable cervical traumatic injury that resulted in quadriplegia.

D   Application of the Halo

Three people are ideal for placement of a halo. In this scenario, one person holds the head and halo while the other two apply the pins. If head holders or positioning pins are available, less people may be necessary. An experienced member of the team should hold the head. This is particularly important in cases with unstable fractures (45,68,69).

Prior to initiating application, a properly sized ring should be selected. It should provide 1 to 2 cm of clearance around the circumference of the head. A proper vest piece should be selected based on chest circumference and a crash cart with resuscitation equipment must be readily available (45,69).

The patient should be alert during application so that the neurological status can be monitored during placement of the halo and manipulation of the head and neck. If an associated procedure is to be performed, general anesthesia can be used, although it is not recommended (45,69).

The patient should be positioned in the supine position with the head slightly beyond the edge so that the ring can be easily applied. If an open ring is used, the head can remain on the bed, although slight elevation with a bump in the midline of the head aids during placement of the posterior pins.

The anterior pin sites should be chosen over the lateral third of the eyebrow and just above the supraorbital ridge. Complimentary sites posteriorly can then be identified. These should be diagonal to the contralateral anterior sites, which should allow allow for placement of the ring below the equator of the skull, but approximately 1 cm above the pinna of the ear.

The skin anteriorly should be cleansed with a povidone–iodine solution, and the skin posteriorly should be shaved and cleansed in a like manner. The skin in the area of pin placement should be infiltrated with lidocaine down to the periosteum of the skull. The ring is then placed over the head and the pins are advanced through the skin to finger tightness. The eyes should be kept shut during advancement of the anterior pins to avoid tenting of the skin. Once the pins are finger tight, opposite pins should be advanced simultaneously in 2 inch-pound increments up to 8 inch-pounds. A calibrated torque wrench is necessary for this step. The lock nuts are then tightened, with care taken not to overtighten, and possibly cause backing out of the pins (45,69).

The vest should then be applied. The posterior portion is positioned first, then the anterior half. The proper position of the neck and head is then maintained as the upright posts are positioned and tightened with the torque wrenches. It is imperative to keep wrenches at the bedside in case the anterior portion of the vest needs to be removed for emergent access to the chest. A radiograph should be obtained after the halo is placed.

The pins should be retightened to 8 inch-pounds 24 to 48 h after application. It is unnecessary to apply dressings to the pins sites, although they should be routinely cleaned every other day, or more frequently, if needed with hydrogen peroxide (45,69).

If loosening of the pins occurs, they should be retightened to 8 inch-pounds if resistance is met within two rotations. If no resistance is met, a new pin site should be sought. To avoid displacement of the halo, the new pin should be placed prior to removal of the loose pin (51).

If drainage develops around a pin site, cultures and appropriate antibiotic therapy should be instituted. Continued drainage or abscess development mandates pin replacement in a different location. Debridement and intravenous antibiotic may be necessary (51).

Placement of the head and neck in excessive extension may cause symptoms of dysphagia. This usually responds to repositioning of the head (51).

If dural leakage occurs, the patient should be hospitalized, placed in an elevated head position, and placed on IV antibiotics. This complication can occur as a result of trauma, a fall, or by excessive retightening of a loose pin.

Because the halo cannot completely immobilize the cervical spine, loss of reduction has been reported (66). This has been more common with fractures of the posterior elements, particularly unilateral facet dislocations. Poor-fitting vests can also lead to loss of position due to inadequate fixation to the thorax (60,66).

V PEDIATRIC CONSIDERATIONS

Cervical spine injuries very rarely occur in children. Evans reported an incidence of 1.2 cases per year over a 20-year period at a major children's hospital, while Rang noted a rate of 1.3 cases per year over 15 years (70). The majority of cervical spine fractures that do occur in younger children occur at the upper cervical spine (70,71). Consequently, the majority of published literature on cervical spine immobilization in the pediatric population addresses issues surrounding halo immobilization in children.

The use of halo bracing in children is complicated by the developing skull. Skull thickness, open cranial sutures, fontanels, and cranial distortion are unique concerns when applying forces to the pediatric skull during halo application. Kopits and Steingrass published the first report on halo immobilization in children (72). Their early series consisted of six children between the ages of three-and-one-half and ten years old. Halos were applied under general anesthesia using a four-pin technique. Pins were placed at the anterolateral and posterolateral aspects of the skull under 1.5 to 5 inch-pounds of torque. The authors cautioned against using greater than 5 inch-pounds of torque in children and discouraged the use of the halo in children younger than three-and-one-half years old. The halo provided excellent immobilization in all six patients, was remarkably well tolerated, and was associated with minimal complications in this series.

Kopits' empiric recommendations for pin placement at the anterolateral and posterolateral positions of the pediatric skull have been validated by CT-derived data on regional skull thickness (55). Garfin et al. found average skull thickness in one- to two-year-olds at the anterolateral and posterolateral regions of the skull to be 3.7 and 3.9 mm, respectively. Average thickness linearly increased to 6.1 and 5.9 mm in 5- to 12-year-olds. However, several authors have recommended the routine use of limited CT scans to help plan pin sites away from suture lines or areas of thin calvarium (55,73,74). This should be strongly considered in children younger than 24 months (before cranial sutures have closed) and in the setting of congenital cranial abnormalities or prior craniosynostosis surgery.

More recently, Mubarak and associates have recommended a low-torque, multiple-pin technique for children less than 2 to 3 years of age (74). By using 10 to 12 pins, less torque is required (2 inch-pounds) and pins can be placed at thinner regions of the skull with less risk of skull penetration. While the hardware design and application techniques are the same as those used for older patients, custom-made components are often required for small children, depending on manufacturer inventory. Using this technique, Mubarak and associates have effectively treated patients as young as 7 months old in halo fixation. They note that concerns about cranial distortion are minimized by short application periods, custom-fitted halo rings, and by multiple-pin–low-torque technique that allows for even distribution of pressure.

Complication rates in children managed with halo immobilization are similar to those in adult series (75). Reported complications include pin-site infection, aseptic drainage, dural penetration, loosening, nerve injury, pressure sores, scarring, and pain (70,72,73,75). In a recent retrospective analysis of 37 patients between 3 and 16 years old, Dormans and associates noted an overall complication rate of 68% (75). Pin-site infections occurred in 59% of patients and loosening in 41%. Other complications included a single case of dural penetration and a single transient supraorbital nerve injury. All patients were able to complete their halo treatment periods. Close monitoring of pin-site interfaces and early treatment of pin-site infections are required for successful halo immobilization in children.

VI CONCLUSIONS

Based on the results of the aforementioned studies, some general recommendations regarding the use of orthoses can be made. While the halo is best at limiting motion below C2, it remains the gold standard for immobilizing the upper cervical spine as well. The thermoplastic Minerva brace appears to have promise in this area, but studies from multiple centers are lacking. Immobilization of the lower cervical spine can be achieved with a halo, CTO, or CO. Among the cervicothoracic orthoses, the Minerva and Yale performed the best. The NecLoc and Miami J collars tested the best among the cervical orthoses.

All of these orthoses have potential complications, not the least of which is the possible loss of reduction of the cervical spine. This point must be kept in mind when deciding between operative or nonoperative management, or between the different types of orthoses. Careful examination of the underlying skin, attention to pin sites, and frequent radiographs are necessary to minimize these complications.

REFERENCES

1. American Academy of Orthopaedic Surgeons. Atlas of Orthotics. St. Louis: CV Mosby, 1975.
2. Smith GE. The most ancient splints. Br Med J 1908; 732–734.
3. American Academy of Orthopaedic Surgeons. Atlas of Orthotics. St. Louis: CV Mosby, 1985.
4. Peltier LF. Orthopedics, a history and iconography. San Francisco: Norman Publishing, 1993.
5. Edwards JW. Orthopaedic appliances atlas. St. Louis: American Academy of Orthopaedic Surgeons, 1952.
6. White AA, Panjabi MM. Physical properties and functional biomechanics of the spine. In: White AA, Panjabi MM, eds. Clinical Biomechanics of the Spine, 2nd ed. Philadelphia: JB Lippincott, 1990:1–83.
7. Chase A, Pearcy M, Bader D. Spinal orthoses. In: Bowker P, Condle DN, Bader DL, Pratt DJ, eds. Biomechanical Basis of Orthotic Management. Oxford: Bteerworth-Heinemann Ltd, 1993.
8. Alberts LR, Mahoney CR, Neff JR. Comparison of the Nebraska Collar, a new prototype cervical immobilization collar, with three standard models. J Orthop Trauma 1998; 12: 425–430.
9. Hannah RE. The canadian collar: A new cervical spine orthosis. Am J Occup Ther 1985; 39:171–177.
10. Hughes SJ. How effective is the Newport/Aspen collar? A prospective radiographic evaluation in healthy adult volunteers. J Trauma 1998; 45:374–378.
11. Fisher SV, Bowar JF, Awad EA, Gullickson G. Cervical orthoses effect on cervical spine motion: Roentgenographic and goniometric method of study. Arch Phys Med Rehabil 1977; 58:109–115.
12. Jones MD. Cineradiographic studies of the collar-immobilized cervical spine. J Neurosurg 1960; 17:633–637.
13. Hartman JT, Palumbo F, Hill J. Cineradiography of the braced normal cervical spine. Clin Orthop 1975; 109:97–102.
14. Colachis SC, Strohm BR, Ganter EL. Cervical spine motion in normal women: Radiographic study of effect of cervical collars. Arch Phys Med Rehabil 1973; 54:161–169.
15. Johnson RM, Hart DL, Simmons EF, Ramsby GR, Southwick WO. Cervical orthoses: A study comparing their effectiveness in restricting cervical motion in normal subjects. J Bone Joint Surg 1977; 59-A:332–339.
16. Benzel EC, Hadden TA, Saulsbery CM. A comparison of the minerva and halo jackets for stabilization of the cervical spine. J Neurosurg 1989; 70:411–414.

17. Barkana Y, Stein M, Scope A, Maor R, Abramovich Y, Friedman Z, Knoller N. Pre-hospital stabilization of the cervical spine for penetrating injuries of the neck—Is it necessary? Injury Int J Care Injured 2000; 21:305–309.
18. Cline JR, Scheidel E, Bigsby EF. A comparison of methods of cervical immobilization used in patient extrication and transport. J Trauma 1985; 25:649–653.
19. Curran C, Dietrich AM, Bowman MJ, Ginn-Pease ME, King DR, Kosnik E. Pediatric cervical-spine immobilization: Achieving neutral position? J Trauma: Injury, Infect Crit Care 1995; 39:729–732.
20. Graziano AF, Scheidel EA, Cline JR, Baer LJ. A radiographic comparison of prehospital cervical immobilization methods. Ann Emerg Med 1987; 16:10:1127–1131.
21. Huerta C, Griffith R, Joyce SM. Cervical spine stabilization in pediatric patients: Evaluation of current techniques. Ann Emerg Med 1987; 16:10:1121–1126.
22. Kaufman WA, Lunsford TR, Lunsford BR, Lance LL. Comparison of three prefabricated cervical collars. Orthot Prosthet 1986; 39:21–28.
23. McCabe JB, Nolan DJ. Comparison of the effectiveness of different cervical immobilization collars. Ann Emerg Med 1986; 15:1:50–53.
24. Perry SD, McLellan B, Mcllry WE, Maki BE, Schwaretz M, Fernie GR. The efficacy of head immobilization techniques during simulated vehicle motion. Spine 1999; 24:1839–1844.
25. Podolsky S, Baraff LJ, Simon RR, Hoffman JR, Larmon B, Ablon W. Efficacy of cervical spine immobilization methods. J Trauma 1983; 23:461–465.
26. Rosen PB, McSwain NE, Arata M, Stahl S, Mercer D. Comparison of two new immobilization collars. Ann Emerg Med 1992; 21:10:1189–1195.
27. Treloar DJ, Nypaver M. Angulation of the pediatric cervical spine with and without cervical collar. Ped Emerg Care 1997; 13:5–8.
28. Chandler DR, Nemejc C, Adkins RH, Waters RL. Emergency cervical-spine immobilization. Ann Emerg Med 1992; 21:10:1185–1188.
29. Askins V, Eismont FJ. Efficacy of five cervical orthoses in restricting cervical motion: A comparison study. Spine 1997; 22:1193–1198.
30. Powers J. A multidisciplinary approach to occipital pressure ulcers related to cervical collars. J Nurs Care Qual 1997; 12(1):46–52.
31. Chendrasekhar A, Moorman DW, Timberlake GA. An evaluation of the effects of semi-rigid cervical collars in patients with severe closed head injury. Am Surg 1998; 64:604–606.
32. Rodgers JA, Rodgers WB. Marginal mandibular nerve palsy due to compression by a cervical hard collar. J Orthop Trauma 1995; 9:177–179.
33. Ferguson J, Mardel SN, Beattie TF, Wytch R. Cervical collars: A potential risk to the head-injured patient. Injury Int J Care Injured 1993; 24:454–456.
34. Plaisier B, Gabram SGA, Schwartz RJ, Jacobs LM. Prospective evaluation of craniofacial pressure in four different cervical orthoses. J Trauma 1994; 37:714–719.
35. Johnson RM, Owen JR, Hart DL, Callahan RA. Cervical orthoses: A guide to their selection and use. Clin Orthop 1981; 154:34–45.
36. Hart DL, Johnson RM, Simmons EF, Owen J. Review of Cervical Orthoses. Phys Ther 1978; 58:857–860.
37. Johnson RM, Hart DL, Owen JR, Lerner E, Chapin W, Zeleznik R. The Yale cervical orthosis: An evaluation of its effectiveness in restricting cervical motion in normal subjects and a comparison with other cervical orthoses. Phys Ther 1978; 58:865–871.
38. Zelenik R, Chapin W, Hart D, Smith H, Southwick WO, Zito M. Yale cervical orthosis. Phys Ther 1978; 58:861–864.
39. Benzel EC, Larson SJ, Kerk JJ, Millington PJ, Novak SM, Falkner RH, Wenninger WJ. The thermoplastic Minerva body jacket: A clinical comparison with other cervical spine splinting techniques. J Spinal Disord 1992; 5:311–319.

40. Perry J, Nickel VL. Total cervical-spine fusion for neck paralysis. J Bone Joint Surg 1959; 41-A:37–60.

41. Millington PJ, Ellingsen JM, Hauswirth BE, Fabian PJ. Thermoplastic Minerva body jacket—A practical alternative to current methods of cervical spine stabilization: a clinical report. Phys Ther 1987; 67:223–225.

42. Maiman D, Millington P, Novak S, Kerk J, Ellingsen J, Wenninger W. The effect of the thermoplastic Minerva body jacket on cervical spine motion. Neurosurgery 1989; 25: 363–368.

43. Sharpe KP, Rao S, Ziogas A. Evaluation of the effectiveness of the Minerva cervico-thoracic orthosis. Spine 1995; 20:1475–1479.

44. Garrett AL, Perry J, Nickel VL. Stabilization of the collapsing spine. J Bone Joint Surg Am 1961; 43:474–484.

45. Botte MJ, Garfin SR, Byrne TP, Woo SL-Y, Nickel, VL. The halo skeletal fixator: Principles of application and maintenance. Clin Orthop 1989; 239:12–18.

46. Clayman DA, Murakami Vines FS. Compatibility of cervical spine braces with MR imaging: A study of nine nonferrous devices. AJNR 1990; 11:385–390.

47. Garfin SR, Lee TQ, Roux RD, Silva FW, Ballock RT, Botte MJ, Katz MM, Woo SL-Y. Structural behavior of the halo orthosis pin-bone interface: biomechanical evaluation of standard and newly designed stainless steel halo fixation pins. Spine 1986; 11: 977–981.

48. Triggs KJ, Ballock RT, Lee TQ, Woo SL-Y, Garfin SR. The effect of angled insertion on halo pin fixation. Spine 1989; 14:781–783.

49. Ballock RT, Lee TQ, Triggs KJ, Woo SL-Y, Garfin SR. The effect of pin location on the rigidity of the halo pin-bone interface. Neurosurgery 1990; 26:238–241.

50. Garfin SR, Botte MJ, Centeno RS, Nickel VL. Osteology of the skull as it affects halo pin placement. Spine 1985; 10:696–698.

51. Garfin SR, Botte MJ, Waters RL, Nickel VL. Complications in the use of the halo fixation device. J Bone Joint Surg 1986; 68-A:320–325.

52. Botte MJ, Byrne TP, Garfin SR. Use of skin incisions in the application of halo skeletal fixator pins. Clin Orthop 1989; 246:100–101.

53. Perry J. The halo in spinal abnormalities: practical factors and avoidance of complications. Orthoped Clin North Am 1972; 3:69–80.

54. Botte MJ, Byrne TP, Garfin SR. Application of the halo fixation device using an increased torque pressure. J Bone Joint Surg 1987; 69-A:750–752.

55. Garfin SR, Roux R, Botte MJ, Centeno R, Woo SL-Y. Skull osteology as it affects halo pin placement in children. J Pediatr Orthop 1986; 6:434–436.

56. Rizzolo SJ, Piazza MR, Cotler JM, Hume EL, Cautilli G, O'Neill DK. The effect of torque pressure on halo pin complication rates. Spine 1993; 18:2163–66.

57. Krag MH, Beynnon BD. A new halo-vest: rationale, design and biomechanical comparison to standard halo-vest designs. Spine 1988; 13:228–235.

58. Mirza SK, Moquin RR, Anderson PA, Tencer AF, Steinmann J, Varnau D. Stabilizing properties of the halo apparatus. Spine 1997; 22:727–733.

59. Triggs KJ, Ballock RT, Byrne T, Garfin SR. Length dependence of a halo orthosis on cervical immobilization. J Spinal Disord 1993; 6:34–37.

60. Wang GJ, Moskal JT, Albert T, Pritts C, Schuch CM, Stamp WG. The effect of halo-vest length on stability of the cervical spine. J Bone Joint Surg 1988; 70A:357–360.

61. Garfin SR, Botte MJ, Triggs KJ, Nickel VL. Subdural abscess associated with halo-pin traction. J Bone Joint Surg 1988; 70-A:1338–1340.

62. Glaser JA, Whitehill R, Stamp WG, Jane JA. Complications associated with the halo-vest: A review of 245 cases. J Neurosurg 1986; 65:762–769.

63. Goodman ML, Nelson PB. Brain abscess complicating the use of a halo orthosis. Neurosurgery 1987; 20:27–30.

64. Kaplan SL, Rocco TP, Silverman DI, Kemper AJ. Acute pulmonary edema following removal of a spinal orthosis: An unusual complication of a halo vest. Arch Phys Med Rehabil 1990; 70:255–257.
65. Lind B, Bake B, Lundqvist C, Nordwall A. Influence of halo vest treatment on vital capacity. Spine 1987; 12:449–452.
66. Whitehill R, Richman JA, Glaser JA. Failure of immobilization of the cervical spine by the halo vest. J Bone Joint Surg 1986; 68-A:326–332.
67. Chan RC, Schweigel JF, Thompson GB. Halo-thoracic brace immobilization in 188 patients with acute cervical spine injuries. J Neurosurg 1983; 58:508–515.
68. Botte MJ, Byrne TP, Abrams RA, Garfin SR. The halo skeletal fixator: current concepts of application and maintenance. Orthopedics 1995; 18:463–471.
69. Vaccaro AR, Lavernia CJ, Botte M, Bergmann K, Garfin SR. Spinal orthoses in the management of spine trauma. In: Levine A, Garfin SR, Eismont F, Zigler, JE, eds. Spine Trauma. Philadelphia: WB Saunders, 1998:171–194.
70. Evans DL, Bethem D. Cervical spine injuries in children. J Pediatr Orthop 1989; 9:563–568.
71. Eleraky MA, Theodore N, Adams M, Rekate HL, Sonntag VKH. Pediatric cervical spine injuries: Report of 102 cases and review of the literature. J Neurosurg (Spine 1) 2000; 92:12–17.
72. Kopits SE, Steingass MH. Experience with the ''halo-cast'' in small children. Surg Clin North Am 1970; 50:935–943.
73. Letts M, Kaylor D, Gouw G. A biomechanical analysis of halo fixation in children. J Bone Joint Surg 1988; 70-B:277–279.
74. Mubarak SJ, Camp JF, Vuletich W, Wenger DR, Garfin SR. Halo application in the infant. J Pediatr Orthop 1989; 9:612–614.
75. Dormans JP, Criscitiello AA, Drummond DS, Davidson RS. Complications in children managed with immobilization in a halo vest. J Bone Joint Surg 1995; 77-A:1370–1373.

22

Surgical Approaches for the Operative Management of Cervical Spine Fractures

HOWARD S. AN

Rush-Presbyterian-St. Luke's Medical Center, Chicago, Illinois, U.S.A.

REX A. W. MARCO

University of Texas M.D. Anderson Cancer Center, Houston, Texas, U.S.A.

I INTRODUCTION

Successful spinal surgery begins with a careful and meticulous surgical approach. The most appropriate approach is dependent on the nature of the fracture, its location, and its extent. This chapter discusses anterior and posterior approaches to the cervical, thoracic, and lumbar spine.

II ANTERIOR APPROACHES

A Upper Cervical Spine

Anterior approaches to the upper part of the cervical spine include transpharyngeal and retropharyngeal approaches (1–8). Each procedure has advantages and disadvantages. Familiarity with the anatomy and potential complications associated with each approach facilitates proper management of upper cervical spinal fractures and related disorders.

The transpharyngeal approach allows exposure of the midline between the arch of the atlas and C2 (Fig. 1). The transpharyngeal procedure is technically demanding and has limited indications (1,9). Any oropharynx or dental infections must be treated

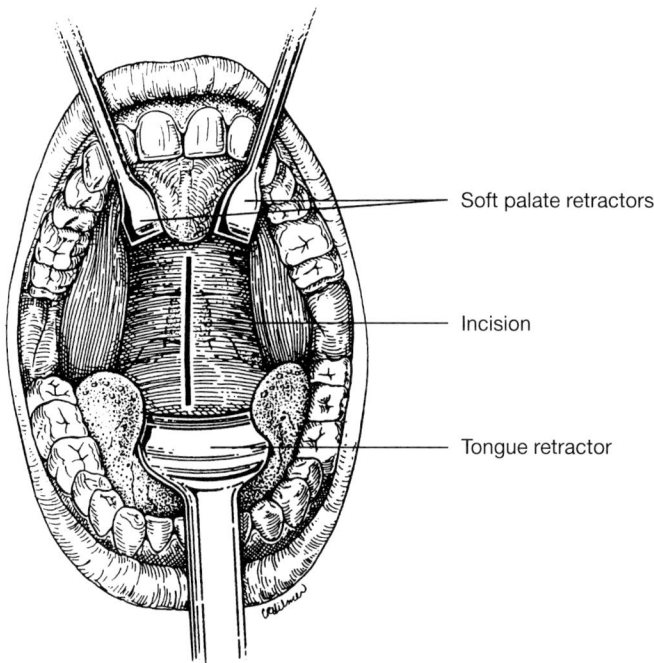

Figure 1 Diagram of the transpharyngeal approach, which allows exposure of the midline between the arch of the atlas and C2. The exposure may be extended cephalad by dividing the soft and hard palate to allow access to the foramen magnum and lower half of the clivus. (Reproduced with permission from Ref. 16.)

prior to elective transoral surgery. Somatosensory-evoked potential monitoring, fiberoptic nasotracheal intubation, and a nasogastric tube are used.

The patient is placed in the supine position with the head held in slight extension using the Mayfield frame. The oral cavity is cleansed with chlorhexidine. Prophylactic perioperative antibiotics, combined with an intravenous cephalosporin and metronidazole, are instituted for 72 h. Transoral retractors are inserted to expose the posterior oropharynx. The key surgical landmark is the anterior tubercle of the atlas to which the anterior longitudinal ligament and longus colli muscles are attached. The vertebral artery is at a minimum of 2 cm from this point in the midline. The area of the incision is infiltrated with 1:200,000 epinephrine. A midline 3-cm vertical incision centered on the anterior tubercle is made through the pharyngeal mucosa and muscle. The mucosa and muscle are later closed in separate layers. The tubercle of the atlas and anterior longitudinal ligament are exposed superiosteally, and the longus colli muscles are mobilized laterally. A high-speed burr may be used to remove the anterior arch of the atlas to expose the odontoid process. The exposure may be extended cephalad by dividing the soft and hard palate to allow access to the foramen magnum and lower half of the clivus. Osteotomy of the mandible can provide additional exposure of the cervical spine. The use of bone graft may be associated with higher infection rates following transpharyngeal approaches. Therefore, anterior bone graft is not usually performed.

Extrapharyngeal approaches are more likely to have a lower incidence of infection than transpharyngeal approaches. The anteromedial extrapharyngeal approach described by DeAndrade and Macnab (3) is an extension of the Smith-Robinson (10) approach to the lower cervical spine. Preoperative voluntary cervical extension is assessed to determine the degree of extension tolerated by the patient. Intraoperative hyperextension is avoided to help prevent the development or worsening of myelopathic signs and symptoms. Gardner-Wells tongs are applied and the neck is extended to the previously determined degree of tolerance. The chin is turned to the opposite side. Either the left- or the right-sided approach is used since the exposure is cephalad to the recurrent laryngeal nerve. A skin incision is made along the anterior aspect of the sternocleidomastoid muscle and curved toward the mastoid process. The platysma and the superficial layer of the deep cervical fascia are divided in line with the incision to expose the anterior border of the sternocleidomastoid. The sternocleidomastoid muscle is retracted anteriorly, and the carotid artery laterally. The superior thyroid artery and lingual vessels are ligated. The external branch of the superior laryngeal nerve is in close proximity to the superior thyroid artery. Excessive retraction of this nerve causes hoarseness or inability to sing high notes, as this nerve innervates the cricothyroid muscle. The facial artery is identified at the upper portion of the incision as it passes under the stylohyoid and the posterior belly of the digastric muscles These muscles are also adjacent to the hypoglossal nerve, which can also be identified. Stripping of the longus colli muscle exposes the anterior aspect of the upper cervical spine and basiocciput.

McAfee et al. (6) described another extrapharyngeal approach via a right-sided (for right-handed surgeons) submandibular transverse incision combined with a vertical limb, which can be extended caudally as necessary (Fig. 2). Division of the platysma exposes the sternocleidomastoid muscle and its deep cervical fascia. The mandibular branch of the facial nerve is identified with the aid of a nerve stimulator, and the retromandibular vein is ligated near its junction with the internal jugular vein. The facial nerve is usually superficial to the retromandibular vein, thus deep dissection to this vein helps protect the mandibular branch of the facial nerve. The anterior border of the sternocleidomastoid muscle is mobilized and the submandibular salivary gland and the jugular digastric lymph nodes are excised if necessary. Care should be taken to ligate the salivary gland duct to prevent a salivary fistula. The digastric tendon is divided and tagged for later repair. The stylohyoid muscle is removed from the hyoid bone, which allows medial retraction of the hyoid and hypopharynx. A nerve stimulator is used to help identify the hypoglossal nerve, which is then mobilized. Arterial and venous branches of the carotid sheath can be ligated to help mobilize the carotid contents laterally. These branches include the superior thyroid, lingual, ascending pharyngeal, and facial arteries and veins. The external branch of the superior laryngeal nerve is identified and mobilized. The prevertebral fasciae is transected longitudinally to expose and dissect the longus colli muscles.

The anterolateral retropharyngeal approach described by Whitesides and Kelley also provides exposure of the upper cervical spine (8). This approach involves dissection anterior to the sternocleidomastoid but posterior to the carotid sheath. The skin incision is made from the mastoid along the anterior aspect of the sternocleidomastoid. The external jugular vein is ligated and, if possible, the greater auricular nerve is spared. The sternocleidomastoid and splenius capitus muscles are detached

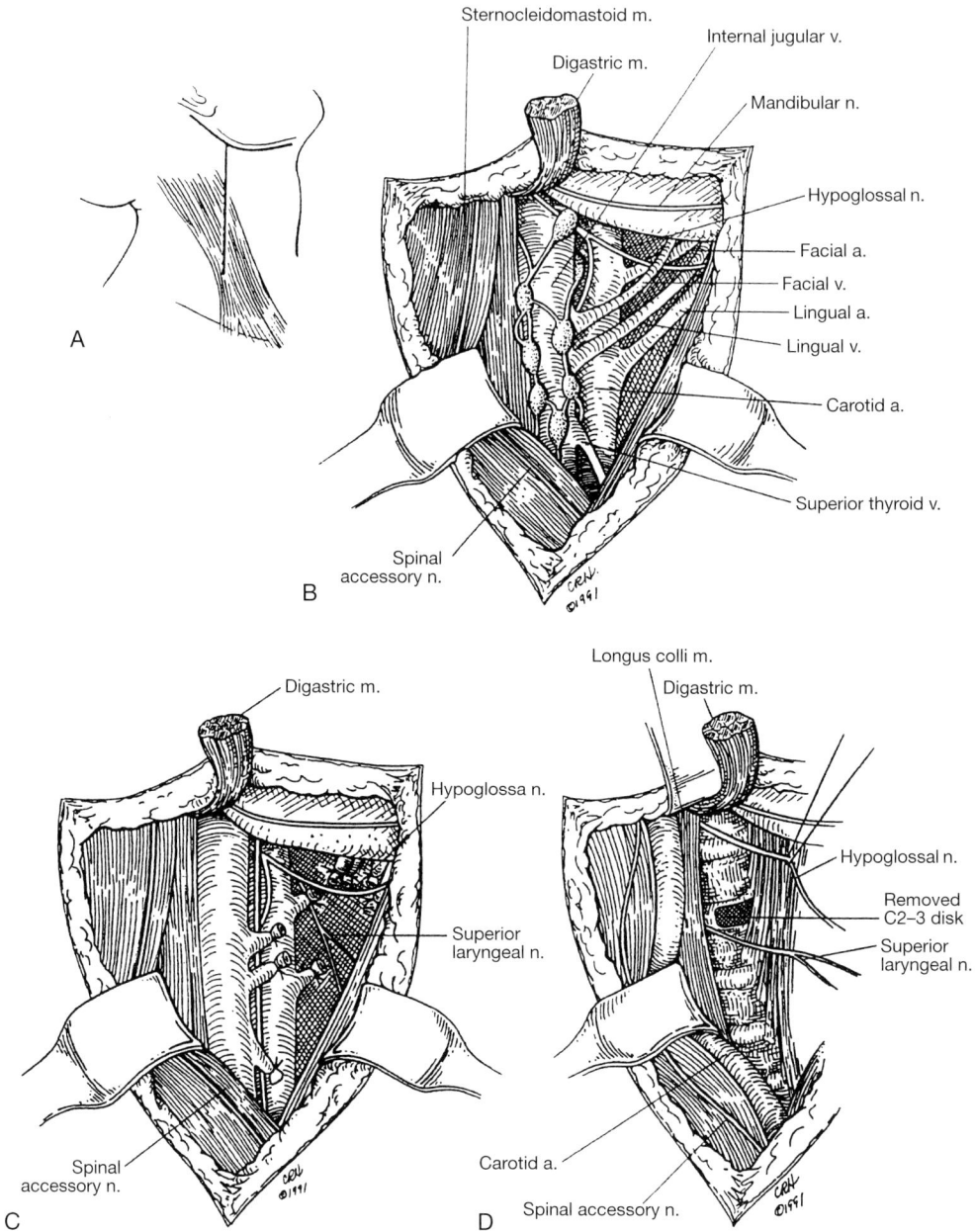

Figure 2   McAfee's retropharyngeal approach to the upper cervical spine. (A) A right-sided submandibular T-shaped incision is made. (B) Division of the platysma leads to the sternocleidomastoid muscle and its deep cervical fascia. The mandibular branch of the facial nerve should be preserved. The digastric tendon is divided and tagged for later repair. The hypoglossal nerve is next identified and mobilized. (C) The carotid contents are mobilized laterally by ligating arterial and venous branches. These include the superior thyroid, lingual, ascending pharyngeal, and facial arteries and veins, beginning inferiorly and progressing superiorly. The external branch of the superior

from the mastoid, leaving a fascial edge for subsequent repair. The spinal accessory nerve should be identified and protected. The carotid sheath contents and the hypoglossal nerve are retracted anteriorly, while the sternocleidomastoid is retracted posteriorly. Blunt dissection leads to the transverse processes and anterior aspect of C1 to C3. Potential complications of this approach include injuries to the spinal accessory nerve, the sympathetic ganglion, and vertebral artery.

B Lower Cervical Spine

The anterior approach to the lower cervical spine is well described in the literature (7,10,11). The patient is placed in a supine and slight reverse Trendelenburg position to minimize venous pooling in the surgical area. Traction is applied to the head using Gardner-Wells tongs or halter device, while caudally directed traction to the shoulders is applied using adhesive tape. The right-handed surgeon often prefers the right-sided approach. On the right side, however, the recurrent laryngeal nerve occasionally leaves the carotid sheath within the neck. Many surgeons thus approach the lower cervical spine from the left side to minimize the risk of injury to the recurrent laryngeal nerve, especially for fractures involving the C6–TI region. Palpable neck structures help identify the proper level. The hyoid bone overlies the third vertebra, the thyroid cartilage spans C4 and C5, and the cricoid cartilage is located at the C6 vertebra (Fig. 3A). Placement of a needle on the skin combined with an intraoperative radiograph or fluoroscopy may also help locate the proper level. A horizontal incision in line with a skin crease at the appropriate level from just lateral to the midline to the midportion of the sternocleidomastoid is used. A vertical incision anterior to the sternocleidomastoid may be necessary if multiple levels of exposure are required. The skin and subcutaneous tissue are undermined, followed by division of the platysma muscle. The sternocleidomastoid muscle is retracted laterally and the strap muscles medially. The deep cervical fascia is divided between the sternocleidomastoid muscle and strap muscles, and blunt finger dissection is performed through the pretracheal fascia along the medial border of the carotid sheath, thereby avoiding injury to the carotid artery, internal jugular vein, or vagus nerve (Fig. 3B). Great caution should also be taken medially, as the strap muscles surround the thyroid gland, trachea, and esophagus. The surgical dissection should not enter the plane between the trachea and esophagus because the recurrent laryngeal nerve lies in this interval. A self-retaining retractor is then positioned to expose the prevertebral fascia and longus colli muscles (Fig. 3C). A sharp self-retaining retractor should be avoided to prevent perforation of the visceral structures. The temporal artery pulse is palpated after the retractor is spread and used as a gauge to determine carotid artery patency. The superior thyroid artery is encountered above C4 and the inferior thyroid artery is seen below C6. These vessels should be identified and ligated as necessary.

The thoracic duct is at risk for injury during the left-sided approach. The thoracic duct ascends into the neck as high as C6 before it descends to empty near the

←——

laryngeal nerve is also identified and mobilized. (D) The prevertebral fasciae are transected longitudinally to expose and dissect the longus colli muscles. (Reproduced with permission from Ref. 15.)

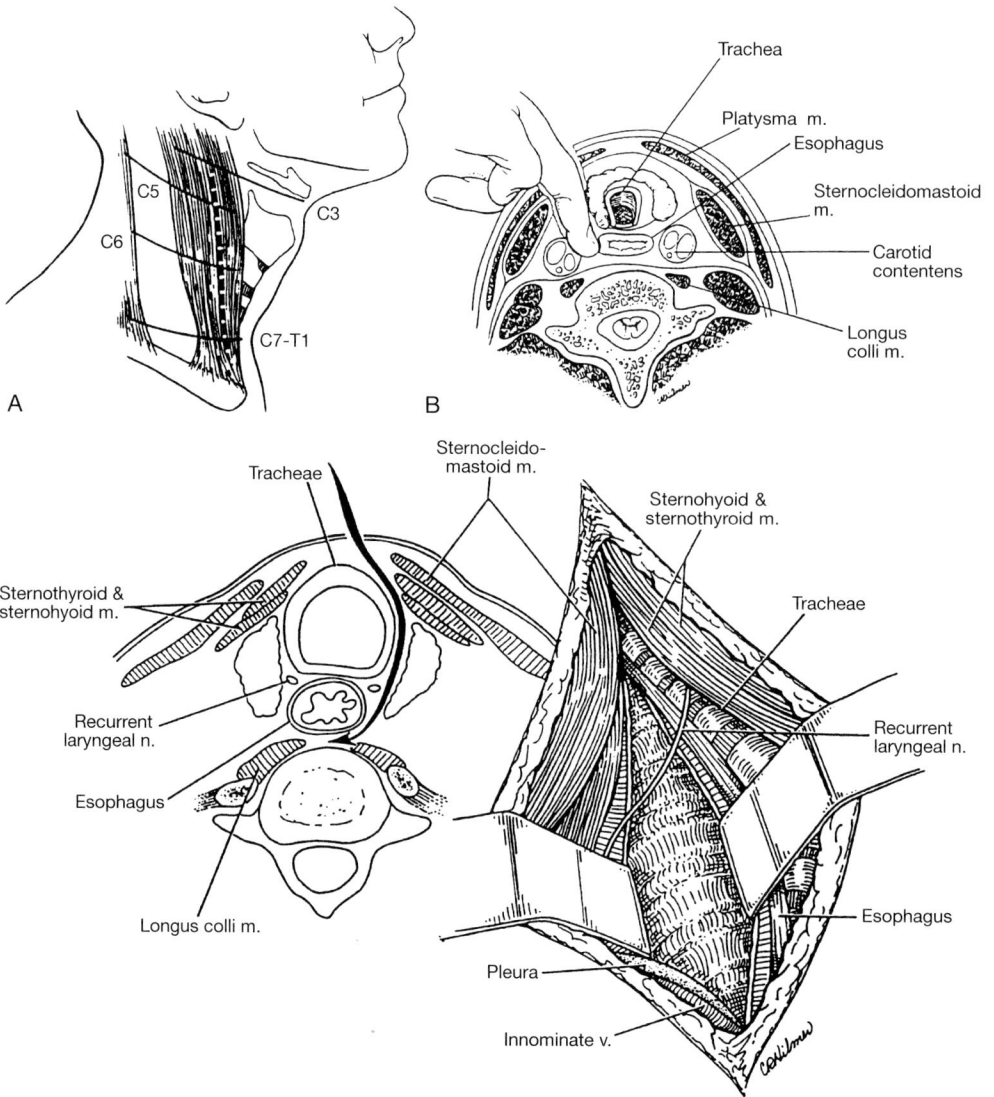

Figure 3 The Smith-Robinson anteromedial approach to the lower cervical spine. (A) Diagram of skin incisions for anterior cervical approaches. A horizontal incision is used at the level of the hyoid bone for C3–C4, the thyroid cartilage for C4–C5, and the cricoid ring for C6. (B) Division of the platysma muscle is followed by lateral retraction of the sternocleidomastoid muscle. The deep cervical fascia is divided between the sternocleidomastoid muscle and strap muscles, and blunt finger dissection is performed through the pretracheal fascia along the medial border of the carotid sheath. (C) A self-retaining retractor is then positioned to expose the prevertebral fascia and longus colli muscles. Vital structures that are vulnerable to injury during this approach include recurrent laryngeal nerve, carotid contents and branches, thoracic duct, trachea, thyroid, and esophagus. (Reproduced with permission from Ref. 15.)

internal jugular and subclavian vein junction. Further dissection is performed by palpating the prominent disk margins ("hills") and concave anterior vertebral bodies ("valleys"). A bent 18-gauge needle is placed in the disk space, and a lateral radiograph is taken to confirm the correct level. The bent needle prevents inadvertent penetration into the spinal cord. The prevertebral fascia and the anterior longitudinal ligament are divided in the midline to minimize bleeding and prevent injury to the sympathetic chain. Subperiosteal mobilization of the longus colli muscles is then completed. This anteromedial approach to the cervical spine is utilized in the majority of cases.

In special circumstances, however, lateral approaches described by Hodgson (12) and Verbiest (13) can be used. Hodgson described an approach to the lower cervical area, dissecting posterior to the carotid sheath to expose the anterior and lateral aspect of the cervical spine. This approach avoids the thyroid vessels, vagus nerve, and external branch of the superior laryngeal nerve. Verbiest modified the approach for the exposure of the vertebral artery and involves dissecting anterior to the carotid sheath and exposing the vertebral artery and nerve roots posterior to the transverse processes. These lateral approaches are preferred in laterally located lesions or if the vertebral artery must be exposed.

Some fractures are stabilized with a vertebrectomy and strut grafting after the anterior approach is performed. Proper diskectomy and fusion techniques are crucial to successful outcomes. The endplates should be flattened with a power burr to maximize contact area with the graft and to enhance vascularity and healing of the graft (14). Drill holes in the middle of the endplate enhance vascular flow without jeopardizing the strength of the endplate (15,16). Distraction of the intervertebral space can be achieved by skull traction and laminar spreader. Graft extrusion can be avoided if the graft is countersunk 2 mm under the anterior cortical margin of the vertebral body. Exact measurement of width and depth of the bone graft slot should be made using a caliper or ruler.

Potential complications associated with anterior approaches of the cervical spine are numerous (Table 1). The most devastating complication is neurological deterioration. Most spinal cord or nerve root injuries are associated with technical mishaps. The first consideration is anesthesia and positioning. Awake intubation with the aid of a fiberoptic light is helpful to prevent excessive manipulation during intubation. Awake intubation and somatosensory-evoked potential monitoring can help prevent the development or worsening of neurological injury. Careful removal of bone or disk material in the lateral corner near the uncovertebral joint may help avoid nerve root injury. The posterior longitudinal ligament is usually left intact. If the posterior longitudinal ligament is perforated by bone or disk material, then decompression to the dura is performed. Proper lighting and loupe or microscopic magnification aids visualization. The depth of grafts should be measured carefully and gentle tapping is utilized for graft insertion. The stability of the graft should be maintained by compressive force on the graft. If neurological complications are discovered postoperatively, then a lateral radiograph is obtained to determine the position of the bone graft and administration of dexamethasone is considered. Computed tomography or magnetic resonance imaging can be helpful in evaluating for signs of a hematoma or cord contusion. If a hematoma or bone graft malalignment is suspected, then expeditious reexploration may be required.

Table 1 Potential Complications of Anterior Cervical Fusion

Neural injury
  spinal cord injury
  nerve root damage
  dural tear
Vascular injury
  carotid artery
  internal jugular vein
  vertebral artery
Vocal cord damage (recurrent laryngeal nerve injury)
Esophageal perforation
Tracheal injury
Homer's syndrome
Thoracic duct injury
Pneumothorax
Bone graft complications
  extrusion
  collapse
  nonunion
  donor site complications
Infection
Wound problems (hematoma, drainage, dehiscence)

Dysphagia after anterior cervical surgery may be caused by edema, hemorrhage, denervation, or infection (17). If persistent dysphagia is present, then obtaining a barium swallow or an endoscopy should be considered. Esophageal perforation is a rare but serious complication of anterior cervical spine operations. Sharp retractors must be avoided and gentle handling of the medial visceral structures is mandatory. Use of a nasogastric tube helps identify the esophagus during surgery. If esophageal perforation is suspected during surgery, methylene blue can be injected in the nasogastric tube to look for dye extravasation from the esophagus. Despite these efforts, esophageal perforations can remain unrecognized until the patient develops an abscess, a tracheoesophagcal fistula, or mediastinitis. The usual treatment consists of intravenous antibiotics, nasogastric feeding, drainage, debridement, and repair. Early consultation with a head and neck or general surgeon is recommended.

Minor hoarseness or sore throat after an anterior cervical approach is usually caused by edema or endotracheal intubation. Occasionally, recurrent laryngeal nerve palsy causes hoarseness (18). The incidence may be as high as 11% (19). The external branch of the superior laryngeal nerve travels along with the superior thyroid artery to innervate the cricothyroid muscle. Damage to this nerve may result in hoarseness, but often produces symptoms such as easy fatiguing of the voice. The inferior laryngeal nerve is a recurrent branch of the vagus nerve, which pierces the cricothyroid membrane and innervates all of the laryngeal muscles except for the cricothyroid. On the left side, the recurrent laryngeal nerve loops under the arch of the aorta and is protected in the left tracheoesophageal groove. On the right side, the recurrent nerve travels around the subclavian artery, passing dorsomedially to the side of the trachea and esophagus. It is vulnerable as it passes from the subclavian

artery to the right tracheoesophageal groove. The nerve usually enters the tracheoesophageal groove where the inferior thyroid artery enters the lower pole of the
thyroid. The right inferior laryngeal nerve is occasionally nonrecurrent, and travels
directly from the vagus nerve and carotid sheath to the larynx. This anomaly results
from the right subclavian artery arising directly from the aortic arch, rather than from
the brachiocephalic artery (20,21). The subclavian artery then passes posterior to the
esophagus and recurrence of the inferior laryngeal nerve does not develop. The
incidence of a nonrecurrent laryngeal nerve on the right side is reported as 1% (22).
If hoarseness persists for more than 6 weeks following anterior cervical surgery,
laryngoscopy should be done to evaluate the vocal cord and laryngeal muscles. Treatment of inferior laryngeal nerve palsy includes observation for 6 months to allow
for spontaneous recovery of function. Further treatment or surgery by an otolaryn-
gologist may be necessary in persistent cases.

Injury to the sympathetic chain can result in a Horner's syndrome. The cervical
sympathetic chain lies on the anterior surface of the longus colli muscles just posterior to the carotid sheath. Subperiosteal dissection helps prevent damage to these
nerves. Horner's syndrome is usually temporary but can be permanent in less than
1% of patients (23). Ophthalmological consultation may be needed for treatment of
ptosis.

Serious bleeding complications following anterior cervical surgery are fortunately rare. A hematoma can cause airway obstruction or spinal cord compression
(22). Meticulous hemostasis, placement of a drain and elevation of the head in the
immediate postoperative period can help prevent these complications. Careful identification and ligation of the superior or the inferior thyroid artery can prevent arterial
bleeding. Avoiding far lateral dissection helps prevent injury to the vertebral artery
and nerve roots (24). The transverse foramen of the more cephalad cervical vertebrae
is more medial and dorsal than the foramina of the lower cervical vertebrae. The
vertebral artery is thus more susceptible to injury in the midcervical region than in
the lower cervical region (25). Tears of the vertebral artery should be repaired by
direct exposure of the vessel in the foramen, if possible. Injuries to the carotid artery
or internal jugular vein are exceedingly rare.

Airway obstruction after extubation may occur in the postoperative period.
Airway exchange is confirmed prior to extubation. Prolonged retraction of the soft
tissues can result in retropharyngeal edema. Postoperative intubation and corticosteroids are considered until the edema decreases.

C   Cervicothoracic Junction

Surgical approaches to the upper thoracic vertebrae are challenging. Anterior exposure of the upper thoracic vertebrae may be accomplished through the low cervical,
supraclavicular, sternum-splitting, or transthoracic approach (26). The low cervical
approach is an extension of the anteromedial approach to the lower cervical spine
(27). The incision is either an oblique incision starting 4 cm below the mastoid
process and extending to the sternoclavicular joint, or a horizontal incision at the
base of the neck. After division of the platysma muscle, blunt dissection between
the sternocleidomastoid muscle laterally and the esophagus and trachea medially is
performed to expose the spine. The inferior thyroid artery and vein are ligated. The
recurrent laryngeal nerve is identified and protected. The midline is identified and a

subperiosteal dissection of the longus colli off the vertebral bodies is performed. Subperiosteal dissection can help prevent injury to the thoracic duct during left-sided approaches. If damaged, the thoracic duct should be doubly ligated both proximally and distally to prevent chylothorax.

The supraclavicular approach utilizes a transverse incision above the clavicle with a dissection posterior to the carotid sheath (28). The platysma muscle is incised and the clavicular head of the sternocleidomastoid is divided. The internal jugular and subclavian veins, as well as the carotid artery, must be protected from injury during division of the sternocleidomastoid muscle. The fascia beneath the sterno-cleidomastoid is divided to release the omohyoid from its pulley. The subclavian artery and its branches, which include the vertebral artery and the thyrocervical trunk, are identified. The suprascapular, transverse cervical, and inferior thyroid arteries are identified and ligated as necessary as they leave the thyrocervical trunk. The phrenic nerve is identified lying on the anterior scalene and gently retracted before division of the scalenus anterior muscle. The supraclavicular nerves are superficial and lateral to the scalenus anterior muscle, while the brachial plexus is deep and lateral to this muscle. Division of the scalenus anterior muscle exposes Sibson's fascia, which covers the dome of the lung. Sibson's fascia is divided transversely using scissors and the visceral pleura and lung should be retracted inferiorly. The trachea, the esophagus, and the recurrent laryngeal nerve must be protected during medial re-traction. The posterior thorax, stellate ganglion, and upper thoracic vertebral bodies are now visible through the thoracic inlet.

The low cervical or supraclavicular approaches usually allow exposure of the lower cervical spine and the first and second thoracic vertebrae. Obese or muscular patients with short necks are generally poor candidates for these approaches due to the limited distal extent of the exposure. The complications discussed in the antero-medial approach to the low cervical spine also apply to these approaches. Injury to the thoracic duct, the lung, or the great vessels can also occur.

Upper thoracic vertebrae can also be approached through a thoracotomy that enters the chest through the bed of the third rib, but access to the low cervical region is restricted by the scapula and remaining ribs (29). The right-sided approach is preferred to avoid the left subclavian artery, which is more curved than the right brachiocephalic artery. The incision is medial and inferior to the scapula. The scapula is retracted laterally by dividing the trapezius, latissimus dorsi, rhomboids, and le-vator scapulae muscles. The posterior 7 to 10 cm of the second, third, fourth, and fifth ribs are removed. If T1 is involved, 2 to 3 cm of the first rib are also excised. Exposure of the vertebrae is accomplished by making an L-shaped incision in the pleura and intercostal muscles. Potential complications of this approach include restriction of scapular movement and paralysis of intercostal muscles due to the muscle-splitting aspects of this dissection.

The sternum-splitting approach provides better access to the cervicothoracic junction from C4 to T4, particularly in the obese patient (Fig. 4) (26,30). The skin incision is made anterior to the left sternocleidomastoid muscle and extends along the midsternal area to the xiphoid process. The platysma muscle and superficial cervical fascia are divided, and blunt dissection is done between the laterally situated neurovascular bundle and medial visceral structures. The retrosternal adipose and thymus tissues are retracted from the manubrium. Median sternotomy is performed, taking care to prevent injury to the pleura. Sternohyoid, sternothyroid, and omohyoid

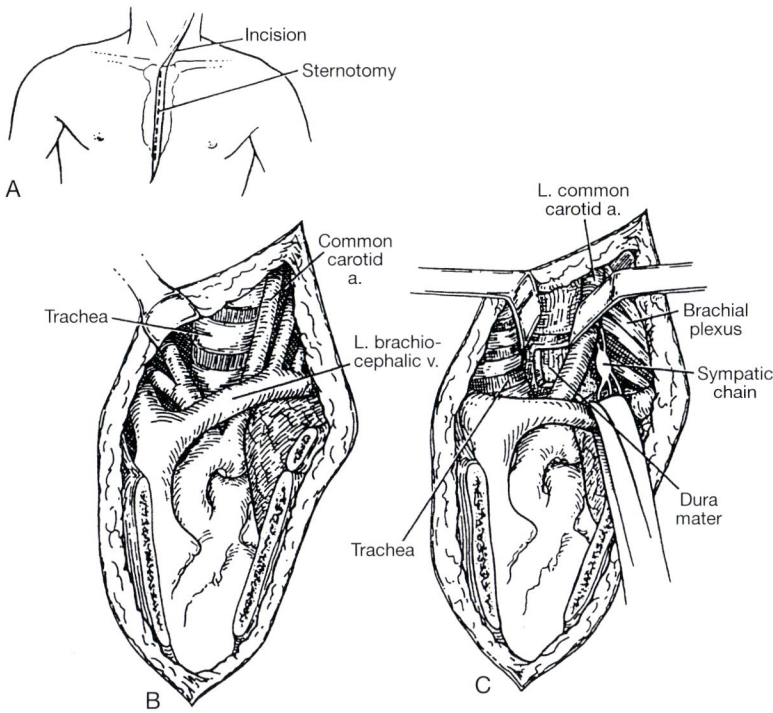

Figure 4   Diagrams of the sternum-splitting approach. (A) The skin incision is made anterior to the left sternocleidomastoid muscle and extends along the midsternal area down to the xiphoid process. (B) The neck dissection is the same for the Smith-Robinson approach. The retrosternal adipose and thymus tissues are retracted from the manubrium. Median sternotomy exposes the left brachiocephalic vein and the common carotid artery. (C) Retraction of the left brachiocephalic vein and common carotid exposes from C4–T4. (Reproduced with permission from Ref. 15.)

muscles are identified and transected as necessary. The inferior thyroid artery is ligated and transected. Blunt dissection is performed from the cranially to caudally until the left brachiocephalic vein is exposed. This vein can be ligated and transected if necessary, but postoperative edema of the left upper extremity can be a problem. The sympathetic nerves, the cupola of the pleura, the great vessels, and the thoracic duct are at risk for injury during this approach.

The perioperative morbidity and mortality associated with the sternum-splitting approach has led to the development of modified approaches to the cervicothoracic junction (31–33). Sundaresan (33) described a less aggressive T-shaped incision to the anterior chest wall (Fig. 5). Dissection is taken down to the manubrium and clavicle with ligation and transection of the anterior jugular venous arch. The medial supraclavicular nerves are also transected. The recurrent laryngeal nerve is less variable on the left side. Therefore, left-sided approach is preferred.

The sternal and clavicular heads of the sternocleidomastoid muscle are detached and retracted. The strap muscles are similarly detached and retracted. After clearing the fatty and areolar tissues in the suprasternal space, the sternal origin of the pec-

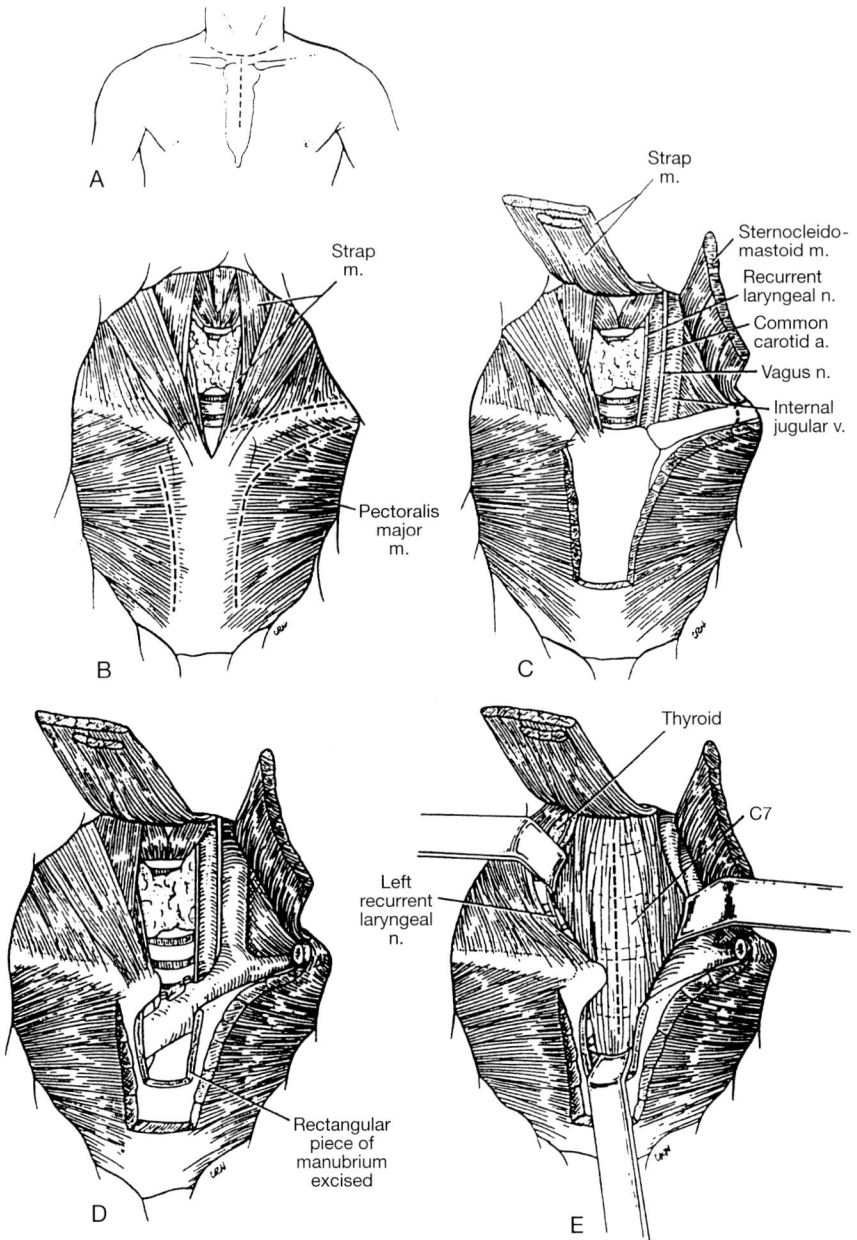

Figure 5 Modified approach to the anterior cervicothoracic junction used by Sundaresan. (A) T-shaped incision on the anterior chest wall. (B) Dissection is taken down to the level of the manubrium and clavicle. (C) The sternal and clavicular heads of the sternocleidomastoid muscle are detached and retracted. The strap muscles on the ipsilateral side of approach are similarly detached and retracted. (D) The sternal origin of the pectoralis major is stripped laterally, and the medial third of the clavicle and a rectangular piece of the manubrium are removed. (E) Dissection is continued between the left carotid artery on the laterally and the innominate artery, trachea, and esophagus medially. (Reproduced with permission from Ref. 15.)

toralis major is stripped laterally. The medial half of the clavicle is then stripped subperiosteally and the medial third of the clavicle is excised with a Gigli saw. A rectangular piece of the manubrium is removed along with its posterior periosteum. At this point, the exposed inferior thyroid vein and, if necessary, the innominate vein are ligated. Dissection is then continued between the left carotid artery laterally and the innominate artery, trachea, and esophagus medially. Special attention must be given to protection of the thoracic duct and left recurrent laryngeal nerve. Kurz and Herkowitz presented a modified anterior approach to the cervicothoracic junction by removing the medial one-third of the clavicle (32). They reported no complications in four patients with tumors. A combined low cervical and transthoracic approach has also been described to gain greater access to the cervicothoracic junction in patients with severe kyphoscoliosis (34).

III POSTERIOR APPROACHES

A Upper Cervical Spine

Posterior approaches to the upper cervical spine are usually performed for occipitocervical junction or atlantoaxial stabilization. A halo vest or Gardner-Wells tong traction is usually applied preoperatively. Careful induction and awake fiberoptic intubation is recommended in patients with unstable fractures to minimize neck manipulation. The use of somatosensory-evoked potential monitoring is routine in myelopathic cases. If traction is not required and preoperative alignment is acceptable, surgery can be performed in the halo vest on the routine operating table. If traction is required or spinal realignment is necessary during the procedure, the halo ring should be attached to a traction device on the Stryker table. To facilitate exposure of the occiput and the upper cervical spine, a halo ring with a posterior opening is recommended.

A reverse Trendelenburg position encourages venous drainage, which decreases intraoperative bleeding. A midline incision is made from the external occipital protuberance to the spinous process of C2. Surgical dissection on the occiput and the ring of the atlas is gently performed as excess pressure may result in a fracture or slippage of the instrument. Dissection of the C1 ring should remain within 12 mm lateral to the midline on the posterior aspect and within 8 mm of the midline on the superior aspect to avoid injury to the vertebral artery (35). Avoiding dissection along the inferior edge of the foramen magnum can help prevent uncontrollable venous bleeding and dural tears.

B Lower Cervical Spine

Exposure of the posterior elements of the lower cervical spine utilizes a Mayfield positioner or Gardner-Wells tongs for positioning. A reverse Trendelenburg position improves venous drainage. A midline incision is made and the midline raphe is identified and split. A subperiosteal dissection is then performed exposing spinous processes, lamina, and facet joints. The spinous processes from C2 to C6 are bifid. Meticulous hemostasis helps prevent hematoma formation.

REFERENCES

1. Crockard HA. Anterior approaches to lesions of the upper cervical spine. Clin Neurosurg 1988; 34:389–416.

2. Crockard HA, Calder I, Ransford AO. One stage transoral decompression and posterior fixation in rheumatoid atlanto-axial subluxation. J Bone Joint Surg 1990; 72 (B):682–685.

3. DeAndrade JR, Macnab I. Anterior occipitocervical fusion using an extra-pharyngeal exposure. J Bone Joint Surg 1969; 51A:1621–1626.

4. Fang HSY, Ong GB. Direct anterior approach to the upper cervical spine. J Bone Joint Surg 1962; 44:1588.

5. Hall JE, Denis F, Murray J. Exposure of the upper cervical spine for spinal decompression. J Bone Joint Surg 1977; 59A:121–123.

7. McAfee PC, Bohlman HH, Riley LH, et al. The anterior retropharyngeal approach to the upper pan of the cervical spine. J Bone Joint Surg 1987; 69A:1371–1383.

9. Riley LH Jr. Surgical approaches to the anterior structures of the cervical spine. Clin Orthop 1973; 91:16–20.

11. Whitesides TE Jr, Kelley RP. Lateral approach to the upper cervical spine for anterior fusion. South Med J 1966; 59:879–883.

13. Scuderi GT, Garfin SR. Anterior approaches to the cervical spine. In: Bradford DS, ed. The Spine. Master Techniques in Orthopaedic Surgery. Philadelphia: Lippincott-Raven, 1997:3–7.

15. Smith GW, Robinson RA. The treatment of certain cervical spine disorders by anterior removal of the intervertebral disc and interbody fusion. J Bone Joint Surg 1958; 40-A: 607.

11. Robinson RA, Walker E, Ferlic DC, Wiecking DK. The results of anterior interbody fusion of the cervical spine. J Bone Joint Surg 1962; 44A:1569–1587.

12. Hodgson AR. An approach to the cervical spine (C3–7). Clin Orthop 1965; 39:129.

13. Verbiest H. Anterolateral operations for fractures and dislocations in the middle and lower parts of the cervical spine. J Bone Joint Surg 1969; 51A:1489–1530.

14. Emery SE, Bolesta MJ, Banks MA, Jone PK. Robinson anterior cervical fusion. Comparison of the standard and modified techniques. Spine 1994; 19:660–663.

15. An HS, Cotler JM. Spinal Instrumentation. Baltimore: Williams and Wilkins, 1992.

16. An HS, Simpson JM, eds. Surgery of the Cervical Spine. London: Martin-Dunitz, 1994: 383.

17. Welsh LW, Welsh JJ, Chinnici JC. Dysphagia due to cervical spine surgery. Ann Otol Rhinol Laryngol 1987; 96:112–115.

18. Bulger RF, Rejowski JE, Beatty RA. Vocal cord paralysis associated with anterior cervical fusion: consideration for prevention and treatment. J Neurosurg 1985; 62:657–661.

19. Heeneman, H. Vocal cord paralysis following approaches to the anterior cervical spine. Laryngoscope 1973; 83:17–21.

20. Anderson JE. Grant's Atlas of Anatomy. 8th ed. Baltimore: Williams & Wilkins, 1983.

21. Sanders G, Uyeda RY, Karlan MS. Nonrecurrent inferior laryngeal nerves and their association with a recurrent branch. Am J Surg 1983; 146:501–503.

22. Sang UH, Wilson CB. Postoperative epidural hematoma as a complication of anterior cervical discectomy. J Neurosurg 1978; 49:288–291.

23. Flynn TB. Neurologic complications of anterior cervical interbody fusion. Spine 1982; 7:536–539.

24. Smith MD, Emery SE, Dudley A, Murray KJ, Leventhal M. Vertebral artery injury during anterior decompression of the cervical spine. J Bone Joint Surg 1993; 75-B:410, 1993.

25. Vaccaro AR, Ring D, Scuderi G, Garfin SR. Vertebral artery location in relation to the vertebral body as determined by two-dimensional computed tomography evaluation. Spine 1994; 19:2637–41.

26. An HS, Vaccaro A, Cotler JM. Spinal disorders at the cervico-thoracic junction. Spine 1994; 19:2557–2564.

27. Fielding JW, Stillwell WT. Anterior cervical approach to the upper thoracic spine. A case report. Spine 1976; 1:158–161.
28. Johnson RM, Murphy MJ, Southwick WO. Surgical approaches to the spine. In: Rothman RH, Simeone FA. The Spine, 3rd ed. Philadelphia: WB Saunders, 1992:1607–1738.
29. Turner PL, Webb JK. A surgical approach to the upper thoracic spine. J Bone Joint Surg 1987; 69B:542–544.
30. Hodgson AK, Stock FE, Fang HSY, et al. Anterior spinal fusion: the operative approach and pathologic findings in 412 patients with Pott's disease of the spine. Br J Surg 1960; 48:172–178.
31. Darling GE, McBroom R, Perrin R. Modified anterior approach to the cervicothoracic junction. Spine 1995; 13:1519–1521.
32. Kurz LT, Pursel SE, Herkowitz HN. Modified anterior approach to the cervicothoracic junction. Spine 1991; 16(suppl 10):S542–547.
33. Sundaresan N, Shah I, Foley KM, et al. An anterior surgical approach to the upper thoracic vertebrae. J Neurosurg 1984; 61:686–690.
34. Micheli JJ, Hood RW. Anterior exposure of the cervicothoracic spine using a combined cervical and thoracic approach. J Bone Joint Surg 1983; 65A:992–997.
35. Ebraheim NA, Xu R, Ahmad M, Heck B. The quantitative anatomy of the vertebral artery groove of the atlas and its relation to the posterior atlantoaxial approach. Spine 1998; 23:320–323.

23

Occipito–Cervical Fusion

THOMAS J. PUSCHAK

Private practice, Seattle, Washington, U.S.A.

PAUL A. ANDERSON

University of Washington, Seattle, Washington, U.S.A.

I INTRODUCTION

Craniocervical junction injuries have traditionally had a high rate of mortality, with most patients dying before making it to a hospital. There is an increasing prevalence of patients surviving these injuries long enough to make it to emergency rooms because of improvements in trauma care in the field by emergency medical services. Also, improvements in diagnostic imaging may lead to more recognition of these injuries, especially in patients with subtle ligamentous injuries and incomplete dislocations (Fig. 1). The instability created by occipitoatlantal dislocations and subluxations, as well as from certain occipital condyle fractures, is best stabilized by occipito–cervical fusion. In 1927, Foerster (1) described the use of a fibula for occipito–cervical fusion, and subsequently many techniques have been described with (2–7) and without (8,9) internal fixation. Internal fixation has included wires and, more recently, plates or rods. The purpose of this chapter is to review some of the more common techniques of occipito–cervical fusion used in the treatment of occipito–cervical instability due to trauma.

II PERTINENT OCCIPITO–CERVICAL ANATOMY

The occiput is a flat bone, which acts as the bony protection for the cerebellum and posterior fossa. It is adjacent to the foramen magnum. The convex occipital condyles border the foramen magnum laterally and articulate with the superior articular facets of the atlas. The external occipital protuberance, or inion, is located in the center of the occiput approximately 6 cm rostral to the foramen magnum. Being the thickest

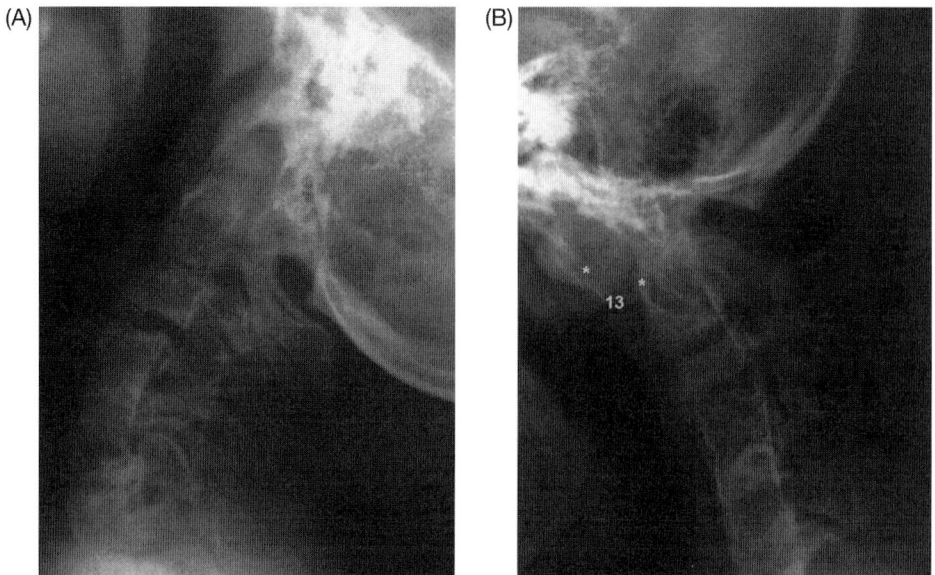

Figure 1   A 17-year-old male with known Klippel–Feil anomaly presents with transient quadriplegia after a MVA. Neurological status returned to normal within 15 min. (A) Extension and (B) flexion lateral radiographs show occipitalization of C1 and 13 mm of instability at C1–C2.

part of the occiput, ranging from 11 to 17 mm thick, it is a good landmark for screw or wire placement (10). The superior and inferior nuchal lines run transversely across the occiput from the external occipital protuberance. The thickness of the occiput decreases caudally from the superior nuchal line. The transverse dural sinus projects 7 mm superior and inferior to the external occipital protuberance (10). The ideal placement of screws in the occiput is near the midline along the external crest. The most cephalad screw should not be directed cranially to minimize injury to the transverse dural sinus.

The vertebral arteries ascend in the transverse foramina of the cervical vertebrae, exit the transverse foramen of the atlas, run medially in the vertebral artery groove, and merge to become the basilar artery. The vertebral artery groove lies on the superior anterior aspect of the posterior ring of the atlas. The vertebral artery and first cervical spinal nerve lie in the groove that is situated posterior to the lateral mass of the atlas, lateral to the spinal canal, and anterior to the atlantooccipital membrane. Ebraheim et al. (11) has reported that the medial edge of the vertebral artery groove ranges from 8 to 18 mm from the midline. Thus, dissection on the superior aspect of the posterior arch of the atlas should not be carried further than 15 mm lateral to midline.

In stabilization techniques, transarticular C1–C2 screw fixation greatly enhances the biomechanical stability of the construct. These screws are placed through the plate, traverse the C2 isthmus and the posterior portion of the C1–C2 articulation, and end in the lateral mass of the atlas. Knowledge of the path of the vertebral artery within the axis is imperative when transarticular screw fixation is incorporated in the fixation construct. The C2 pedicle lies anterior to the articular process of the axis and is often confused with the isthmus of the pars interarticularis. The vertebral artery takes an oblique course through the axis. As it enters the C2 lateral mass inferiorly, it courses 45 degrees laterally forming a groove within the axis. Reports in the literature indicate that placement of a transarticular screw is not anatomically possible in 10 to 18% of the population because of aberrant vertebral artery anatomy or erosion of the C2 lateral mass (12,13). Preoperative CT scans with sagittal reconstruction should be used to evaluate the vertebral artery and C2 isthmus. Recently, Mandel et al. (12) reported that when the C2 isthmus measures less than 5 mm in height or width on CT scan, the placement of a 3.5-mm transarticular screw increases the risk of penetration of the vertebral artery (Fig. 2).

The size of the spinal canal and presence of spinal cord compression should be determined preoperatively by MRI and/or CT imaging. Intraoperatively, after positioning, radiographs should be used to confirm anatomical reduction. Sublaminar wire fixation of the C1–C2 complex can maintain reduction and make transarticular screw placement safer and easier. In general, placement of C1 and C2 sublaminar wires is safe as long as anatomical position is present and there is no stenosis. In the presence of stenosis a C1 laminectomy, posterior occipital decompression, and/or C2 laminotomy should be considered.

III WIRE FIXATION

Numerous techniques (4,5,7) of wire fixation have been described. The wires can be used to stabilize the occipito–cervical junction as well as to hold the bone graft in place. Robinson and Southwick (5) described a wiring technique in 1960. Wertheim and Bohlman (7) described a modification of the Robinson technique in 1984. Their triple-wiring technique uses thick bicortical iliac crest strips and avoids intracranial passage of wires. Their report followed 13 patients for over 3 years. All of the

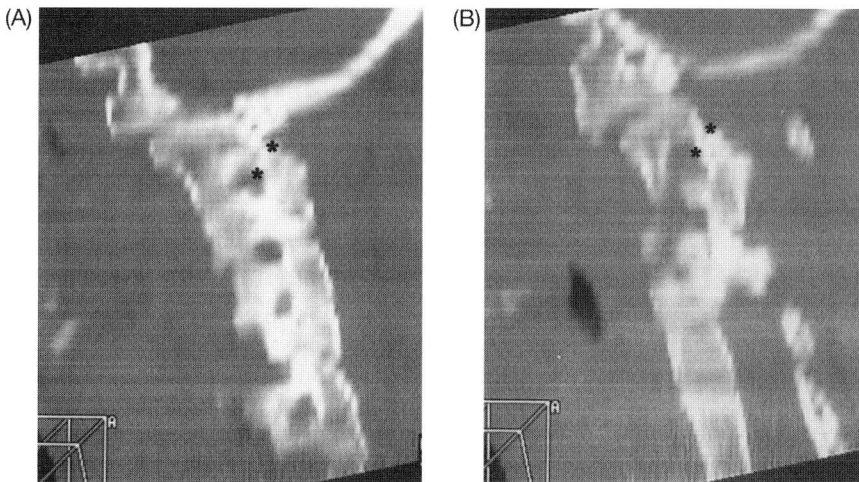

Figure 2 Sagittal CT reconstruction illustrates the C2 isthmus on the (A) left and (B) right. The isthmus on the right is insufficient for placement of a transarticular C1–C2 screw.

patients had successful fusion and all 10 of their myelopathic patients had an improvement in neurological function. Several authors (4,14–16) have described a modification of the wiring technique, where wires are secured to a contoured rod, Steinman pin, or circular rod-frame.

A Bohlman Technique

General anesthesia is usually performed and awake fiberoptic nasotracheal intubation is optimal. The patient is positioned prone and the head is stabilized in Mayfield tongs or a halo-vest. Care must be taken not to distract occipito–cervical dislocations. A lateral radiograph must be obtained immediately after positioning to ensure maintenance of reduction. Spinal cord monitoring with motor-evoked and somatosensory-evoked potentials is recommended in cases of significant instability or high-grade stenosis.

After sterile preparation of the skin and draping, the subcutaneous tissue is infiltrated with a 1:500,000 epinephrine solution. A midline incision is made from the external occipital protuberance to approximately C4. Dissection is carried sharply down to the spinous processes in the ligamentum nuchae to minimize bleeding. The posterior elements are stripped subperiosteally to the lateral margins of the facets at C2 and, if needed, C3. The posterior arch of C1 is exposed. Care must be taken not to carry the dissection further than 15 mm lateral on the posterior arch, especially on the superior edge of the posterior arch, to avoid injuring the vertebral artery as it emerges from the vertebral artery groove (11). The occiput is also exposed cranially to the external occipital protuberance.

A 5-mm groove is placed with a high-speed burr on each side of the external occipital crest 2 cm rostral to the foramen magnum. A tunnel is then created between these holes with a Lewin clamp taking care not to enter the cranium. A 20-gauge wire is passed through the tunnel and looped on itself. A separate 20-gauge wire is passed under the arch of C1. The burr and Lewin clamp are used to make a transverse hole in the spinous process of the axis and a third 20-gauge wire is passed and looped.

The posterior iliac crest is exposed and a 7- to 10-mm-thick bicortical rectangular plate is harvested with an osteotome and mallet. The graft is divided and three holes are placed in each graft with a drill or burr. Curettes are used to harvest separate pieces of cancellous graft. The occiput, posterior C1 arch, and C2 are decorticated with a high-speed burr. The wires are passed through the holes in the graft on each side and tightened on each other. The additional cancellous bone is packed in between the two grafts. The wounds are closed in layers with or without a drain based on the preference of the surgeon.

Postoperative immobilization is dependent on the amount of preoperative instability and the intraoperative assessment of the stability of the fixation. For occipito–cervical dislocations, immobilization for at least 12 weeks in a halo-vest is recommended.

B Rod and Wire Technique

In this modification of the traditional wiring technique, burr holes are made in the occiput 1 cm lateral and rostral to the foramen magnum. A dural elevator or angled curette is used to separate the dura from the inside of the occiput. Double-stranded

20-gauge wire or titanium cables are passed intracranially and exit the foramen magnum. Sublaminar wires are passed at C1 and C2. The wires are then secured to a Steinman pin or Luque rod that has been contoured using plate or rod benders. Precontoured constructs such as the Ransford loop can also be used with this technique. The spine is decorticated and a corticocancellous graft is placed and the wound is closed in layers.

Recently Moskovich et al. (17) described using the Ransford loop with wiring for occipito–cervical stabilization without fusion in patients with craniocervical instability due to rheumatoid arthritis. They reported no difference in neck pain, radiographic cranioverteral motion, Ranawat class, vertical subluxation, or survival than in those managed with stabilization and fusion. While this technique may avoid donor-site morbidity without compromising the outcome in patients with rheumatoid arthritis and vertical instability, further studies are needed to prove whether it will be an effective treatment of traumatic craniocervical instability.

IV PLATE FIXATION

Recently, several authors (2,6,18) have described plate and screw fixation of the occipito–cervical junction. There are several advantages to plating. The increased rigidity of plating constructs may decrease postoperative immobilization requirements. Passage of intracranial and sublaminar wires is avoided. The plates can be extended into the subaxial cervical and thoracic spine, if needed (6). The stability of the construct and success of the fusion are less dependent on the size of the iliac graft, allowing for less invasive posterior iliac crest harvests. Also, transarticular screws can be placed at the atlantoaxial articulation through the plate. Transarticular screws significantly increase the rigidity of the construct, especially in rotation and extension, as well as eliminate the need for sublaminar wiring at C1 to stabilize the atlas.

Roy-Camille first described the use of plate and screw fixation for occipito–cervical fusion (19). Plating techniques have been described using pelvic reconstruction plates (6,20). Now several plates specially designed for posterior cervical fusions are available. There are also systems with plates for occipital fixation that taper into rods that can be attached to transarticular and lateral mass screws in the cervical spine. Usually contoured plates are placed bilaterally (6,20,21), although single-plate constructs have been described (18). Grob et al. (21) reported on the use of a Y-shaped plate that allows the occipital screws to be placed along the thicker bone of the external occipital crest. The AO Cervifix system (Fig. 3) uses a 3.5-mm rod that can be segmentally fixed to screws in the occiput, atlas, and axis. The rod is easier to contour than plates and may make it easier to place occipital screws in the thicker areas of the external crest. Fixation of the atlas can be obtained by a wire looped around the posterior arch secured over the plate or by a transarticular screw placed through the plate. Fixation of C2 can also be provided by a transarticular, or by a C2 pedicle screw. If the fusion needs to be extended into the subaxial spine, lateral mass screws are used for fixation. The use of titanium implants can improve the quality of postoperative imaging.

A Occipito–Cervical Plating Technique

The patient is intubated and positioned as previously described. If transarticular screws are going to be placed, C-arm fluoroscopy should be arranged so that biplanar

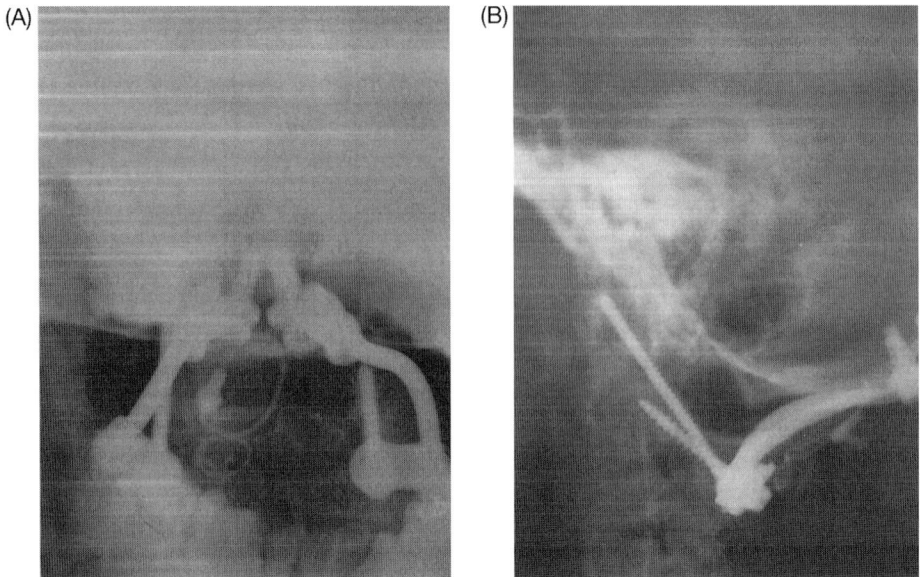

Figure 3 Postoperative (A) anteroposterior and (B) lateral radiographs show an occiput–C2 fusion. Morscher screws were placed in the occiput, a transarticular C1–C2 screw was placed on the left, and a C2 pedicle screw was placed on the right.

intraoperative images can be obtained. The operative exposure is the same as for the wiring technique. A plate or rod template is used to choose the appropriate plate length and to aid in determining the proper contouring. The plate or rod is then sectioned to length and bent to the proper contour. Two or three screws in the occiput are needed for each plate.

The transarticular screw, or C2 pedicle screw, should be prepared and placed first as these screws are the most technically demanding and have the most specific requirements for starting point and trajectory. If lateral mass screws in the subaxial spine are needed, they should be placed next followed by the occipital screws last. For the placement of a transarticular screw, the superior and medial border of the C2 isthmus is identified with a Penfield elevator or an angled 4–0 curette. The starting point for the screw is 3 to 5 mm above the C2–C3 facet joint and as medial as possible without breaking through the medial aspect of the C2 pedicle. A 3-mm burr can be used to make a starting notch to avoid skiving with the drill. We have found that a 2.5-mm AO Dynamic Hip Screw (DHS) threaded guide pin works well as a drill for these screws. The guide pin is placed percutaneously through stab incisions 1 cm lateral to T1 and advanced cranially through the paraspinous muscles to obtain the appropriate screw angle while minimizing the length of the surgical dissection. Using biplanar fluoroscopic guidance, the guide pin is advanced straight toward the center of the C1 lateral mass on the anteroposterior view and toward the middle of the anterior C1 arch on the lateral view. The drill should be placed bilaterally to aid in maintenance of the reduction. The screw length is measured, and a fully threaded self-tapping 3.5-mm cortical screw is placed through the contoured plate. Other authors have advocated caution regarding this technique and have recommended individual drilling of each screw site with removal of the drill to assess for possible vertebral artery injury. This would avoid potential injury to both vertebral arteries during screw placement. Preoperative CT scans with sagittal reconstruction are critical because, in approximately 10 to 18% of patients, the location of the vertebral artery or dimensions of the isthmus prevent the safe placement of transarticular screws (12,13,22).

If a C2 pedicle screw is to be placed, the starting hole is 5 mm superior to the C2–C3 facet joint and just medial to the midpoint of the facet. The pedicle axis runs 10 to 20 degrees medial and 25 degrees cranial. A 2-mm Steinman pin is used to drill. The pin should be advanced gradually and the hole palpated with the blunt end of a 1-mm K-wire to make sure the pedicle has not been penetrated. The hole is drilled to a depth of 20 to 24 mm, tapped, and a 3.5-mm fully threaded cortical screw is placed through the contoured plate. If the fusion is to be extended into the subaxial spine, lateral mass screws should be placed next. There are numerous methods (20,23,24) of lateral mass screw placement that are discussed in detail in other chapters.

The occipital screws are placed last. Preferably two to three screws are placed in each plate along the external occipital crest as close to midline as possible. Screws should not be placed rostral to the superior nuchal line to avoid injury to the transverse dural sinus. We prefer drilling with a 2-mm diamond-tip burr and then measuring depth. Traditionally, bicortical purchase is recommended, although a recent study (25) suggests that unicortical purchase in the region of the external occipital protuberance is sufficient. If CSF leaks after drilling, the hole should be packed with bone wax and the screw placed. Screw lengths are usually 8 to 10 mm. Bicortical screws should not be placed above the external occipital protuberance to avoid penetration of the transverse dural sinus. Also, the most cranial screw should not be directed cephalad for the same reason.

We have recently used 8-mm Morscher screws for fixation in the occiput with the AO Cervifix. The pilot hole is drilled with a 2-mm diamond burr and then overdrilled with a 3.0-mm drill. The hole is tapped, and an 8-mm Morscher screw is placed through a neutral connector that attaches to a 3.5-mm rod. The rod is easy to contour and allows placement of the Morscher screws in the thickest bone along the external occipital crest. A set screw expands the head of the Morscher screw to rigidly link the screw to the rod connector. Rigidly locking the screws to the rod significantly increases the stiffness of the construct. The use of rigid locking screws in the lateral masses with the AO Cervifix system has recently been shown to provide significantly greater stiffness than traditional plate–screw constructs in the treatment of traumatic subaxial instability (26).

After the hardware is placed, the exposed bone of the occiput, atlas, and axis are decorticated with a burr and corticocancellous strips are placed to bridge the occipito–cervical junction. If the fusion is to be extended into the subaxial spine, the involved facet joints are decorticated and packed with cancellous bone graft. A corticocancellous graft may also be wired to the occiput and spinous process of C2 as described in the Bohlman wiring technique (7). The wound is then closed in layers.

Postoperative immobilization is in a hard collar or Minerva brace for 8 to 12 weeks, depending on the amount of preoperative instability and the intraoperative assessment of the strength of the construct. If there is concern over the strength of the fixation, a halo-vest should be used for 12 weeks.

V CONCLUSION

Fortunately, patients are increasingly surviving occipital cervical injuries. When instability is present, patients should be treated by posterior occipital to C2 fusion. Traditional wiring techniques are highly efficacious, but require postoperative halo vest immobilization and may not sufficiently maintain reduction. More rigid fixation using screw techniques allows rapid patient mobilization and decreases postoperative bracing requirements. Reports suggest excellent fusion success and low complication rates (2,6,19–21). Proper preoperative planning, especially to gain knowledge of the course of the vertebral artery is required. These techniques are technically demanding and meticulous attention to detail is required for safe placement.

REFERENCES

1. Foerster O. Die Leitungsbahnen des Schmerzgefuhls und die chirurgische Behandlung der Schmerzzustande. Berlin: Urban and Schwarzenberg, 1927.
2. Grob D, Crisco JJ, Panjabi M, Wang P, Dvorak J. Biomechanical evaluation of four different posterior atlantoaxial fixation techniques. Spine 1992; 17:480–490.
3. Hamblin DL. Occipital-cervical fusion: indication, technique and results. J Bone Joint Surg 1967; 49B:33–45.
4. Itoh T, Tsuji H, Katoh Y, Yonezawa T, Kitagawa H. Occipito-cervical fusion reinforced by Luque's segmental spinal instrumentation for rheumatoid diseases. Spine 1988; 13: 1234–1238.
5. Robinson RA, Southwick WO. Indications and techniques for early stabilization of the neck in some fracture dislocations of the cervical spine. South Med J 1960; 53:565–579.
6. Smith MD, Anderson P, Grady MS. Occipitocervical arthrodesis using contoured plate fixation: an early report on a versatile fixation technique. Spine 1993; 18:1984–1990.
7. Wertheim SB, Bohlman HH. Occipitocervical fusion: indications, technique and long-term results in thirteen patients. J Bone Joint Surg 1987; 69A:833–836.
8. Clark CC, White AA III. Fractures of the dens. J Bone Joint Surg 1985; 67A:1340–1348.
9. Newman P, Sweetnam R. Occipito-cervical fusion: an operative technique and its indication. J Bone Joint Surg 1969; 51B:423–431.
10. Ebraheim NA, Lu J, Biyani A, Brown JA, Yeasting RA. An anatomic study of the thickness of the occipital bone. Implications for occipitocervical instrumentation. Spine 1996; 21(15):1725–1729.
11. Ebraheim NA, Xu R, Ahmad M, Heck B. The quantitative anatomy of the vertebral artery groove of the atlas and its relation to the posterior atlantoaxial approach. Spine 1998; 23:320–323.
12. Mandel IM, Kambach BJ, Petersilge CA, Johnstone B, Yoo JU. Morphologic considerations of C2 isthmus dimensions for the placement of transarticular screws. Spine 2000; 25:1542–1547.
13. Paramore CG, Dickman CA, Sonntag VK. The anatomical suitability of the C1-2 complex for transarticular screw fixation. J Neurosurg 1996; 85:221–224.
14. Apostolides PJ, Dickman CA, Golfinos JG. Threaded Steinman pin fusion of the craniovertebral junction. Spine 1996; 21:1630–1637.
15. Ransford AO, Crockard HA, Pozo JL. Craniocervical instability treated by contoured loop fixation. J Bone Joint Surg 1986; 68B:173–177.
16. Sakou T, Kawaida H, Morizino Y. Occipitoatlantoaxial fusion utilizing a rectangular rod. Clin Orthop 1989; 239:136–144.

17. Moskovich R, Crockard HA, Shott S, Ransford AO. Occipitocervical stabilization for myelopathy in patients with rheumatoid arthritis. Implications of not bone-grafting. J Bone Joint Surg 2000; 82A:349–365.
18. Heywood AWB, Learmonth ID, Thomas M. Internal fixation for the occipito-cervical fusion. J Bone Joint Surg 1988; 70B:708–711.
19. Roy-Camille R, Saillant G, Mazel C. Internal fixation of he unstable cervical spine by a posterior osteosynthesis with plates and screws. In: Sherk HH, Dunn EJ, Eismont FJ, et al., eds. The Cervical Spine, 2nd ed. Philadelphia: JB Lippincott, 1989:390–403.
20. Anderson PA, Henley MB, Grady MS. Posterior cervical arthrodesis with AO reconstruction plates and bone graft. Spine 1991; 16:S72–S79.
21. Grob D, Dvorak J, Panjabi M, Froehlich M, Hayek J. Posterior occipitocervical fusion: a preliminary report of a new technique. Spine 1991; 16:S17–S24.
22. Solanki GA, Crockard HA. Peroperative determination of safe superior transarticular screw trajectory through the lateral mass. Spine 1999; 24:1477–1482.
23. Jeanneret B, Magerl F, Ward EH, Ward J. Posterior stabilization of the cervical spine with hook plates. Spine 1991; 16:S56–S63.
24. Roy-Camille R, Mazel C, Saillant G, Benazet JP. Rationale and techniques of internal fixation in trauma of the cervical spine. In: Errico J, Bauer RD, Waugh T, eds. Spinal Trauma. Philadelphia: JB Lippincott, 1990:163–191.
25. Haher TR, Yeung AW, Carusso SA, Merola AA, Shin T, Zipnick RI, Gorup J, Bono C. Occipital screw pullout strength: A biomechanical investigation of occipital morphology. Spine 1999; 24:5–9.
26. Mirza SK, Chapman JR, Newell DW, Grady MS, Schimbo GT, Tencer AF. Posterior cervical lateral mass fixation with a rigid locking implant. Proceedings of the 26th Annual Meeting of the Cervical Spine Research Society, December 3–5, 1998, Atlanta, Georgia.

24

Odontoid Screw Fixation

RICK C. SASSO

Indiana University School of Medicine, Indianapolis, Indiana, U.S.A.

I INTRODUCTION

The rationale for direct anterior fixation of odontoid fractures is to improve the chance of healing in an anatomically reduced position while avoiding restrictive bracing and the complications associated with bone grafting techniques. By providing stable internal fixation, these goals may be met while preserving motion at the C1–C2 articulation. It is rare that spine surgeons are able to perform direct fixation of a spinal fracture to allow primary healing, rather than fuse a motion segment across an injury. Direct anterior osteosynthesis of the odontoid fracture with anterior odontoid screw fixation is an alternative to atlantoaxial arthrodesis for management of odontoid fractures that are at risk for nonunion which avoids halo immobilization. Although the success rate of posterior C1–C2 fusion is very high for these fractures, this "success" results in significant loss (50%) of axial rotation (1). Especially in a young person, this may be quite debilitating. The loss of neck motion, as a result of these surgical procedures, led to the development of direct methods of internal fixation for odontoid fractures.

II ANATOMY

Because of the complex anatomy of the occipitocervical junction, C2 fractures should not be considered isolated bony injuries. The intricate interconnecting array of anterior ligaments requires the occipitocervical junction (occiput, C1, and C2) to be regarded as a unit. The strong, paired alar ligaments attach the tip of the odontoid process to the occipital condyles. The tectorial membrane (a continuation of the posterior longitudinal ligament) connects the odontoid process to the foramen magnum. The transverse atlantal ligament is a posterior odontoid sling attached to the lateral masses of the atlas, preventing anterior dislocation of C1 on C2. The C1–C2 articulation is a unique, flat joint that allows an average rotational range of motion of 47° on each side. This range of motion represents approximately 50% of the axial rotation of the entire cervical spine (1).

Very dense, thick trabecular bone is present in the center of the tip of the dens, and cortical bone at the anterior base of the body of C2 (where the anterior longitudinal ligament attaches) is uniformly thick. High-density trabecular bone also is present in the lateral masses beneath the superior facets. Hypodense bone, however, consistently is present beneath the odontoid process at the upper portion of the body of C2 (2). The quality of bone is critical for optimal screw purchase. Anterior odontoid screws obtain strong fixation at their entrance site (the anteroinferior aspect of the C2 body) and exit site (the tip of the dens) but traverse the very weak hypodense bone in the body of C2.

The most variable dimension of the axis is the dens angle in the sagittal plane, which can range from −2° (leaning slightly anterior) to 42° (leaning posterior) (3). This extremely variable angle can make assessment of fracture reduction challenging. All odontoid dimensions, in fact, show considerable variability, and patient body size has been shown to be a poor predictor of the size of the odontoid process (4). The diameter of the odontoid process in a significant percentage of people is less than 6 mm, which is not sufficient to accommodate the passage of two 3.5-mm screws (3,5).

III INDICATIONS

Acute type II or high (with a shallow base) type III odontoid fractures are appropriate for direct internal fixation. Fracture patterns that portend a high rate of nonunion such as initial displacement greater than 6-mm are especially suitable. Patients who initially fail a halo trial due to instability of the fracture where fracture reduction can be obtained but not maintained and those unable to tolerate a halo are also fitting candidates. Odontoid screw fixation provides a reasonable approach to odontoid fractures with a concomitant C1 Jefferson burst fracture and especially in multiple trauma patients, in whom immediate mobilization has proven beneficial.

IV CONTRAINDICATIONS

Inability to anatomically reduce the fracture is an absolute contraindication for direct internal fixation. The stability of the construct is dependent upon the interdigitation of the lagged fracture fragments (6). Displacement of even 1 mm significantly reduces the contact surface area and thus weakens the internal fixation. If anatomic reduction cannot be achieved, posterior C1–C2 arthrodesis should be considered. Relative contraindications to anterior screw fixation include transverse atlantal ligament disruption, osteopenia, nonunion, and an oblique fracture in an anteroinferior to posterosuperior plane. With this type of oblique fracture in the same plane as the screw, the odontoid fragment may shear anteriorly at the fracture site during lag compression. This shearing could cause iatrogenic translation of C1 anterior on C2.

V IMAGING

A comprehensive, diagnostic approach in evaluating suspected upper cervical spine injuries remains controversial, particularly in the presence of polytrauma or for obtunded patients. The standard, initial cervical spine radiographic series in trauma patients includes a cross table lateral view, an anteroposterior view, and an open mouth view. The usefulness of the anteroposterior view has been questioned because it provides little additional information (7). Although this 3-view screening series can detect 65 to 95% of axis injuries, (8–12) the C2 vertebra often is obscured by overlying bony maxillary, mandibular, and dental structures; therefore, C2 fractures may be missed. Thin-section CT is the best study for evaluating C2 bony fractures (13). Sagittal reconstruction of CT images is important because axial images may not detect a transverse odontoid fracture.

Although CT is excellent in evaluating bony injuries, it can miss soft-tissue and significant ligamentous injuries. Recently, therefore, dynamic flexion extension lateral fluoroscopic evaluation has been advocated in polytrauma patients to identify occult ligamentous instabilities and confirm that the cervical spine is uninjured (14). Magnetic resonance imaging (MRI) also is helpful in assessing the spinal cord in those with neurologic deficit and is becoming increasingly important in evaluating the status of ligamentous structures such as the transverse atlantal ligament (TAL) (Fig. 1).

The assessment of transverse atlantal ligament integrity with odontoid fractures is an important consideration in selecting appropriate treatment options (15). Injuries of the TAL can result in atlantoaxial instability after odontoid fracture osseous healing, and the chance of odontoid fracture nonunion is increased with TAL disruption (16). Furthermore, anterior odontoid screw fixation will not provide C1–C2 stability if the TAL is not competent. Transverse atlantal ligament disruption occurs in 10% of patients with odontoid fractures (16). The combination of MRI, CT, and plain

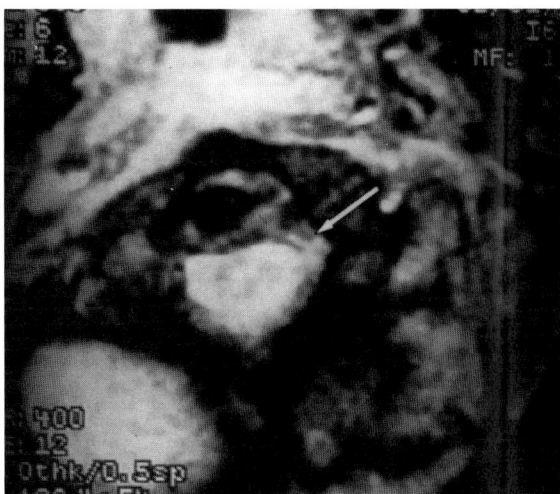

Figure 1   MRI of transverse atlantal ligament disruption identified by the high signal on the T2-weighted axial image.

radiographs, therefore, is important for evaluating unstable C2 fractures and planning a rational treatment course. When a C2 fracture is identified, it is necessary to evaluate the subaxial spine carefully because 16% of patients will have a noncontiguous fracture (17).

VI TECHNIQUE

Odontoid screw fixation is a technically demanding procedure that requires thorough preoperative planning and adequate surgical training. The entry point is critical at the anterior margin of the inferior endplate. If started more cephalad, the proper angle of inclination for fracture fixation cannot be achieved with resultant short screw fixation in the dens fragment and anterior gapping of the fracture is common. Also, poor proximal fragment purchase with subsequent screw cutout may occur since the screw head is seated in relatively poor bone (2). It is important to engage the far cortex of the odontoid tip to ensure adequate purchase and it is mandatory to lag the fracture fragments either through screw design or by creating a gliding hole through the body fragment. AP and lateral fluoroscopy is essential for constant monitoring during all stages of this procedure.

The goal of this procedure is to safely place a lag screw across an acute type II odontoid fracture resulting in stable, direct fixation of this injury. The patient is positioned supine with a Mayfield pin headrest. Under biplane fluoroscopy, anatomical reduction is obtained. Excellent visualization of the odontoid in both planes is mandatory. Depending upon the amount of flexion required for reduction, the AP view might be best shot through the mouth. If appropriate, a radiolucent bite block or a wad of gauze in the mouth can facilitate the visualization of the odontoid. The occipitocervical junction is flexed or extended to anatomically reduce the fracture.

A Steinman pin is placed alongside the neck to assure proper trajectory under lateral fluoroscopy while clearing the sternum before the incision is made. If it does not clear, anterior translation of the entire head and neck may allow a free path. A transverse skin incision is made at the C5–C6 level. Dissection is accomplished cephalad to the C2–C3 disk. The proper entry point is in the anterior aspect of the inferior endplate of C2 with the screw exiting the tip of the odontoid (Fig. 2). A 2.5-mm drill bit is directed through the center of the odontoid, exiting the cortical tip of the dens (Fig. 3). The body fragment is then over-drilled with a 3.5-mm bit up to, but not across, the fracture (Fig. 4). A 3.5-mm tap is placed through the gliding hole to the fracture and the dens fragment is tapped including the strong cortex at the tip. One 3.5-mm fully threaded cortical screw is pushed through the gliding hole, engaging the dens fragment. The proper screw length is important to accomplish a lag effect. As the screw head contacts the strong cortical inferior endplate, pulling the dens fragment down, compression occurs across the fracture.

Intraoperative difficulties may include inability to anatomically reduce the fracture, nonvisualization of the odontoid on fluoroscopy because of osteopenia, and inability to position your hand for ideal drill trajectory. Proper drill trajectory is usually hindered by a barrel chest, short neck, fixed thoracic kyphosis, and fracture patterns that require a flexed position to obtain reduction. If resistant anterior displacement is a problem, pushing on the anterior arch of C1 by an assistant through the mouth, or pushing up on the posterior spinous process of C2 may be helpful. Shearing, binding and driving the K-wire into the spinal canal can occur if a can-

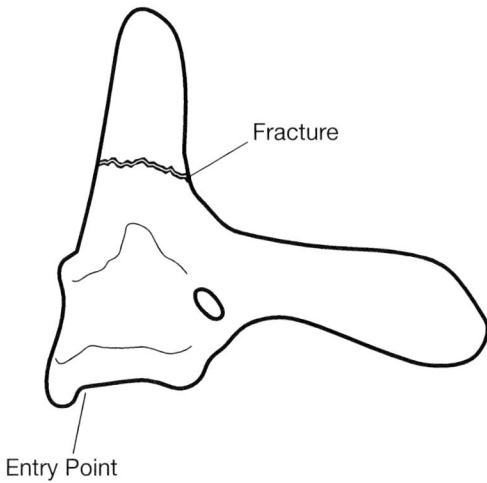

Figure 2 Proper entry point at the anterior aspect of the inferior endplate of C2.

nulated technique is used. If a partially threaded ''lag'' screw is used, a high fracture may not allow the threads to be completely contained in the dens fragment. These threads across the fracture site will keep the fracture distracted. Cutting the tip of a partially threaded screw to shorten the length of threads if too long can remedy this situation.

Postoperatively, a cervical collar is worn for 6 weeks. Biomechanically, the odontoid screw construct is 50% as stiff as the intact dens (6).

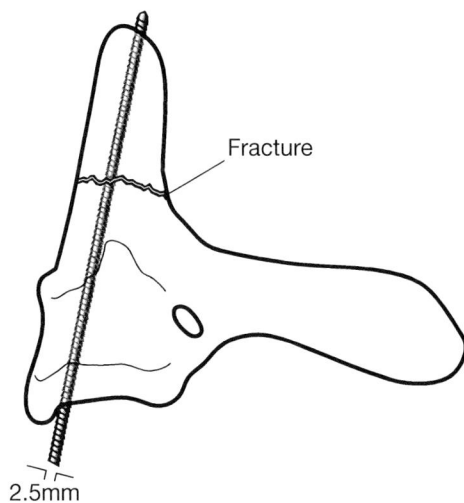

Figure 3 The 2.5-mm drill bit is driven across the fracture site in the middle of the odontoid process, exiting the hard cortical bone at the tip of the dens.

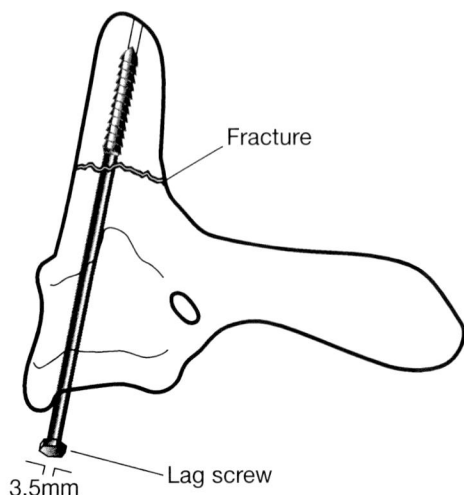

Figure 4   The body fragment is over-drilled with the 3.5-mm bit to create the gliding hole.

VII   OUTCOME

Direct anterior fixation of an odontoid fracture results in very high primary healing rates without requiring fusion of C1–C2, or the need for a bone graft donor site. Odontoid screw fixation limits the complications of halo immobilization and the further morbidity of the loss of 50% of cervical axial rotation by C1–C2 arthrodesis if the halo fails. This technique has demonstrated a high success rate similar to posterior atlantoaxial arthrodesis (92%–100%), with a similarly low complication rate (8,18–21). A theoretical advantage of this technique over posterior methods is the preservation of atlantoaxial motion (8,18,22). Anterior screw stabilization of the odontoid allows preservation of axial rotation. Jeanneret (23) found normal atlantoaxial joint motion in about 40% of patients who underwent anterior screw fixation of a dens fracture. In the other patients, rotation was diminished but still possible as documented in a postoperative dynamic CT study.

Overall, the literature has established this technique as an efficacious treatment of odontoid fractures (24–28). Complications and their incidence reported in clinical series as a result of direct anterior odontoid screw fixation include the following: screw malposition, 2%; screw breakout, 1.5%; neurological or vascular injury, 0%. The series has an aggregate fusion rate of 94.5% (20,21,24). Controversy, however, does exist regarding selection of patients, whether or not to use the technique in nonunions, and whether one or two screws should be applied.

The placement of two screws is technically more difficult, often not anatomically possible, and offers no biomechanical advantage, as compared to one-screw fixation (3,5,6,18,29,30). Sasso et al. compared the use of one or two screws for stabilization of the odontoid (6). Mechanically produced type II odontoid fractures were stabilized with either one or two 3.5-mm screws. After internal fixation, the stability was restored to one half that of the unfractured odontoid. The use of two screws did not significantly enhance the stability in testing to refailure. Graziano et al. also found no difference between one and two screws in bending and torsional stiffness of the instrumented odontoid (30). Clinically, the high healing rate has not been found to be dependent upon the number of screws used (18).

Traditionally, the first-line treatment of type II odontoid fractures after prompt closed reduction has been halo-vest immobilization for 3 months with the knowledge that a significant percentage will require subsequent surgery for established nonunion. Since the results of delayed posterior C1–C2 fusion is as good as primary atlantoaxial arthrodesis; this initial nonoperative plan has been reasonable. With increased clinical and basic science literature on anterior odontoid screw fixation, its role in our traditional treatment plan is uncertain because it is not a reliable procedure in the setting of a nonunion. Thus, if initial nonoperative treatment is chosen and it fails, then C1–C2 arthrodesis is the only viable surgical option with concomitant decreased range of motion.

Type II odontoid fractures with greater than 6 mm of initial radiographic displacement have a very high incidence of nonunion despite immobilization in a halo for 3 months. If anatomical closed reduction is possible, it is reasonable to consider direct fixation of the fracture. Since anterior odontoid screw stabilization is not highly effective for established nonunions, if halo treatment fails then the only surgical alternative is posterior C1–C2 arthrodesis with subsequent loss of axial rotation.

Another group of patients who have a high incidence of failure of halo treatment for type II odontoid fractures is the elderly. Age greater than 50 years is a highly significant risk factor for failure of halo immobilization with a 21 times higher risk of nonunion (31). Halo complications are also more frequent in older patients (32).

At present, the Food and Drug Administration (FDA) consider anterior odontoid screws class III devices. They are off-label uses for FDA approved bone screws. Screws and plates are commercially available in the US and Canada to fix other bone fractures in the intended manner (lag), and to be placed in the cervical vertebral bodies. However, no specific screw is commercially available for treatment of odontoid fractures.

Although the data for the use of an anterior odontoid screw for the treatment of acute type II fractures is compelling, there does not exist a prospective study critically assessing the results of treatment. A prospective, controlled study is needed to definitively solve this dilemma.

REFERENCES

1. Penning L. Normal movements of the cervical spine. Am J Roentgenol 1979; 130:317–319.
2. Heggeness MH, Doherty BJ. The trabecular anatomy of the axis. Spine 1993; 18:1945–1949.
3. Doherty BJ, Heggeness MH. Quantitative anatomy of the second cervical vertebra. Spine 1995; 20:513–517.
4. Schaffler MB, Alson MD, Heller JG, Garfin SR. Morphology of the dens: a quantitative study. Spine 1992; 17:738–743.
5. Heller JG, Alson MD, Schaffler MB, Garfin SR. Quantitative internal dens morphology. Spine 1992; 17:861–866.
6. Sasso RC, Doherty BJ, Crawford MJ, Heggeness MH. Biomechanics of odontoid fracture fixation: comparison of the one- and two-screw technique. Spine 1993; 18:1950–1953

7. Freemyer B, Knopp R, Piche J, Wales L, Williams J. Comparison of five-view and three-view cervical spine series in the evaluation of patients with cervical trauma. Ann Emerg Med 1989; 18:818–821.

8. Marchesi DG. Management of odontoid fractures. Orthopaedics 1997; 20:911–916.

9. Schaffer MA, Doris PE. Limitation of the cross table lateral view in detecting cervical spine injuries: A retrospective analysis. Ann Emerg Med 1981; 10:508–513.

10. Spain D, Trooskin S, Flancbaum L, Boyarsky A, Nosher J. The adequacy and cost effectiveness of routine resuscitation-area cervical spine radiographs. Ann Emerg Med 1990; 19:276–278.

11. Vandemark RM. Radiology of the cervical spine in trauma patients: Practice pitfalls and recommendations for improving efficiency and communication. Am J Roentgenol 1990; 155:465–472.

12. Walter J, Doris P, Shaffer M. Clinical presentation of patients with acute cervical spine injury. Ann Emerg Med 1984; 13:512–515.

13. Blacksin MF, Lee HJ. Frequency and significance of fractures of the upper cervical spine detected by CT in patients with severe neck trauma. Am J Roentgenol 1995; 165: 1201–1204.

14. Harris MB, Waguespack AM, Kronlage S. 'Clearing' cervical spine injuries in poly-trauma patients: Is it really safe to remove the collar? Orthopedics 1997; 20:903–907.

15. Dickman CA, Mamourian A, Sonntag VKH, Drayer BP. Magnetic resonance imaging of the transverse atlantal ligament for the evaluation of atlantoaxial instability. J Neurosurg 1991; 75:221–227.

16. Greene KA, Dickman CA, Marciana FF, Drabier J, Drayer BP, Sonntag VKH. Transverse atlantal ligament disruption associated with odontoid fractures. Spine 1994; 19:2307–2314.

17. Vaccaro AR, An HS, Lin SS, Sun S, Balderston RA, Cotler JM. Noncontiguous injuries of the spine. J Spinal Disord 1992; 5:320–329.

18. Jenkins JD, Coric D, Branch CL. A clinical comparison of one and two-screw odontoid fixation. J Neurosurg 1998; 89:366–370.

19. Aebi M, Etter C, Coscia M. Fractures of the odontoid process: treatment with anterior screw fixation. Spine 1990; 14:1065–1070.

20. Bohler J. Anterior stabilization for acute fractures and nonunions of the dens. J Bone Joint Surg 1982; 64A:18–26.

21. Montesano PX, Anderson PA, Schehr F, Thalgott JS, Lowery G. Odontoid fractures treated by anterior odontoid screw fixation. Spine 1991; 16:533–537.

22. Apfelbaum RI. Screw fixation of the upper cervical spine: indications and techniques. Contemp Neurosurg 1994; 16:1–8.

23. Jeanneret B, Vernet O, Frei S, Magerl F. Atlantoaxial mobility after screw fixation of the odontoid: A computed tomographic study. J Spinal Disord 1991; 4:203–211.

24. Nakanishi T, Sasaki T, Tokita N, Hirabayashi K. Internal fixation for the odontoid fracture. Orthop Trans 1982; 6:176.

25. Fujii E, Kobayashi K, Hirabayashi K. Treatment in fractures of the odontoid process. Spine 1988; 13:604–609.

26. Lesoin F, Autricque A, Franz K, Villette L, Jomin M. Transcervical approach and screw fixation for upper cervical spine pathology. Surg Neurol 1987; 27:459–565.

27. Borne GM, Bedou GL, Pinaudeau M, Cristino G, Hussen A. Odontoid process fracture osteosynthesis with a direct screw fixation technique in nine consecutive cases. J Neurosurg 1988; 68:223–226.

28. Geisler FH, Cheng C, Poka A, Brumback R. Anterior screw fixation of posteriorly displaced type II odontoid fractures. Neurosurgery 1989; 25:30–38.

29. Nucci RC, Seigal S, Merola AA, et al. Computed tomographic evaluation of the normal adult odontoid. Spine 1995; 20(3):264–270.

30. Graziano G, Jaggers C, Lee M, Lynch W. A comparative study of fixation techniques for type II fractures of odontoid process. Spine 1993; 18:2383–2387.
31. Lennarson PJ, Mostafavi H, Traynelis VC, Walters BC. Management of type II dens fractures: A case-control study. Spine 2000; 25:1234–1237.
32. Seybold EA, Bayley JC. Functional outcome of surgically and conservatively managed dens fractures. Spine 1998; 23:1837–1846.

25

Operative Techniques: Anterior Cervical Decompression and Fusion

ROBERT H. BOYCE

Vanderbilt University Medical Center, Nashville, Tennessee, U.S.A.

ALAN S. HILIBRAND

Thomas Jefferson University Hospital and the Rothman Institute, Philadelphia, Pennsylvania, U.S.A.

I INTRODUCTION

The purpose of this chapter is to describe the indications, techniques, and results of anterior decompression and fusion in the management of cervical spine trauma. The anterior approach to the cervical spine has become widely accepted for the treatment of degenerative conditions, including radiculopathy and myelopathy (1). Using this approach, disk and bone that compress the spinal cord may be safely removed. Many traumatic injuries to the cervical spine also result in damage to the intervertebral disk and/or vertebral body. For such patients, the anterior approach provides a safe and effective direct route to achieving the goals of decompression of neural tissue and stabilization of the spine. It provides the best access to anterior pathology, allows for restoration of anterior column support, and provides stability in the setting of intact posterior structures.

II INDICATIONS

A Historical

Anterior decompression and fusion of the cervical spine was first described almost 50 years ago for the treatment of degenerative conditions of the cervical spine (2). Numerous studies have described the efficacy of anterior decompression and fusion for degenerative conditions such as radiculopathy and myelopathy (3,4). In the late 1950s, the anterior approach gained usefulness in the management of tuberculous abscesses and neoplastic conditions involving the anterior cervical spine (5,6). In 1960, Bailey and Badgley first described the anterior approach as a technique of stabilizing the traumatized cervical spine using anterior bone grafting and fusion (7). Cloward reported on the use of interbody fusion using a cylindrical bone dowel for fracture/dislocations of the cervical spine in 11 patients (8). However, in that era, anterior procedures were developed and refined primarily for the management of degenerative conditions such as spondylotic radiculopathy and myelopathy. Traumatic conditions, however, were typically treated with laminectomy and posterior fusion, which did not address the anterior compression of the spinal cord from bone and disk material (9). In addition, many reports of cervical laminectomy for trauma described increased neurological deficit and increased mortality (10,11). Since nonoperative treatment seemed to result in a lower incidence of late instability and better neurological outcome, many surgeons advocated nonoperative treatment of cervical spine injuries (12–14).

In 1979, Bohlman reported on the long-term experience at Johns Hopkins University, which included the outcomes of 300 patients treated for acute cervical injury from 1950 to 1972 (15). Treatment included nonoperative closed management, laminectomy with and without posterior fusion, and anterior decompression and fusion. At that institution, a significant number of patients treated with laminectomy had additional loss of neurological function, whereas no patient treated with an anterior procedure had worsened function. In addition, chronic instability was seen in 42% of patients treated nonoperatively. The study also included an analysis of autopsy specimens, which found disk protrusion in 26 of 64 cases of fracture subluxation and that protruding disk material remained anterior to the posterior longitudinal ligament. Based upon the results of this analysis, Bohlman advocated anterior decompression and stabilization for spinal injuries with anterior spinal cord compression and intact posterior ligaments.

In 1992, Anderson and Bohlman reported on the efficacy of late anterior decompression and fusion for patients with residual anterior compressive pathology (16,17). It was one of the first studies to evaluate anterior decompression and fusion in terms of neurological outcome in both incomplete and complete spinal injuries. The theory behind the use of an anterior approach was based upon fundamental concepts demonstrated by animal studies (18–21): (1) mechanical compression of the spinal cord contributes to injury beyond the initial cord contusion and trauma; (2) the continued presence of compression can prevent neurological improvement; and (3) late decompression may result in further improvement even after a plateau in neurological status has been observed. Subsequent studies have continued to demonstrate the superiority of anterior decompression and fusion over other means of treatment (22–24) in terms of neurological improvement, as well as the prevention of late deformity and early mobilization via spinal stabilization.

More recently, one-stage anterior decompression and fusion combined with posterior fusion has been demonstrated to be safe and effective in treating certain injury patterns. In 1989, McAfee reported substantial improvement in 22 of 24 patients who had combined anterior decompression and posterior stabilization for either tumor or trauma (25). In 1995, McAfee and Bohlman reported on a series of 100 patients managed with single-stage anterior decompression and posterior stabilization

(26). The indication in 31 of these patients was cervical spine trauma. Mean operation time was 4.5 h. Twenty-one of 35 patients who were nonambulatory became community ambulators; 57 of 75 patients who had an incomplete neurological deficit recovered at least one Frankel grade of neurological function. Similarly, McNamara observed neurological improvement of at least one grade and solid fusion in a series of six patients undergoing single-stage anterior decompression and posterior fusion (27). The only complications were two posterior wound infections, which were successfully treated by irrigation and debridement.

B   Contemporary Indications

The selection of anterior versus posterior approaches to the cervical spine rests upon the location of the primary compressive pathology. Certain injury patterns are more commonly associated with anterior spinal cord compression. These patterns are compressive flexion, vertical compression, compressive extension, and distractive extension patterns of injury, as described by Ferguson and Allen (28). In general terms, the anterior approach is indicated in the presence of a traumatic disk herniation (Fig. 1) and vertebral body fracture with retropulsed fragments causing spinal cord compression (Fig. 2). Other indications for anterior decompression and fusion alone or in combination with posterior fusion include injuries with anterior instability and kyphosis across the fracture site and unstable injuries with vertebral body fracture, retrolisthesis of the involved vertebrae, and bilaminar fractures or posterior ligamentous injuries (29).

In cases of anterior cord syndrome, anterior decompression is best suited to address the primary pathology that is usually bone or disk fragments compressing the anterior aspect of the spinal cord. In central cord syndrome, nonoperative treatment was originally advocated (30), although several more recent authors have demonstrated further neurological improvement in these patients despite reaching a plateau in terms of neurological recovery (17,30–32). Currently we advocate waiting 1 to 6 weeks in the setting of an acute central cord injury without evidence of ligamentous injury or spinal instability prior to surgical intervention.

Several of these articles advocate an indication for late decompression up to 1 year from injury (16,17). In most cases, such patients must have demonstrable residual anterior compressive pathology. Improvement in neurological function drops off precipitously at greater than 12 months postinjury (17); however, the efficacy of anterior decompression and fusion performed more than 12 months after the traumatic injury in alleviating spasticity and refractory pain at the involved root level (upper extremities) has also been observed (16).

III   TECHNIQUE

As described in previous chapters, the treatment of fracture/dislocation of the cervical spine begins with prompt skeletal traction and spinal realignment (33), as well as administration of high-dose steroids to patients seen within 8 h of their injury. We advocate the use of reduction techniques with high weights (>50 pounds), if necessary, to achieve spinal column alignment preoperatively. Additional preoperative preparation includes obtaining advanced imaging studies following closed reduction, including CT, MRI, and MRA.

After the administration of anesthesia, the patient is placed in Gardner-Wells tongs with the head resting on a Mayfield horseshoe. Five to 10 pounds of traction are applied. Care is taken to tuck the arms and tape the shoulders in order to visualize the operative levels on intraoperative lateral radiographs. Loupe magnification and a head lamp or the use of an operating microscope are essential for adequate visualization.

The anterior approach as described by Smith and Robinson is used. Once exposure and localization of the appropriate levels has been obtained, the procedure will proceed according to the need for diskectomy versus corpectomy. Diskectomy is carried out via the standard described techniques. A No. 15 blade is directed at a 15° cephalad angle and passed along the vertebral endplates to a depth of 5 mm to incise the annulus. Progressively smaller curettes are then placed into the disk space and used to remove all nucleus pulposus tissue from anterior to posterior. Once the posterior annulus is reached, a Cloward intervertebral spreader or a Caspar distractor may be applied to open the disk space and better expose the posterior annulus. Care must be taken to avoid overdistraction of the disk space. Remaining annulus may then be removed to expose the underlying neural elements. If a traumatic disk herniation was identified on preoperative imaging studies, it should be localized and removed. We advocate the use of the operating microscope for this portion of the procedure.

Once the decompression is complete, the vertebral endplates are denuded of any remaining cartilage and decorticated to the point of achieving punctate bleeding with a 5-mm high-speed carbide-tipped burr. After decortication of adjacent endplates, a trough is created with the burr, taking care to leave a posterior lip of endplate to prevent posterior dislodgement of the graft. We advocate the use of autogenous iliac crest bone graft to facilitate rapid, reliable healing, especially in the setting of trauma. Many types of bone graft have been described for reconstruction following anterior cervical diskectomy. These include the horseshoe-shaped graft (Robinson), dowel graft (Cloward), iliac strut (Bailey and Badgely), and keystone graft (Simmons). Biomechanical testing has shown the Robinson horseshoe-shaped graft to be the strongest and most resistive to compressive forces (34). In an attempt to eliminate donor-site morbidity (pain, hematoma, infection) some authors have reported reasonably good experience with allografts (35,36). Young and Rosenwasser observed fusion rates of 92% using fibular allograft in 23 patients for nontraumatic pathology

$\longrightarrow$

Figure 1   Patient S.S., a 42-year-old female who presented with bilateral upper extremity weakness and numbness following a motor vehicle accident. (A) Lateral radiograph demonstrating a unilateral facet dislocation of C6 on C7. (B) Follow-up lateral radiograph after application of Gardner-Wells tongs and 50 pounds of axial traction demonstrating reduction of the dislocation. (C,D) Sagittal and axial MR images following reduction demonstrating a herniated disk at the C6–C7 level resulting in spinal cord compression. (E) Pictorial depiction of the anterior cervical diskectomy and interbody grafting technique used in this patient. (F) Postoperative lateral radiograph demonstrating early consolidation of the interbody graft. Care was taken *not* to overdistract the disk space with a large graft (an 8-mm graft was used). As a result, the posterior elements at the C6–C7 level are not widened.

(A)

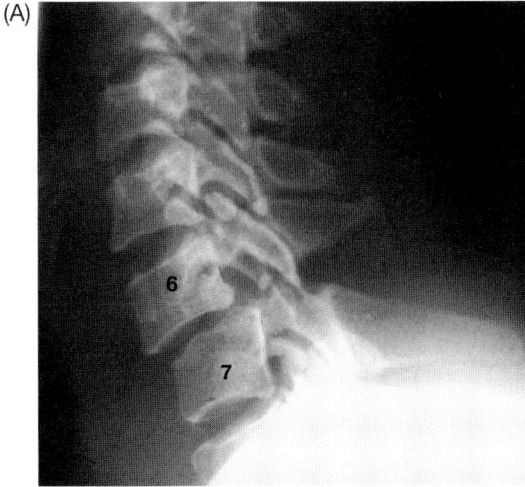

(B)

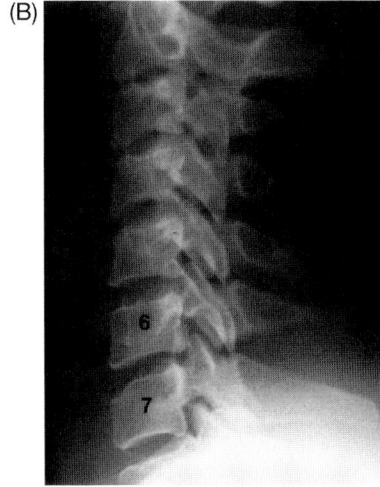

(C)

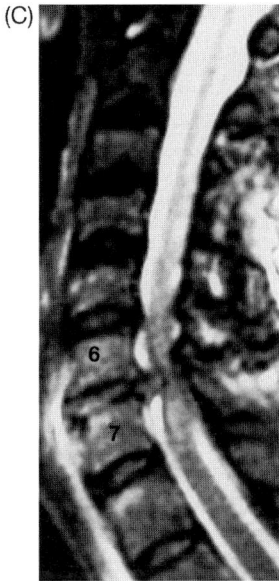

(D)

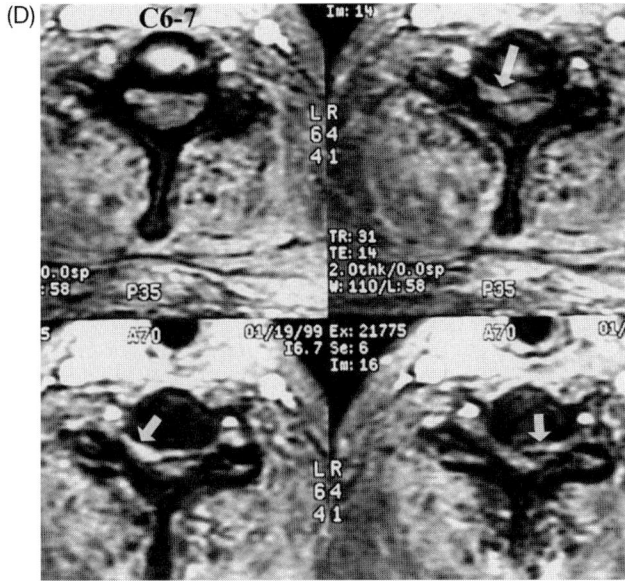

(E)

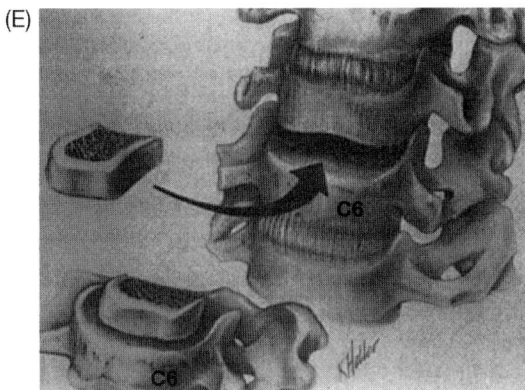

(F)

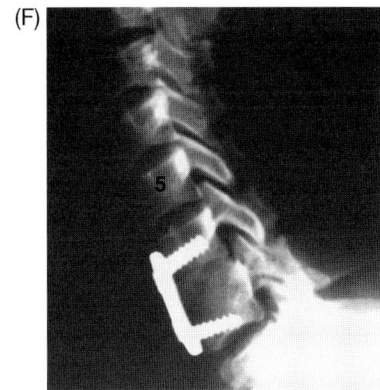

(A)
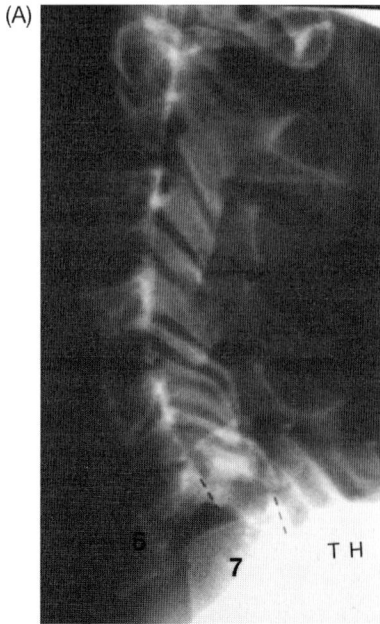

(B)
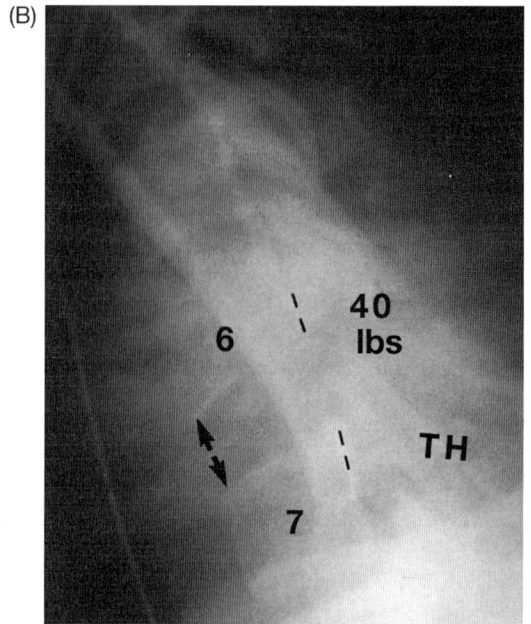

(C)
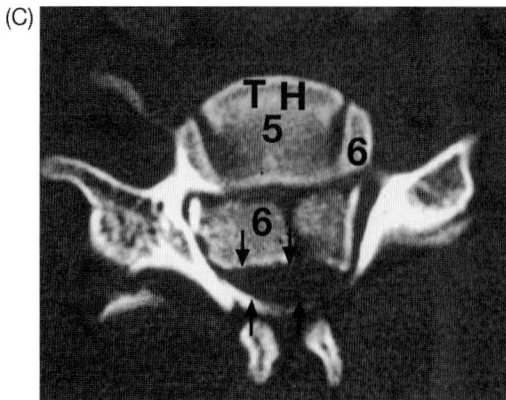

(D)
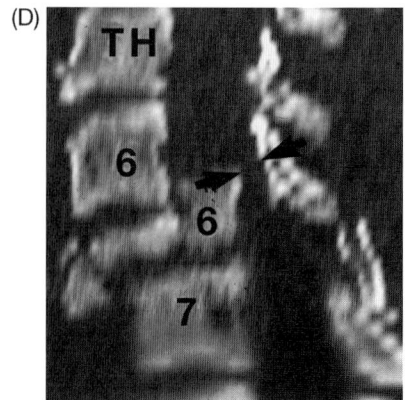

(E)
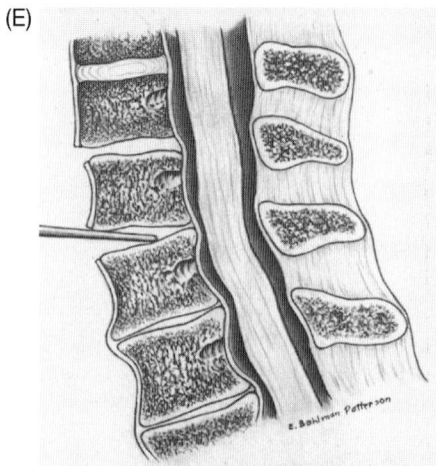

(F)
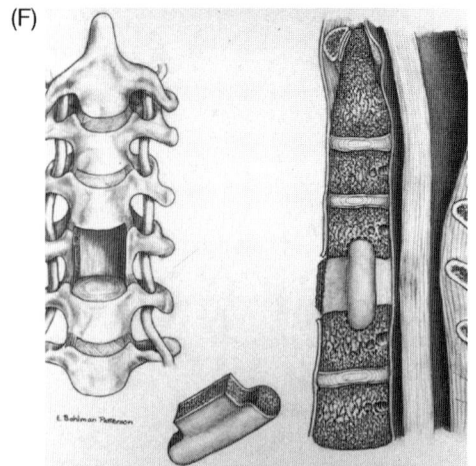

(G)

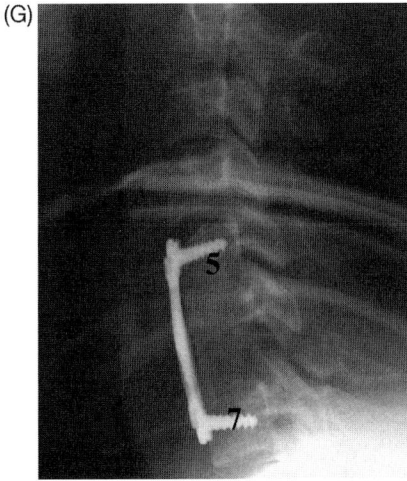

Figure 2   Patient T.H., a 20-year-old male admitted following a motorcycle accident who presented with a C6 ASIA A quadriplegia. (A) Lateral radiograph obtained in the emergency room demonstrating a flexion compression injury with a fracture dislocation of C6 on C7. (B) Lateral radiograph following application of a halo ring and reduction with 40 pounds of axial traction demonstrating restoration of overall anatomical alignment. (C,D) Axial and sagittal images of the cervical spine following reduction with traction, demonstrating comminution of the C6 vertebral body with retropulsion of fragments into the spinal canal. (E,F) Schematics of the technique of anterior cervical corpectomy and strut grafting, demonstrating removal of all disk and soft tissue from the disk spaces (Fig. 2E) followed by removal of the middle third of the vertebral body and placement of an iliac crest strut graft spanning the decompression site (Fig. 2F). (G) Postoperative lateral radiograph demonstrating reconstruction of the C6 vertebral body with a strut graft spanning from C5 to C7.

(37). Care must be taken to harvest an appropriate-sized graft that will not overdistract the disk space. In general, the appropriate dimensions for an interbody bone graft are 2 mm greater than the preoperative disk height (38). Most commonly, this requires a graft height of 7 or 8 mm.

Following placement of the graft, anterior plating is recommended to decrease the possibility of graft extrusion and to increase stability of the construct. In degenerative conditions, the use of an anterior plate has also been demonstrated to improve the fusion rates for multilevel interbody grafts (39,40). In 1989, Coe evaluated the biomechanics of different fixation systems and concluded that anterior plating was inferior to other techniques although the study did not involve bone graft (41). Current practice in both degenerative and traumatic conditions of the cervical spine supports the use of unicortical as opposed to bicortical fixation screws with anterior titanium plating (42). For patients with intact posterior structures, the added stability from the plate may obviate the need for halo immobilization postoperatively.

In cases of a traumatic herniated disk with an irreducible facet dislocation, An recommends beginning with anterior decompression and diskectomy (43). If the diskectomy does not effect a reduction, he describes placement of a bone graft in the disk space, followed by turning the patient and performing an open posterior reduction and fusion. If the graft migrates during the posterior procedure, or if anterior plating is desired, the patient may require repositioning and a return to the anterior aspect of the cervical spine (a so-called "540 fusion").

In the presence of vertebral body fracture, subtotal corpectomy is indicated. This procedure follows the same approach as an anterior diskectomy. Once the anterior annulus and the nucleus pulposus of the adjacent disks have been evacuated, attention is directed to the uncovertebral joints, which are completely cleaned of all disk material and soft tissue. Using these as a guide to the lateral margins of a safe decompression, the intervening fractured vertebral body or bodies may be safely removed. The corpectomy is initiated with a large Leksell rongeur (the cancellous bone may be saved if a concomitant posterior fusion is planned) and continued with a high-speed, 5-mm, carbide-tipped burr. The posterior cortical wall may be safely removed using either a diamond-tipped burr or curved microcurettes. In case of a sagittal slice-type vertebral body fracture, there may be a laceration of the dura. If cerebrospinal fluid is encountered, care should be taken to elevate bone fragments without removing any of the remaining dura. Direct repair with small sutures may not be possible, but a lumbar drain should be applied to allow control of the CSF volume while the defect heals over. Corpectomy must be performed wide enough to allow adequate decompression, although dissection should not proceed lateral to the joints of Lushka to minimize the risk of injury to the vertebral arteries (44). There should be no adjacent vertebral body injury. Again, it is important to avoid overdistraction and to appropriately size the bone graft.

A concomitant posterior stabilization procedure may also be indicated, especially in the setting of a posterior ligamentous injury or posterior element fracture. Certain authors have questioned the ability of anterior fusion alone to provide adequate stability to the acutely injured cervical spine because of the potential for unrecognized, but significant, posterior ligamentous disruption (45–47). Consideration for a posterior procedure should also be given to those patients in whom two- or three-level corpectomy has been performed even without evidence of obvious ligamentous injury.

IV RESULTS

Since Bohlman's 1979 report of the treatment of 300 patients with acute cervical spine injury, several authors have reported on their success with anterior decompression and fusion. In Bohlman's series, there were 229 subaxial cervical spine injuries. Of 33 patients with anterior cord syndrome, nine were treated nonoperatively, 15 underwent laminectomy with or without posterior fusion, four had anterior decompression and fusion, two had laminectomy and anterior as well as posterior fusion, and one had anterior and posterior fusion alone. A total of seven patients had anterior decompression with removal of disk or bone fragments. Three of these seven recovered completely and the other four experienced partial recovery. In the 15 patients who had laminectomy, only one patient recovered completely, two recovered partially, and the remaining patients were unchanged, worsened, or died. Of 53 patients with complete cord lesions, 11 were treated nonoperatively, 32 by laminectomy, and 5 underwent anterior decompression and fusion. In the laminectomy group, seven patients lost motor function or died. In the anterior decompression and fusion group, one patient had slight root return, three were no better, and one died. In patients without neurological injury, 7 of 62 patients had an anterior fusion (15).

A 1984 review by Capen of 212 patients undergoing cervical fusion compared the results of anterior (59 patients) and posterior (98 patients) fusion. They found a high rate of graft dislodgement (6 patients), loss of reduction (32 of 59 patients) and esophageal perforation (2 patients). The authors concluded that anterior fusion alone was inferior to posterior fusion and that the absence of posterior element widening could not be considered absolute evidence that the posterior ligamentous structures are intact. However, in this series no anterior plate was used and the majority of grafts used were fibular strut grafts (46).

For the most convincing evidence that anterior decompression reliably improves neurological outcomes in both incomplete and complete spinal cord injuries, one must refer to Bohlman and Anderson's two-part paper published in 1992 (16,17). Of 58 patients with incomplete injuries who underwent anterior decompression and fusion, half became functional ambulators while the other half had root improvement. Average interval to decompression was 13 months. Less improvement was seen in patients decompressed at greater than 12 months. In a second study of 51 patients with complete lesions, 32 patients recovered at least one cervical root level. Average interval to decompression in this group of patients was 15 months and average follow-up 5 years. Less improvement was seen in this group when decompression was performed at greater than 18 months postinjury and in patients older than age 58.

Other authors have continued to report similar promising results with anterior decompression and fusion for cervical spine injury. Randle reported on 54 patients who all had stable fusion at 6 months' follow-up (48). Half of these demonstrated significant neurological improvement. Aebi reported on 86 patients followed for an average of 40 months (49). On average, patients with incomplete cord injuries recovered at least one Frankel grade and successful fusion occurred by 3 to 4 months postoperatively. Garvey reported on 13 patients with acute cervical fracture and/or dislocations with associated posterior ligamentous disruption (23). Average follow-up in this series was 30 months. All patients obtained solid arthrodesis and were satisfied with the procedure.

A recent study by Dai showed an average increase in the ASIA motor score from 47 to 86 in a group of 24 patients with central cord syndrome treated with anterior decompression and fusion. Advanced age was a poor prognostic sign (50).

Complications of anterior decompression and plating include neurological injury, vertebral artery injury, dural tear, failure of the plate or graft, and late kyphosis. Minor complications include sore throat, hoarseness, and dysphagia. Graft-related complications include migration and collapse. Without plating, graft migration has been reported to be as high as 50% (47). Stauffer and Kelly reported a 30% incidence of recurrent deformity and graft migration which they attributed to impaired spinal stability as a result of an anterior procedure; however, no anterior plating was used in their series (45). Anterior decompression and fusion in the treatment of degenerative, neoplastic, and traumatic conditions with two- and three-level corpectomy has shown a graft dislodgement rate of 9% and 50%, respectively (51). Late kyphosis may also occur secondary to overdistraction and failure to recognize posterior injury.

The vertebral artery may be injured in the initial traumatic insult to the cervical spine. The integrity of the vertebral arteries should be ascertained following any trauma to the cervical spine that results in vertebral body fracture; injuries to a vertebral artery have been identified after trauma in 20 to 40% of cases (52,53). Although up to 50% of patients with a damaged vertebral artery show no evidence of brain ischemia because of collateral circulation, we recommend preoperative MRA where suspicion for this injury exists, particularly if CT scan shows bone fragments or fracture into the transverse foramen.

Dural tears are unusual with anterior decompression, except in the setting of OPLL. However, they may occur secondary to fracture of the vertebra. Direct repair should be performed, if possible, although this will usually require the application of a fascial or muscle patch. We also recommend application of a topical sealant as well as the use of a lumbar drain.

Other, less common complications associated with the anterior approach to the cervical spine include tracheal and esophageal injuries and recurrent laryngeal nerve injury, which is more commonly associated with the use of the right-sided approach given the different course of this nerve on the right compared to the left.

In summary, anterior decompression and fusion is an excellent method for the treatment of traumatic injuries to the cervical spine causing anterior spinal cord compression. This procedure is best applied in cases of disruption of the anterior column such as vertical compression and compressive flexion. There are few major complications for anterior decompression and fusion, although the greater degree of instability in traumatic rather than degenerative conditions should be appreciated and the surgeon should have a low threshold for providing further stability via concomitant posterior fusion. Most importantly, the anterior approach provides direct decompression of the neural elements and the existing literature describes improved neurological outcomes relative to nonoperative and posterior operative treatment approaches.

REFERENCES

1. Emery SE, Bohlman HH, Bolesta MJ, Jones PK. Anterior cervical decompression and arthrodesis for the treatment of cervical spondylotic myelopathy. Two to seventeen-year follow-up. J Bone Joint Surg Am 1998; 80:941–951.
2. Smith G, Robinson R. The treatment of certain cervical spine disorders by anterior removal of the intervertebral disc and interbody fusion. J Bone Joint Surg 1958; 40A: 607–624.
3. Herkowitz HN. The surgical management of cervical spondylotic radiculopathy and myelopathy. Clin Orthop 1989:94–108.
4. Herkowitz HN, Kurz LT, Overholt DP. Surgical management of cervical soft disc herniation. A comparison between the anterior and posterior approach. Spine 1990; 15: 1026–1030.
5. Southwick W, Robinson R. Surgical approaches to the vertebral bodies in the cervical and lumbar regions. J Bone Joint Surg 1957; 39A:631–644.
6. Kirkady-Willis W, Thomas T. Anterior approaches in the diagnosis and treatment of infections of the vertebral bodies. J Bone Joint Surg 1965; 47A:87.
7. Bailey R, Badgley RF. Stabilization of the cervical spine by anterior fusion. J Bone Joint Surg 1960; 42A:565–594.
8. Cloward R. Treatment of acute fractures and fracture-dislocations of the cervical spine by vertebral-body fusion: Report of eleven cases. J Neurosurg 1961; 18:201–209.
9. Holdsworth F. Fractures, dislocations and fracture-dislocations of the spine. J Bone Joint Surg 1970; 52A:1534–1551.

10. Comarr A, Kaufman A. A survey of the neurological results of 858 spinal cord injuries. A comparison of patients treated with and without laminectomy. J Neurosurg 1956; 13: 95–106.

11. Bohlman H. Complications of treatment of fractures and dislocations of the cervical spine. In: Epps CHJ, ed. Complications in Orthopaedic Surgery, vol. 2. Philadelphia: J.B. Lippincott, 1978:1871–1892.

12. Cheshire D. The stability of the cervical spine following the conservative treatment of fractures and fracture-dislocations. Paraplegia 1969; 7:193–203.

13. Bedbrook G. Pathological principles int the management of spinal cord trauma. Paraplegia 1966; 4:43–56.

14. Burke D, Berryman D. The place of closed manipulation in the management of flexion-rotation dislocations of the cervical spine. J Bone Joint Surg 1971; 53B:165–182.

15. Bohlman HH. Acute fractures and dislocations of the cervical spine. An analysis of three hundred hospitalized patients and review of the literature. J Bone Joint Surg [Am] 1979; 61:1119–1142.

16. Bohlman HH, Anderson PA. Anterior decompression and arthrodesis of the cervical spine: long-term motor improvement. Part I—Improvement in incomplete traumatic quadriparesis. J Bone Joint Surg [Am] 1992; 74:671–682.

17. Anderson PA, Bohlman HH. Anterior decompression and arthrodesis of the cervical spine: long-term motor improvement. Part II—Improvement in complete traumatic quadriplegia. J Bone Joint Surg [Am] 1992; 74:683–692.

18. Tarlov I. Acute spinal cord compression paralysis. J Neurosurg 1972; 36:10–20.

19. Dolan E, Tator C, L E. The value of decompression for acute experimental spinal cord compression injury. J Neurosurg 1980; 53:749–755.

20. Ducker T, Salcman M, Daniell H. Experimental spinal cord trauma, III: Therapeutic effect of immobilization and pharmacologic agents. Surg Neurol 1978; 10:71–76.

21. Ducker T. Experimental injury of the spinal cord. In: Vinken P, Bruyn GW, eds. Handbook of Clinical Neurology. Injuries of the Spine and Spinal Cord. Part I. Vol. 25. New York: American Elsevier, 1976:9–26.

22. Dai L, Ni B, Yuan W, Jia L. Radiculopathy after laminectomy for cervical compression myelopathy. J Bone Joint Surg Br 1998; 80:846–849.

23. Garvey TA, Eismont FJ, Roberti LJ. Anterior decompression, structural bone grafting, and Caspar plate stabilization for unstable cervical spine fractures and/or dislocations. Spine 1992; 17:S431–S435.

24. Kiwerski JE. Early anterior decompression and fusion for crush fractures of cervical vertebrae. Int Orthop 1993; 17:166–168.

25. McAfee PC, Bohlman HH. One-stage anterior cervical decompression and posterior stabilization with circumferential arthrodesis. A study of twenty-four patients who had a traumatic or a neoplastic lesion. J Bone Joint Surg [Am] 1989; 71:78–88.

26. McAfee PC, Bohlman HH, Ducker TB, Zeidman SM, Goldstein JA. One-stage anterior cervical decompression and posterior stabilization. A study of one hundred patients with a minimum of two years of follow- up. J Bone Joint Surg Am 1995; 77:1791–1800.

27. McNamara MJ, Devito DP, Spengler DM. Circumferential fusion for the management of acute cervical spine trauma. J Spinal Disord 1991; 4:467–471.

28. Rizzolo S, Cotler J. Unstable cervical spine injuries: Specific treatment approaches. J Am Acad Orthopaed Surg 1993; 1:57–66.

29. Ripa DR, Kowall MG, Meyer PR, Jr., Rusin JJ. Series of ninety-two traumatic cervical spine injuries stabilized with anterior ASIF plate fusion technique. Spine 1991; 16:S46–S55.

30. Schneider R, Knighton R. Chronic sequalae of acute trauma to the spine and spinal cord. Part III. The syndrome of chronic injury to the cervical spinal cord in the region of the central canal. J Bone Joint Surg 1959; 41A.

31. Bose B, Northrup BE, Osterholm JL, Cotler JM, DiTunno JF. Reanalysis of central cervical cord injury management. Neurosurgery 1984; 15:367–372.

32. Brodkey JS, Miller CF, Jr., Harmody RM. The syndrome of acute central cervical spinal cord injury revisited. Surg Neurol 1980; 14:251–257.
33. Frankel H, Hancock D, Hyslop G, Melzak J, Michaelis L, Ungar G, Vernon J, Walsh J. The value of postural reduction in the initial management of closed injuries of the spine with paraplegia and tetraplegia. Part I. Paraplegia 1969; 7:179–192.
34. White A, Hirsch, C. An experimental study of the immediate load bearing capacity of some commonly used iliac bone grafts. Acta Orthop Scand 1971; 42:482–490.
35. Zdeblick T, Ducker, TD. The use of freeze dried allograft bone for anterior cervical fusions. Spine 1991; 16:726–729.
36. Bishop RC, Moore KA, Hadley MN. Anterior cervical interbody fusion using autogeneic and allogeneic bone graft substrate: a prospective comparative analysis. J Neurosurg 1996; 85:206–210.
37. Young W, Rosenwasser, RH. An early comparative analysis of the use of fibular allograft versus autologous iliac crest graft for interbody fusion after anterior cervical discectomy. Spine 1993; 18:1123–1124.
38. An H, Evanich C, Nowicki B, Haughton V. Ideal thickness of Smith-Robinson graft for anterior cervical fusion. A cadaveric study with computed tomographic correlation. Spine 1993; 18:2043–2047.
39. Wang JC, McDonough PW, Endow KK, Delamarter RB. Increased fusion rates with cervical plating for two-level anterior cervical discectomy and fusion. Spine 2000; 25: 41–45.
40. Connolly PJ, Esses SI, Kostuik JP. Anterior cervical fusion: outcome analysis of patients fused with and without anterior cervical plates. J Spinal Disord 1996; 9:202–206.
41. Coe J, Warden, KE, Sutterlin, CE, McAfee, PC. Biomechanical evaluation of cervical spinal stabilization methods in a human cadaveric model. Spine 1989; 14:1122–1131.
42. Sidhu K, Herkowitz, HN. Surgical management of cervical disc disease. In: Herkowitz H, ed. Rothman-Simeone the Spine. Vol. 1. Philadelphia: Saunders, 1999:497–528.
43. An H. Cervical spine trauma. Spine 1998; 23:2713–2729.
44. Cosgrove G, Theron, J. Vertebral arteriovenous fistula following anterior cervical spine surgery. Report of two cases. J Neurosurg 1987; 66:297.
45. Stauffer E, Kelly E. Fracture-dislocations of the cervical spine. Instability and recurrent deformity following treatment by anterior interbody fusion. J Bone Joint Surg 1977; 59A:45–48.
46. Capen DA, Garland DE, Waters RL. Surgical stabilization of the cervical spine. A comparative analysis of anterior and posterior spine fusions. Clin Orthop 1985:229–237.
47. Van Peteghem PK, Schweigel JF. The fractured cervical spine rendered unstable by anterior cervical fusion. J Trauma 1979; 19:110–114.
48. Randle MJ, Wolf A, Levi L, Rigamonti D, Mirvis S, Robinson W, Bellis E, Greenberg J, Salcman M. The use of anterior Caspar plate fixation in acute cervical spine injury. Surg Neurol 1991; 36:181–189.
49. Aeibi M, Zuber, K, Marchesi. Treatment of cervical spine injuries with anterior plating: Indications, techniques, and results. Spine 1990; 16:S38–S45.
50. Dai L, Jia L. Central cord injury complicating acute cervical disc herniation in trauma. Spine 2000; 25:331–335; discussion 336.
51. Vaccaro A, Falatyn S, Scuderi G, Eismont F, McGuire R, Singh K, Garfin S. Early failure of long segment anterior cervical plate fixation. J Spinal Disord 1998; 11:410–415.
52. Giacobetti FB, Vaccaro AR, Bos-Giacobetti MA, Deeley DM, Albert TJ, Farmer JC, Cotler JM. Vertebral artery occlusion associated with cervical spine trauma. A prospective analysis. Spine 1997; 22:188–192.
53. Willis BK, Greiner F, Orrison WW, Benzel EC. The incidence of vertebral artery injury after midcervical spine fracture or subluxation. Neurosurgery 1994; 34:435–441; discussion 441–442.

26

Posterior Cervical Fixation

STEVEN C. LUDWIG and MUSTASIM N. RUMI

The Milton S. Hershey Medical Center of the Pennsylvania State University College of Medicine, Hershey, Pennsylvania, U.S.A.

ALEXANDER R. VACCARO and TODD J. ALBERT

Thomas Jefferson University Hospital and the Rothman Institute, Philadelphia, Pennsylvania, U.S.A.

I INTRODUCTION

Prior to the widespread utilization of surgical fusion for the treatment of unstable cervical spine injuries, conservative treatment was the cornerstone of managing such injuries. Long-term cast immobilization and traction comprised the armamentarium of treatment options for the unstable cervical spine. While this procedure is advantageous in that it spares the patient an operation, it is problematic for several reasons. The degree of stability conferred by conservative treatment is variable and unpredictable. Also, it may subject patients to prolonged traction and immobility, thereby further compromising their overall care by the morbidities associated with prolonged bedrest. The goals of rigid internal fixation are to allow early mobilization and rehabilitation as well as to predictably stabilize the cervical spine.

Berthold Hadra is credited with the first successful surgical stabilization of the cervical spine in 1891 by utilizing interspinous wires. Various materials have subsequently been used for surgical stabilization, including fascia, bone struts, and celluloid material. Rogers popularized his technique of interspinous wiring for posterior cervical stabilization (1). Alternate techniques to wire fixation of the cervical spine, such as lateral mass plates and pedicle screw fixation, have been introduced and utilized over the past two decades. Each of these techniques have unique characteristics that affect their indications for use. Specific anatomical considerations and biomechanical properties render them advantageous in certain injury patterns, but risky in other situations.

Conditions that may necessitate surgical stabilization of the cervical spine include trauma, degenerative disease, neoplasm, infection, deformity correction, congenital abnormalities, and skeletal dysplasias. Iatrogenic instability secondary to extensive laminectomies may also require mechanical fixation. The specific fusion and instrumentation technique depends upon the pathoanatomy and nature of the instability. The goals of spinal stabilization include the maintenance of cervical alignment, biological fusion, decreased need for postoperative bracing, and early rehabilitation. There are several different methods of posterior stabilization of the cervical spine, each with their own inherent advantages and disadvantages. Thus, spine surgeons must determine the most appropriate technique for each particular clinical scenario.

II BIOMECHANICS

Cervical spine instability is defined as segmental hypermobility under physiological loads leading to mechanical displacement or neurological compromise (2). The cervical spine can be divided into two columns. The anterior column extends from the anterior longitudinal ligament to the posterior longitudinal ligament and includes the vertebral bodies and disks. The posterior column involves spinal structures posterior to the posterior longitudinal ligament. Disruption of both columns renders the cervical spine unstable (3).

Deforming forces on the cervical spine include flexion, extension, anterior and posterior shear, and axial rotation primarily at the atlantoaxial junction. The instantaneous axis of rotation determines the location of flexion and extension in the sagittal plane. It is this plane that divides tension and compression forces during flexion and extension. Disruption of the posterior elements displaces the instantaneous axis of rotation anteriorly, therefore rendering the spine unstable in flexion. In such a situation, posterior instrumentation is more stable by reconstructing the disrupted anatomical tension band posteriorly. The converse is true of anterior column insufficiency and anterior instrumentation (4–6). Additionally, it is important to maintain or reestablish physiological cervical lordosis in order to avoid neurological compromise from anterior cord compression that occurs in cases of cervical kyphosis (7).

The goals of cervical stabilization are to maintain alignment, provide stability, and promote healing. Cervical vertebrae are biomechanically unique in that the alignment of the facets and disks more evenly distribute compressive forces and provide a greater range of motion compared to the thoracolumbar spine. Techniques of posterior stabilization are designed to recreate the tension band of the posterior column of the cervical spine. This can be achieved by combinations of wiring techniques, screws, plates, and rods. The overall stability of the posteriorly reconstructed cervical spine depends upon tension through the instrumentation that is reinforced by tension in the intact ligamentous structures combined with compression through the disks or bone graft (8:148). The design of the final construct must reflect the pattern of instability.

III TECHNIQUES

A Posterior Cervical Wiring

Posterior cervical fusion by spinous process wire fixation is feasible when the posterior osseous elements are intact, without rotational or extension instability, and the anterior column is capable of bearing weight (9). Such a construct acts as a tension band to simulate the function of the posterior bony elements. Spinous process wires can be used to stabilize single or multiple cervical motion segments. Techniques that are commonly used include the Rogers technique, the Bohlman technique, and facet wiring. The Rogers technique of interspinous wiring was first described in 1942. Bohlman's modification includes a triple wire technique that provides superior flexural and torsional stiffness to Rogers' original method (9:488). Facet wiring allows for posterior fixation at cervical motion segments following laminectomy.

Monofilament stainless steel wire is the most common type used for posterior spinal fixation, although cable fixation may be used in the same manner. In the cervical spine, 20-gauge wire is used for fixation of the spinous processes, laminae, and facet joints. The strength of wire fixation is determined by (1) the handling of the wire and the manner in which it is applied; (2) the integrity of the bone structure; (3) the strength of the wire–bone interface; (4) the fatigue characteristics of the wire; and (5) the extent of the injury (10,11). If the underlying bone stock is osteoporotic, the wire fixation is tightened excessively, or the spine is excessively loaded, the wire will fail. The mechanical failure will be due either to cutting out through the bone or to the wire breaking. Repetitive loading can cause any wire to fatigue and break. The frustrations of problems inherent in wire fixation led to the development of cable fixation. Unlike wires, cables are flexible and easier to insert or remove, and stronger than wires in fatigue strength. Furthermore, their flexibility leads to safer passage during insertion (12).

For the Rogers technique, a standard posterior approach to the cervical spine is performed. The levels of instrumentation are selected. Drill holes are made in the spinous processes at the junction of the laminae. A wire is passed through the superior hole and looped around the spinous process once. It is then looped through the hole of the inferior spinous process and secured. The spinous processes, laminae, and facet joints are decorticated and bone graft is packed in the appropriate area to be fused (13).

Bohlman's approach is similar to that of Rogers. Drill holes are made in the spinous processes of the selected levels. A single 22-gauge wire is passed through both the superior and inferior spinous processes so that the free ends are on the same side of the spinous process. The first wire is then tightened to stabilize the injury. An additional two wires are passed through the holes and used to compress two large corticocancellous iliac struts against the laminae and spinous processes after decortication (Fig. 1).

Facet wires are placed into the inferior articular facets of the cervical vertebrae. Holes are drilled into the middle of the inferior facet joints while they are held open with a Penfield dissector. Wires are pulled through the holes. The facet wires are attached to corticocancellous struts. Since the facet joints are thin, wires can pull out of the facets if overtightened or if the bone is osteoporotic. Facet wiring is biomechanically weaker than spinous process wiring (6) (Fig. 2).

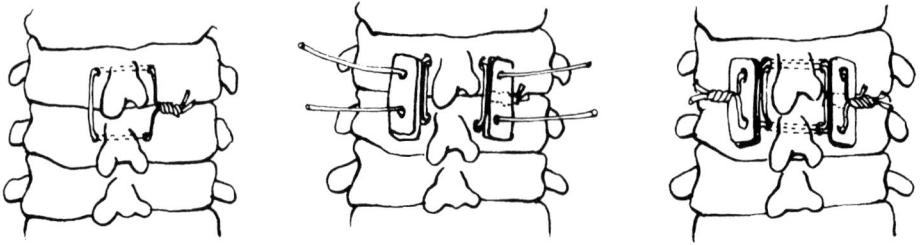

Figure 1 Triple-wire technique with interspinous process wires. A 20-gauge wire is passed through the superior aspect of the spinous process, looped around, and passed through the inferior aspect of the spinous process, looped around, and then tightened. The second and third wires are passed through the same holes in the superior and inferior spinous processes. The lamina and facet joints are then decorticated. Wires are then placed through corticocancellous autogenous bone grafts and tightened down.

Patients who undergo a posterior cervical fusion with wiring techniques require a postoperative cervical orthosis to control excessive motion and reduce the loads on the fixation until a biological fusion is achieved. The choice of orthotic is dependent upon the degree of deformity, quality of the bone, strength of the fixation, and patient compliance.

B Lateral Mass Plating

Most patients with cervical spine instability can be treated with wiring techniques. However, specific clinical situations require more rigid internal fixation. Lateral mass plating is useful in the absence of intact posterior spinous processes or in instances in which the anterior column is incapable of weight bearing (9). Roy-Camille orig-

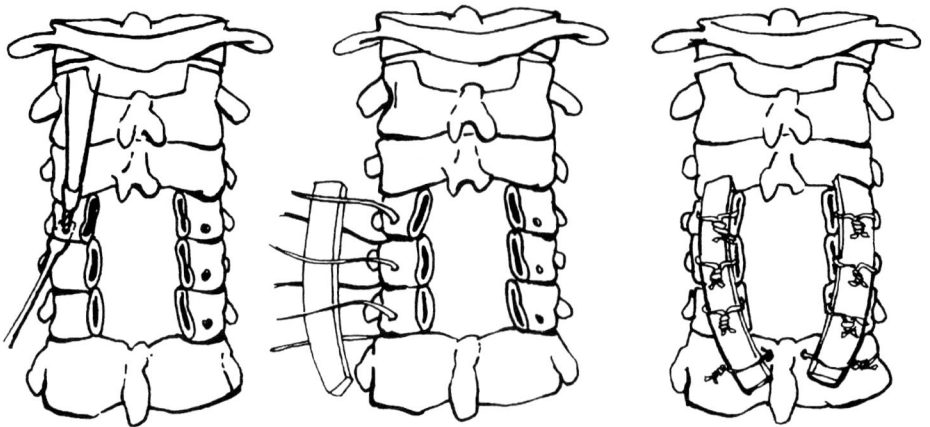

Figure 2 Multilevel facet wiring. Drill holes are created in the facet. A penfield No. 4 is used to slightly elevate the facet joint to facilitate drilling. Wire is then passed into the facet from cranial to caudad and passed around corticocancellous autogenous bone grafts. Final tightening is then performed.

inally described placement of these screws. The technique of posterior plate and screw fixation requires attention to anatomical details. Malposition of the screw may pose serious risk to the nerve root, vertebral artery, and spinal cord. Advantages of lateral mass plating include additional stability at the time of fixation, less loss of spinal reduction, and decreased postoperative immobilization. Unlike wiring techniques that require compression of a potentially injured disk space, lateral mass plating allows reduction and stabilization without significant compression.

Several modifications of the technique originally described by Roy-Camille have been made in an attempt to reduce the risk of neurovascular injury. Proper screw placement requires identification of the proper starting point for screw insertion and correct screw trajectory. A preoperative CT scan to study the relationship of the neural foramen, vertebral artery, and lateral masses is important in each case.

A thorough knowledge of the posterior cervical anatomy is paramount when utilizing the lateral mass plating technique. The third through the sixth cervical vertebrae are well suited for the lateral mass screw plate technique. However, because of the thin transitional C7 lateral mass, an attempt to place a screw at this level poses a danger to the underlying nerve root and facet joint. For this reason, if stabilization at C7 is required, we prefer to utilize pedicle screw fixation at this level if the anatomy is suitable.

Roy-Camille described the original technique for screw placement (Fig. 3), which involves angling the screw 10 degrees lateral and perpendicular to the plane of the facet joint. The starting point is directly in the center of the facet so that the screw achieves bicortical purchase (14). The technique was modified by Magerl to angle the screw 30 degrees superiorly to direct it parallel to the articular surface of the superior facet (15). The starting point is 1 to 3 mm medial to the center of the lateral mass, with a lateral trajectory of 30 degrees to avoid injury to the vertebral artery. This trajectory also allows the longest possible screw path within bone (screw length is usually 16 to 22 mm in size). Anderson further modified the technique with the use of AO reconstruction plates. The starting point was determined to be 1 mm medial to the center of the lateral mass and angled superiorly 30 degrees and laterally 15 to 20 degrees. An localized the entry point for screw insertion at 1 mm medial to the midpoint of the lateral mass. The trajectory is directed 15 degrees superiorly and 30 degrees laterally.

The techniques of lateral mass screws differ biomechanically. The Magerl technique is superior in load to failure and in stiffness. This is thought to be due to the longer screw utilized for the Magerl technique which results in a stronger construct than the Roy-Camille technique (16). No significant difference has been shown in biomechanical strength between screws inserted with bicortical versus unicortical purchase (17). Anatomically, the Magerl technique directs the screw away from neurovascular structures, whereas the Roy-Camille technique directs the screw toward these structures. In the sagittal plane, the vertebral artery is located directly anterior to the laminofacet junction. Thus, with the laterally oriented screw, the vertebral artery is located medial to the screws. The foramina and nerve roots are avoided by angling the screws cranially and laterally (18,19). It is important to realize the few contraindications to posterior plating. The technique should not be used in patients with osteopenic bone or metabolic bone disease due to the significant risk of screw pullout and loss of reduction.

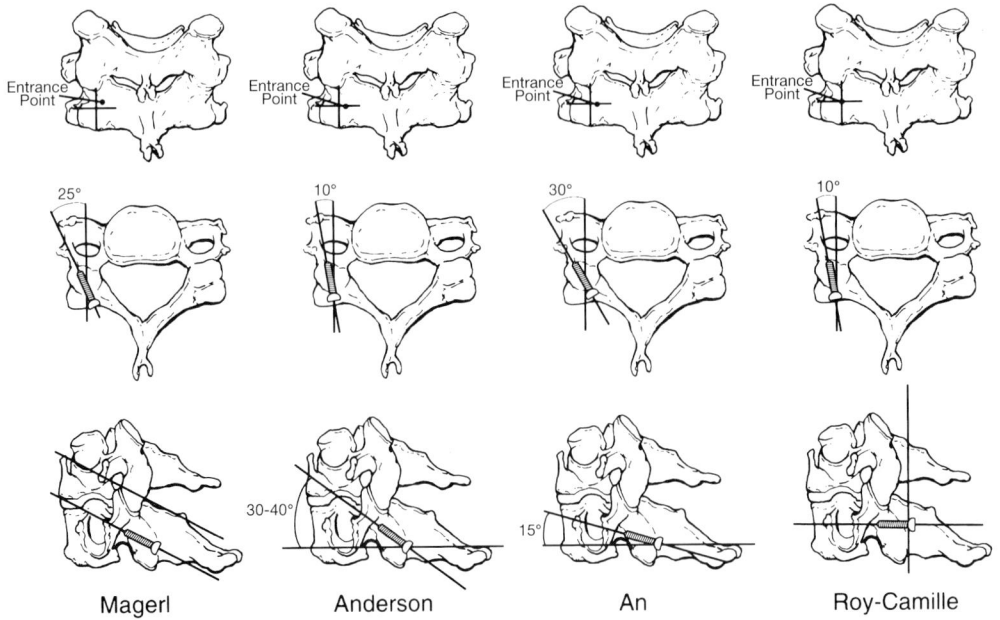

Figure 3 Lateral mass fixation: techniques of screw placement. (1) Roy-Camille technique: starting point is in the middle of the lateral mass, the trajectory is perpendicular to the facet joint and 10 lateral. (2) Magerl technique: starting point is slightly medial and cranial to the midpoint of the lateral mass, the trajectory in the sagittal plane is parallel to the facet joint and 25 laterally in the axial plane. (3) Anderson technique: starting point is 1 mm medial to the midpoint of the lateral mass, the trajectory is 30 to 40 degrees superior and 10 lateral. (4) An technique: starting point is 1 mm medial to the midpoint of the lateral mass, the trajectory is 15 superior and 30 lateral.

Roy-Camille reported his results in 221 patients who had lateral mass plating without a biological fusion. Eighty-five percent maintained their cervical alignment and 39% showed an increase of 10 degrees or more in sagittal plane angulation (20). Fehlings et al. reported their long-term outcome (4 years) in patients treated with cervical lateral mass plating. They reported a fusion rate of 92.7%, 3.8% screw loosening, and a preoperative kyphosis of 24.4 degrees which had improved to 5.5 degrees postoperatively (21). Anderson et al. reported their results in 30 patients with lateral mass fixation with comparable excellent results (22).

C Pedicle Screw Fixation

Dissatisfaction with lateral mass fixation, especially at the cervicothoracic junction, has led spine surgeons to utilize cervical pedicle screw fixation for reconstruction in a number of different cervical spine disorders. The biomechanical advantage of a three-column fixation device implanted to secure an unstable cervical spine has proven to be a valuable tool in the spine surgeon's armamentarium (23). Successful placement of a pedicle screw in the cervical spine requires a sufficient three-dimensional understanding of pedicle morphology to allow accurate identification of the ideal screw axis. Variability in cadaveric-based morphometric measurements used to guide the surgeon in the placement of a pedicle screw has raised legitimate concerns as to whether transpedicular fixation can be applied without significant neurovascular complications (24,25).

Transpedicular screws can be applied as a posterior stabilization device in cases of cervical laminectomy, burst fracture, spinal tumor, and infective spondylitic processes of the cervical spine involving the anterior spinal elements (i.e., tuberculosis). Pedicle screws can be a useful adjunct in situations with multilevel instability patterns, postlaminectomy kyphotic reconstructions, and other cases that require longer fixation (i.e., fixation from the upper to lower cervical spine, or from the middle to the upper thoracic spine).

Description of transpedicle fixation in the cervical spine has been confined to the relatively large C2 pedicle or isthmus. Transpedicular screw placement at C2 was first described by Leconte, for the management of traumatic spondylolisthesis of the axis (26). Roy-Camille described the technique and indications for the placement of a transpedicle screw at C2 for Hangman's fractures (14,27). Anatomically, Panjabi et al. studied the human morphometry of the C2 pedicle and reported the height ranging from 9 to 11 mm and the width ranging from 7 to 9 mm (28). The diameter of the C2 pedicle is larger than those of C3–C7. Therefore, screw insertion into the C2 pedicle is generally easier than insertion in the C3–C7 pedicles. According to Xu et al., the point of entry for screw placement is approximately 5 mm inferior to the superior border of the C2 lamina and 7 mm lateral to the lateral border of the spinal canal. The drilling is directed 10 to 15 degrees medially and 35 degrees superiorly to avoid injury to the vertebral artery (18,19). Ebraheim et al. determined the safest method for C2 pedicle screw placement, which employed drilling guided by palpation of the medial and superior aspect of the individual C2 pedicle (16). C2 pedicle fixation improves plate screw fixation from the occiput to C2 or C2 through the subaxial spine.

D   Laminoforaminotomy Technique

At our institution, we routinely use C2 and C7 pedicle screw fixation as well as upper thoracic spine pedicle fixation. Our preferred technique includes placing all pedicle screws following direct palpation of the pedicle with a right angle nerve hook after performing a small laminoforaminotomy (Fig. 4).

It is of paramount importance for the surgeon to review all preoperative radiographic studies to ensure that no destruction of the pedicle or vertebral body exists that may preclude the placement of a pedicle screw. Moreover, the structural size of the pedicle and the quality of the bone may prevent the safe placement of a transpedicle screw.

A 2-mm burr is used to start the pedicle hole and a drill with an automatic stop at 18 mm is used to further sound the pedicle. A power drill is used because the pedicle is too hard for a hand drill or awl. In this region of the spine, the authors feel the use of an awl or hand drill will create too much force, have too great a chance for surgical slippage, and therefore present more of a danger. All screws should be 3.5 mm in diameter and placed with intraoperative neurophysiological monitoring. This technique is especially useful for complex reconstructions in which long fusions to the cervicothoracic junction are required. This open laminotomy

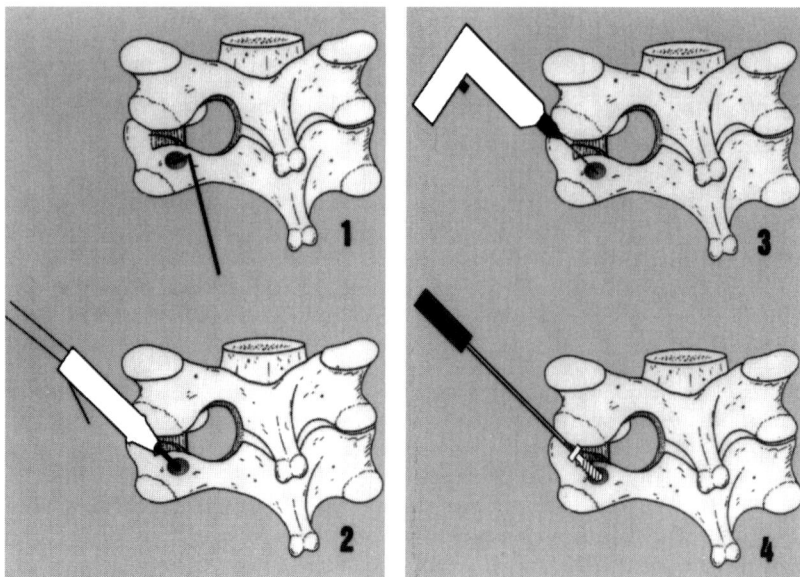

Figure 4 Laminoforaminotomy technique for placing pedicle screws. (1) A keyhole foraminotomy is performed at the correct interval and a nerve hook palpates the pedicle both superiorly and medially. (2) A 2-mm burr is used to create a starting hole in the previously palpated pedicle. (3) A power drill is utilized with a stop set at 18 mm to drill through the pedicle into the body through the starting hole previously created with the burr. (4) After tapping the screw hole, a 20-mm screw is placed through the plate and into the pedicle.

technique is readily reproducible and excellent fusion results can be expected. It is important to obtain a preoperative CT scan to delineate the bony anatomy and course of the vertebral artery.

In the majority of patients, the vertebral artery will be absent from the foramen transversarium of C7 (Fig. 4). Studies have shown that the foramen transversarium of C7 will contain the vertebral artery, vein, and associated nerve fibers in approximately 5% of patients (29). Therefore, CT imaging prior to pedicle screw placement in the seventh vertebrae is necessary (Fig. 5).

Albert et al. reported on 21 patients in which cervical pedicle screw fixation was used at C7 with or without upper thoracic pedicle screw fixation (30). All pedicle screws were placed after direct palpation of the pedicle with a right-angle nerve hook following a laminoforaminotomy at C6–7. The authors reported no neurological complications related to pedicle screw placement and no patient was symptomatically worse following the operation. At 1-year follow-up, no failures of fixation or complications related to pedicle fixation occurred. Albert concluded that pedicle screws in C7, placed with a laminoforaminotomy and palpation technique, appeared to be safe and efficacious while offering excellent fixation.

E Image-Guided Surgical Technique

In order for a stereotactic tracking system to be helpful in the placement of transpedicular screws, the device should meet certain stringent criteria (31). First, the in-

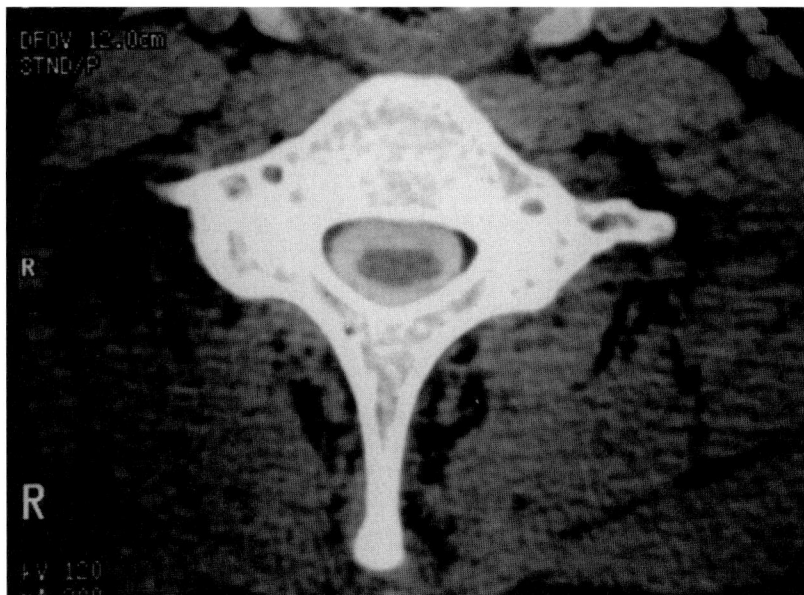

Figure 5 CT scan through the C7 pedicle showing no evidence of the foramen transversarium. A CT scan through the C7 level is mandatory to identify a vertebral artery entering the C7 pedicle prior to the placement of the pedicle screw.

strumentation should be easy to use. The computer should not interfere with and require only slight modifications of standard surgical procedures and principals. The computer should provide sufficient accuracy over more conventional means in directing the surgeon to the correct entry point, trajectory, and depth of insertion. The system should be fast enough to allow real-time instrument control and visualization. Last, the total surgical time should not be significantly affected.

The authors utilize the Stealthstation (Sofamor Danek, Memphis, Tennessee). This system can facilitate insertion of pedicle screws through the application of these stereotactic principles. Stereotaxis is an evolving technology currently used to locate positions in a body without direct access to its interior.

Preoperative cervical spine computed axial tomograms are obtained of the patients and are loaded into the Stealthstation™ (Fig. 6). During an intraoperative session, each spine is registered at the level to be instrumented so that the virtual-world data of the computer screen can communicate with the real-world data of the operating room. Registration utilizes the paired-point (PointMerge™) as well as the surface-mapping (SurfaceMerge™) procedure, which enhances the accuracy of the registration. Once the matching process is completed, the surgeon locates and marks the predefined entry points with the space pointer. A drill guide that is mounted with an emitting diode can relay drill-tip position and orientation to an optical reader. This allows transformation of the real-world data from the operative site into the virtual-world image on the Stealthstation™. Under computerized image guidance, the screw hole is then drilled along the chosen trajectory. During the actual drilling, guidance functions assist the surgeon in matching the chosen trajectory. These guidance functions include a display of colored lines representing the preoperatively

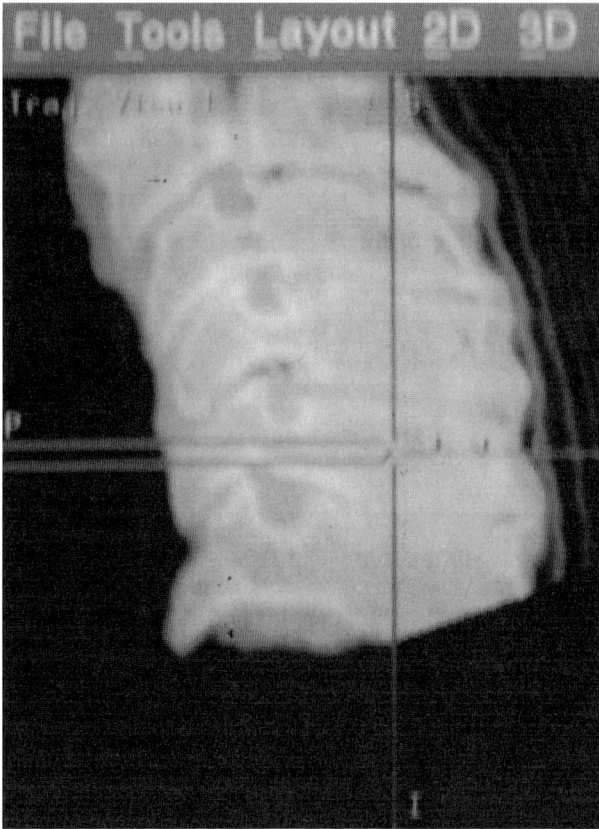

Figure 6 Axial imaging of the trajectory of a pedicle screw using the computer-assisted image-guided surgical system (Stealthstation™, Sofamor Danek, Memphis, TN).

planned trajectory relative to the real-time trajectory of the drill bit in the sagittal, transverse, and coronal planes. An image of a colored circle representing the screw diameter within the coronal cuts through the pedicle can also allow the surgeon to identify any impending cortical breach. Once the pilot hole has been prepared, a 3.5-mm diameter screw can be inserted without additional visualization.

F Abumi Technique

The first report of cervical pedicle screws successfully employed in humans to manage subaxial traumatic injury was published in 1994 by Abumi et al. (26). In this report, 13 patients with destabilizing cervical spine injuries were treated with transpedicular plate-screw constructs. In his study, Abumi was also the first to report a method for identifying the entry point of screw penetration in the posterior aspect of the lateral mass using topographic landmarks combined with lateral fluoroscopy (Fig. 7A,B).

The point of screw penetration at the posterior cortex of the lateral mass facet was found to be slightly lateral to the center of the lateral mass and close to the

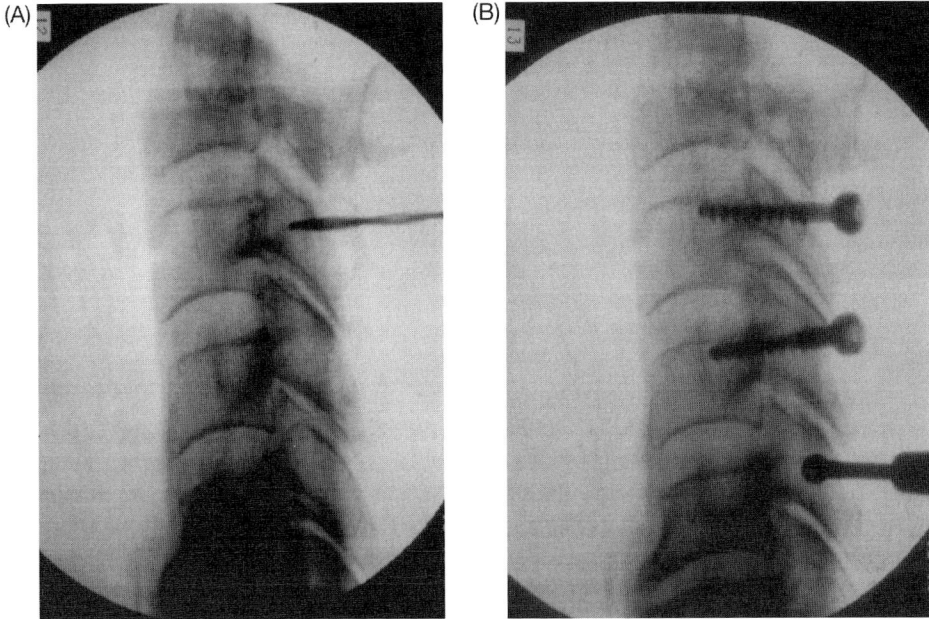

Figure 7 (A) Abumi technique lateral fluoroscopic view of the cervical spine. Sounding the cervical pedicle using a 1.25-mm hand-held drill bit. (B) Lateral fluoroscopic view of the cervical spine: 3.5-mm pedicle screw placement at C3 and C4 with 2-mm burr decorticating the C5 lateral mass to obtain the starting position.

posterior proximal margin of the superior articular surface. After creating an insertion hole with a 2-mm burr, the surgeon could then directly visualize the bleeding cancellous bone indicating the entrance to the pedicle. The pedicle is then probed utilizing a hand-guided 1.25-mm drill bit, thus enhancing visual and tactile sensory feedback cues. Laminotomies are not performed. Based on measurements from preoperative CT images, the intended angle of the screw was 30° to 40° medial to the midline in the transverse plane. The angular orientation in the sagittal plane, prior to sounding the pedicle with the probe, is determined using intraoperative fluoroscopy. The pilot hole is then tapped under fluoroscopic guidance with a 3.5-mm tap followed by insertion of the screw. This technique requires a thorough knowledge of the cervical spine anatomy, careful preoperative planning, and excellent intraoperative fluoroscopic guidance.

Transpedicular cervical spine screw insertion is associated with obvious risks to major neurovascular structures, including the spinal cord, nerve root, and vertebral arteries. In previous human cadaveric in vitro studies comparing the accuracy of different pedicle insertion screw methods, critical structures were injured between 11 to 66%, depending upon which technique was used (24,25). Regardless of the method employed, the vertebral artery is the structure most likely to be injured followed by the exiting nerve root (Fig. 8).

In clinical series of pedicle screw fixation for degenerative or traumatic lesions of the middle and lower cervical spine, neither Abumi nor Albert reported any neurovascular complications with the placement of pedicle screws (26,28,30–32). Direct

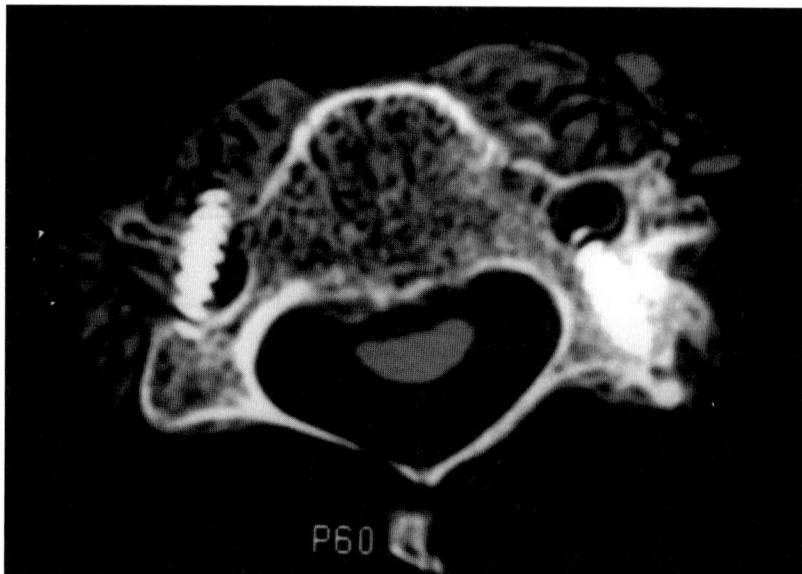

Figure 8 Postoperative CT scan performed in a human cadaveric study. Note bilateral violation of the foramen transversarium. Open dissection revealed complete transection of the vertebral artery on the right side and perforation of the vertebral artery on the left side.

exposure of the pedicle cavity prior to screw placement, and the aid of an image intensifier, adequately confirmed screw insertion. In their series, no pseudoarthroses were demonstrated at a 12- to 22-month follow-up. Abumi reported a rate of screw penetration of the pedicle wall between 5.3 to 6.7% (26,28,31,32). Even in those cases with lateral wall perforation, no complication of the vertebral artery was clinically apparent. Since the vertebral artery does not occupy the whole part of the foramen transversarium, minimal violations of the foramen transversarium may not be as risky as initially thought.

Kramer and Ludwig et al. performed a two-part study on the topographic characteristics of the posterior cervical elements and the safety and efficacy of various pedicle insertion techniques (24,25). The second part of the study compared the accuracy of pedicle screw placement using topographic guidelines alone, a laminoforaminotomy technique with manual palpation of the pedicle, and computer-assisted image guidance (Stealthstation, Sofamor Danek, Memphis, TN). They concluded that topographic guidelines alone were unsafe for screw placement in the subaxial spine. Their success rate improved following laminoforaminotomy, with no vital structures injured at the C7 level. However, the greatest accuracy was achieved using the computer-assisted image-guided surgical system, in which 89.4% of the screws were placed within the pedicle without injuring a vital structure. No critical structures were injured at the C4, C6, or C7 level.

Abumi et al. has the greatest clinical experience with the placement of pedicle screws in the subaxial cervical spine (26,28,31,32). His group has reported on 58 patients with their technique of cervical spine pedicle screw placement in patients with both traumatic and nontraumatic injuries of the cervical spine. With his fluoroscopic-assisted technique, he has reported no neurovascular complications despite a 5.3 to 6.7% pedicle wall perforation rate (26,28,31,32).

Ludwig et al. compared the safety of pedicle screw placement using the most accurate in vitro technique (image-guided surgical system) to the most accurate clinical technique (Abumi method) (33). No significant differences were detected between the two methods of pedicle screw placement. Further analysis determined that no injuries to critical structures, such as the spinal cord, nerve root, or vertebral artery, occurred when pedicles greater than 4.5 mm were instrumented with a 3.5-mm pedicle screw. Based on their analysis, when no other reconstructive options are available for stabilization, pedicle screws should be considered a viable option and should only be placed in those pedicles greater than 4.5 mm in transverse width.

Spine surgeons attempting to place pedicle screws in the cervical spine should employ specific methods to avoid misinsertion. These include a thorough understanding of the patient's cervical spine anatomy, exact preoperative measurements of the pedicle diameter (>4.5 mm), excellent intraoperative imaging techniques, and close attention to the registration process if an image-guided surgical system is to be utilized.

When circumstances do arise in which wire, cable, or lateral mass screw fixation are not applicable for posterior cervical reconstructive procedures, the cervical pedicle screw may be a practical alternative point of fixation. Numerous clinical reports attest to the effectiveness and success of pedicle fixation at the C2 and C7 levels. Elsewhere in the subaxial cervical spine, pedicle screw insertion poses a more significant challenge. The dimensions of the pedicles are smaller, and thus the margins for error are less.

G   C1–C2 Fusion

Acute or chronic instability at the atlantoaxial junction can result in severe neurological injury or death. Progressive anterior translation of the atlas on the axis may be secondary to disruption of the transverse ligament, odontoid fractures, nonunion of odontoid fractures, as well as atraumatic causes of instability such as rheumatoid arthritis. Sublaminar wiring is the posterior instrumentation method of choice for C1–C2 instability. In this region, the area for the spinal cord is greater than in the more caudal segments of the cervical spine. This unique anatomical feature allows for the safe passage of sublaminar wires (8). An anatomical prerequisite for utilizing this method is that the posterior arch of C1 and C2 are intact.

Passage of sublaminar wires must be done with spinal cord monitoring. The neck is placed in slight flexion in the prone position. The occipitoatlanto and atlantoaxial membranes and the insertion of the ligamentum flavum along the inferior border of C3 are elevated transversely in a subperiosteal manner off their respective cervical lamina insertion sites. A sublaminar suture is passed with the aid of a vascular needle to guide passage of the wire (tied to the suture) to be utilized in the fixation. Care is taken to avoid injury to the dura mater during this process. Bone graft is then applied and stabilized by the sublaminar wires. Variations in this basic technique of sublaminar wire placement involve the manner in which bone graft is secured to complete the fusion.

Gallie describes a technique of sublaminar wire fixation at the atlantoaxial junction in which a single sublaminar wire is doubled and passed under the posterior

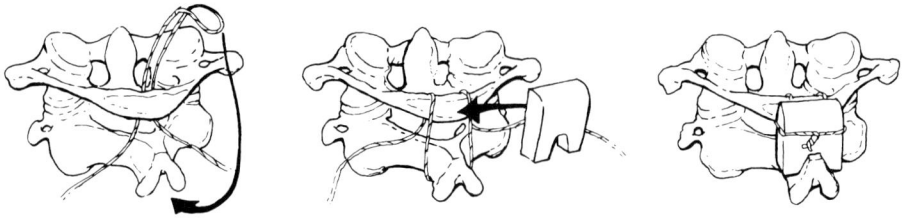

Figure 9 Gallie fusion. A sublaminar wire is passed under C1 and looped around the C2 spinous process. A corticocancellous graft is notched to fit in the C1–C2 region. The free wire ends are then tightened around the bone graft.

arch of C1 (Fig. 9). The doubled end is secured to the spinous process of C2, while the two arms of the wire are joined posteriorly over a corticocancellous bone graft to secure its placement (34,35). Brooks describes passage of two sublaminar wires at C1 and C2 that are tied individually and separately over bilateral struts of bone graft (36,37) (Fig. 10). While the Gallie method is safer because a sublaminar wire is passed only under C1 and not C2, the Brooks method provides superior torsional stability (35).

Callahan's modification of the standard Brooks technique enables utilization of "intralaminar" wires at C1 in the event of neural canal compromise at the C1 level. While the wire is passed in a sublaminar fashion at C2, drill holes are placed through the posterior arch of C1 through which the wires are passed. Struts of bone graft are then secured posteriorly in the standard Brooks fashion. This technique avoids passage of true sublaminar wires at C1 to avoid further neural canal compromise (8: 1733). Magerl advocates transarticular screws at the C1–C2 facet joint to provide additional rotational stability. The entry point is the inferior facet of the axis and 2 to 3 mm lateral to the medial border of the C2–C3 facet joint (Figs. 11,12). The direction in the sagittal plane is guided by the image intensifier. The target is the middle to upper part of the ventral arch of the atlas. The drill is guided by a micro-

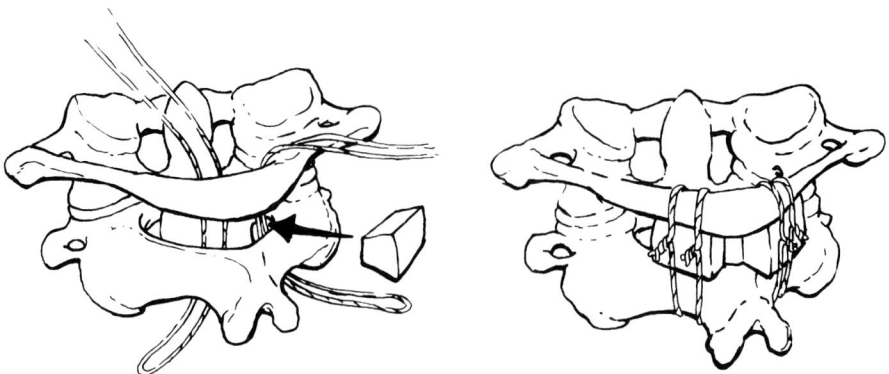

Figure 10 Brooks fusion. Two looped wires are passed sequentially beneath C2 and C1. The looped ends of the wires are then cut. Corticocancellous bone graft are fitted into the C1–C2 region. The wires are then twisted to compress the bone graft to the host bone.

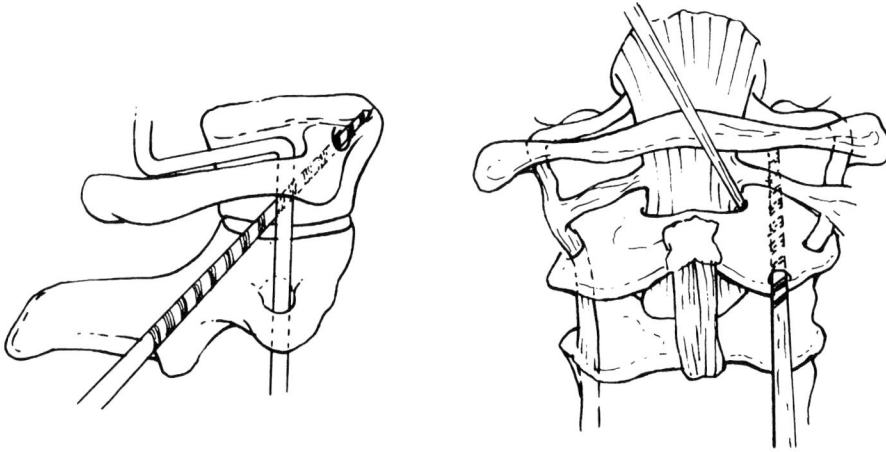

Figure 11 Magerl's technique of C1–C2 transarticular screw fixation. Prior to drilling, the medial aspect of the C2 pedicle is visualized with a micronerve hook, following subperiosteal dissection. The lateral aspect of the C2 pedicle with the foramen transversarium and vertebral artery are not dissected. The drill trajectory is guided strictly in the sagittal plane by intraoperative fluoroscopy aiming toward the upper portion of the anterior ring of the atlas.

nerve hook placed along the medial aspect of the C2 isthmus. Lateral deviation may endanger the vertebral artery. After screw insertion, coupling of the C1 and C2 vertebrae must be examined to exclude any possibility of movement. Sublaminar wiring and bone graft fusion in addition to this construct are then performed (35). While obviating the need for postoperative halo-vest immobilization, such a technique increases the risk of neurovascular injury and may be best indicated in the event of a deficient C1 posterior ring (35).

Knowledge of the anatomy of the C1–C2 region is mandatory for the successful placement of transarticular screws. The relationship of the C2 transverse foramen to the C1–C2 facet joint, lateral spinal cord, and vertebral artery is critical to determine the correct trajectory for the screw or to decide if transarticular screw placement is a viable option. With the evolution of reformatted CT images, the intricacies of the C1–C2 complex are better appreciated and allow determination of whether the patient's anatomy will support the placement of the screws.

Magerl (15) and Grob (11) et al. did not report any vertebral artery injuries in their retrospectively reviewed series of 180 patients (11). All of these patients had bilateral screw placement. Sonntag et al. (38) revealed that 18% of patients had a high riding transverse foramen on at least one side of the C2 vertebrae that would preclude the placement of transarticular screws. The fusion rate with transarticular screw placement is very high. Grob (39) reported only 1 patient out of 126 with detectable motion on flexion extension radiographs between C1 and C2. Marcotte (40) reported fusion in all 17 patients. No screw loosening or failure was reported in either group. Grob also reported an injury to the hypoglossal nerve in one patient in which the screw was too long. Nerve paresis resolved after screw removal (39).

The C1–C2 articulation accounts for 50% of axial rotation in the cervical spine. Biomechanical comparisons of the Brooks versus the Gallie technique of posterior

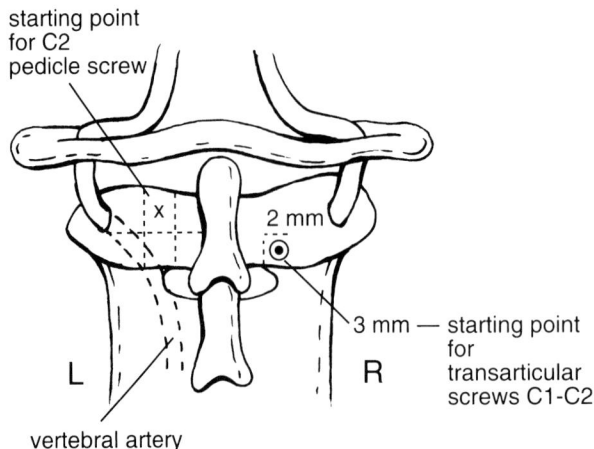

Figure 12 Starting point C2 pedicle screw versus C1–C2 transarticular screw placement. The starting point for the Magerl transarticular screw technique is approximately 2 mm lateral to the lateral aspect of the spinal canal and 3 mm superior to the C2–C3 facet joint. Note the difference in starting point for the C2 pedicle screw in the superomedial corner of the C2 lateral mass.

C1–C2 wiring demonstrate that the Brooks method is a stiffer construct in flexion, extension, and rotational stress. Comparing the Brooks, Gallie, and Magerl methods shows the biomechanical inferiority of the Gallie method compared to the others. Of the three methods, the Magerl technique is the stiffest, especially in rotational strength, but also poses the greatest potential for neurovascular complications due to the proximity of the transarticular screw to the spinal cord medially and to the vertebral artery laterally (35).

The main advantage of transarticular screw fixation is to prevent postoperative translational movements that may occur with the Gallie and Brooks techniques. It also allows early mobilization of the patient with major cervical injuries. A Gallie- or Brooks-type fusion is added when possible to the transarticular screw fixation to strengthen the stability of the construct and to optimize the bone graft to host bone interface.

IV CONCLUSION

When the need arises to operate upon an instability of the cervical spine, it is wise to tailor the operation to the particular pathoanatomy and biomechanical requirements of the situation. From the available techniques, the surgeon should select that method of instrumentation which will adequately resist the deforming forces while imparting the least technical difficulty and morbidity risk. Time-tested wiring configurations will suffice for most posterior cervical procedures. When wire or cable fixation is either inadequate or not applicable, screws may be employed to gain purchase of the vertebrae. Lateral mass screw fixation has been useful in managing some of the more complex instability patterns in recent years. Unfortunately, circumstances do arise in which the lateral masses are not suited for screw insertion. In such instances, the cervical pedicle may be a practical alternative point of fixation.

REFERENCES

1. Murphy MJ, Daniaux H, Southwick WO. Posterior cervical fusion with rigid internal fixation. OCNA 1986; 17(1):55–65.
2. White AA, Johnson RM, Panjabi MM, Southwick WO. Biomechanical analysis of clinical stability in the cervical spine. CORR 1975; 109:85.
3. Panjabi MM, White AA, Johnson RM. Cervical spine mechanics as a function of transection of components. J Biomech 1975; 8:327.
4. Haher TR, O'Brien M, Felmly WT, et al. Instantaneous axis of rotation as a function of the three columns of the spine. Spine 1992; 17(6 Suppl):149.
5. Saito T, Yamamuro T, Shikata J, Oka M, Tsutsumi S. Analysis and prevention of spinal column deformity following cervical laminectomy I. Pathogenetic analysis of postlaminectomy deformities. Spine 1991; 16(5):494.
6. Ulrich C, Woersdoerfer O, Kalff R, Claes L, Wilke HJ. Biomechanics of fixation systems to the cervical spine. Spine 1991; 16(3 Suppl):4.
7. Zdeblick TA, Bohlman HH. Cervical kyphosis and myelopathy: treatment by anterior corpectomy and strut grafting. J Bone Joint Surg 1989; 71A:170.
8. Bridwell KH, DeWald RL, eds. Textbook of Spinal Surgery, 2nd ed. Philadelphia: Lippincott-Raven, 1997.
9. Clark CR, ed. The Cervical Spine, 3rd ed. Philadelphia: Lippincott-Raven, 1998.
10. Furgeson RL, Allen BL. Biomechanical principles of spinal correction. In: Cotler JM, Cotlar HB, eds. Spinal Fusion. Berlin: Springer-Verlag, 1992.
11. Grob D, Crisco JJ, Panjabi MM, et al. Biomechanical evolution of four different posterior atlantoaxial fixation techniques. Spine 1992; 17:480–490.
12. Songer MN, Spencer DI, Meyer PR. The use of sublaminar cable to replace Luque wires. Spine 1991; 16(Suppl):418–421.
13. Rogers WA. Treatment of fracture dislocation of the cervical spine. J Bone Joint Surg 1942; 24A:245–258.
14. Roy-Camille R. Early fixation of the unstable cervical spine by posterior osteosynthesis with plates and screws. In: Cervical Spine Research Society, ed. The Cervical Spine, 2nd ed. Philadelphia: J.B. Lippincott, 1985:390–403.
15. Magerl F, Seemann PS. Stable posterior fusion of the atlas and axis by transarticular screw fixation. Kehr P, Weidman A, eds. Cervical Spine I. Berlin: Springer-Verlag, 1987.
16. Ebraheim NA, Klausner T, Xu R, Yeasting RA. Safe lateral mass screw lengths in the Roy-Camille and Magerl techniques. Spine 1998; 23(16):1739–1742.
17. Jones EL, Heller JG, Silcox DH, Hutton WC. Cervical pedicle screws versus lateral mass screws. Spine 1997; 22(9):977–982.
18. Xu R, Ebraheim NA, Klausner T, Yeasting RA. Modified Magerl technique of lateral mass screw placement in the lower cervical spine: an anatomic study. J Spine Disord 1998; 11(3):237–240.
19. Xu R, Haman SP, Ebraheim NA, Yeasting RA. The anatomic relation of lateral mass screws to the spinal nerves. Spine 1999; 19:2057–2061.
20. Roy-Camille R, Scillant G, Berteaux D, et al. Early management of spinal injuries. In: McKibbon B, ed. Recent Advances in Orthopaedics. New York: Churchill Livingstone, 1979:57–87.
21. Fehlings MG, Cooper PR, Errico TJ. Posterior plates in the management of cervical spine instability: Lone term results in 41 patients. J Neurosurg 1994; 81:341–349.
22. Anderson PA, Healey MR, Gudy MS, et al. Posterior cervical arthrodesis with AO reconstruction plates and bonegraft. Spine 1991; 16:572–579.
23. Kotani Y, Cunningham BW, Abumi K, McAfee PC. Biomechanical analysis of cervical stabilization systems. An assessment of transpedicular screw fixation in the cervical spine. Spine 1994; 19:2529–2539.

24. Kramer DL, Ludwig SC, Balderston RA, Foley KF, Vaccaro AR, Albert TJ. Placement of pedicle screws in the cervical spine. Comparative accuracy of cervical pedicle screw placement using three techniques. Orthop Trans 1997; 21:496.

25. Ludwig SC, Kramer DL, Vaccaro AR, Albert TJ. Transpedicle screw fixation of the cervical spine. CORR 1999; 359:77–88.

26. Abumi K, Itoh H, Taneichi H, Kaneda K. Transpedicular screw fixation for traumatic lesions of the middle and lower cervical spine: Description of the techniques and preliminary report. J Spinal Disorders 1994; 7:19–28.

27. Roy-Camille R. Rationale and techniques of internal fixation in trauma of the cervical spine. In: Errico T, Bauer RD, Waugh T, eds. Spinal Trauma. Philadelphia: J.B. Lippincott, 1991:163–191.

28. Abumi K, Kaneda K, Shono Y, Fujiya M. One stage posterior decompression and reconstruction of the cervical spine by using pedicle screw fixation systems. J Neurosurg 1999; 90:19–26.

29. Jovanoic MS. A comparative study of the foramen transversarium of the sixth and seventh cervical vertebrae. Surg Radiol Anat 1990; 12:167–172.

30. Albert T, Klein G, Joffe D, Vaccaro A. Use of cervicothoracic junction pedicle screws for reconstruction of complex cervical spine pathology. Spine 1998; 23:1596–1599.

31. Abumi K, Kaneda K. Pedicle screw fixation for nontraumatic lesions of the cervical spine. Spine 1997; 22:1853–1863.

32. Abumi K, Shono Y, Ito M, Taneichi H, Kotani Y, Kaneda K. Complications of pedicle screw fixation in reconstructive surgery of the cervical spine. Spine (in press, reported in AAOS at Anaheim, 1999).

33. Ludwig SC, Kowalski J, Edwards C, Heller JG. Comparative accuracy of pedicle screw placement in the cervical spine: Abumi versus image guided surgical technique. Spine (in press, presentation at NASS at Chicago, 1999).

34. Gallie WE. Fractures and dislocations of the cervical spine. Am J Surg 1939; 46:495.

35. An HS. Internal fixation of the cervical spine: current indications and techniques. JAAOS 1995; 3(4):194–206.

36. Brooks AL, Jenkins EB. Atlantoaxial arthrodesis by the wedge compression method. J Bone Joint Surg 1978; 60A:279.

37. Meyer PR. Surgery of Spine Trauma. New York: Churchill Livingstone, 1988.

38. Paramore CG, Dickman CA, Sonntag VKH. The anatomical stability of the C1–C2 complex for transarticular screw fixation. J Neurosurg 1996; 85:221–224.

39. Grob D, Jeannenet B, Achi M, et al. Atlantoaxial fusion with transarticular screw fixation. J Bone Joint Surg 1991; 73B:972–976.

40. Marcotte P, Dickman CA, Sonntag VKH, et al. Posterior atlantoaxial facet screw fixation. J Neurosurg 1993; 79:234–237.

27

Posterior Cervical Decompression Techniques

SETH M. ZEIDMAN

University of Rochester, Rochester, New York, U.S.A.

MARCO T. SILVA, PAUL T. RUBERY, and ALEXANDER R. VACCARO

Thomas Jefferson University Hospital and the Rothman Institute, Philadelphia, Pennsylvania, U.S.A.

I INTRODUCTION

Cervical decompressive procedures (i.e., laminectomy, foraminotomy) are rarely indicated in the context of acute cervical trauma (1,2). Rare exceptions are patients with depressed laminar fractures and patients with multilevel spondylosis suffering hyperextension injuries with a resultant central cord syndrome (3–5).

Laminectomy was routinely the procedure of choice for many anterior compressive lesions, but laminectomies fail to address the responsible pathology and their use was often poorly tolerated and generally unsuccessful (6–8). The classic analogy is removing the top of your shoe in an attempt to stop the pain of stepping on a rock. Furthermore, laminectomies destabilize an already unstable spine, precipitating the development of progressive kyphotic deformity, often with an associated further compromise of neural function (9,10).

A concomitant arthrodesis will stabilize the spine with either lateral mass plates or facet wiring for any traumatic spinal injury that requires a laminectomy. In the spondylotic spine with preserved lordosis, a multilevel laminectomy will often produce a significant degree of posterior spinal cord displacement. Cord displacement can produce cervical nerve root tension with consequent radiculopathy. The C5 nerve root is the most tethered of the cervical roots and the most susceptible to a tethering injury when the spinal cord displaces posteriorly. The short length of the C5 nerve root and its straight course within the canal are secondary reasons for its suscepti-

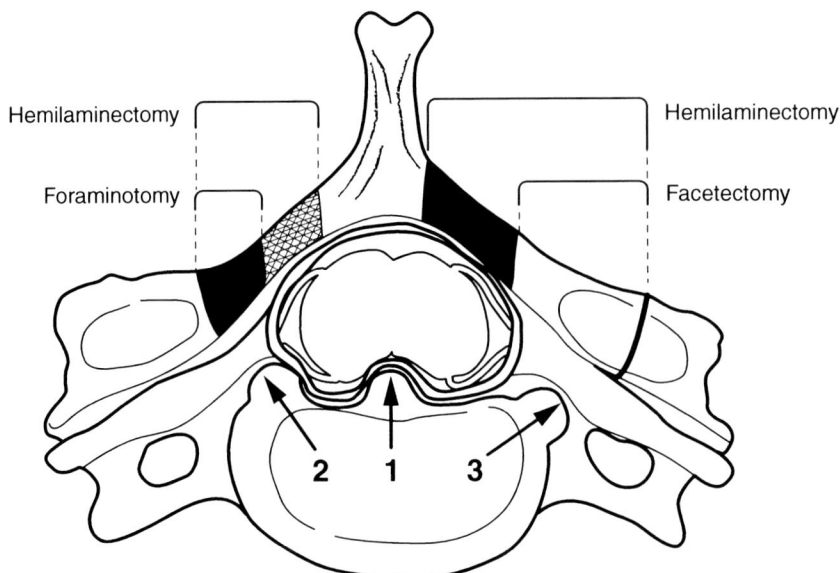

Laminectomy

Figure 1   Schematic representation of the cervical spine with nomenclature demonstrating various types of decompression(s).

bility to a tethering injury. We advise completion of a foraminotomy to minimize the potential for iatrogenic neural injury. Foraminotomy is also indicated for those patients with fractured facets and resultant nerve root injury (Fig. 1).

II   LAMINECTOMY: PROCEDURE

Patients are placed in a prone position on an operative wedge frame, a Jackson spinal table, or a turning frame with the head held firmly by Gardner-Wells tongs or halo ring traction. The neck is maintained in a neutral position without any hyperflexion or hyperextension. After placing the head in traction, a portable radiograph or fluoroscopic image should confirm alignment and exclude the possibility of over-distraction.

Once the patient is prepared for surgery, a midline skin incision is followed by subperiosteal exposure of the lamina and spinous processes up to the medial edge of the facet capsules (Fig. 2). We routinely attempt to maintain the integrity of the facet capsules until the levels of dissection are confirmed. If a posterolateral arthrodesis using lateral mass plates is anticipated, the dissection is extended to the lateral edge of the lateral masses. Using small 5-0 and 4-0 curettes, we usually strip the articular cartilage from joints that must be fused and drill out the remaining cartilaginous material to improve the probability of solid arthrodesis.

One of two methods that is used to complete laminectomies requires piecemeal removal of the spinous processes and lamina with a Leksell rongeur, followed later with Kerrison punches. This procedure is time consuming and requires placement of

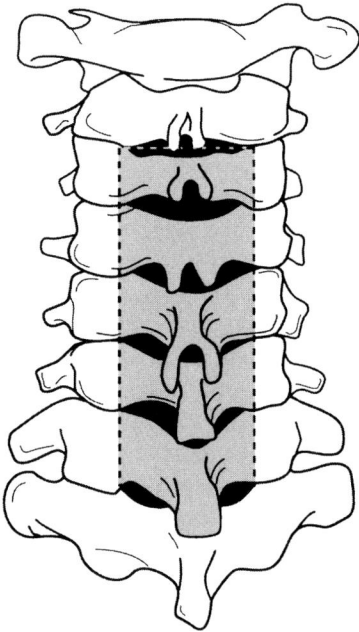

Figure 2 View of posterior cervical spine. Dotted line represents laminofacet border where trough placement is used for laminectomy.

instrument footplates below the lamina, which increases the possibility of injury to the spinal cord. In experienced hands, this is a safe and effective method that has been used for many years without injury. We prefer the second method, which consists of an en bloc resection of the laminae.

After radiographic confirmation of the operative level, the interspinous ligaments—both cranial and caudal to the levels of interest—are divided sharply with either a scalpel or scissors. Two lateral troughs are created at the medial edge of the lateral mass using a high-speed cutting burr (Fig. 3). The lateral bone can be thinned significantly using a high-speed air drill with great care to avoid entry into the canal or downward pressure upon the neural elements that are already compromised. Some surgeons prefer to use a diamond burr because of its less aggressive cutting head, but this instrument generates tremendous heat and is very slow and tedious. The use of loupe magnification and the operative headlight facilitates visualization of the operative field.

The lamina has three distinct layers that are encountered with the drill. The outer layer is cortical and rapidly penetrated, the middle layer is cancellous, red, and bleeds readily, while the innermost layer is cortical bone, white in color, and relatively avascular. We try to avoid any downward pressure and let the mechanics of the drill do the work. Most of the outer cortical layer and the middle cancellous bone are removed safely but rapidly; the inner cortical layer is thinned but not intentionally penetrated. Overaggressive drilling can result in plunging through the bone into the canal with damage to the dura and potentially the spinal cord (Fig. 4). We intermittently irrigate the operative field to decrease the heat buildup

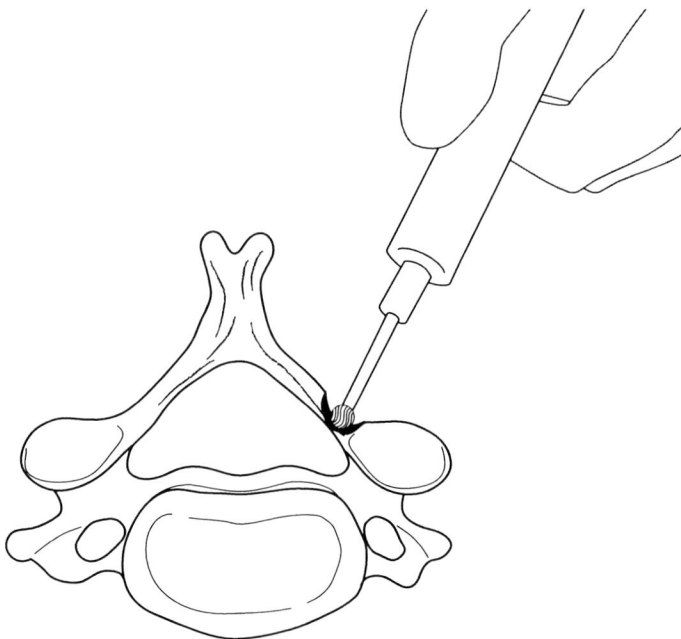

Figure 3   A 3- to 4-mm burr (airdrill) is used for trough drilling. Note the 15-degree angle.

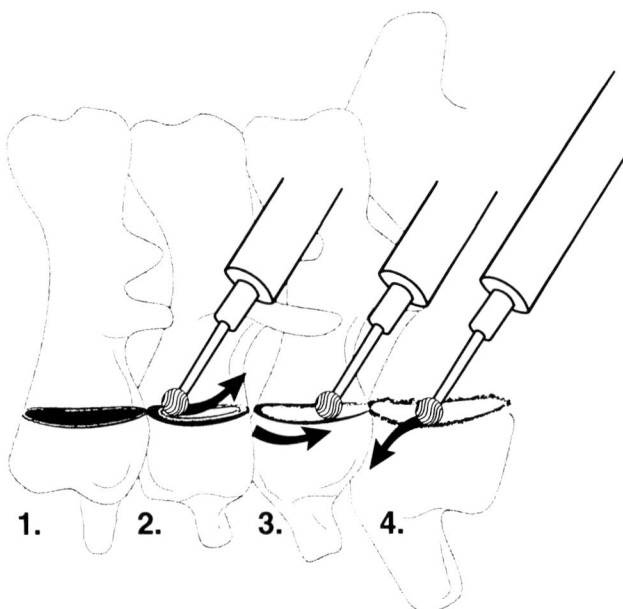

Figure 4   Technique used for drilling. Drilling is performed in a rostrocaudal direction to avoid injury or plunging into neural elements.

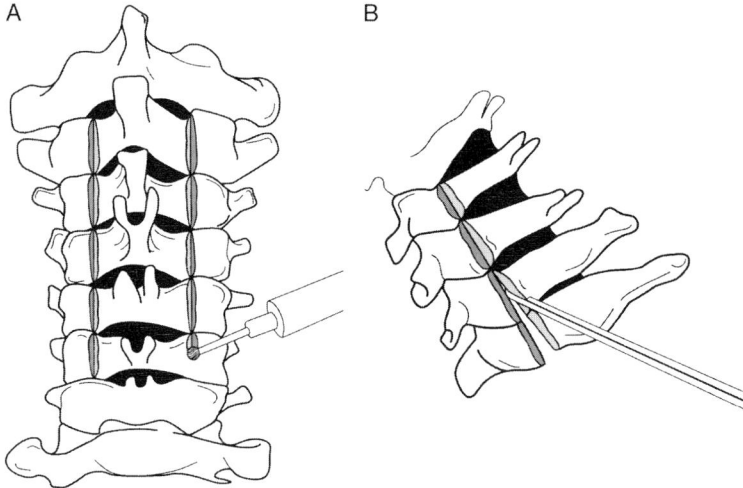

Figure 5 (A) Drilling of troughs is demonstrated. (B) A 1-mm Kerrison is used in a caudal-rostral direction to release the lamina from its facet articulation.

and thermal injury and to prevent obscuring the operative field with bone dust and blood.

Lateral trough laminectomies are then performed using the 1- or 2-mm Kerrison punch once the lateral troughs are completed and thinned. The 1- or 2-mm Kerrison completes the laminectomy and the spinous process is stabilized using an Allis, Kocher, or penetrating towel clamp. Once the channels have been completed bilaterally, each lamina can be lifted free of the spinal cord and the tethering ligamentum flavum can then be sharply divided. The laminae are teased away to unroof the canal. Any lateral compression can then be excised with the careful use of the 2-mm Kerrison punch.

Resection of the block of laminae should be carefully and precisely controlled. The lamina should be held in place without excessive tension to keep them from dipping into the spinal canal and compress the spinal cord. Once the ligamentum flavum is divided, the entire block of lamina can then be excised as a unit (Figs. 5,6). The lateral margin of the thecal sac will be visible and lateral epidural veins can be identified and coagulated as necessary using the bipolar coagulator under low power. The surgeon should avoid coagulating any of the dural surface or packing hemostatic agents into the lateral gutters when attempting to achieve hemostasis.

The presence of depressed laminar fractures may be associated with torn or entrapped dura and potentially trapped neural elements. After exposure of the margins of the lamina, the ligamentum flavum insertion is excised sharply while avoiding any downward pressure on the depressed laminar segment. Small, angled cervical curettes are useful to facilitate elevation of the depressed segment. Careful attention must be paid to any dural adherence. The remaining jagged fracture ends should be smoothed with the Kerrison rongeurs and the dura should be inspected and repaired.

(A)

(B)

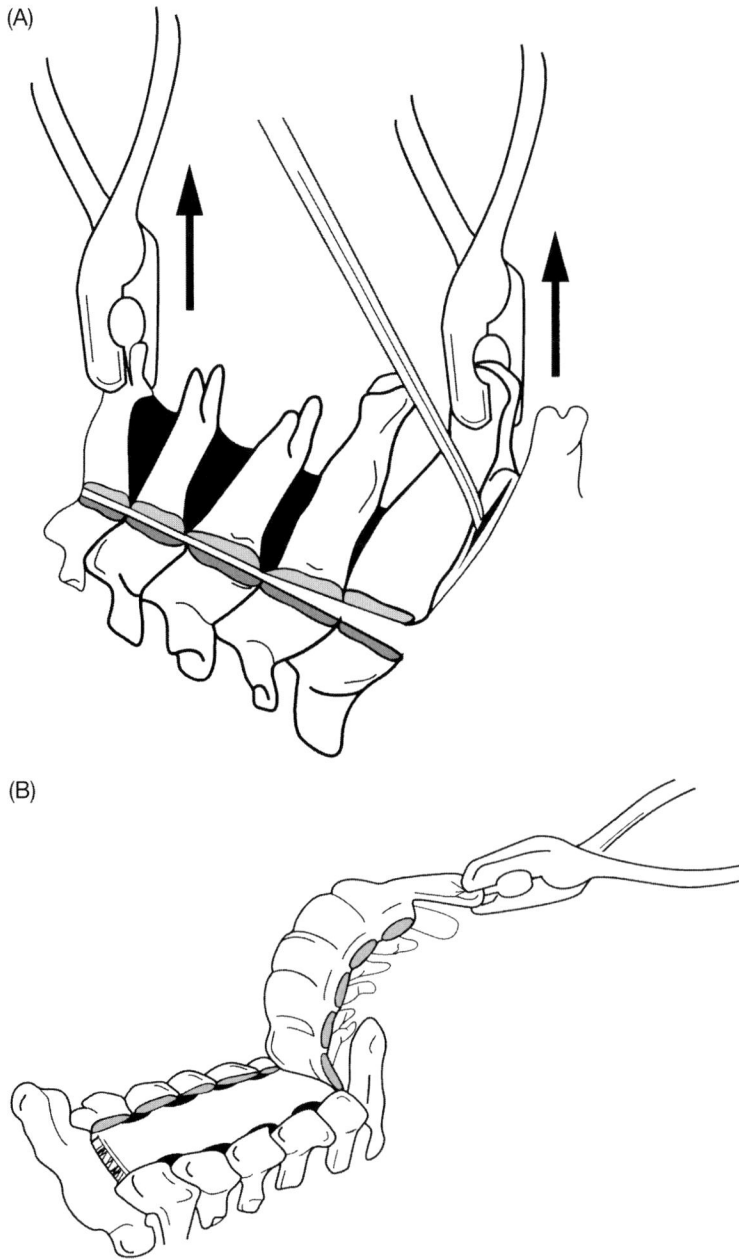

Figure 6   (A) After completion of troughs, towel clips are placed on each spinous process. The ligamentum flavum is separated at the lateral and superior/inferior borders with a 1- to 2-mm Kerrison. (B) The lamina are then removed en bloc in a caudal-rostral direction.

III FORAMINOTOMY: PROCEDURE

While mechanical studies have shown that up to 50% of the facet joints can be removed without developing instability, the possibility of instability increases in trauma cases and any decompressive foraminotomy in this setting should include an arthrodesis. The cervical neural foramen is located directly below and slightly cranial to the facet joint. If a laminectomy is unnecessary, a 1- or 2-mm Kerrison rongeur is used to create a circular laminotomy approximately 10 mm in size, which should be centered relative to the superior and inferior lamina.

We prefer a high-speed drill to carefully thin the bone of the facet joint directly overlying the nerve root. The foramen can be palpated with a fine dental probe to facilitate identification of site of decompression. Once again, the three distinct layers of bone are encountered with rapid removal of the outer cortical and middle cancellous layers and more cautious thinning of the inner cortical layer. To protect the spinal cord, drilling should be performed working from a medial to lateral direction. Continuous irrigation while drilling prevents thermal damage and renders the field clean and bloodless.

Once the inner cortical layer has been thinned sufficiently, the last layer of thinned cortical bone is chipped off with a fine 3-0 or 4-0 curette. The surgeon should use the curette with a pulling motion away from the spinal cord and the nerve root. The lateral extent of the foraminotomy is determined by passing a thin, blunt dental probe out the lateral foramen and feeling the tightness of the nerve. Proper lateral decompression requires approximately 5 mm of nerve root exposure. Cranial-to-caudal decompression should extend from pedicle to pedicle (Fig. 7).

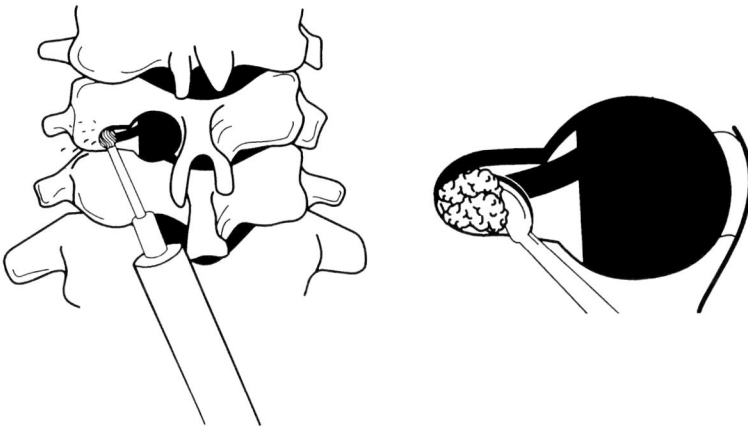

Figure 7 After exposure of the lamina and facet, the inferior aspect of the superior lamina is removed with a 1- to 2-mm Kerrison in a keyhole fashion. A 3-mm burr (airdill) is then used to drill along the foramen over the nerve. A dental or ball-dissector instrument is used to define the foramen and extent of decompression. One must define the inferior aspect of the superior pedicle and superior aspect of the inferior pedicle. The decompression is accomplished with a combination of drill, 1-mm Kerrison, and curved curette. Once the decompression is complete, the nerve may be gently retracted for removal of disk or drilling of osteophyte.

REFERENCES

1. Fehlings MG, Tator CH. An evidence-based review of decompressive surgery in acute spinal cord injury: rationale, indications, and timing based on experimental and clinical studies. J Neurosurg 1999; 91(1 Suppl):1–11.
2. Zeidman SM, Ducker TB, Raycroft J. Trends and complications in cervical spine surgery: 1989–1993. J Spinal Disord 1997; 10(6):523–526.
3. Chen TY, Lee ST, Lui TN, Wong CW, Yeh YS, Tzaan WC, Hung SY. Efficacy of surgical treatment in traumatic central cord syndrome. Surg Neurol 1997; 48(5):435–440; discussion 441.
4. Hardy RW. The posterior surgical approach to the cervical spine. Neuroimaging Clin N Am 1995; 5(3):481–490.
5. Rosenfeld JF, Vaccaro AR, Albert TJ, Klein GR, Cotler JM. The benefits of early decompression in cervical spinal cord injury. Am J Orthop 1998; 27(1):23–28.
6. McAfee PC, Bohlman HH, Ducker TB, Zeidman SM, Goldstein JA. One-stage anterior cervical decompression and posterior stabilization. A study of one hundred patients with a minimum of two years of follow-up. J Bone Joint Surg Am 1995; 77(12):1791–1800.
7. Mirza SK, Krengel WF, Chapman JR, Anderson PA, Bailey JC, Grady MS, Yuan HA. Early versus delayed surgery for acute cervical spinal cord injury. Clin Orthop 1999; (359):104–114.
8. Tator CH, Fehlings MG, Thorpe K, Taylor W. Current use and timing of spinal surgery for management of acute spinal surgery for management of acute spinal cord injury in North America: results of a retrospective multicenter study. J Neurosurg 1999; 91(1 Suppl):12–18.
9. Collins WF. Surgery in the acute treatment of spinal cord injury: a review of the past forty years. J Spinal Cord Med 1995; 18(1):3–8.
10. Waters RL, Adkins RH, Yakura JS, Sie I. Effect of surgery on motor recovery following traumatic spinal cord injury. Spinal Cord 1996; 34(4):188–192.

28

Intraoperative Neurophysiological Monitoring During Post-Traumatic Spine Surgery

DANIEL M. SCHWARTZ

Surgical Monitoring Associates, Bala Cynwyd, Pennsylvania, U.S.A.

Neurological deficit is the most feared complication of spine surgery. Although infrequent in the general spine surgery population, there is significant opportunity for neurological insult in patients undergoing corrective spine surgery for post-traumatic injury. Neurological injury is not simply a by-product of the surgery itself; rather, it can occur presurgically during transfer of the patient to the operating room table, neck extension for airway management during intubation or patient positioning for adequate operative exposure. From a surgical perspective, appropriate preoperative preparation, careful surgical planning, surgical execution, and constant surgical vigilance can minimize risk for neurological complications. An additional increasingly important means of injury prevention is continuous neurophysiological monitoring of spinal cord and spinal nerve root function. Development of better-defined methods for assessing spinal cord motor and nerve root integrity essentially in real time makes intraoperative neurophysiological monitoring (IONM) a particularly attractive means of reducing the prevalence of new or additional neurological impairment in this select patient population. It behooves the spine surgeon, therefore, to have at least basic understanding of neuromonitoring methodology and how best to apply the information presented in order to facilitate prompt reversal of impending neurological injury.

I WHEN SHOULD MONITORING COMMENCE?

The post-traumatic spine-injured patient is particularly challenging for all involved, including the neurophysiologist. For patients with spinal instability, spinal cord compression injury from displaced vertebral subluxation/dislocation or migrating bone or disk fragments can occur following neck extension for intubation, placement of halo fixation, and/or positioning. Likewise, excessive counter traction of adhesive tape applied to the shoulder(s) and fastened to the foot of the operating table can result in brachial plexus stretch injury. Consequently, IOMN must begin immediately following anesthesia induction before neck extension for asleep endotrachial intubation. In the case of fiberoptic awake intubation, IONM should begin immediately after anesthesia induction, but only after a clinical neurological examination verifies intact motor function.

The strategy for monitoring intubation and positioning should include recording of both upper and lower extremity somatosensory (SSEP) and transcranial electrical motor-evoked potentials (TcMEP), respectively. Transcranial electrical motor-evoked potentials using multipulse electrical stimulation (Digitimer Ltd, Hertfordshire, UK) are recorded over distal hand, leg, and foot muscles for all cervical and thoracic spine surgeries. In patients who have significant preexisting spinal cord injury, it is not uncommon for both SSEPs and TcMEPs from hand and lower extremity muscles to be absent. Because these patients typically have at least intact deltoid or bicep function, we have found it possible to monitor TcMEPs from these muscle groups, thereby facilitating preservation of this small, but definite, level of residual spinal cord function.

Particular care is given to TcMEPs in the presence of an unstable cervical spine to ensure that there is no forceful head movement upon initiating the stimulating voltage across the cortex. Partial neuromuscular blockade (i.e., 2/4 twitches) usually will eliminate head "bucking." It is also prudent practice to begin at a low-voltage level and increase that level gradually until a response is recorded. If the risk of additional spinal cord injury is too great with any sudden head movement, it is best to monitor intubation only with bilateral or interleaving upper extremity somatosensory-evoked potentials. Once the head is securely fixed in a head-holder, then TcMEP monitoring can be safely accomplished for patient positioning. These same restrictions do not apply, of course, for thoracic spine instability since whole-body movement does not typically occur with controlled cortical stimulation.

Since TcMEPs are recorded over muscle, it is imperative that the neuromuscular junction not be entirely blocked. It is preferable for neurophysiologists to monitor the level of neuromuscular blockade by recording a nerve conduction response series to "train of four" electrical pulses. In patients who have no worse than minor motor weakness, TcMEPs usually can be recorded in the presence of 1 to 2 twitches. It is very important that the level of neuromuscular block remain stable from the time of intubation through positioning so as not to cause significant TcMEP amplitude variability. If more partial paralysis is needed, it is best to wait until after final positioning. Such stability in level of relaxant should also resume after exposure and during the "high-risk" segments of the procedure. In cases with more clinically obvious motor weakness, almost any dose of paralytic agent will ablate a motor-evoked potential, and thus it is best to avoid any blocking of the neuromuscular junction.

Once the intubation is completed and pre- versus postintubation upper extremity sensory and/or transcranial motor-evoked potentials show no significant change, then prepositioning lower extremity SSEPs should be recorded. Immediately following patient positioning, recording of all sensory and motor responses should be repeated and continued until final positioning of the head and torso.

Time-locked the TcMEP amplitude changes $\geq$50% occurring alone, or coupled with like amplitude degradation in SSEPs after turning the patient from supine to prone, represent the neurophysiological signature of spinal cord injury "in-the-making" and demand immediate intervention, as illustrated in Figure 1. Immediately upon turning this patient prone, there was complete loss of the right cortical (left ulnar nerve) SSEP and the left hand and foot muscle TcMEP. Because of the rapidity and magnitude of these changes, the patient was re-turned supine with complete restoration of sensory and motor response amplitude within about 3 min. Regardless of whether the neurophysiological change is due to cord compression or vascular insult, the patient should be re-turned supine and reevaluation of TcMEPs with intermittent SSEP testing should be conducted over the next 20 min. If there are no signs of improvement within 15 min after raising MAP to at least 90 mmHg, then a spinal cord injury protocol of methylprednisolone should be initiated. If improvement in TcMEP amplitude of at least 50% is not noted, then we recommend that surgery be canceled and rescheduled for a second attempt on another day allowing at least a 48-h recovery period. If, on the other hand, TcMEP amplitude shows recovery, then positioning can recommence at a very deliberate rate with continuous IONM to ensure stable motor function while maintaining an elevated mean arterial blood pressure.

Ulnar nerve SSEPs are particularly sensitive to impending brachial plexopathy and should be rerecorded immediately after application of counter traction of the shoulder(s) with adhesive tape for anterior positioning or after the patient is turned prone and arms outstretched on arm boards for posterior approaches (1). If the unilateral ulnar nerve SSEP is noted to change $\geq$30%, then the tape should be released or axilla/shoulders adjusted.

While it is true that IONM during intubation and positioning may delay incision time by 5 to 10 min, the benefits of this small time cost are far too great to proceed without it. We have had numerous cases over the years that identified impending brachial plexus or spinal cord injury during positioning that were easily reversed with rapid intervention. Had such monitoring not been initiated until after positioning, then either reduced amplitude or completely absent responses would have been used to define baseline without ever revealing the presence of new injury. Assuming no further intraoperative events, evidence of neurological deficit observed postoperatively would be attributed to some type of surgical insult and IONM would be held responsible for being insensitive to injury detection. Similarly, it is entirely possible that postpositioning baseline IONM shows complete absence of any monitorable responses simply because complete injury occurred during the unmonitored positioning. In this case, the surgeon would be falsely misled into thinking that IONM was precluded when, in fact, a new, undetected insult had occurred. Again, when the patient emerges from anesthesia and the deficit is revealed, the surgeon would attribute cause inappropriately to a surgical maneuver. Obviously, the medical–legal implications of these two scenarios are significant.

II NEUROPHYSIOLOGICAL MONITORING DURING SURGERY

IONM is a dynamic process and clinically significant changes can occur almost any time during the operative procedure. Table 1 presents a partial list of surgical events

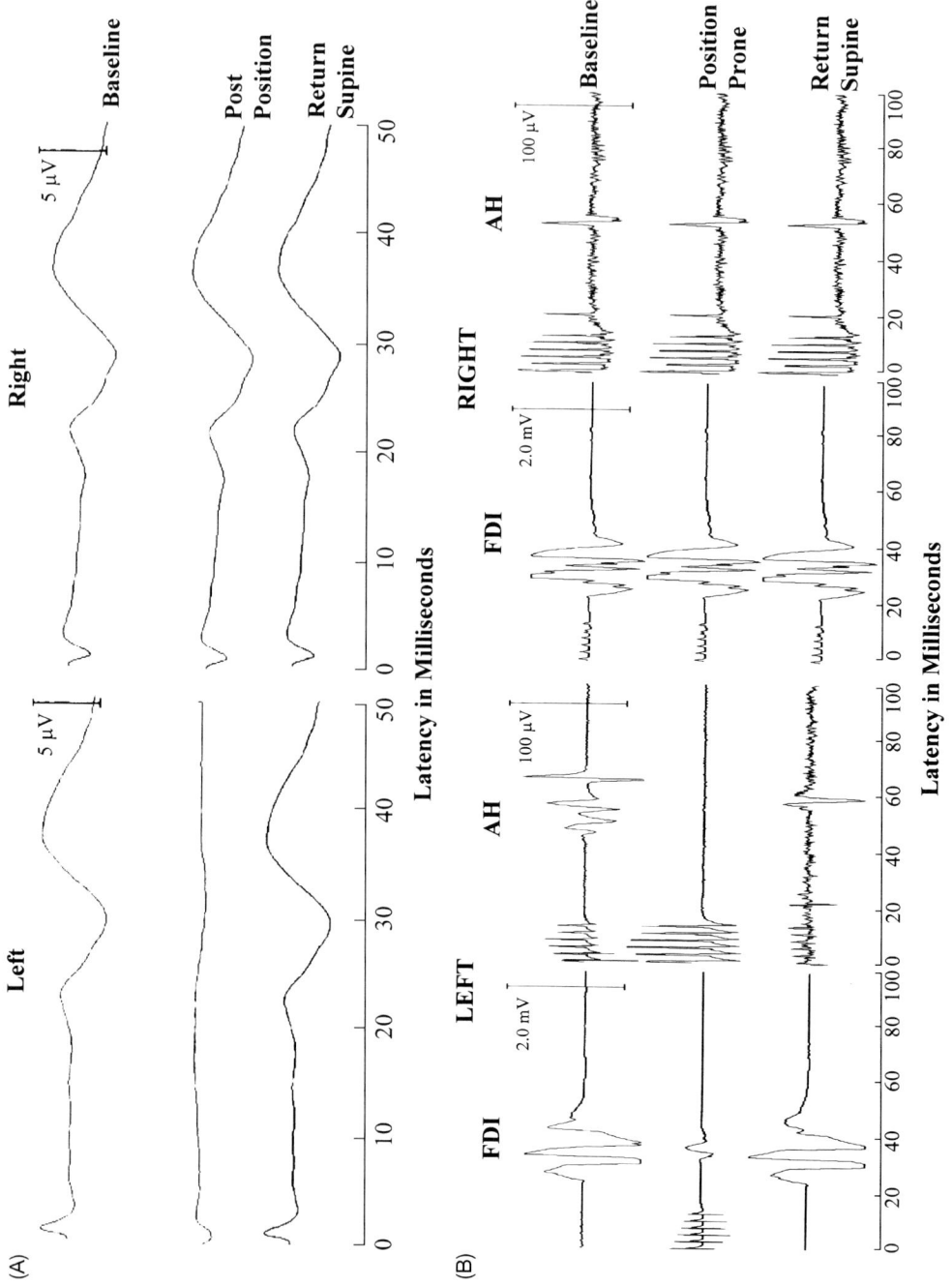

Figure 1 Exemplary IONM results illustrating unilateral loss of ulnar nerve cortical somatosensory- and transcranial motor-evoked potentials after positioning a patient prone.

Table 1 Summary of Surgical Events or Maneuvers That Can Cause Neurophysiological Change

Cause of injury	SSEP	TcMEP	EMG
Excess cervical weight	✓	✓	
Vertebral body distraction	✓	✓	
Cervical decompression		✓	✓
Foraminotomy		✓	✓
Root traction		✓	✓
Pass sublaminar wire/cable	✓	✓	
Tighten wires/cables	✓	✓	✓
Vertebral artery injury	✓		
Deeply impacted bone graft	✓	✓	
Surgical instrument contusion	✓	✓	✓
Malpositioned cervical screw			✓
Migrating bone or disk fragment	✓	✓	
RLN traction			✓
Dural patty compression	✓	✓	
Hook shoe encroachment	✓	✓	
Rod distraction/derotation	✓	✓	✓
Lumbar pedicle cortex fracture			✓
Thecal sac retraction		✓	✓
Overdistraction–fusion cage		✓	✓
Lumbar root retraction			✓

that can lead to neurophysiological alert along with the specific modality (modalities) that best detect neural injury. A multimodality approach to IONM is necessary to assess functional integrity of spinal cord, nerve root, brachial plexus, and, at times, the recurrent laryngeal nerve (2,3).

Technological advances in neurophysiological instrumentation permit the neurophysiologist to monitor SSEPs, TcMEPs, and both spontaneous and stimulated electromyography (EMG) in a single test protocol all displayed simultaneously. Limited IONM based on recording SSEPs alone is inadequate today. Not only does the SSEP represent an indirect measure of motor tract integrity, but it is effectively insensitive to root traction injury as illustrated in Figure 2. Observe that while cortical SSEPs remained entirely stable and unchanged throughout the C4/5 decompression, sustained spontaneous EMG activity was detected over the left deltoid muscle recording site, thereby prompting surgical alert of excessive C5 nerve root traction. Parenthetically, there was a concomitant TcMEP amplitude loss also over the left deltoid muscle supporting altered left C5 root function. Had upper extremity mixednerve SSEPs alone been monitored, this root injury would have gone unrecognized. Furthermore, there would not have been any timely intervention.

For anterior cervical procedures, we rely heavily on TcMEPs for injury detection, prior to and following the application of weight to achieve vertebral body distraction, following placement of vertebral body distracters, impaction of bone graft and plate fixation, as well as during other salient elements of the operation. Figure 3 is an example of TcMEP identification of impending spinal cord injury seemingly

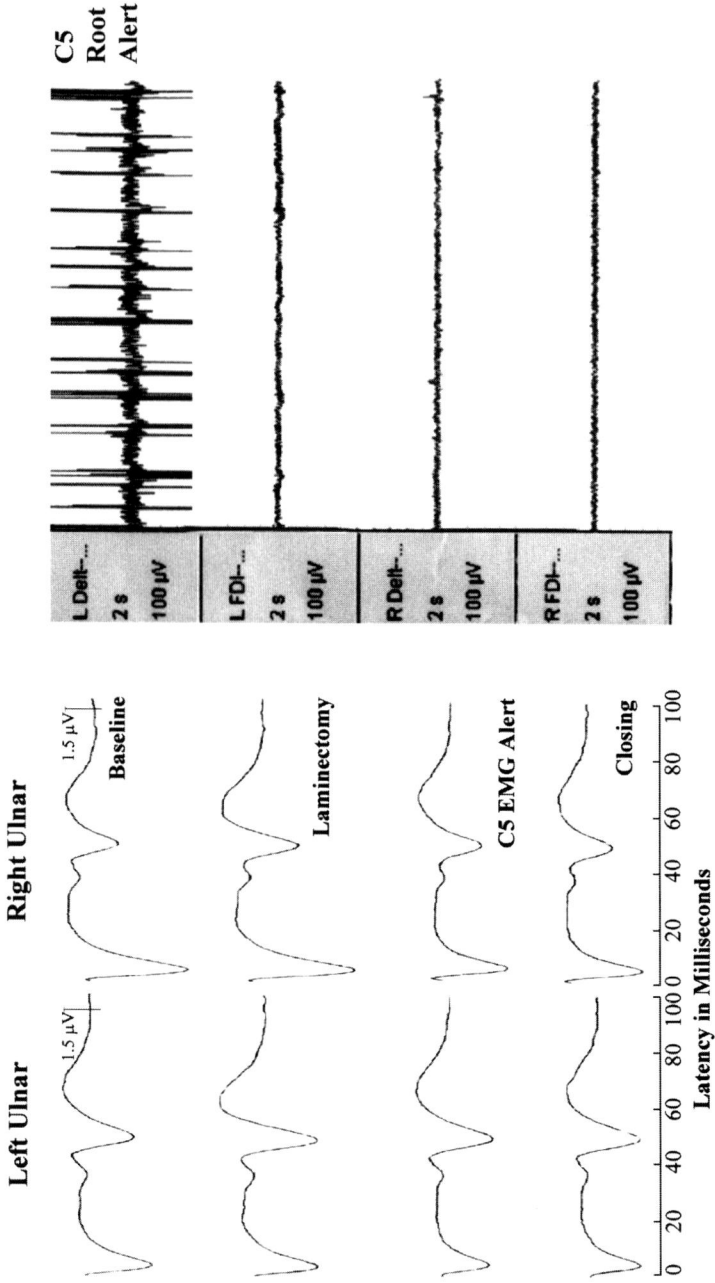

Figure 2 Detection of excessive C5 nerve root traction by sustained spontaneous EMG activity from left deltoid muscle. Note the insensitivity of ulnar nerve cortical and subcortical SSEPs toward root injury detection.

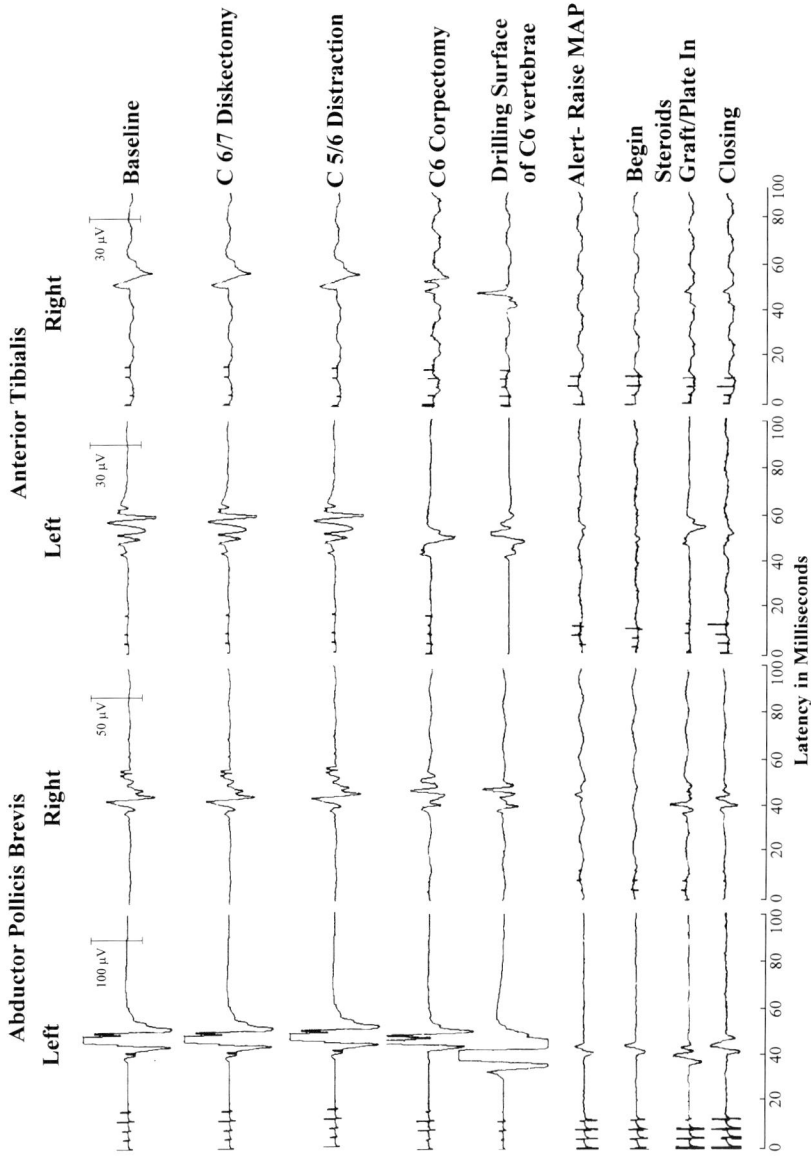

Figure 3 TcMEP identification of spinal cord injury attributed to migration of a bony fragment while drilling the body of C6.

due to migration of a dislocated bone fragment while drilling the surface of the C6 body during corpectomy. Clearly, the complete bilateral loss of upper and lower motor-evoked potentials represented the harbinger of neurological disaster. Consistent with our intervention protocol, a spinal cord injury dose of methylprednisolone was administered immediately and mean arterial blood pressure was raised to ≥90 mmHg. Because of the obvious spinal instability, the decision was made to graft, plate, and then close rapidly without delay. By the end of closing, there appeared the beginning of functional TcMEP return. This was a welcomed prognostic indicator for at least partial recovery. Expectedly, the patient awakened with motor deficit but continued to gain functional improvement over the postoperative course.

Spinal cord injury during thoracic spine surgery often occurs as a result of mechanical or ischemic insult. Ischemic injury usually results from stretching of spinal cord vascular supplies following distraction and is a primary factor leading to spinal cord shock. Mechanical injury can result from direct spinal cord contusion or concussion during placement or adjustment of instrumentation. Passing sublaminar wires or cables are particularly problematic because they can inadvertently be pushed forward against the cord. Likewise, wire/cable overtightening can also lead to "lifting" and, therefore, stretching of the cord as depicted in Figure 4. Note that there was complete bilateral loss of TcMEPs from leg muscles and 50% loss of the bilateral SSEP. Moreover, the SSEPs showed more rapid amplitude return following higher perfusion levels and steroid therapy. Conversely, the TcMEPs took considerably longer to show reemergence of at least a left leg response, which led to the decision to remove all hardware and to close. It is possible that had SSEPs alone been monitored, surgery may have continued based on the response amplitude improvement. This patient also awakened with transient lower extremity weakness, with complete recovery within 48 hs.

An infrequent but possible complication of lumbosacral spine surgery and associated instrumentation is injury to spinal nerve roots, which result in postoperative sensory and/or motor deficits. IONM is applicable to placement of interbody fusion cages or femoral rings, strut graft, and internal fixation devices. For L1–L2 burst fractures, it is necessary to monitor both spinal cord and spinal nerve root function. For surgery below L2, the best mode of IONM is EMG with augmentation by TcMEPs. SSEPs are essentially insensitive to most nerve root injuries and therefore are of little or no value, particularly if used as the sole monitoring modality.

Spontaneous electromyography is used to minimize neural trauma to lumbosacral spinal nerve roots during decompression, pedicle screw insertion, removal of bony fragments, tumor resection, distraction, or traction. Abrupt traction of a spinal nerve root or mechanical contact by a surgical instrument will elicit intermittent burst or sustained train activity, respectively. In general, elicitation of brief synchronized burst activity is not considered to indicate an injury-related potential. On the other hand, sustained neural "trains" that mimic motorboat, popcorn, or dive bomber sounds are warnings of potential nerve root injury. At this time all surgical maneuvers accounting for this response should be discontinued.

Improper trajectory of a pedicle screw for lumbosacral fixation can result in a medial breach of the pedicle cortex and possible spinal nerve root injury. The efficacy of applying an electrical current to the head or shaft of a pedicle screw and recording a compound muscle action potential over innervated muscle is now well established and need not be reviewed again (2–6). The underlying premise is that if the screw

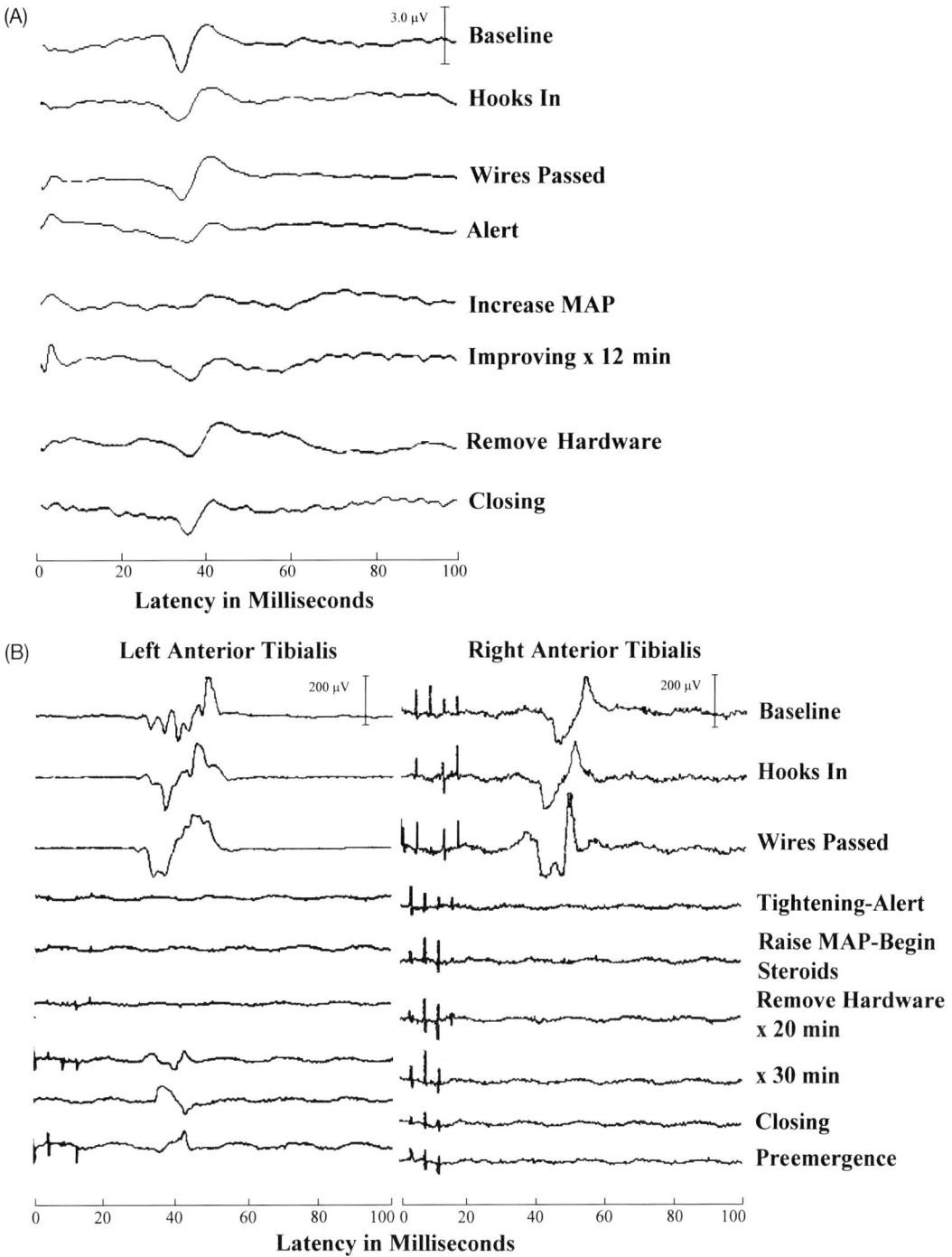

Figure 4 Neurophysiological evidence of spinal cord stretch injury caused by over-tightening of sublaminar wires.

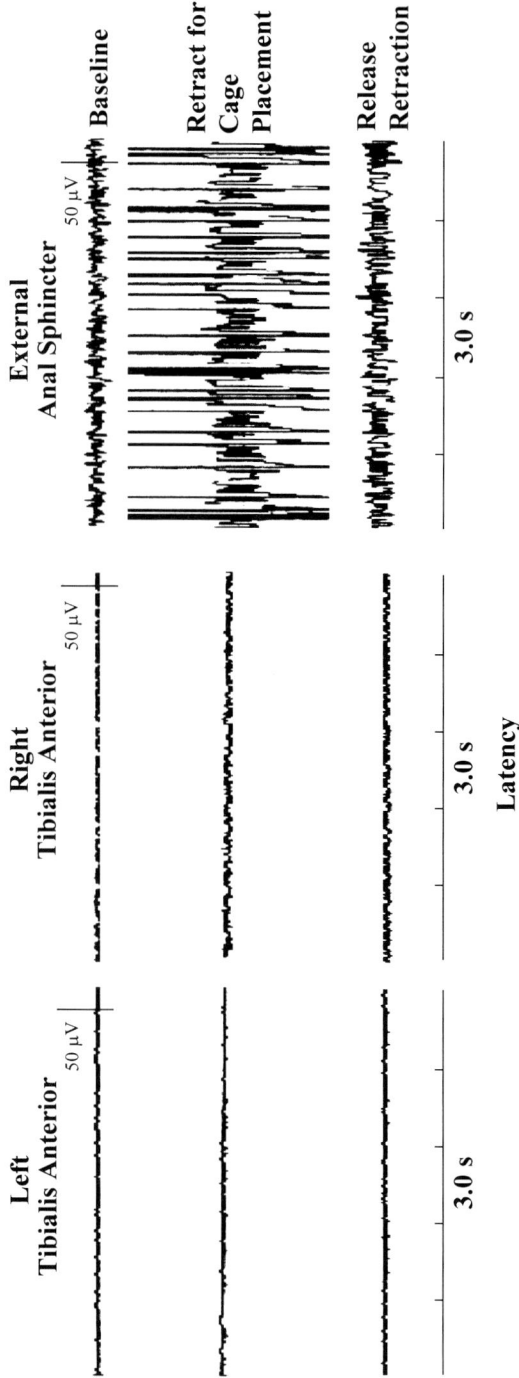

Figure 5 Example of excessive sustained spontaneous EMG activity signifying impending low sacral nerve root injury during retraction for fusion cage placement.

inadvertently perforates the pedicular cortex, the resistance of the formerly intact bone would be significantly lowered from normal. Since current follows the path of least resistance, it would flow through the medial breach to the nerve root. The current then would provoke ion depolarization in the adjacent nerve root resulting in a compound muscle action potential from a muscle innervated by that specific nerve root.

Spontaneous EMG neuromonitoring is also warranted whenever a fusion cage is used because of the high potential for nerve root or thecal sac retraction as represented in Figure 5. Observe the excessive "sustained EMG train" during distraction for cage placement. Following release, the train activity subsided and returned to a "quiet" background.

III CONCLUSIONS

Intraoperative neurophysiological monitoring has proven its efficacy over the past decade when performed by experienced neurophysiologists. It plays a particularly important role for monitoring the spinal cord during intubation, positioning, and halo or weight application prior to surgery. As such, IONM should be considered an integral adjunct to the surgical management of the spine-injured patient. The literature and textbooks are now replete with publications and book chapters illustrating the efficacy of IONM. To ignore its value as a safeguard against new or additional neurological deficit, particularly in light of the increased risk associated with post-traumatic spine injury, would not be prudent. While it certainly should not be the spine surgeon's responsibility to interpret neurophysiological data, he or she should develop a working appreciation of the neurophysiological armamentarium available, as well as how best to utilize the information disseminated. The time has come for spine surgeons to make greater demands of monitoring personnel to utilize all of the modalities available to monitor neural elements at risk for injury in this specialized population.

REFERENCES

1. Schwartz DM, Drummond DS, Hahn M, et al. Prevention of positional brachial plexopathy during surgical correction of scoliosis. J Spinal Disord 2000; 13:178–182.
2. Schwartz DM, Sestokas AK, Turner LA, et al. Neurophysiological identification of Iatrogenic neural injury during complex spine surgery. Semin Spine Surg 1998; 10:242–251.
3. Schwartz DM, Wierzbowski LR, Fan DF, Sestokis AK. Intraoperative neurophysiological monitoring during spine surgery. In: Vaccaro A, ed. Spine Surgery. New York: Thieme, 1999.
4. Schwartz DM, Sestokas AK, Wierzbowski LR. Intraoperative neurophysiological monitoring during surgery for spinal instability. Semin Spine Surg 1996; 8:3182–3331.
5. Schwartz DM, Drummond DS, Schwartz JA, et al. Neurophysiological monitoring during scoliosis surgery: A multimodality approach. Semin Spine Surg 1997; 9:97–111.
6. Toleikis JR, Skelly JP, Carlvin, AO, Toleikis SC, et al. The usefulness of electrical stimulation for assessing pedicle screw placement. J Spinal Disord 2000; 13:283–289.

29

Classification of Thoracic and Lumbar Fractures

DANTE G. MARCHESI

McGill University, Montreal, Quebec, Canada

The management of a patient with a spinal fracture—from the scene of the accident to definitive treatment—is dependent on several variables, one of which is a thorough understanding of the fracture pattern and its degree of stability. This is accomplished by an appropriate clinical and radiological evaluation of the patient.

A fracture classification should not be seen only as a complicated, tedious, and useless exercise to identify injuries with a specific name or code. It should help us to better analyze the fracture, identify its severity, and give guidelines for its management and prognosis. A unanimously accepted classification would also have a scientific value to appreciate and report results. Attempts to classify thoracolumbar fractures have been proposed since the beginning of this century, based on clinical (mainly neurological) criteria and mechanism of injury, or through progressive development of new radiological methods based on morphological criteria (1–11) In 1949, Nicoll described two basic groups of injuries, stable and unstable fractures, and provided us with the first valid classification (10). Holdsworth recognized the importance of the injury mechanism and proposed to classify the various injury patterns into five categories (7,12). He further identified the significance of the posterior ligament complex in the stability of the spine. Whitesides also defined a mechanistic classification based on a two-column concept with the vertebral bodies and the disks forming the pressure-resistant anterior column and the posterior vertebral elements and ligaments forming the tensile-resistant posterior column (13). Louis introduced a morphological classification with a three-column concept consisting of the vertebral bodies and the two rows of the articular processes (14). Concern regarding the relationship of the spinal injury with the neural structures was expressed by Roy-Camille and Denis who described a second, three-column classification

(1,2,9,15,16). This newer classification introduced the concept of the third column which is represented by the structures that must be torn in addition to the posterior ligament complex in order to create acute instability. Each of these classifications has added to a better understanding of spinal injuries; however, none can be considered all-encompassing with unanimous consensus.

More recently, Magerl and coworkers tried to resolve this situation by proposing a comprehensive classification primarily based upon the pathomorphological criteria of the injuries (17). Using easily recognizable radiological criteria, three main categories, or "types," have been identified as having a typical, fundamental injury pattern—common denominators of the various types of injury (18). This pattern also reflects the effect of the three main forces acting on the spine, as described by White and Panjabi. Compressive forces cause compression and burst fractures (type A); tensile forces produce transverse disruption injuries (type B); and axial torque creates rotational injuries (type C). Morphological criteria are used to further classify each main type into distinct "groups" and eventually "subgroups" to provide the most accurate description of almost any spinal injury. The classification is hierarchically organized according to progressive severity and instability (19).

I TYPE A: VERTEBRAL BODY COMPRESSION

Vertebral body compression (Table 1) includes injuries caused by axial compression with or without flexion (Fig. 1). The vertebral body is almost exclusively affected, with loss of height. The posterior elements either are not, or are only insignificantly, injured, and there is no translation in the sagittal plane. Neurological deficits are extremely rare.

A Group A1: Impaction Fractures

These are the less severe and the more stable spinal fractures. Minor injuries of an endplate (A1.1—endplate impaction), more severe compression injuries with angu-

Table 1 Type A Injuries: Groups and Subgroups

Type A   Vertebral Body Compression
A1   Impaction fractures
A1.1   Endplate impaction
A1.2   Wedge impaction fracture
A1.3   Vertebral body collapse
A2   Split fractures
A2.1   Sagittal split fracture
A2.2   Coronal split fracture
A2.3   Pincer fracture
A3   Burst fractures
A3.1   Incomplete burst fracture
A3.2   Burst-split fracture
A3.3   Complete burst fracture

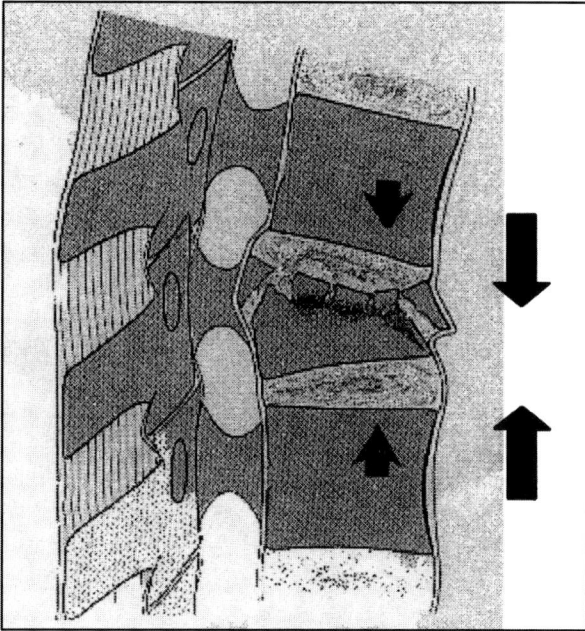

Figure 1 Type A injuries are caused by axial compression with or without flexion.

lation over 5 degrees (A1.2—wedge impaction fracture) or complete vertebral body collapse as observed in osteoporotic bone (A1.3—vertebral body collapse) are included in this group. Common characteristics of these injuries are the intact posterior elements, intact posterior vertebral body wall, and no violation of the spinal canal (Fig. 2).

Osteoporotic fractures may be more severe with pronounced collapse of the vertebral body and of the posterior wall (fish vertebra). In these cases, extruded bone fragments are found in the spinal canal and these injuries show characteristics of burst fractures (A3).

B   Group A2: Split Fractures

The vertebral body can be split in the coronal (A2.1) or the sagittal (A2.2) plane with a variable degree of displacement of the main fragments (Fig. 3). When the main fragments are significantly displaced (A2.3), the gap is filled with disk material that may result in higher incidence of fracture nonunion (also called Pincer fracture). In this group of injuries, the posterior elements are not affected and neurological deficits are uncommon.

C   Group A3: Burst Fractures

The vertebral body is partially or completely comminuted and fragments of the posterior wall are retropulsed into the spinal canal, occasionally causing neural injuries. A minor vertical split through the posterior arch may also be found in these

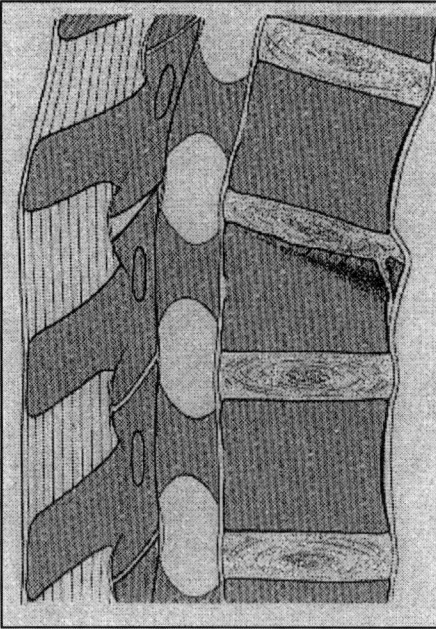

Figure 2 Impaction fractures present with intact posterior elements, intact posterior wall, and no violation of the spinal canal as in this type A1.2 injury.

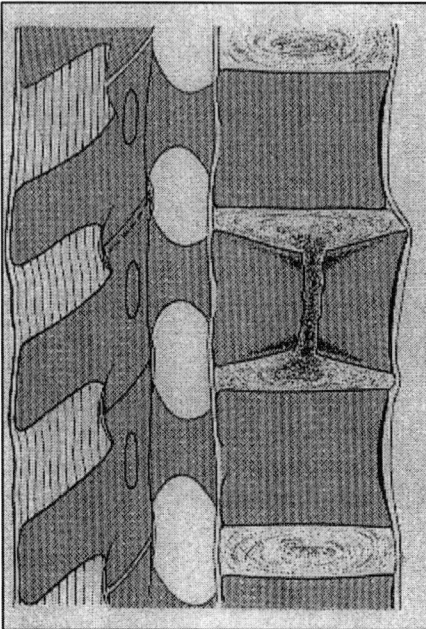

Figure 3 Coronal split fracture (A2.2).

injuries; however, its contribution to instability is negligible because the posterior ligamentous complex is intact. Flexion and compression applied to these fractures may result in an additional loss of vertebral body height and spinal canal encroachment with risk of neurological damage.

In incomplete burst fractures (A3.1) only the upper or the lower half of the vertebral body presents with a burst component, while the other half of the vertebra remains intact (Fig. 4). In burst–split fractures (A3.2), one-half of the vertebra, most often the upper part, has a burst component whereas the other half is split sagittally (Fig. 5). In complete burst fractures (A3.3), the entire vertebral body is comminuted. The spinal canal is often significantly narrowed by posterior wall fragments and the frequency of neurological injuries is higher than in incomplete and burst–split fractures (Fig. 6).

D   Common Clinical and Radiological Signs of Type A Injuries

Type A injuries may produce only moderate pain, even in the standing position, or they may be very painful, as in cases of severe burst fractures. Visible gibbus deformity due to marked wedging of the vertebral body can be observed. No posterior swelling or subcutaneous hematoma is present due to the absence of relevant injuries of the posterior elements.

Common radiological findings include widening and loss of vertebral body height, local kyphotic deformity, shortening of the posterior wall, and increase in the interpedicle distance. The distance between spinous processes should not (or only

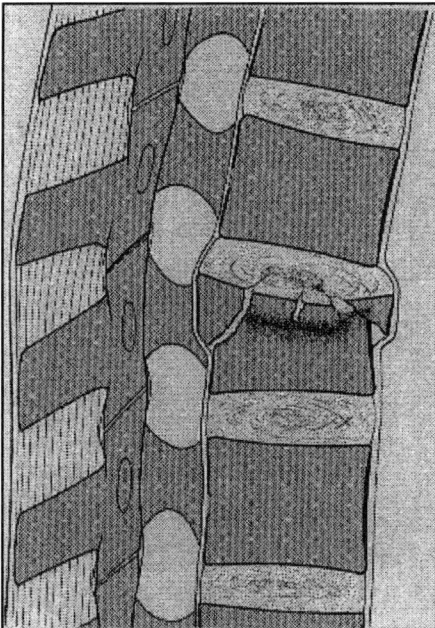

Figure 4   Superior incomplete burst fracture (A3.1).

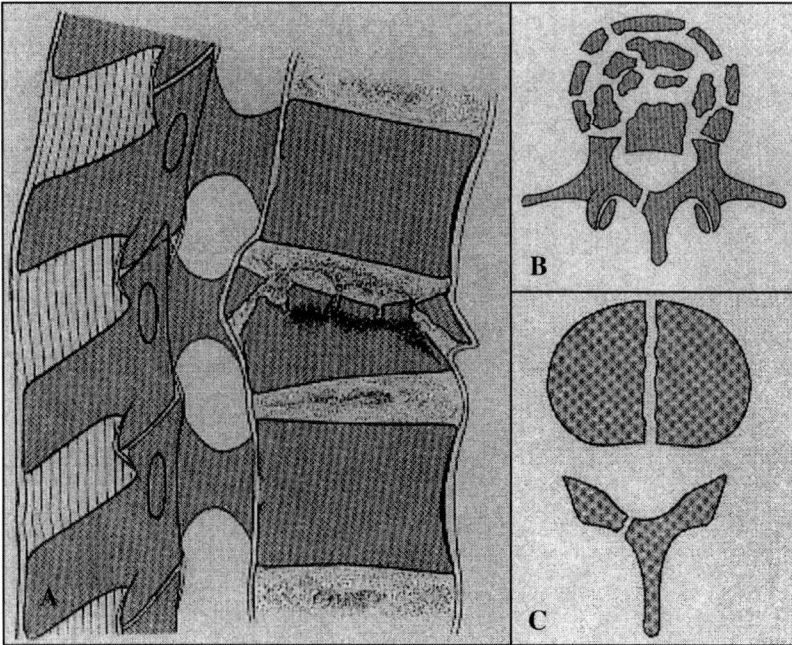

Figure 5   (A) Lateral view of a burst-split fracture type A3.2. (B, C) CT scan of the upper and lower part of the vertebral body.

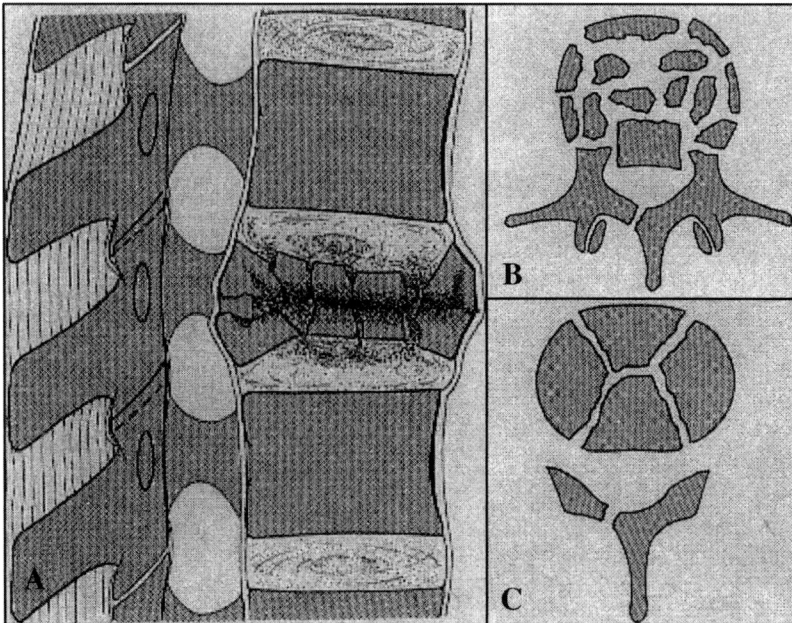

Figure 6   (A) Lateral view of a complete burst fracture type A3.3. (B, C) CT scan of the upper and lower part of the vertebral body.

minimally) increase, even in kyphotic injuries. Displaced fragments into the spinal canal are better visualized on CT or MRI.

II TYPE B: ANTERIOR AND POSTERIOR ELEMENT INJURIES WITH DISTRACTION

Fractures presented with injuries of both anterior and posterior structures of the spine result in transverse disruptions with elongation of the distance between the posterior or anterior vertebral elements (Table 2). They can result from a flexion distraction mechanism initiating posterior elongation (groups B1 and B2), or from hyperextension causing anterior elongation (B3) (Fig. 7).

Type B injuries are diagnosed by the presence of a posterior injury but are further subdivided by the description of the anterior lesion going through the disk or involving the vertebral body, as in type A fractures. Translation or dislocation in the sagittal direction may be present, and, if not seen on radiographs, the potential for sagittal translation should always be suspected. The degree of instability ranges from partial to complete and the rate of neurological deficits is significantly higher than in type A injuries.

A Group B1: Posterior Disruption Predominantly Ligamentous

Common findings are the disruption of the posterior ligamentous complex with bilateral subluxation, dislocation, or facet joint fractures. The posterior lesion is associated with either a transverse disk disruption (B1.1) (Fig. 8) or a fracture of the vertebral body (B1.2) (Fig. 9). Further subdivision is based upon the degree of dislocation and the morphology of the vertebral body fracture as previously described for type A injuries (Table 2).

B Group B2: Posterior Disruption Predominantly Osseous

In this group, the posterior injury is represented by a fracture through the laminae and pedicles or the isthmi. Interspinous and/or supraspinous ligaments are torn. As

Table 2 Type B Injuries: Groups and Subgroups

Type B   Anterior and Posterior Element Injury with Distraction
B1   Posterior disruption predominantly ligamentous (flexion distraction injury)
B1.1   With transverse disruption of the disk
B1.2   With type A fracture of the vertebral body
B2   Posterior disruption predominantly osseous (flexion distraction injury)
B2.1   Transverse bicolumn fracture
B2.2   With transverse disruption of the disk
B2.3   With type A fracture of the vertebral body
B3   Anterior disruption through the disk (hyperextension shear injury)
B3.1   Hyperextension subluxation
B3.2   Hyperextension spondylolysis
B3.3   Posterior dislocation

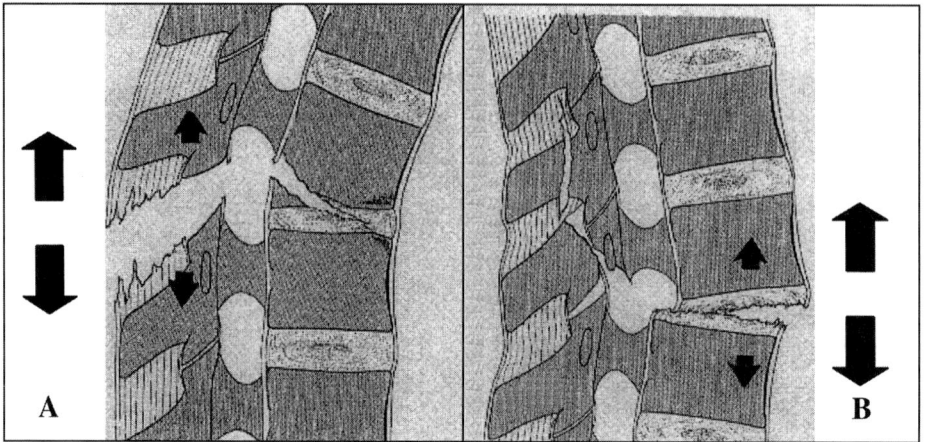

Figure 7 Type B, two-column injury with either (A) posterior or (B) anterior transverse disruption.

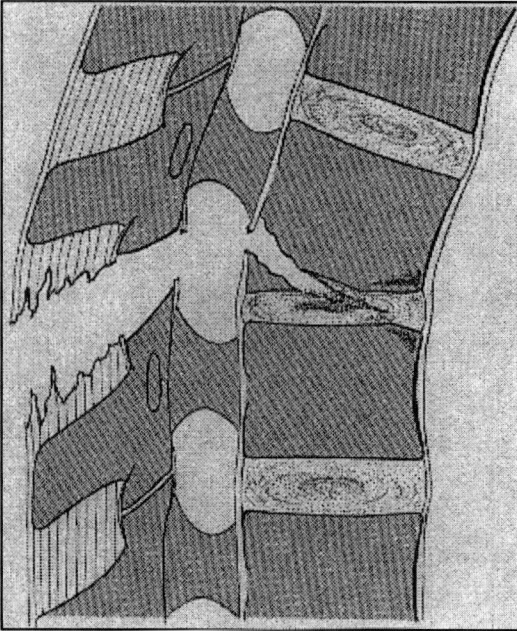

Figure 8 Injury with posterior disruption (predominantly ligamentous) associated with an anterior lesion through the disk (type B1.1).

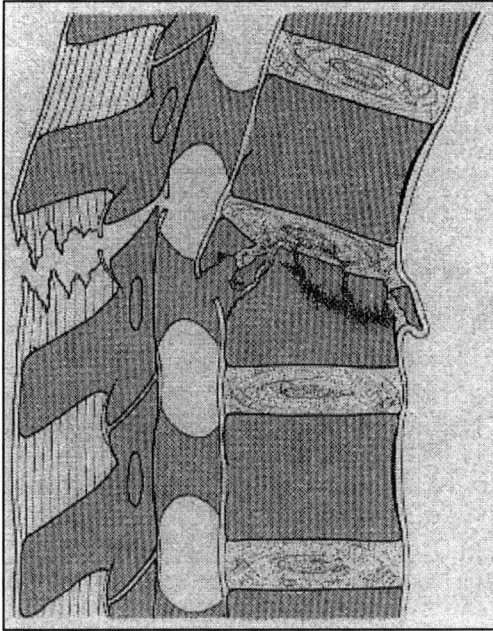

Figure 9 Posterior, predominantly ligamentous disruption with subluxation of the facet joints associated with an incomplete superior burst fracture (type B1.2 + A3.1).

described for the B1 injuries, the posterior lesion is associated with either a transverse disk disruption (B2.1) (Fig. 10) or a fracture of the vertebral body (B2.2) (Fig. 11).

1 Common Clinical and Radiological Findings of B1 and B2 Injuries

Marked tenderness, swelling, and subcutaneous hematoma at the fracture site or the palpation of a gap between the spinous processes are highly indicative of a distractive type of injury. Kyphotic deformity may be present.

Typical radiological findings include increased interspinous process distance with possible kyphotic deformity. Bilateral facet subluxation, dislocation, fracture of the articular processes, or other posterior vertebral elements are other typical signs. The radiological findings of the vertebral body fracture are the same as in type A injuries. In rare instances, it is possible to identify on CT a bony fragment, which is 180 degrees rotated, and the cortex of the spinal canal is now inside the vertebral body (also called reverse cortical sign). MRI may help to individualize the posterior soft tissue injuries.

C Group B3: Anterior Disruption Through the Disk

These particular and rare injuries are caused by a hyperextension–shear mechanism. The transverse disruption originates anteriorly and extends posteriorly to various extents (Fig. 7B). These lesions are seen particularly in patients with previously multilevel spinal ankylosis or diffuse idiopathic skeletal hyperostosis.

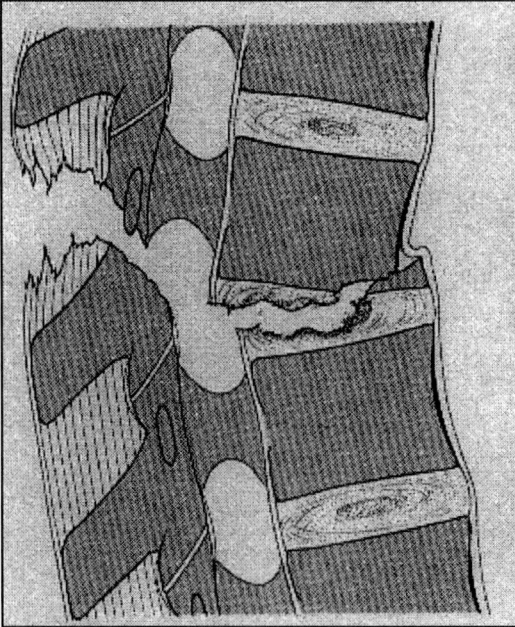

Figure 10 Posterior disruption predominantly osseous associated with an anterior lesion through the disk (type B2.1).

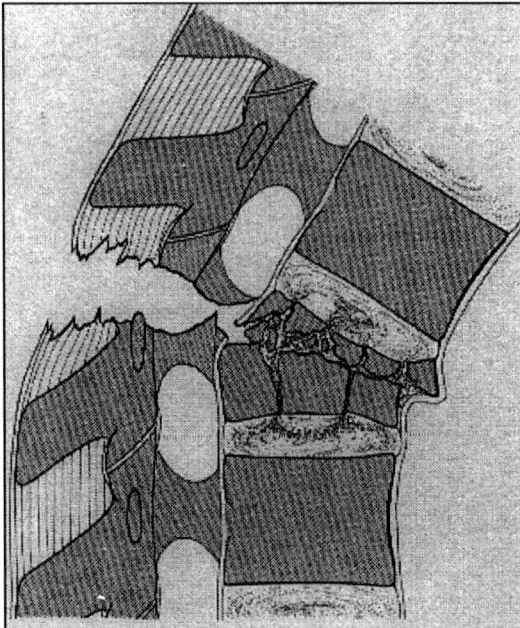

Figure 11 Posterior disruption predominantly osseous combined with a complete burst fracture (type B2.2 + A3.3).

III TYPE C: ANTERIOR AND POSTERIOR ELEMENT INJURIES WITH ROTATION

Type C of fractures includes a variety of severe injuries of both the anterior spinal column and posterior elements showing a common morphological pattern resulting from axial torque (Table 3) (Fig. 12). These can be type A lesions with superimposed rotation (C1); type B injuries with rotation (C2); or rotation–shear fractures (C3).

Common characteristics of these very unstable fractures are the injury of both the anterior and posterior spinal columns. This includes rotational displacement, fracture of the articular processes, usually unilateral, fracture of the transverse processes, rib dislocation, and asymmetrical fractures of the vertebral body. Due to severe instability, there is potential for translational displacement in all directions of the horizontal plane. With few exceptions, rotational injuries represent the most severe lesions of the thoracolumbar spine and are associated with the highest rate of neurological deficit.

A Group C1: Type A Fractures with Rotation

Both vertebral body and posterior elements are injured and signs of rotation are present in this group. Vertebral body fracture may be a simple wedge where one lateral vertebral wall often remains intact, resulting in almost a normal-appearing lateral x-ray (C1.1, rotational wedge fracture). Other injuries are represented by rotational split fractures (C1.2) or more comminuted lesions as rotational burst fractures (C1.3).

B Group C2: Type B Injuries with Rotation

The complete spinal injuries are caused by distraction and rotation. These include flexion distraction injuries with posterior ligamentous lesions combining with rotational abnormalities (C2.1); flexion distraction injuries combining with a posterior osseous lesion and rotational abnormalities (C2.2); and hyperextension shear injuries with rotation (C2.3).

Table 3 Type C Injuries: Groups and Subgroups

Type C   Anterior and Posterior Element Injury with Rotation

C1 Type A injuries with rotation (compression injuries with rotation)
   C1.1 Rotational wedge fracture
   C1.2 Rotational split fracture
   C1.3 Rotational burst fracture
C2 Type B injuries with rotation
   C2.1 B1 injuries with rotation (flexion distraction injuries with rotation)
   C2.2 B2 injuries with rotation (flexion distraction injuries with rotation)
   C2.3 B3 injuries with rotation (hyperextension shear injuries with rotation)
C3 Rotational shear injuries
   C3.1 Slice fracture
   C3.2 Oblique fracture

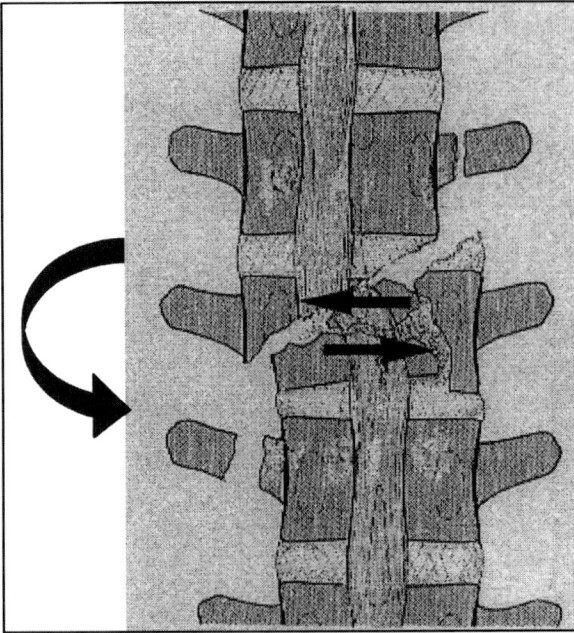

Figure 12 Two-column injury with rotation.

C   Group C3: Rotational Shear Injuries

These are probably the most unstable of all injuries of the spine (20). They are
mainly localized in the thoracic spine and include slice fractures (C3.1) and oblique
fractures (C3.2).

1   Common Clinical and Radiological Signs

Local clinical findings are the same as those described for type B injuries. Radiologically, signs of rotational lesions include transverse process fractures and should
alert the physician to suspect a more severe rotational mechanism. Other signs will
consist of asymmetrical findings mainly on the AP radiographs.

   The radiological evaluation and the perfect understanding of spinal injury
mechanisms are crucial for their correct management. The concepts reported in this
comprehensive fracture classification should provide for a more careful assessment
of radiological images, and the choice of further examinations in order to provide
the most accurate fracture analysis. This in essence will inform us about the severity
of the injury and guide further treatment.

   This classification appears to be very complicated, but this is mainly for scientific purposes of reporting, for example, specific treatment results for a particular
group of injuries. For practical use, many of its subdivisions are unnecessary and a
simplified form can be used without impairment of the information most essential
for clinical practice. Emphasis must be placed on the extent of involvement of the
anterior and posterior spinal elements, with particular attention to soft-tissue injuries
as well as ancillary bony lesions.

On AP radiographs, attention should be placed on the vertebral body height and diameter, pedicle and spinous processes alignment, interpedicular and interspinous process distance, the integrity of laminae, pars interarticularis, facet joints and especially the transverse processes. On plain lateral films, the evaluation must include the height of disk spaces, anterior, middle, and posterior aspect of the vertebral bodies, continuity of facet joints and posterior arches, distance between spinous processes, and maintenance of sagittal curves. Additional information regarding the integrity of the spinal canal, congruency of facets joints, and soft-tissue integrity is provided by the CT or MRI scan.

The analysis of the injury pattern provides information on the pathomechanics of the injury, at least regarding the main mechanisms. Loss of vertebral body height implies a compressive force or transverse disruption; increased distance in the posterior elements suggests distraction or shear; and rotational displacement in the vertical axis indicates torsion. Each of these mechanisms produces injuries with its own characteristic pattern.

The application of the classification can be facilitated by using the simple algorithm presented in Figure 13. The first observation will be directed to the analysis of the vertebral body injury (impaction, wedge, partial or complete burst, osteoporotic). If no additional signs of posterior column injury are present, the fracture is classified as a "type A." If posterior column injuries (fracture, interspinous ligament disruption) without rotational signs are seen, the fracture is a "type B." If rotational changes are present, it is a "type C."

During the last decade, this classification system has gained progressive popularity throughout the world. Experience has demonstrated that to a great extent the

Thoracolumbar Fracture Classification - Algorithm

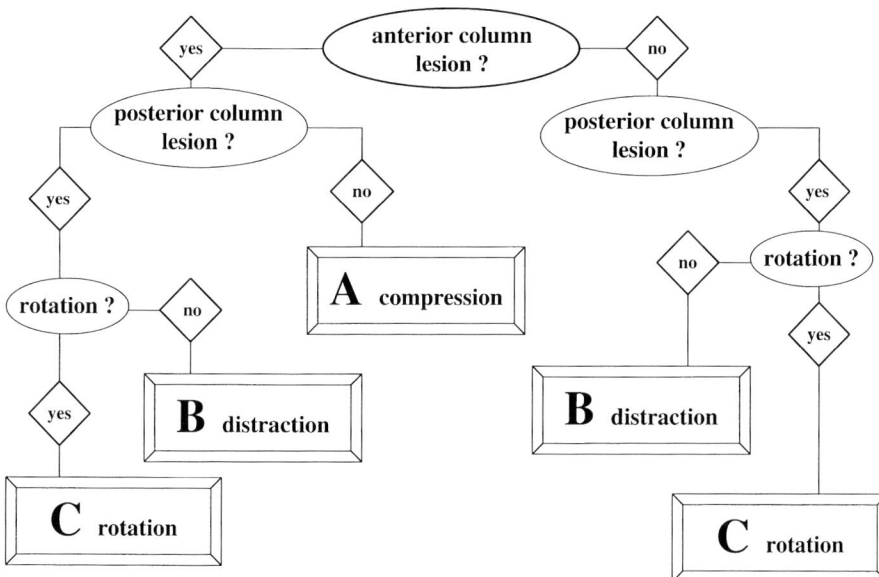

Figure 13 Algorithm for the determination of the injury types.

classification meets the previously outlined requirements. The injuries are logically grouped into different categories according to the main mechanisms of injury and pathomorphological uniformity. This organization presents a progressive scale of morphological damage by which the degree of instability may be determined. Thus, the severity of the injury in terms of instability is expressed by its ranking within this classification system. The degree of instability and prognostic aspects direct the treatment to be applied.

REFERENCES

1. Denis F. Updated classification of thoracolumbar fractures. Orthop Trans 1982; 6:8–9.
2. Denis F. The three column spine and its significance in the classification of acute thoracolumbar spinal injuries. Spine 1983; 8:817–831.
3. Ferguson RL, Allen BL Jr. A mechanistic classification of thoracolumbar spine fractures. Clin Orthop 1984; 189:77–88.
4. Gertzbein SD, Court-Brown CM. Flexion/distraction injuries of the lumbar spine. Mechanisms of injury and classification. Clin Orthop 1988; 227:52–60.
5. Gertzbein SD, Court-Brown CM. The rationale for management of flexion/distraction injuries of the thoracolumbar spine, based on a new classification. J Spinal Disord 1989; 2:176–183.
6. Gumley G, Taylor TKF, Ryan MD. Distraction fractures of the lumbar spine. J Bone Joint Surg [Br] 1982; 64:520–525.
7. Holdsworth FW. Fractures, dislocations, and fracture-dislocations of the spine. J Bone Joint Surg [Br] 1963; 45:6–20.
8. Jeanneret B, Ho PK, Magerl F. "Burst-shear" flexion/distraction injuries of the lumbar spine. J Spinal Disord 1993; 6:473–481.
9. McAfee PC, Yuan HA, Fredrickson BE, Lubicky JP. The value of computed tomography in thoracolumbar fractures. An analysis of one hundred consecutive cases and a new classification. J Bone Joint Surg [Am] 1983; 65:461–479.
10. Nicoll EA. Fractures of the dorso-lumbar spine. J Bone Joint Surg [Br] 1949; 31:376–394.
11. Rennie W, Mitchell N. Flexion distraction injuries of the thoracolumbar spine. J Bone Joint Surg [Am] 1973; 55:386–390.
12. Holdsworth FW. Review article: Fractures, dislocations, and fracture-dislocations of the spine. J Bone Joint Surg [Am] 1970; 52:1534–1551.
13. Whitesides T. Traumatic kyphosis of the thoracolumbar spine. Clin Orthop 1977; 128:78–92.
14. Louis R. Les théories de l'instabilité. Rev Chir Orthop 1977; 63:423–425.
15. Denis F. Spinal instability as defined by the three-column spine concept in acute spinal trauma. Clin Orthop 1984; 189:65–76.
16. Roy-Camille R, Gagnon P, Catonne Y, Benazet JB. La luxation antéro-latérale du rachis lombo-sacré. Rev Chir Orthop 1980; 66:105–109.
17. Magerl F, Aebi M, Gertzbein S, Harms J, Nazarian S. A comprehensive classification of thoracic and lumbar injuries. Eur Spine J 1994; 3:184–201.
18. White A, Panjabi M. Clinical biomechanics of the spine. Philadelphia: Lippincott, 1978.
19. Müller ME, Nazarian S, Koch P. Classification AO des fractures. 1 Les os longs. Springer: Berlin, 1987.
20. Denis F, Burkus JK. Shear fracture dislocation of the thoracic and lumbar spine associated with forceful hyperextension (lumbar-jack paraplegia). Spine 1992; 17:156–161.

30

Thoracolumbar Spine Stability

**JONATHAN N. GRAUER, TUSHAR CH. PATEL,
and MANOHAR M. PANJABI**

Yale University School of Medicine, New Haven, Connecticut, U.S.A.

I INTRODUCTION

An accepted classification of thoracic and lumbar spine injuries allows clinicians to work from a common ground when managing the traumatized patient. Several perplexing questions plague the treating physician when evaluating a patient with a thoracolumbar fracture, such as: Which injuries can be managed conservatively? Which patient will require surgery, and what should be performed? These decisions require an understanding of when the spine should be considered clinically unstable.

Biomechanical instability of a motion segment (two adjacent vertebrae with interconnecting disk, ligaments, and facet joints) can be objectively studied with cadaveric experiments. Once these principles are established, they can be extrapolated to the clinical setting. An understanding of clinical instability can then be used to direct patient care.

II BIOMECHANICAL PRINCIPLES

The intact spine must be characterized before understanding the changes produced by trauma. The load displacement curve is the standard means of measuring the physical properties of a spinal segment (Fig. 1A). It becomes readily apparent that such load displacement curves are nonlinear because the spine, which is flexible at low loads, stiffens with increasing loads. In order to characterize this response to loading, two parameters have been described: range of motion (ROM) and neutral zone (NZ).

ROM is the displacement of a motion segment, or functional spinal unit, from one extreme to the other when physiological loads are applied in any of the six

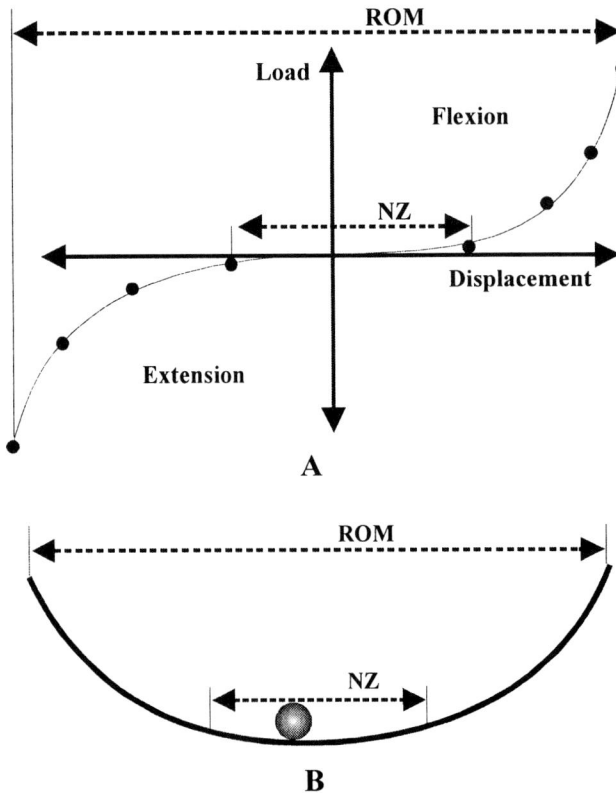

Figure 1 (A) Nonlinear response of a spine segment loaded in flexion (positive load) and extension (negative load). Range of motion (ROM) is the total displacement observed under physiological loading. Neutral zone (NZ) is the component of the ROM before the change in stiffness is observed. (B) A ball in a bowl analogy is shown. The ball can move easily in the bottom of the bowl, but encounters increased resistance at the limits of motion. (Adapted from Ref. 2.)

degrees of freedom. NZ, on the other hand, is the central portion of the ROM for which no significant resistance is met (1). NZ is thus a measure of laxity.

An image of a ball in a bowl has been used as an analogy to clarify the NZ/ROM concept (2) (Fig. 1B). The load displacement curve is transformed into a bowl by flipping the extension portion of a flexion/extension curve around the displacement axis. An imaginary ball moves easily within the bottom of the bowl (NZ), but requires greater effort to push up the sloping sides of the bowl (ROM).

These motion parameters exist for each of the three planes of motion: flexion/extension, lateral bending, and axial rotation. However, it is important to remember that each region of the spine has distinct characteristics. For example, the thoracic spine is the least mobile region of the spine, because it is stabilized by the costovertebral articulations and the rib cage. Consequently, normal motions have been defined for each level of the human spine and serve as benchmarks from which traumatic changes can be studied (3).

III BIOMECHANICAL INSTABILITY

Biomechanical instability is noted when supraphysiological motions are observed with physiological loading, perhaps because of factors such as traumatic injury, degenerative changes, or postoperative destabilization.

Several trauma classification schemes exist, including the three-column theory of thoracolumbar fractures. This was initially described by Denis after reviewing over 400 radiographs, and it stressed the importance of the middle column for spinal stability (4). However, it was not until later that this was objectively studied in the laboratory (5,6). Alterations in NZ and ROM were evaluated in cadaveric specimens before and after experimentally produced fractures. The results of these studies did, in fact, support the concept that the middle column is a crucial bony determinant of mechanical stability.

We can now link clinical trauma to alterations in biomechanical characteristics. Along these lines, other trauma modeling has been performed to evaluate the stabilizing role of other aspects of the spinal motion segment. For example, facets have been shown to be the principal stabilizers for axial rotation (7,8).

The effective stabilization of lumbar spinal ligaments was studied in a transection model (9). Specimens loaded in flexion were most affected when ligaments were sequentially transected from posterior to anterior. Specimens loaded in extension were most affected when ligaments were sequentially transected from anterior to posterior. This can be extrapolated to instabilities that can be expected with traumatic rupture of spinal ligaments.

The role of muscles in stabilizing the spine is more difficult to quantitate. The cross-sectional area of the muscles around the spine, and the relatively long moment arms over which the muscles act, provide significant potential stability to the spine. In fact, it has been shown that osteoligamentous thoracolumbar and lumbar spine segments are not able to support the weight above them without the stabilizing effect of the surrounding muscles (10,11).

Further, cadaveric experiments have simulated muscle forces around intact and injured osteoligamentous spine segments. Panjabi found that by adding such muscle forces to the injured spine, the ROM decreased in extension and axial rotation but increased in flexion, whereas NZ decreased in flexion and extension (12). Quint found that simulated muscle forces decrease lateral bending and axial rotation ROM but increase flexion/extension ROM. This study did not evaluate NZ (13). These ambiguous results may suggest that muscle forces lead to variable responses of ROM, but more consistent decreases in NZ. This certainly requires further investigation.

IV CLINICAL INSTABILITY

The extrapolation of biomechanical instability to clinical instability is controversial. White and Panjabi defined clinical instability as the loss of the spine's ability to maintain patterns of displacement under physiological loads so that there is no major deformity or progression of deformity, no initial or additional neurological deficit, and no incapacitating pain (3). It follows from this definition that clinical instability requires mechanical instability plus a propensity to progress or involvement of a neurological component.

Table 1 Checklist for the Diagnosis of Clinical Instability in the Lumbar and Lumbosacral Spine (L1–S1)

Element	Point value[a]
Anterior elements destroyed or unable to function	2
Posterior elements destroyed or unable to function	2
Radiographic criteria	4
Flexion extension radiographs	
Sagittal plane translation >4.5 mm or 15% (2 pt)	
Sagittal plane rotation	
5° at L1–L2, L2–L3, and L3–L4 (2 pt)	
>20° at L4–L5 (2 pt)	
>25 at L5–S1 (2 pt)	
OR	
Resting radiographs	
Sagittal plane displacement >4.5 mm or 15% (2 pt)	
Relative sagittal plane angulation >22° (2 pt)	
Cauda equina damage	3
Dangerous loading anticipated	1

[a]A point value total of 5 or more indicates clinical instability.
Source: Ref. 15.

The first systematic approach to the analysis of clinical stability was in the cervical spine. A checklist of factors to diagnosis clinical instability was developed (3) based on cadaveric experiments (14,15). This helped provide the clinician with a systematic approach to the assessment of clinical instability. Similar checklists were developed for the thoracic and lumbar spine (3). These were largely based on the ligament transection experiments discussed previously in the biomechanical instability section (9). Nevertheless, clinical validation of these checklists has yet to be performed.

Table 2 Checklist for the Diagnosis of Clinical Instability in the Thoracic and Thoracolumbar Spine (T11–L1)

Element	Point value[a]
Anterior elements destroyed or unable to function	2
Posterior elements destroyed or unable to function	2
Radiographic criteria	4
Sagittal plane displacement >2.5 mm (2 pt)	
Relative sagittal plane angulation >5° (2 pt)	
Spinal cord or cauda equina damage	2
Disruption of costovertebral articulations	1
Dangerous loading anticipated	1

[a]A point value total of 5 or more indicates clinical instability.
Source: Ref. 15.

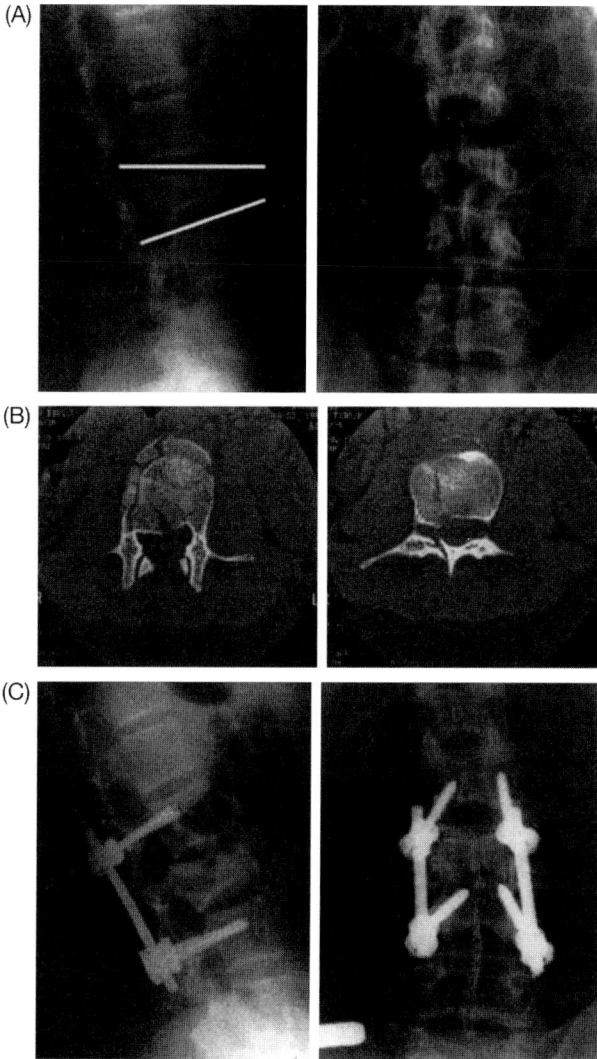

Figure 2 Example of clinical instability. This 14-year-old back-seatbelted passenger was involved in a motor vehicle accident when her car struck a pole at approximately 35 miles per hour. She presented after this hyperflexion injury neurologically intact with back pain. (A) Plain films revealed a L3 compression fracture with a 23 degree relative flexion deformity (2 pt). (B) CT scan showed anterior disruption (2 pt) with approximately 10% canal compromise and laminar fracture posteriorly (2 pt). (C) With a total of six points, this was consistent with instability per the grading scale presented and was fixed posteriorly with a L2 and L4 screw and rod construct.

The lumbar spine checklist uses several elements, such as biomechanical parameters, neurological damage, and anticipated loading on the spine (Table 1). A point-value system is used to determine stability or instability. The anterior elements include the posterior longitudinal ligament and all anatomical structures anterior to it (two points). The posterior elements are all anatomical structures posterior to the

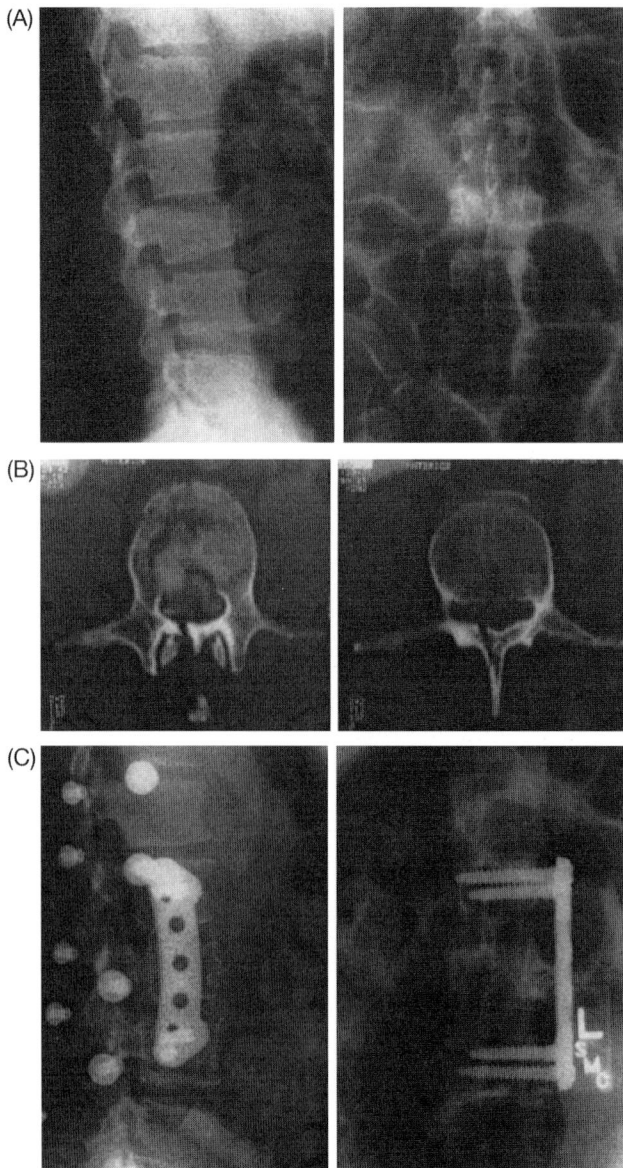

Figure 3   Another example of clinical instability. This 40-year-old front-seatbelted passenger was involved in a motor vehicle accident. He presented with back pain and bilateral anterior thigh paresthesias (3 pt) but was otherwise neurologically intact. (A) Plain films revealed a compression fracture with a 5 degree relative flexion deformity. (B) CT scan showed anterior disruption (2 pt) with approximately 90% canal compromise and a laminar fracture (2 pt). (C) With a total of seven points, this was consistent with instability per the grading scale presented. Anterior decompression was performed and an anterior plate was applied from L2 to L4 after a strut graft was placed.

longitudinal ligament (two points). The intervertebral translations and rotations are measured either on flexion/extension or resting radiographs (two points each). Damage to the cauda equina is given three points, and the anticipated exposure to high loading on the spine is given one point. If the sum of the points is five or more, then the spine is considered to be clinically unstable.

Thoracic instability is a less common entity, but has a separate checklist because of the differences in anatomy at these levels (Table 2). Anterior or posterior element injury, sagittal plane displacement of >2.5 mm, relative sagittal plane angulation of >5°, and spinal cord or cauda equina damage are each worth two points. Disruption of costovertebral articulations and anticipated exposure to dangerous loading are each worth one point. As with the lumbar spine, if the sum of the points is five or more, then the spine is considered to be clinically unstable.

V APPLICATION OF PRINCIPLES

The principles discussed in this chapter are applied to sample cases in Figures 2 and 3. Each of these patients presented with greater than five points using the grading scale described above and were thus consistent with clinical instability and stabilized as shown.

In summary, there are circumstances where instability will be obvious, but the principles outlined here are directed to the circumstances where the question of stability is less clear. Basic concepts can be applied to specific spinal injuries as shown in Figures 2 and 3 as well as in the following chapters.

REFERENCES

1. Panjabi MM. The stabilizing system of the spine: Part II. Neutral zone and instability hypothesis. J Spinal Disord 1992; 5: 390–397.
2. Panjabi MM. Low back pain and spinal instability. In: Weinstein J, Gordon S, eds. Low back pain: A scientific and clinical overview. Rosemont: American Academy of Orthopedic Surgeons, 1996: 367–384.
3. White AA III, Panjabi MM. Clinical Biomechanics of the Spine, 2nd ed. Philadelphia: J.B. Lippincott Company, 1990.
4. Denis F. The three column spine and its significance in the classification of acute thoracolumbar spinal injuries. Spine 1983; 8: 817–831.
5. Panjabi MM, Oxland TR, Kifune M, Arand M, Chen A. Validation of the three-column theory of thoracolumbar fractures: a biomechanical investigation. Spine 1995; 20: 1122–1127.
6. Panjabi MM, Oxland TR, Lin RM, McGowen TW. Thoracolumbar burst fracture: A biomechanical investigation of its multidirectional flexibility. Spine 1994; 19: 578–585.
7. Farfan HF, Cossette JW, Robertson GH, Wells RV, Kraus H. The effects of torsion on the lumbar intervertebral joints: The role of torsion in the production of disc degeneration. J Bone Joint Surg 1970; 52A: 468–497.
8. Abumi K, Panjabi MM, Kramer KM, Duranceau J, Oxland T, Crisco JJ. Biomechanical evaluation of lumbar spinal stability after graded facetectomies. Spine 1990; 15: 1142–1147.
9. Posner I, White AA III, Edwards WT, Hayes WC. A biomechanical analysis of the clinical stability of the lumbar and lumbosacral spine. Spine 1982; 7: 374–389.
10. Lucas DB, Bressler B. Stability of the ligamentous spine. Technical report No. 40, Biomechanics Laboratory, University of California San Francisco, The Laboratory, 1961.

11. Crisco JJ, Panjabi JJ, Panjabi MM, Yamamoto I, Oxland TR. Euler stability of the human ligamentous lumbar spine. Part II Experiment. Clin Biomech 1992; 7: 27–32.
12. Panjabi M, Abumi K, Duranceau J, Oxlan T. Spinal stability and intersegmental muscle forces: a biomechanical model. Spine 1989; 14: 194–200.
13. Quint U, Wilke HJ, Shirazi-Adl A, Parianpour M, Loer F, Claes LE. Importance of the intersegmental trunk muscles for the stability of the lumbar spine. A biomechanical study in vitro. Spine 1998; 23: 1937–1945.
14. Panjabi MM, White AA III, Johnson RM. Cervical spine biomechanics as a function of transection of components. J Biomech 1975; 8: 327–336.
15. White AA III, Johnson RM, Panjabi MM, Southwick WO. Biomechanical analysis of clinical stability in the cervical spine. Clin Orthop 1975; 109: 85–96.

31

Thoracic Fractures

**G. MICHAEL LEMOLE, Jr., JEFFREY S. HENN,
and VOLKER K.H. SONNTAG**

Barrow Neurological Institute, Phoenix, Arizona, U.S.A.

JUAN BARTOLOMEI

Yale University School of Medicine, New Haven, Connecticut, U.S.A.

This chapter addresses the diagnosis and management of thoracic fractures from T1 to T10. Fractures of the thoracolumbar (T11–L1) junction are considered separately because the biomechanics of this transitional segment between a hypermobile and relatively immobile region differ from the rest of the thoracic spine. Much of our understanding of thoracic fractures is derived from series that include both thoracic and thoracolumbar fractures. An attempt is made to differentiate the data pertinent to thoracic fractures from those involving the transitional segments.

I EPIDEMIOLOGY

Fractures of the thoracic spine are less common than those involving the cervical, thoracolumbar, and lumbar regions. In a study by Hanley and Eskay (1), thoracic fractures (T2–T10) represented only 16.4% of all fractures involving the thoracic and lumbar vertebrae. These numbers (T1–T10) were comparable in larger case series examining all spinal fractures by Frankel et al. (26.8%) (2) and Magerl et al. (23.7%) (3). Given that more than 150,000 Americans injure their spinal columns each year, these percentages are significant (4).

The demographics of thoracic spinal fractures tend to follow those for trauma in general. In Hanley and Eskay's series (1) of 57 patients with thoracic fractures, 45 were male and average age was 29.9 years (range, 13–58). Sex distributions for thoracic fractures alone could not be gleaned from the larger studies; however, most thoracolumbar fracture series suggest a male predominance and age of presentation in the second through fourth decades of life (2,5).

The thoracic spine is more rigid than its cervical or lumbar counterparts, because of the structural stability supplied by the ribs, facet orientations, and vertebral body configurations. The force required to disrupt the thoracic spine is reflected in the commonly reported mechanisms of injury, including motor vehicle accidents, falls, diving from heights, or direct forceful back blows (1,2). Most fractures tend to involve the kyphotic apex around T6–T8 (1,3). It should be noted, however, that up to 23% of cases will have multisegmental injuries of the thoracolumbar spine (3) and 5% may be noncontiguous (4).

Considerable force is required to fracture the thoracic spine. This fact and the small spinal canal relative to the spinal cord diameter may explain why thoracic fractures are more often associated with neurological injury when they do occur. Hanley and Eskay (1) noted that 52.6% of their patients with thoracic fractures suffered neurological injury. Of those, 76.6% sustained complete (Frankel grade A) injuries. Rogers et al. (6) found, in contrast, that only 17% of patients with upper thoracic spine injury suffered paraplegia. Another way to consider thoracic injury and neurological impairment is to observe that 15 to 16% of spinal cord injuries result from thoracic spine injury (7,8). These numbers were even higher in a study by Roberts and Curtis (9) in which 50% of patients with traumatic paraplegia suffered injury to the upper thoracic spine.

Clearly, injury to the thoracic spine tends to result in certain injury patterns. Why these trends occur has very much to do with biomechanics specific to the thoracic spine.

II THORACIC BIOMECHANICS

The biomechanical properties of the thoracic spine help explain the nature and frequency of associated fracture patterns. The overall stability of the thoracic spine is imparted by the interaction of the bony and soft-tissue elements including ligaments, disks, and muscles. The thoracic spinal column (T1–T9) articulates with the thoracic rib cage and through the rib cage to the sternum. Costovertebral and radial ligaments secure the vertebral bodies and transverse processes to the ribs (4). Cadaveric studies have demonstrated that the rib cage significantly increases the stability and immobility of the thoracic spinal column, most notably during extension, by as much as 70%. During flexion and rotation, the effect of the rib cage is less significant. A thoracic column with an intact rib cage may resist compressive forces four times better than without an intact rib cage (10).

The considerable tensile strength of the anterior and posterior longitudinal ligaments, the paraspinous musculature insertions, and the facet articulations also contribute to the stability of the thoracic spinal column. The facets and lamina in the upper thoracic spine are rotated toward a coronal orientation much as shingles on the roof of a house. This configuration allows some rotational movement but significantly inhibits extension. In the lower thoracic spine, particularly in the junctional areas, the facets assume a more sagittal orientation, as in the lumbar spine, which facilitates flexion and extension (11).

The unique kyphosis of the thoracic spine also has ramifications for its patterns of injury. Proceeding caudally, the thoracic vertebral bodies increase in all dimensions. However, the height of a vertebral body is 2 to 3 mm less anteriorly relative to its posterior dimension (12). This difference results in an overall kyphosis from T1 to T10 and shifts the instantaneous axis of rotation forward. Vertical loading then causes a disproportionate amount of the force to be borne by the anterior vertebral body and partially explains why simple anterior wedge fractures occur commonly in the thoracic spine (11).

Another way to consider the biomechanics of the thoracic spine is to analyze which structural features resist different force vectors. Extension, for example, is resisted by the orientation of the thoracic lamina and facets, the presence of an intact rib cage, and the anterior longitudinal ligament. In contrast, flexion is prevented by the posterior tension band, which consists of the interspinous, interlaminar, facet, and posterolongitudinal ligaments as well as the ligamentum flavum. The rib cage also limits flexion (11,13). Because much of the posterior tension band is composed of ligaments, these elements can be disrupted by hyperflexion without a bony injury occurring.

Resistance to compressive forces is largely borne by the bony vertebral bodies and articular interactions at the facet joints. The instantaneous axis of rotation of a particular vertebral body determines what portion of the vertebral body bears the brunt of a vertical load (4). Distracting forces are most often opposed by the host of thoracic spinal ligaments, including the anterior and posterior spinal ligaments, posterior tension band, and the rib cage. Rotational stability in the thoracic spine is provided by the anterior and posterior longitudinal ligaments as well as by the rib cage. The facet joints and disks provide rotational stability, especially in the caudal thoracic spine (11).

Finally, translational or shear forces are countered by the anterior and posterior longitudinal ligaments as well as by the disk components, including the annulus fibrosis. Furthermore, the vertebral facets and their ligamentous attachments inhibit forward translation of one vertebral body upon another (4). Fractures involving significant dislocation of one vertebral body upon another imply a variety of ligamentous and bony injuries over almost all of the stabilizing elements at the level of injury.

The end result of all biomechanical considerations is ultimately the concept of spinal stability. The spine must have the intrinsic ability to support itself and the body, without compromise, under normal physiological conditions.

III SPINAL STABILITY

The most comprehensive definition of clinical spinal stability is that of White and Panjabi (10): "the ability of the spine under physiologic loads to maintain relationship between vertebrae in such a way that there is neither initial damage nor subsequent irritation to the spinal cord or nerve roots; and in addition, there is no development of incapacitating deformity or pain due to structural changes." Conversely, spinal instability results when the spine is unable to maintain the vertebral relationships or prevent deformity or pain under physiological loads. In the early 1960s, Holdsworth (14) suggested a two-column concept of the spine, emphasizing the importance of the posterior ligamentous elements (intraspinous and supraspinous ligaments and ligamentum flavum) in providing a tension band for stability. Whitesides (15) further refined this concept by modeling the spine after a construction

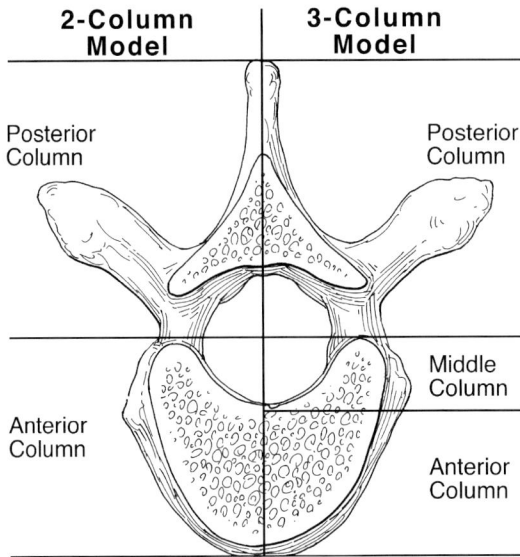

Figure 1 In the two-column spine model, the posterior column is composed of all structures posterior to the pedicles. The anterior or load-bearing column is composed of the vertebral body. The three-column model includes a middle column composed of the posterior portion of the vertebral body, the posterior longitudinal ligament, and posterior annulus. This osteoligamentous column is often assessed to determine structural stability. (Reprinted with permission from Barrow Neurological Institute.)

crane with columns resisting compression (anterior) and tension (posterior). This concept served as a simple and mechanistic model for defining and organizing fractures and for providing a framework to develop management strategies. However, the model had conceptual limitations, and subsequent biomechanical studies failed to support it (16). Some of the fractures considered stable by this model were later associated with structural deformities, suggesting some form of chronic mechanical insufficiency. For example, under the Holdsworth classification, burst fractures were deemed stable regardless of vertebral height loss (14).

With the advent of diagnostic imaging, all elements of the spine could be assessed more thoroughly. In the early 1980s, Denis (5) and McAfee et al. (17) independently proposed a three-column model of spinal stability. In this model, the anterior column consists of the anterior half of the vertebral body, annulus fibrosus, and anterior longitudinal ligament. The middle, or osteoligamentous, column is formed by the posterior half of the vertebral body, annulus fibrosus, and posterior longitudinal ligament. The posterior column is composed of the supra- and infraspinous ligaments, facets with their respective ligaments, articular process, lamina, spinous process, and interspinous ligament. McAfee (17) emphasized the role of the middle column in determining the degree of instability. Also according to Denis, the failure mode of the middle column provides a method for distinguishing between stable and unstable injuries. Disruption of two or more columns creates an unstable fracture. This model is now widely used to define clinical stability (Fig. 1).

IV DIAGNOSTIC IMAGING

The diagnostic modalities that can be used to identify thoracic fractures range from simple plain radiography to CT and MR imaging. Each imaging modality has its advantages and drawbacks. In all likelihood, the complete evaluation of a patient with a thoracic injury will include a combination of various imaging techniques. Typically, plain radiographs in AP and lateral planes can be used as a screening test, particularly when mechanisms of injury suggest the possibility of spinal column compromise. CT is used to assess suspicious areas, and CT with myelography or MR imaging is often used to correlate fracture level or level of neurological impairment with SCI and ligamentous injury. Depending on the mechanism of injury, the presence of localized pain, and focal neurological injury, the threshold for performing diagnostic studies at any suspected level must be low.

A Plain Radiography

At each level, plain radiographs should be analyzed in a systematic and organized fashion (Fig. 2). Radiographs should be inspected for disruptions in spinal alignment or severe changes in angulation associated with translational motion. In lateral plain radiographs, spinal alignment is determined by identifying the margins of the anterior and posterior vertebral bodies, orientation of facets, and posterior spinous process line. On AP views, rotational injuries can be determined by inspecting pedicular alignment, position of the transverse processes, and spinous process alignment. Changes in vertebral body height with antero- or retropulsion of fragments should alert clinicians to the potential of spinal cord compression.

If no bony injuries are evident on radiographs, ligamentous injuries can be assessed by carefully studying changes in the facet joint space and interspinous process distance. Subtle changes in the superior or inferior articular facets can denote significant ligamentous disruption from flexion distraction injuries (18). Loss in disk height with minimal vertebral body change can suggest a compression-type fracture. Likewise, increased disk height might suggest a distracting-type injury. Associated abnormalities in the soft tissue, such as loss of the psoas' stripe, paraspinal soft-tissue swelling, hemo- or pneumothorax, and rib fractures, should also raise suspicion of associated vertebral body fractures.

B CT

When plain radiographs suggest bony or ligamentous injury at any level, further evaluation with CT is necessary (Fig. 3). The area of interest should be imaged up to and including one vertebral level above and below. CT offers the best resolution of bony anatomy. CT also visualizes the cervicothoracic junction, which is difficult to assess by plain radiography. This imaging modality also shows small fractures extending through bony elements that might be missed by plain radiography. CT has been shown to be particularly useful when assessing the degree of spinal instability as defined by anterior, middle, and posterior column compromise (17). Axial CT images cannot accurately visualize neural elements or axially oriented injuries such as Chance fractures. This limitation, however, can be partially overcome with computer-aided sagittal reconstructions, which can demonstrate spinal canal compromise and axially oriented fractures. The sensitivity of this imaging modality can be in-

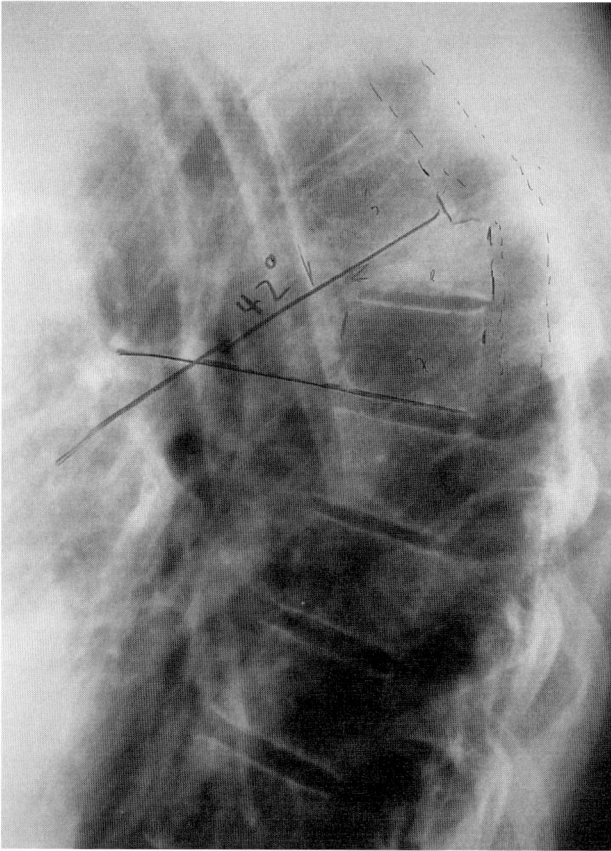

Figure 2   Lateral radiographs of a 55-year-old patient involved in a motor vehicle accident showing a T6 burst fracture with 42 degrees of kyphotic angulation.

creased by refining the thickness of axial imaging from 3 to 1 mm. In conjunction with intrathecal myelography, CT can be used to assess compromise of the spinal canal elements, including the nerve roots and spinal cord itself.

CT myelography should be considered in patients who are not candidates for MR imaging. CT myelography delineates the intrathecal compartment and subtle changes within the spinal cord itself that may manifest with spinal cord edema (19,20). CT myelography can adequately assess extra-axial lesions such as epidural hematomas, traumatic disk herniations, and dural lacerations presenting with pseudo-meningoceles. CT also offers the ability to obtain three-dimensional reconstructions that might play a role in preoperative surgical planning.

C   MR Imaging

MR imaging is the imaging modality of choice for assessing soft tissues, including the spinal cord, and should be used as a complementary diagnostic modality (Fig. 4). Using specialized imaging weightings, MR shows ligamentous injuries and disruptions that may have otherwise been missed by CT or plain radiography. If the

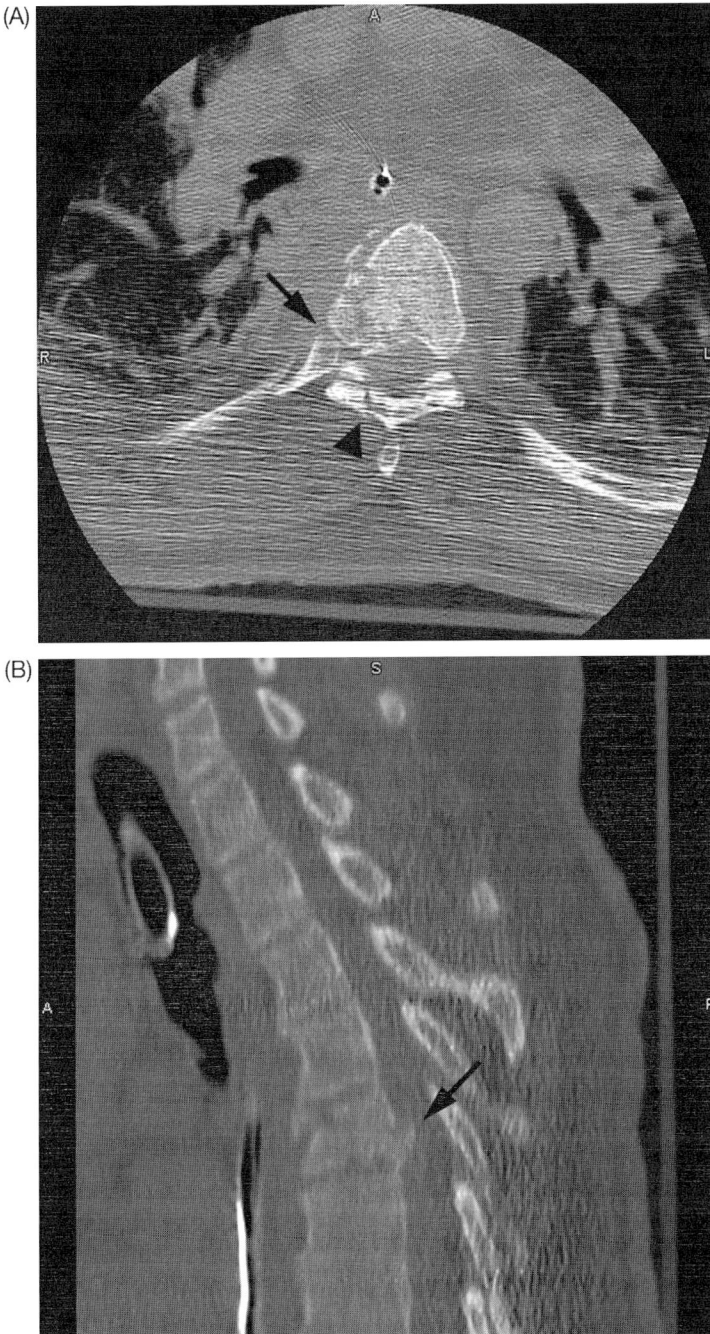

Figure 3 (A) Axial computed tomographic image showing a lateral (burst) fracture of the body of T6 (*arrow*) and involvement of posterior structures including the spinal lamina (*arrowhead*). A small amount of bone is retropulsed in the spinal canal. (B) Sagittal reconstruction image showing that more height has been lost anteriorly than posteriorly. The small amount of bone retropulsed into the canal (*arrow*) is again apparent.

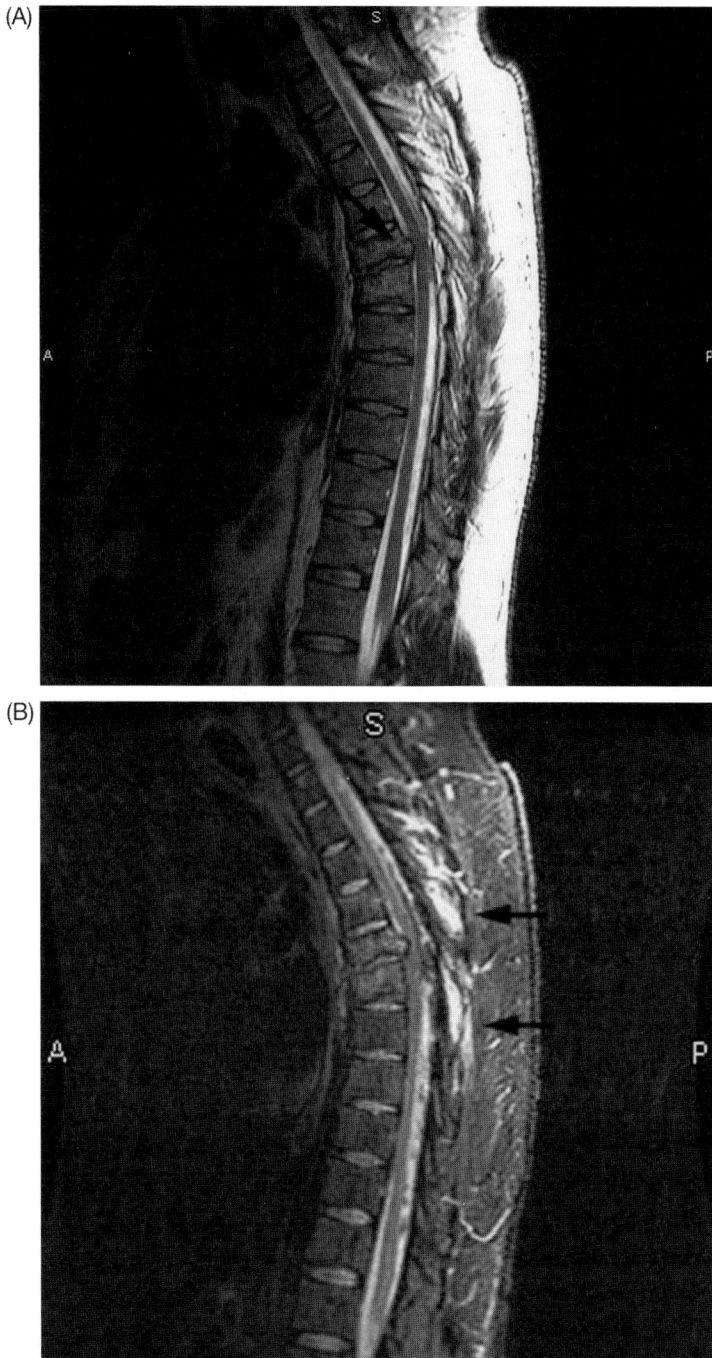

Figure 4 (A) Sagittal T2-weighted magnetic resonance image from the patient shown in Figure 3A. The burst fracture and the bone retropulsed into the spinal canal and impinging on the spinal cord are visible (*arrow*). (B) Sagittal fat-suppressed magnetic resonance image showing significant ligamentous and soft-tissue injury over the dorsal spine as indicated by the hyperintense signal (*arrows*).

bony vertebral column is intact, significant instability may be present due to ligamentous disruption alone. For example, MR imaging demonstrates Chance fractures because they cause an enormous amount of ligamentous disruption and, in some instances, have no osseous component. Ligamentous disruptions appear as increased signal intensity on T2-weighted, fat-suppressed images.

MR imaging offers the best resolution of the spinal canal and reveals mass intrusions into that space, including disk herniations, bony protrusions, and hematomas. Changes in signal intensity within the spinal cord parenchyma can provide evidence of neural injury that should correlate with neurological dysfunction. Several patterns of signal abnormalities follow acute SCI. Spinal cord hemorrhage is usually denoted by a hyperintense signal on T1-weighted images, whereas spinal cord edema and contusion usually appear hyperintense on T2-weighted images. Evidence of acute hemorrhage on MR imaging is associated with worse outcomes (21–24).

MR imaging can also provide information about pathological fractures caused by tumors, osteoporosis, or infection. MR imaging can complement CT when a compression fracture is present on CT and plain radiography but the acuity or chronicity cannot be determined. Acute, recent, or subacute fractures usually have a high signal intensity on T2-weighted images.

The disadvantages of MR imaging include its slower acquisition time, the possibility of metal artifacts, and the relatively poor delineation of bony structures. MR imaging is inappropriate for patients who are claustrophobic, who have large body habitus, or who have cardiac pacemakers or ferromagnetic implants.

V FRACTURE TYPES

Classifications of spinal fractures should be simple and complete, and they should reflect a thorough understanding of the mechanisms implicated in the etiology of the fracture. The ability to assess spinal fractures with CT is partially responsible for the development of classification systems (5,17,25). Thoracic fractures have been classified by the anatomical area involved, the morphology of the fracture, and the forces involved. Only the most widely used classification schemes are discussed below.

The extent of injury depends on the orientation of the force vector in relation to the instantaneous axis of rotation for each vertebral body. The location of the instantaneous axis of rotation within the vertebral body, in conjunction with the force vector, creates a bending moment. The magnitude of the force vector and the distances of the bending moment, in turn, delineate the extent of the fracture. According to Denis's classification, and applying the basic concepts of force vectors and location of the instantaneous axis of rotation, four major types of spinal fractures can be identified: (1) compression fractures; (2) burst fractures; (3) seat-belt fractures; and (4) fracture dislocations (5).

With his three-column classification system, McAfee (17) defined three vector forces acting to produce injury in the thoracolumbar spine: axial compression, axial distraction, and translation. The injuries produced by these vectors included (1) wedge compression fractures; (2) stable burst fractures; (3) unstable burst fractures; (4) Chance fractures; (5) flexion distraction injuries; and (6) translational injuries.

With Holdworth's (14) original model, several injury types could be defined, including (1) simple wedge fractures; (2) dislocations; (3) rotational fracture dislocations; (4) extension injuries; (5) burst injuries; and (6) shear fractures. Hanley and

Eskay (1) added the subgroup of burst dislocation to this list while condensing the remainder into compression fractures, fracture dislocations, and burst fractures, as applicable to the thoracic spine.

Magerl et al. (3) proposed a comprehensive classification of fractures based on the forces generating them and on their morphological characteristics. Fractures result from three basic types of forces that are present during injury: compression, distraction, and rotation. This classification has been applied to all levels in the spine and is further divided into subtypes 1, 2, and 3, depending on the severity. A major advantage of this type of classification is its comprehensive and descriptive nature. The type of injury can be conceptualized clearly, leading to a logical treatment plan. The model's detail and complexity, however, make it difficult to remember for all the fractures and their subdivisions.

Although there is significant overlap with each of these models, perhaps the simplest and most descriptive is that given by Denis et al. (5). Each subtype in that schema is described in detail below.

A Compression Fractures

Compression fractures that do not involve the middle column are considered stable (Fig. 5). Compression fractures result from an axial load with flexion or, in some cases, with a slight lateral bend. In these fractures, the anterior portion of the vertebral body collapses, disrupting the anterior column. These fractures are the consequence of the natural kyphotic curvature of the thoracic spine, applying a bending moment ventral to the instantaneous axis of rotation with almost no involvement of the middle and posterior columns. Various fracture patterns can include disruption of the superior or inferior endplates or both. When a lateral bending moment with axial forces is imposed on the spine, a lateral wedge-compression fracture results. These fractures are identified on plain radiography; however, CT is sometimes necessary to quantify the extent of the fracture and to assess the involvement of the middle column.

Two different subtypes of compression fractures have been identified: IA and IB (4). Vertebral body compression is less than 50% and angular deformity is less

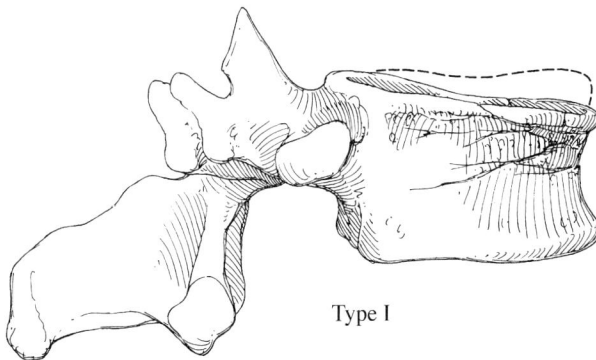

Type I

Figure 5 Illustration of an anterior wedge compression fracture showing collapse of the anterior vertebral column and sparing of the middle column. (Reprinted with permission from Barrow Neurological Institute.)

than 30° in type IA fractures. Type IA fractures tend to be stable. Type IB fractures have more than 50% vertebral body compression and more than 30° of angulation. These fractures tend to involve the middle and posterior columns. They are usually unstable and require some form of stabilization. About 88% of patients with compression fractures will be neurologically intact (1).

B   Burst Fractures

Burst fractures result from a direct axial load without the presence of a bending moment (Fig. 6). The failure of the middle column, along with the anterior column, is the key to their instability. The two-column involvement renders these fractures unstable. Various degrees of bony retropulsion into the spinal canal may be present. Plain radiography reveals loss of vertebral body height, widened interpedicular distance, and fragments retropulsed into the spinal canal. Given the kyphotic curvature of the spine, these fractures are rare in the upper thoracic region. The posterior elements are compromised bilaterally in 50% of cases and unilaterally in 40% (26). Burst fractures are usually associated with some degree of neurological compromise, depending on how severely the spinal canal is compromised and on the spinal level

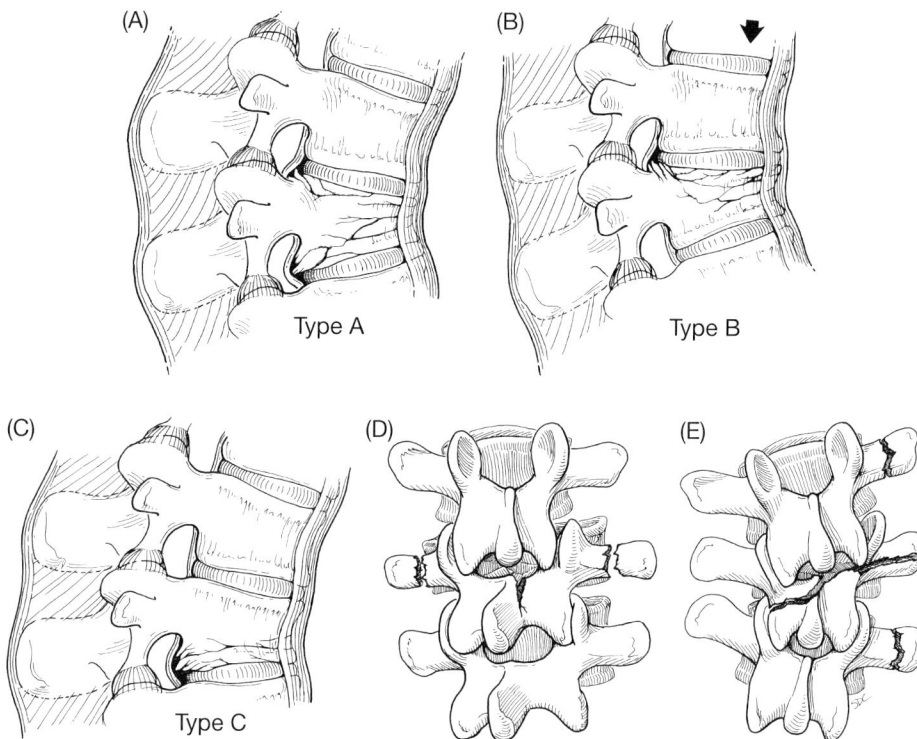

Figure 6   According to the Denis classification of burst fractures, there are five specific morphologies. (A) Fractures may involve both endplates; (B) the superior endplate; (C) the inferior endplate; (D) they may have an associated rotational deformity or; (E) a lateral flexion component. (Reprinted with permission from Barrow Neurological Institute.)

involved (27). A combination of axial compression and translational forces may result in burst dislocation fractures, in which the burst fracture is coupled with destruction of the inferior vertebral body posterior elements as described by Hanley and Eskay (1). Compared to the inferior vertebral body, the superior vertebral body exhibits anterolisthesis. Destruction of the posterior elements of the inferior vertebra decompresses the spinal canal, decreasing the risk of neurological impairment. With three-column destruction and a translational component, these types of fractures are extremely unstable (1).

C   Flexion Distraction (Seat-Belt) Fractures

Seat-belt-related fractures are caused by shearing and distractive forces that disrupt the middle column, making these unstable fractures (Fig. 7). These fractures occur when flexion is coupled with a fulcrum located anterior to the vertebral column. Because of the rigidity and stiffness afforded by the rib cages, these injuries seldom occur in the upper thoracic spine. Typically, they are located in the lower thoracic region near or at the transitional zone with the lumbar spine. This type of injury was described by Chance (28) and bears his name. The stability of this fracture depends on the magnitude of the force applied to the fulcrum as well as the involvement of the anterior column. These injuries can involve purely osseous structures, purely ligamentous structures, or both. When a purely osseous component is present, these injuries may heal by bony union. Ligamentous or combined injuries that lack the potential for self-repair may require internal stabilization.

D   Fracture Dislocations

Thoracic fracture dislocations represent up to 50% of all fractures (1) (Fig. 8). The failure of all three-column fractures makes them unstable. The middle column often fails during rotation, shearing, or both. One vertebral body is usually displaced with

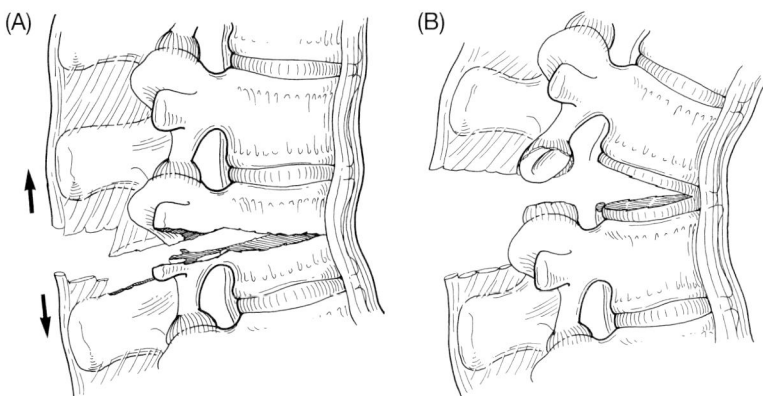

Figure 7   Seat-belt-type injuries result from significant distracting forces. Flexion distraction fractures may manifest by primary failure of (A) osseous structures or (B) purely ligamentous structures such as the facets or disk spaces. The latter rarely heals without surgical stabilization and fusion. (Reprinted with permission from Barrow Neurological Institute.)

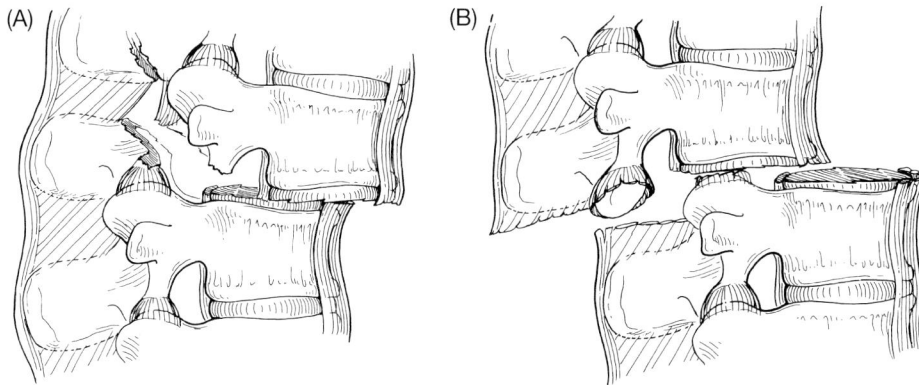

Figure 8 Fracture dislocation injuries result from the failure of all three spinal columns, often in response to shearing forces. Depending on the force vectors applied, vertebral bodies may be displaced (A) anteriorly or (B) posteriorly.

respect to another, compromising the spinal canal with resulting severe SCI. An anteroposterior translational component is usually present due to the lateral rigidity provided by the rib cage. In some instances, however, several forces, including rotation, distraction, compression, and shearing, are all involved. Regardless of the forces involved, these fractures are unstable. Of patients with fracture dislocations, 90% will have a SCI, and 84% of these will have complete SCI (1).

E Miscellaneous Fractures

Isolated posterior element fractures (spinous process, transverse process) can occur as a result of direct blunt trauma. These fractures are assessed with CT imaging through the region of interest. They are stable and seldom require an external orthosis unless significant pain is present. Occasionally, they can present with radicular injury or reflect underlying cord contusion (5). Unlike the thoracolumbar region, extension–distraction fractures of the upper thoracic spine are extremely rare. The normal kyphotic curvature of the thoracic spine, which places the center of gravity anteriorly, and the rigidity from the rib cages, prevent these injuries from occurring. In transitional zones, these fractures occur because of the lever effect generated by the thoracic spine and rib cage acting as a unit over a mobile, adjacent segment during forceful extension.

VI MANAGEMENT

The management of thoracic fractures can be considered in both the acute and definitive care phases. Acute care is usually beyond the scope of practice for most surgeons and relies upon the institution of appropriate EMS and trauma protocols for care of patients with suspected spinal injury. Once the patient has been stabilized and a definitive diagnosis is made with appropriate imaging, indications for conservative or surgical treatments must be decided upon. If surgery is entertained, the issues of decompression and stabilization must be addressed. These considerations are among the most contentious in spine surgery. We present a review of generally accepted guidelines and practices.

A   Acute Management

Management of thoracic fractures begins immediately at the scene of injury. These priorities are guided toward maintenance of airway and circulatory support. Once these systems are secured, the patient can be moved while maintaining complete spinal alignment. Traumatic injuries should increase suspicion for potential unstable fractures. Consequently, log-rolling techniques and cervical spine precautions must be instituted immediately at the scene. Fortunately, paramedics in this country are well trained to follow these precautionary measures by using long-board immobilization and cervical collars while they transfer patients to the hospital.

Once patients arrive at the emergency room, a dedicated trauma team institutes the first line of care by evaluating the patient's condition through a primary survey, as recommended by the American College of Surgeons for Advanced Trauma Life Support (29). During this survey, careful attention is again directed toward airway patency, perfusion pressure, and maintenance of circulation. If the patient requires endotracheal intubation, in-line traction technique must be used to avoid cervical injuries. The patient should then be turned in a log-rolling fashion to maintain in-line spinal alignment. When examining the patient's back, the midline is palpated carefully to examine for tenderness or evidence of gross deformity.

To minimize further neurological deficits in patients with a SCI, hypoxia must be avoided during the acute phases of trauma. Volume status is important because it can affect spinal cord perfusion in cases of SCI. Reasons for hypovolemic shock need to be determined and addressed in an expedient fashion. Aggressive fluid resuscitation should be instituted for spinal shock to avoid hypoxic injury of neural tissue. Inotropic support must be considered carefully in trauma patients because concomitant abdominal injuries could be exacerbated by the use of pressors. In a recent study, Vale et al. (30) implemented and adhered to a strict protocol maintaining a mean arterial pressure above 85 mmHg for 7 days in patients with SCI. They used a combination of pressors, methylprednisolone, and early reduction (closed or operative, when indicated). Outcomes exceeded previous reports (31–33). Patients who had prolonged and significant spinal shock did not do as well as those who received aggressive measures. These clinical observations are consistent with experimental reports employing aggressive hemodynamic treatment after SCI.

Once the primary survey is completed, suspected spinal injuries can be assessed in an expeditious manner. A graded neurological examination is performed from the head to the lower extremities. Motor and sensory functions are graded (ASIA) (34). Serial examinations are necessary to detect any deterioration during the course of management and permit a more aggressive and directed course of treatment, if needed. Portable AP, lateral, and odontoid views of the cervical spine are obtained, and if the trauma mechanism or examination suggests thoracic or lumbar injuries, plain radiographs are obtained of these regions. Once a final assessment of spinal injuries is established, the patient should be removed from the rigid board to prevent pressure sores, particularly SCI patients with impaired sensory and motor functions. If spinal cord injury is identified, early institution of steroid therapy can improve outcome.

Pharmacological therapies for the treatment of acute SCI include a bolus dose of methylprednisolone (30 mg/kg) with a continuous infusion (5.4 mg/kg/h) over 24 to 48 h as recommended by the National Acute Spinal Cord Injury Study (NASCIS) trials (35,36). In the most recent NASCIS trial, a continuous infusion was given for 24 h if the methylprednisolone bolus was started within 3 h of injury. If the 3-h window was missed or the SCI occurred within 8 h, a 48-h infusion followed the initial bolus (36). Another pharmacological therapy that has been tested clinically but not implemented widely is the use of GM-1 gangliosides. GM-1 infusion after acute SCI improves motor deficits, particularly in the lower extremities (37).

B Indications for Conservative or Surgical Treatment

The appropriate management of thoracic fractures depends on a clear conceptualization of the underlying pathomechanics. Mechanisms of injury and their interaction with regional anatomy to produce specific fracture morphologies must be understood. The goals of treatment are to (1) avoid further neurological injury; (2) decompress neural elements indirectly or directly; (3) reduce and stabilize the spine to prevent further acute or delayed deformity; (4) achieve early mobilization to prevent medically related complications; (5) alleviate pain; and (6) minimize the cost of treatment. To achieve these goals, the surgeon must recognize the nature of specific fracture types and consider the potential for acute or possible delayed neurological injury.

Conservative treatment of thoracolumbar fractures through postural reduction and immobilization has historically been as effective as surgery for most fractures. Guttman (38) and Frankel et al. (2) used postural reduction and immobilization and found that, with rare exception, vertebral stability was achieved. A further study by Young et al. (39) suggested no significant difference in neurological recovery after SCI, comparing conservative vs. surgical interventions. Burke and Murray (40) showed a small, but significant, difference in neurological recovery with surgery over conservative management (38 vs. 35%). However, the surgery subset included more patients with an incomplete SCI with a better prognosis. In addition, the surgical series suffered more chronic pain than the conservatively treated group.

More recent literature expanded the goals of treatment to include postinjury pain, kyphosis, time to mobilization and rehabilitation, and economic impact. Leidholt et al. (41) noted that some patients with thoracolumbar injury developed progressive deformity despite postural reduction and bracing. Denis et al. (5) devised a relative index of pain and postinjury employment and found that surgically treated patients suffer less severe pain overall and have increased rates of return to work. Most importantly, several authors (5,17,42) noted a significant occurrence of late neurological deterioration in conservatively treated patients. The development of alternative routes of access to the spinal column and improved forms of spinal stabilization and fusion have made surgery more feasible. Decreasing surgical morbidity and mortality have lessened historical biases against surgery. Nonetheless, the treatment of thoracic fractures remains controversial, especially in cases of complete SCI and in the neurological intact patient.

The indications for surgical decompression during acute SCI continue to be refined, and several prognostic indicators of poor outcomes may help guide the surgeon's decision to perform an acute surgical decompression. One of these factors is the extent of neurological injury at presentation. The presence of severe spinal shock and a complete SCI may indicate severe anatomical or physiological transection of the spinal cord. Such patients have a low percentage of neurological recovery (31). MR imaging also provides evidence for the potential of neurological recovery. The presence of spinal cord parenchymal hemorrhage on T2-weighted images represents a very poor prognosticator (43). Age is another factor that seems to predict the prognosis of patients with acute SCI. Patients older than 50 years who sustain a SCI have a much poorer prognosis for neurological recovery and survival than younger patients (44).

C   Timing of Surgery

The timing of treatment depends on the patient's status, which is determined systematically with the trauma team or medical intensivists. Experimental data suggest that neurological recovery is directly related to the duration of spinal compression (45–47). Several anecdotal retrospective studies also report favorable outcomes after acute decompression in SCI patients (48). In contrast, others have found no significant improvements after acute decompression for SCI (32). Unfortunately, no randomized studies have addressed the role of acute surgical decompression of traumatic SCI. Series of patients with some form of cauda equina syndrome or incomplete SCI have claimed neurological improvements after acute reduction and decompression (49,50).

Early surgery decreases the complications caused by prolonged immobilization: pneumonia, pulmonary embolism, deep venous thrombosis, and decubiti ulcers (50). Surgery within 24 to 72 h of SCI decreases the length of hospitalization and increases the rate of early mobilization (51,52). Moreover, early surgery also reduces hospitalization costs (53). Some authors have reported that early surgery has not been associated with an increase in neurological deterioration or other complications (50–53).

Advances in spinal instrumentation, intraoperative monitoring, and neuroanesthesia have made spinal surgery during the acute phases of trauma a much safer endeavor. Experienced spine surgeons and an anesthesiologist are needed during these procedures to minimize intraoperative time and hypoxic events. Several studies, however, have questioned the safety of early surgery, citing an increased risk of neurological deterioration (54–56) due to increased blood loss, hemodynamic instability, multiple organ injuries, and vulnerability of spinal cord during the acute phase of edema.

VII   TREATMENT BY FRACTURE TYPE

A   Compression Fractures

Type IA compression fractures can be associated with some element of neurological deficit. The compression usually results from a herniated disk, which can easily be assessed with MR imaging. Early decompression may be of some benefit for patients with an incomplete neurological deficit and evidence of spinal cord compression. If neurological injury is present without compression, careful examination of CT and MR imaging is warranted to rule out ligamentous injuries. In the absence of ligamentous injury, there are no surgical indications.

The dilemma arises when a neurologically intact patient has some compression of the spinal cord. It is reasonable for these patients to be evaluated and treated conservatively. If supine and upright films reveal evidence of segmental instability with resultant neurological symptoms, including either weakness or pain, some form of surgical decompression and stabilization is reasonable. If there is no evidence of gross instability or clinical symptoms, the patient is placed in an external orthosis and followed closely with outpatient radiography to monitor the potential for the development of a deformity. Surgical decompression and stabilization might also be necessary in patients who develop a kyphotic deformity or evidence of a neurological compromise.

Patients with type IA fractures wear a thoracolumbosacral orthosis (TLSO) brace for 8 to 12 weeks. Afterward, patients undergo a period of back-strengthening and hyperextension exercises. Conservative treatment achieves early mobilization and minimizes hospitalization. The overall recommendation for patients with type IA fractures is conservative management unless spinal cord compression is associated with a neurologically incomplete injury. If surgery is required, the posterior elements should be preserved, if possible. If the posterior elements are resected through a laminectomy, stabilization will be necessary.

Stronger arguments can be made for the surgical correction of type IB compression fractures, which are usually unstable and can cause significant pain during follow-up (57). There is no indication for surgical decompression during the acute phase of injury in patients with type IB compression fractures and a complete SCI. Acute surgical decompression, however, might benefit patients with an incomplete SCI and evidence of spinal cord compression.

The treatment for neurologically intact patients or those with incomplete SCI and no evidence of cord compression with a type IB compression fracture is controversial. In these patients, as in those with type IA fractures, careful radiographic examination is necessary to rule out segmental instability. Given the higher likelihood that these fractures will cause future kyphotic deformities with further compression of neural elements, early correction of a surgical deformity might prevent these delayed consequences and thus justify surgery during the subacute phase of injury. Although the exact type of fractures (type IA or IB) presented in a report by Bradford et al. (58) is unclear, they noted that patients with compression fractures who were treated conservatively developed delayed kyphotic deformity over 6 months to 8.5 years. Similarly, Nash et al. (42) reported two patients with stable compression fractures who were neurologically intact and subsequently developed severe kyphosis with neurological deficits.

An advantage of surgical decompression and correction of compression type IB fractures is the potential for early mobilization. Regardless of the patient's neurological condition or type of fracture, increasing mobilization appears to reduce postoperative complications (51,52). The question of timing of surgical intervention in neurologically intact patients is difficult. If conservative treatment is chosen, very close follow-up is needed to monitor the potential development of deformity. If patients experience pain or neurological deterioration, diagnostic imaging, including plain lateral and AP radiographs and MR imaging and/or CT, should be obtained and the possibility of surgical correction entertained.

B   Burst Fractures

The acute management of thoracic and lumbar burst fractures is perhaps one of the most controversial. Numerous authors have advocated different criteria for the conservative or surgical management of burst fractures, depending on the amount of deformity, spinal compromise, and neurological impairment. Neurologically intact patients with fractures that do not involve the posterior column can be treated conservatively with external orthosis and early mobilization. The absence of both posterior midline tenderness and widening interspinous ligaments on lateral plain radiographs suggest that the posterior ligamentous structures are intact and that the posterior column is not impaired. However, Cantor et al. (59) concluded that patients with a kyphosis of more than 30°, more than 50% loss of vertebral body height, and a concomitant facet fracture had an incompetent posterior column. Surgical stabilization might be indicated to achieve alignment and to prevent a deformity from developing.

Patients who are neurologically intact with continued radiographic evidence of cord compression present a management dilemma. According to Denis' (5) classification scheme, burst fractures are unstable because two columns are injured. It would seem reasonable to follow these patients closely with radiography to try to identify the development of pain, neurological symptoms, or radiographic evidence of instability. Some evidence suggests that retropulsed fragments will be resorbed over time and therefore surgery should not be considered in this patient population (60–62). In contrast, Brown et al. (63) advocated surgical decompression and stabilization in patients with more than 40% spinal canal compromise because of the small diameter of the thoracic spinal canal compared to the thoracolumbar region. In 1984 Denis et al. (64) reported that as many as 17% of patients with acute burst fractures and a normal neurological examination deteriorated after conservative treatment. There is no straightforward answer regarding the management of neurologically intact patients with burst fractures and fragments retropulsed into the spinal canal. If conservative management is chosen, careful follow-up examinations and diagnostic imaging are needed to prevent a progressive kyphotic deformity from developing as well as subsequent neurological deterioration.

Patients with incomplete neurological injuries after a burst fracture who have residual spinal cord compression may benefit from acute surgical decompression and stabilization (49,65,66). Patients who suffer a complete neurological injury after burst fractures do not require immediate surgical decompression, regardless of the presence of spinal cord compression. Patients with an incomplete SCI or who are neurologically intact with no evidence of spinal compression have no need for surgical decompression. However, if an external orthosis does not appropriately immobilize the spine, a fusion is indicated.

The surgical goals of treating burst fractures are to decompress the spinal canal, if needed, and to restore spinal alignment. Neuronal elements can be decompressed either through indirect reduction, posterior or anterior approach. Sometimes retropulsed fragments can be reduced indirectly by the application of distractive forces (ligamentotaxis) and realignment of the kyphotic curvature. This procedure is successful as long as the posterior longitudinal ligament is intact during the application of distractive forces across the affected segment. Several studies support this technique (67,68). Others have reported that this procedure is ineffective in the subacute setting, particularly when soft tissue healing prevents adequate reduction and realignment (69). When the posterior longitudinal ligament is injured, direct reduction is possible through a posterior or posterolateral approach by performing a decompressive laminectomy with a transpedicular or extracavitary approach. Retropulsed fragments can be impacted using a tamp or reverse curette. Intraoperative ultrasonography permits visualization of retropulsed fragments that cannot be seen through the operative exposure. The transthoracic anterolateral approach in which the burst fracture is removed under direct vision appears the most logical. The vertebral column is reconstructed with allograft/autograft or with a cage and a laterally placed plate.

C Flexion Distraction Injuries

Typically, flexion distraction injuries involve the lower thoracic region and one or two motion segments. Their management primarily depends on the injury patterns and tissues involved. An external orthosis such as a TLSO brace is sufficient to treat strictly osseous injuries because they tend to have a high rate of fusion. Lesions that involve a ligamentous and/or osseous component are best treated by operative stabilization. These injuries are primarily caused by distraction; therefore, compressive constructs such as interspinous wiring or segmental fixation using pedicle or laminar hooks or pedicle screws should be used (57,70). Disk or bone fragments that might further compromise the spinal canal must be assessed carefully before compressive forces are applied with instrumentation.

D Fracture Dislocations

There is no indication to proceed with emergent surgery in patients with a complete neurological injury. However, conservative management of these patients is associated with significant delayed complications (9). Patients with spinal cord compression and evidence of incomplete neurological injury might benefit from acute surgical decompression and segmental stabilization. Early decompression and segmental stabilization should be entertained for neurologically intact patients with some element of spinal canal compression.

Regardless of the patient's neurological condition, the inherent instability of these fractures necessitates surgical consideration to correct alignment and to provide segmental, long-term stabilization. Unlike burst or extension injuries, fracture dislocations require complex corrective forces. Simple compression or distraction forces alone may fail to reduce and reestablish alignment. A posterior approach is usually advantageous for these fractures. It provides access to injured facets and access for inserting pedicle screws and laminar hooks to correct deformity through multiple planes of force vectors (68,71). An anterior decompression provides a full view of the anterior spinal canal when fracture dislocations are associated with either a burst fracture or significant compromise of the spinal canal. However, anterior surgical decompression without posterior stabilization is not recommended because of the severe disruption of the posterior column. Timely surgical decompression and reduction allow patients to be mobilized in a more effective fashion to decrease the length of hospitalization and to institute effective physical rehabilitation (30,51).

VIII SURGICAL APPROACHES

Once a decision to proceed with surgery has been determined, the choice of surgical approach is guided by the location and characteristic features of the fracture. The surgical goals are to decompress the neural elements and to reconstitute sagittal alignment and segmental stability when needed. The two main surgical corridors available for the repair of thoracic fractures are the posterior and the anterior routes.

A Posterior Approaches

Surgeons usually prefer posterior approaches because they are simple and familiar. Through a posterior approach, the surgeon has access to posterior elements that might impinge on the spinal canal and can perform a fusion and stabilization procedure to correct spinal alignment. Posterior access can be divided into the dorsal midline or posterolateral approaches. The dorsal midline approach can be divided into a straight laminectomy or a transpedicular approach. The posterolateral approach can be divided into a costotransversectomy or lateral extracavitary approach.

1 Dorsal Midline Laminectomy

Earlier surgical series used a straightforward laminectomy to treat thoracic fractures and were associated with significant rates of morbidity (72). When the anterior or middle column is involved, an isolated laminectomy is not indicated unless it is supplemented with some form of arthrodesis. The main advantages of this procedure are the ease and familiarity of the anatomy. The patient is placed in a straight prone position, and the deep tissue is accessed through a midline incision. Posterior elements causing significant spinal canal compromise are an indication for this approach. Laminar fractures with foraminal encroachment are easily accessed through this route. If posterior epidural hemorrhage or dural tears are present, this approach provides wide access for evacuation and repair. This route also permits the placement of posterior instrumentation. This approach, however, does not provide adequate visualization of the anterior portion of the dura, and the site of pathology in most thoracic fractures is ventral (Fig. 9). Moreover, when the anterior column is involved, this procedure destabilizes the spine and instrumentation and fusion are required.

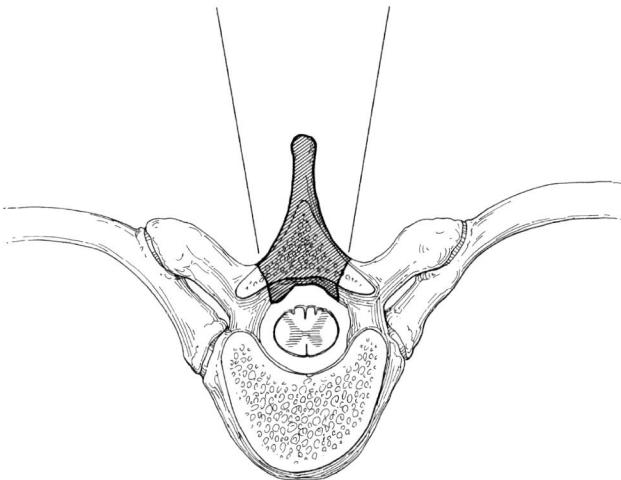

Figure 9   Laminectomy. Removal of the posterior lamina and spinous process allows access to the dorsal spinal cord. The lateral and ventral spinal cord are not well visualized. (Reprinted with permission from Barrow Neurological Institute.)

2 Transpedicular Approach

The dorsal midline approach can be combined with the transpedicular approach when large retropulsed bone fragments impinge on the thecal sac (Fig. 10). The position of the patient and the incision are the same as those used in a laminectomy. To visualize the pedicles in the thoracic region, a portion of the facet needs to be dissected and removed to gain lateral access. Drilling the pedicles bilaterally provides a more ventral view of the thecal sac and access to the vertebral body. For burst fractures, the transpedicular approach, combined with drilling the vertebral body, allows the surgeon to place reverse curettes anterior to the thecal sac and to impact some of the fragments back into the vertebral body. An obvious disadvantage is the inability to visualize the thecal sac anteriorly. Intraoperative ultrasonography may be effective in assessing persistent anterior compression. Because this route offers limited exposure, it can be difficult to safely place a curette anteriorly without significantly retracting the thecal sac or nerve roots. A kyphotic deformity can also develop if an anterior strut graft is not placed. This risk increases when much of the vertebral body is drilled away to permit anteriorly retropulsed fragments to be impacted. Like a laminectomy, this technique is highly destabilizing, particularly when the anterior elements are involved with the injury. Consequently, a posterior instrumented fusion is usually performed at the same sitting.

3 Costotransversectomy Approach

A costotransversectomy provides a more lateral view of the bony anatomy and better access to the anterior portion of the thecal sac than a midline laminectomy (Fig. 11). The patient is placed prone and a median or paramedian incision is made. The approach is indicated when a retropulsed fragment compresses the thecal sac in a more lateral, eccentric position. It provides a more lateral view of the vertebral body

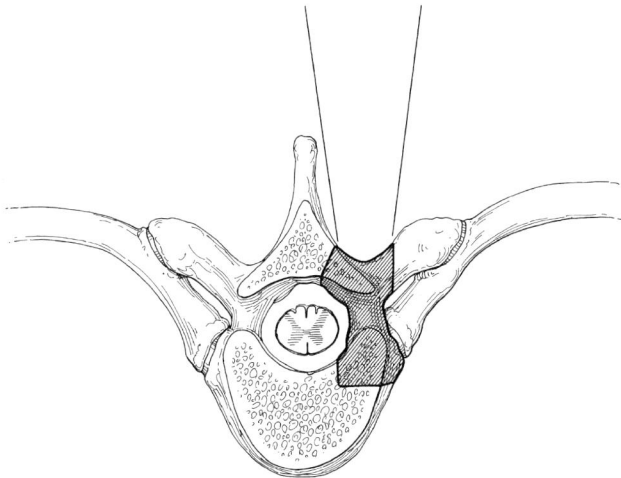

Figure 10 Transpedicular approach. Removal of the posterior lamina and ipsilateral pedicle provides excellent access to the dorsal and lateral spinal cord. The ventral spinal cord is not well visualized or accessed. (Reprinted with permission from Barrow Neurological Institute.)

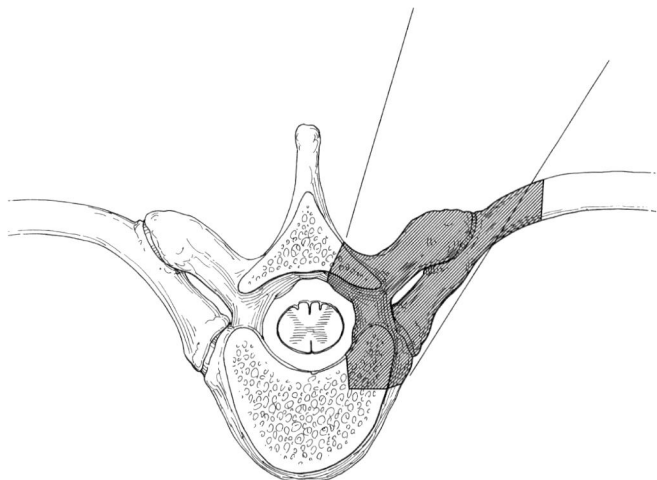

Figure 11   Costotransversectomy approach. Removal of ipsilateral lamina and pedicle as well as the transverse process and proximal rib allows a more lateral trajectory to the spinal cord. As a result, this approach offers excellent exposure of the lateral thecal sac and some exposure of the ventral vertebral body. Midline or contralateral structures are difficult to access, and vertebral body grafts cannot be placed through this approach. (Reprinted with permission from Barrow Neurological Institute.)

because the proximal portion of the rib and the transverse process are resected. However, large ventral retropulsed fragments cannot be removed and an anterior strut graft cannot be placed. Therefore, it is difficult to assess the degree of anterior decompression using this technique. A posterior instrumented construct can also be placed through this approach.

4   Lateral Extracavitary Approach

The lateral extracavitary approach permits a wider view of the lateral aspect of the vertebral body and therefore provides better access to the ventral thecal sac (73,74) (Fig. 12). The patient is placed in a prone position, and a modified hockey-stick paramedian or median incision is made to gain lateral access to the paraspinous muscles. The paraspinous muscles are dissected in the midline as usual, as well as along a more lateral plane so the erector spinae muscles can be mobilized laterally to medially. The ribs and lateral portion of the vertebral body are then exposed. The proximal portion of the ribs are removed. The pleura is not violated, but an ample view of the lateral aspect of the vertebral body is provided. Using a high-speed drill, the surgeon can safely remove the pedicle and visualize the thecal sac ventrally. The lateral extracavitary approach permits anterior decompression with minimal retraction of the neural elements and avoids the morbidity associated with the transthoracic approach. If necessary, an anterior strut graft can be placed, and a segmental stabilization can be performed through the same incision.

Considerable muscle retraction and dissection, with associated complications, are required with this approach, which also make it difficult to visualize the contralateral pedicle. In some instances, depending on the patient's body habitus, a clear view of the anterior portion of the thecal sac is not possible. From T1 to T4, it is

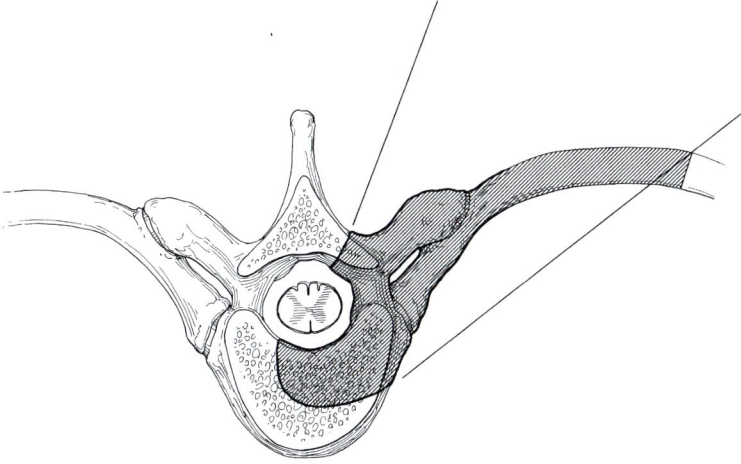

Figure 12   Lateral extracavitary approach. Resecting the ipsilateral lamina, pedicle, transverse process, and rib and approaching the vertebral body through the extracavitary thoracic space provide greater visualization of the ventral spinal canal, which is augmented further by performing a partial corpectomy just anterior to the spinal canal. (Reprinted with permission from Barrow Neurological Institute.)

difficult to mobilize the scapula without causing significant morbidity. Sometimes, during surgery, the patient must be repositioned and the arms manipulated to improve the view obscured by the overlying scapula.

B   Anterior Approaches

Anterior approaches to the thoracic spine offer the benefit of full exposure and visualization of the injured vertebral body and disks. These approaches are ideally suited for burst fractures associated with a significant amount of spinal canal compression. Through an anterior approach, the entire vertebral body can be removed and the thecal sac can be visualized without manipulating the neural elements. When the posterior elements of the thoracic spine are intact, an anterior decompression and fusion may be enough to manage burst or compression fractures. If more complex translational forces are present, the anterior approach should be performed for decompression, if needed, followed by the staged placement of a posterior stabilizing construct. Before an anterior approach is undertaken, the great vessels should be evaluated to rule out the presence of a traumatic lesion. Anterior approaches are also recommended for the treatment of late symptomatic post-traumatic kyphosis that causes pain or neurological deficits (75). Several routes of access, as described below, can be used to expose the anterior elements of the spine.

1   Transsternal Approach

The transsternal route is used if an anterior approach is required for fractures between T1 and T4 (Fig. 13). Numerous vital anatomical structures are present, and the transitional zone between the cervical and thoracic region creates a kyphosis. The transsternal approach has been modified to improve access to the upper thoracic region and to minimize its associated morbidity (76). The transsternal approach can

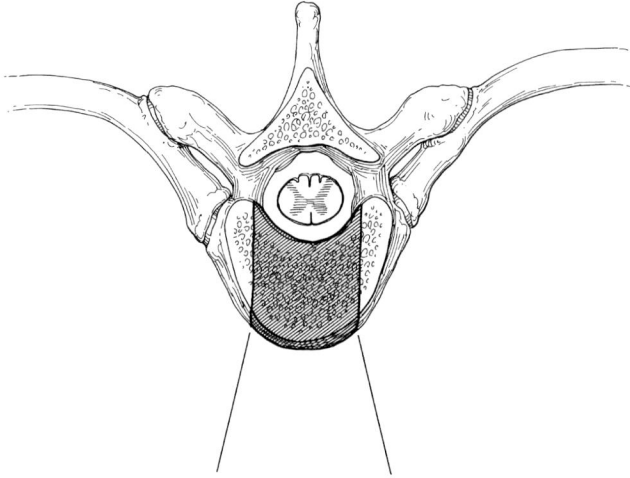

Figure 13 Transsternal approach. By spreading the sternum and gently retracting mediastinal structures, an axis to the upper thoracic spine (T1–T4) is obtained. The vertebral body is removed in the midline to provide access to the ventral spinal canal and spinal cord. (Reprinted with permission from Barrow Neurological Institute.)

be augmented by resecting the medial third of the clavicle or by performing a limited sternotomy with biclavicular resection (77). This procedure, however, is associated with the risk of bilateral pleural injury, pneumothorax, hemothorax, avulsion of the brachiocephalic vein, and transient laryngeal nerve palsy (78). Depending on the patient's anatomy, a supraclavicular anterior sternocleidomastoid approach may provide access to the upper thoracic vertebra without the use of a transsternal or transmanubrial approach (76). The changing curvature of the cervicothoracic junction makes the placement of a graft and plating extremely challenging.

2 Transthoracic Approach

The transthoracic approach can be performed for fractures caudal to T4 (Fig. 14). The patient is placed in a lateral decubitus position, and an extended thoracotomy incision is centered along the region of interest. The approach is ideally suited for fractures associated with a significant amount of compression and retropulsion into the thecal sac. The approach is usually from the left side for fractures between T7–T10 because it is easier to mobilize the aorta and to repair inadvertent arterial injuries. The right-sided approach is used for fractures between T3–T6 to avoid the heart and large vessels. A thoracic CT shows the overlying vascular structures (heart and liver), the presence of the liver on the right, and their relationship to the vertebral bodies, assisting with selection of the appropriate surgical corridor. Anterior exposure and the ability to decompress the vertebral body from pedicle to pedicle are excellent with this approach. Ventrally kyphotic deformities can also be accessed for correction.

The lung is retracted to expose the vertebral column. The overlying parietal pleura, segmental vessels, and periosteum are mobilized to provide a full ventral view of the fracture. Disk spaces are usually removed above and below the fracture

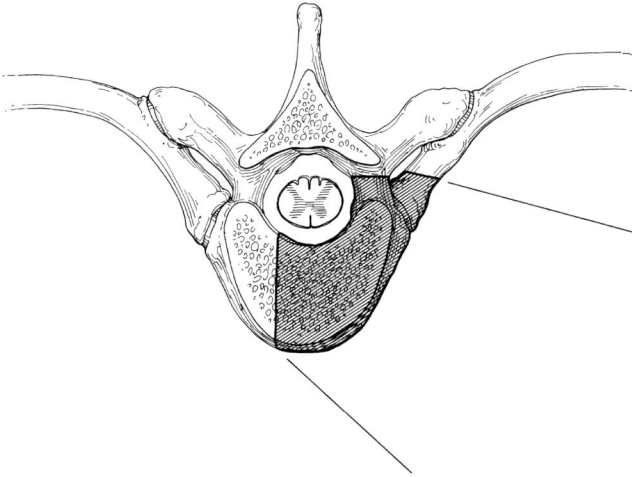

Figure 14 Transthoracic approach. By using the pleural space through a thoracotomy or with thoracoscopy, the lateral aspect of the thoracic vertebral spine can be accessed. Removal of the ipsilateral rib head, pedicle, and vertebral body fully exposes the ventral and lateral spinal canal. This approach is often useful when retropulsed bone fragments from a thoracic fracture occupy this space. (Reprinted with permission from Barrow Neurological Institute.)

site to gauge the depth to the thecal sac. The vertebral body is removed using a combination of osteotomes and a high-speed drill. A bone strut graft or cage is then placed. When T10 is involved, the diaphragm is mobilized. The risks of this procedure include pneumothorax, post-thoracotomy pain syndrome, impaired pulmonary function, and injury to the soft-tissue organs. Depending on the involvement of the posterior column, a second-stage posterior approach might also be needed to provide segmental stabilization through the region.

IX INSTRUMENTATION

A Anterior Instrumentation

After an anterior decompression, an interbody graft (bone graft or cage) is placed for load bearing and to provide anterior support. Before anterior instrumentation was available, an anterior approach was routinely followed by posterior instrumentation to provide compression and to prevent pseudarthrosis. New, commercially available plating systems provide inline compression that prevents graft dislodgement and enhances fusion rates (Fig. 15): the Z-plate for thoracic vertebrae (Sofamor Danek, Memphis TN), VentriFix (Synthes, Paoli, CA), the M2 plates, the Profile plating system, and the Kaneda system (DePuy AcroMed, Cleveland OH). These newer systems have a low profile, and some have in situ adaptable heights to provide a better fit to the patient's anatomy. Depending on the fracture type, posterior instrumentation may not be indicated.

An advantage of performing an anterior decompression and fusion is the limited amount of segments required for fusion. In compression or burst fractures, the bend-

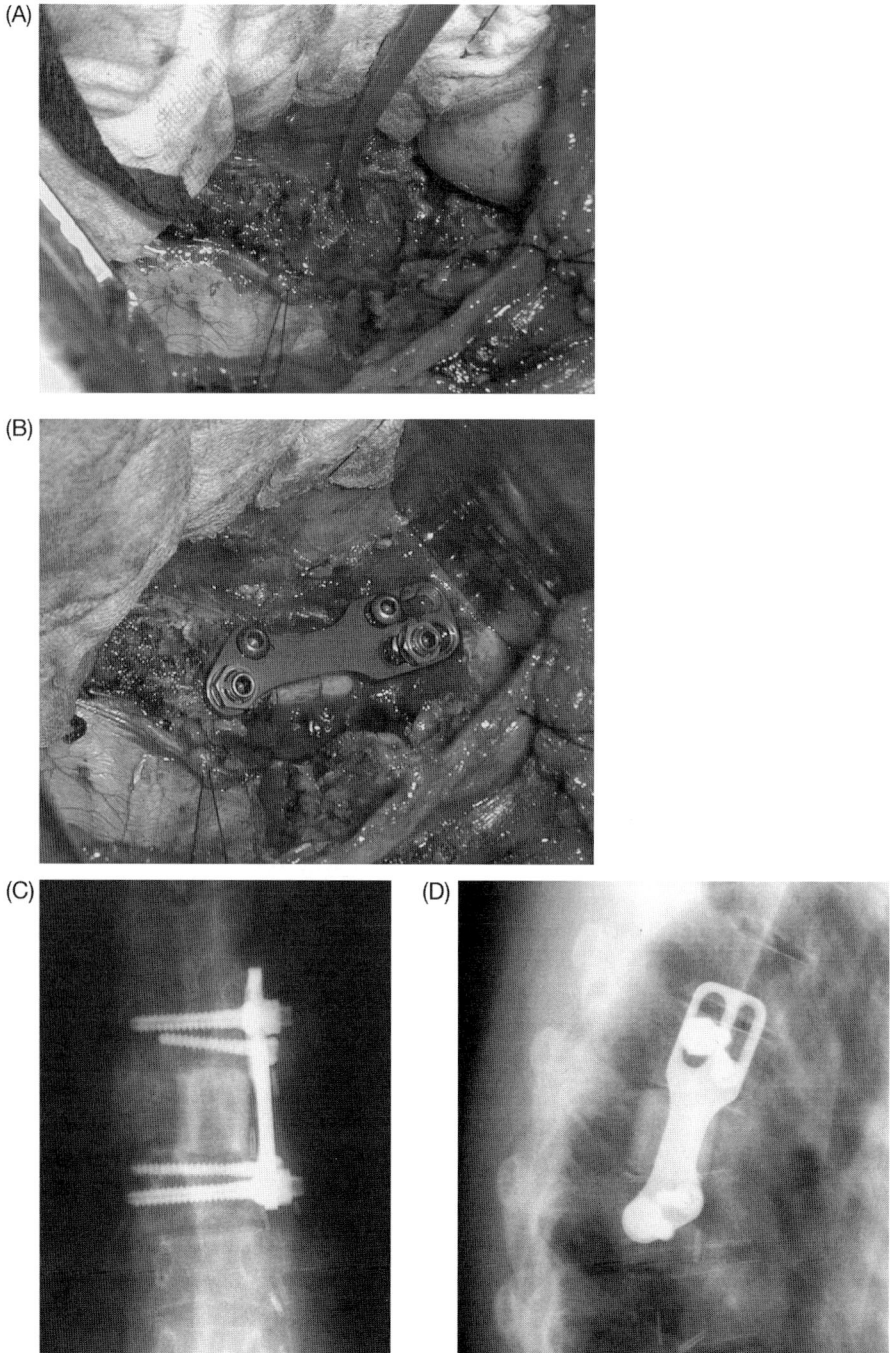

Figure 15   A left-sided thoracotomy centered at T6 was performed in the same pa-
tient as shown in Figure 2. (A) Intraoperative photograph showing a T6 vertebrectomy.
(B) Reduction and stabilization with bone graft and Z-Plate (Sofamor-Danek, Memphis,
TN). Postoperative (C) anteroposterior and (D) lateral radiographs.

ing (flexing) moment is great enough, so that in the absence of an anterior load-bearing construct, a posterior construct would require multiple levels of fixation to resist the bending moment. This posterior construct would have to involve normal adjacent levels with a high risk of failure with pull out of the hook or pedicle construct.

B Posterior Instrumentation

As described by McCullen et al. (79), the development of posterior instrumentation dates to the late 1940s when Harrington began using spinal instrumentation to treat post-polio scoliosis. The Harrington distraction rods anchor into the lamina and span two or more levels above and below the injured segment (Fig. 16A). This system provides local distraction for burst or compression fractures, but it requires long lever arms involving normal segments and is less effective when the anterior column is involved. This system also does not effectively restrict rotational and shearing forces.

Luque developed the technique of segmental fixation by securing contoured rods with sublaminar wires (80) (Fig. 16B). This technique restricts segmental rotation efficiently, but provides no axial support. It is also associated with the potential for neural compromise when the sublaminal wires are placed. Because the wires around the cable cannot be manipulated effectively, this technique neither provides compression nor maintains corrective distraction.

In the mid-1980s, Cotrel et al. (81) introduced a system that merged Harrington's hook-like system with segmental fixation. Multiple hooks are secured to the

(A)   (B)

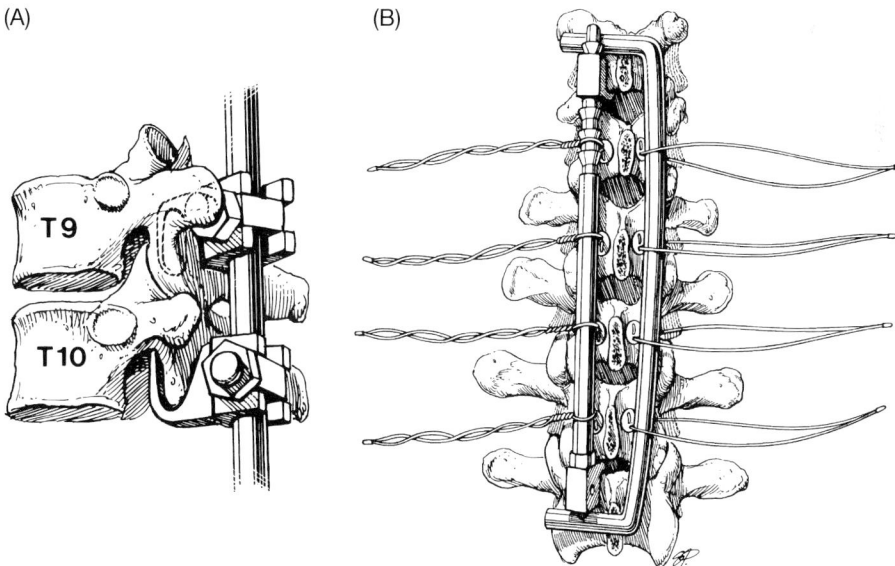

Figure 16   Multiple techniques are available for instrumenting the spine posteriorly: (A) hook–rod constructs as described by Harrington and Cotrel-Dubousset and (B) rod–interspace wiring techniques as described by Luque. (Reprinted with permission from Barrow Neurological Institute.)

lamina, transverse processes, or pedicles along a rod to provide segmental distraction and compression. Bilateral constructs can be cross-linked for improved resistance to torque. This internal construct thus resists compression distraction, shearing, and rotational forces, providing an osteogenic environment for bone fusion. A persistent disadvantage of these constructs is the need to incorporate multiple levels to create sufficient leverage, as a significant moment arm is required to stabilize at increasing distance from the instantaneous axis of rotation. Neurological injury can also be incurred when sublaminar hooks are placed. Newer systems, however, have a much lower profile.

Due to the high stress loads placed on the extreme (cephalad and caudal) poles of the construct, the risk of hook–rod pullout is high, particularly in patients with osteoporosis. Consequently, pedicle screws have been incorporated into these hook–rod constructs. Compared to the lumbar pedicles, midthoracic (T3–T8) pedicles tend to be small. Incorporating the pedicles into the construct in other regions of the thoracic spine provides a biomechanical advantage from the stronger bone–construct interface.

Pedicle screw fixation crosses all three columns of the vertebral axis, facilitating application of corrective forces in all vectors by using a cantilever construct. Fusion segments can be shorter and segmental motion at adjacent levels preserved. Ideally, this technique is suited to treat fracture dislocations. Pedicle screw fixation does not require intact posterior elements, but the status of the anterior columns needs to be assessed carefully. If vertebral body collapse and kyphotic angulation are significant, an anterior strut graft should be placed to prevent hook–pedicle rod failure and to provide a mechanically sound load-sharing construct (82,83).

Inserting screws into thoracic pedicles can be associated with significant morbidity. The anatomy of thoracic pedicles is obscured by the overlying costotransverse and articular facets. In addition, the thecal sac cannot be retracted in the thoracic canal to and with medial pedicle visualization as it can in the lower lumbar canal. Careful radiological examination is needed to determine the feasibility of screw placement. Image-guided surgery might provide some assistance in determining both the feasibility and a safe trajectory. All posterior instrumented constructs need to be supplemented with lateral decortication and some form of bone grafting.

X   OUTCOMES

Over time, the prognosis for patients with thoracic fractures with or without neurological impairment has improved significantly. Much of this improvement is due to advances in the care of persons with paraplegia. Still, little can be done to improve the neurological outcomes of patients with complete neurological injuries and paraplegia below their level of injury once it has occurred. Methylprednisolone given within 8 h of SCI may improve outcome (35,36). Multiple studies have failed to demonstrate significant improvements in such patients even after prompt surgical decompression and stabilization (32,84). Nonetheless, rare patients have improved after early decompression (49).

In summary, complete SCIs due to thoracic fractures offer little hope of recovery below the level of injury, while emergent decompression of incomplete injuries when indicated does appear to be of benefit. The rate of morbidity associated with instrumentation ranges from 1 to 3% in contrast to the complications associated with conservative treatment and prolonged bedrest: deep venous thrombosis, pneumonia, pulmonary embolus, decubitus ulceration, muscle wasting and contractures, urinary tract infections, sepsis, and delayed mobilization and rehabilitation (8,13,53). Long-term failures of stabilization include hardware failures and pseudarthroses. These failures must be factored into any assessment of the efficacy of thoracic stabilization.

XI CONCLUSION

Because of the unique anatomical and biomechanical properties of the thoracic spine, fractures there are less common than other spinal segments. More force may be required to produce an injury in the thoracic spine than at other levels. Because more force is required to injure the thoracic spine and the ratio of spinal canal size to spinal cord size is small, patients with significant thoracic fractures tend to be impaired neurologically. Characteristic injury patterns also occur in the thoracic spine. Prompt diagnosis of thoracic fractures assists with early treatment, which should include immobilization and institution of accepted steroid protocols. Classification schemes of thoracic spinal injury help to determine stability and the need for stabilization procedures. The decision to decompress compromised neural elements will most likely depend on the patient's neurological status and the time elapsed from the initial injury. Anterior and posterior surgical approaches allow access to the compromised spinal canal for decompression and concomitant spinal instrumentation, stabilization, and fusion. Overall, the prognosis of patients with thoracic fractures depends on their neurological status at presentation and the complications associated with the treatments undertaken.

REFERENCES

1. Hanley EN, Jr., Eskay ML. Thoracic spine fractures. Orthopedics 1989;12:689–696.
2. Frankel HL, Hancock DO, Hyslop G, et al. The value of postural reduction in the initial management of closed injuries of the spine with paraplegia and tetraplegia. Paraplegia 1969;7:179–192.
3. Magerl F, Aebi M, Gertzbein SD, Harms J, Nazarian S. A comprehensive classification of thoracic and lumbar injuries. Eur Spine J 1994;3:184–201.
4. Fessler RG, Masson RL. Management of thoracic fractures. In: Menezes AH, Sonntag VK, eds. Principles of Spinal Surgery. New York: McGraw-Hill, 1996:899–918.
5. Denis F. The three column spine and its significance in the classification of acute thoracolumbar spinal injuries. Spine 1983;8:817–831.
6. Rogers LF, Thayer C, Weinberg PE, Kim KS. Acute injuries of the upper thoracic spine associated with paraplegia. Am J Roentgenol 1980;134:67–73.
7. Calenoff L, Chessare JW, Rogers LF, Toerge J, Rosen JS. Multiple level spinal injuries: Importance of early recognition. Am J Roentgenol 1978;130:665–669.
8. Tator CH. Epidemiology and general characteristics of the spinal cord injured patient. In: Benzel EC, Tator CH, eds. Contemporary Management of Spinal Cord Injury. Park Ridge, IL: American Association of Neurological Surgeons, 1994:9–13.
9. Roberts JB, Curtiss PH, Jr. Stability of the thoracic and lumbar spine in traumatic paraplegia following fracture or fracture-dislocation. J Bone Joint Surg Am 1970;52:1115–1130.
10. White AAI, Panjabi MM. Clinical Biomechanics of the Spine. Philadelphia: J.B. Lippincott, 1978.

11. Resnick DK, Weller SJ, Benzel EC. Biomechanics of the thoracolumbar spine. Neurosurg Clin North Am 1997;8:455–469.
12. Lauridsen KN, De Carvalho A, Andersen AH. Degree of vertebral wedging of the dorsolumbar spine. Acta Radiol Diagn (Stockh) 1984;25:29–32.
13. Madsen PW, Lee TT, Eismont FJ, Green BA. Diagnosis and management of thoracic spine fractures. In: Youmans JR, ed. Neurological Surgery. A Comprehensive Reference Guide to the Diagnosis and Management of Neurosurgical Problems, 4th ed. Philadelphia: W. B. Saunders, 1996:2043–2078.
14. Holdsworth FW. Fractures, dislocation, and fracture-dislocations of the spine. J Bone Joint Surg Am 1970;52:1534–1551.
15. Whitesides TE, Jr. Traumatic kyphosis of the thoracolumbar spine. Clin Orthop 1977; 128:78–92.
16. Willen JA, Gaekwad UH, Kakulas BA. Burst fractures in the thoracic and lumbar spine. A clinico-neuropathologic analysis. Spine 1989;14:1316–1323.
17. McAfee PC, Yuan HA, Fredrickson BE, Lubicky JP. The value of computed tomography in thoracolumbar fractures. J Bone Joint Surg Am 1983;65:461–473.
18. O'Callaghan JP, Ullrich CG, Yuan HA, Kieffer SA. CT of facet distraction in flexion injuries of the thoracolumbar spine: The "naked" effect. Am J Roentgenol 1980;134: 563–568.
19. Cooper PR, Cohen W. Evaluation of cervical spinal cord injuries with metrizamide myelography-CT scanning. J Neurosurg 1984;61:281–289.
20. Keene JS. Radiographic evaluation of thoracolumbar fractures. Clin Orthop 1984;189: 58–64.
21. Bondurant FJ, Cotler HB, Kulkarni MV, McArdle CB, Harris JH Jr. Acute spinal cord injury. A study using physical examination and magnetic resonance imaging. Spine 1990; 15:161–168.
22. Blumenkopf B, Juneau PA, 3rd. Magnetic resonance imaging (MRI) of thoracolumbar fractures. J Spinal Disord 1988;1:144–150.
23. Brightman RP, Miller CA, Rea GL, Chakeres DW, Hunt WE. Magnetic resonance imaging of trauma to the thoracic and lumbar spine. The importance of the posterior longitudinal ligament. Spine 1992;17:541–550.
24. Tracy PT, Wright RM, Hanigan WC. Magnetic resonance imaging of spinal injury. Spine 1989;14:292–301.
25. McAfee PC, Yuan HA, Lasda NA. The unstable burst fracture. Spine 1982;7:365–373.
26. Kostuik JP, Huler RS, Eesses SI, Stauffer ES. Thoracolumbar spine fractures. In: Frymoyer JW, ed. The Adult Spine: Principles and Practice. New York: Raven Press, Ltd., 1991:1269–1327.
27. Hashimoto T, Kaneda K, Abumi K. Relationship between traumatic spinal canal stenosis and neurologic deficits in thoracolumbar burst fractures. Spine 1988;13:1268–1272.
28. Chance CQ. Note on a type of flexion fracture of the spine. Br J Radiol 1948;21:452.
29. American College of Surgeons. Advanced Trauma Life Support Manual. Chicago: American College of Surgeons, 1992.
30. Vale FL, Burns J, Jackson AB, Hadley MN. Combined medical and surgical treatment after acute spinal cord injury: Results of a prospective pilot study to assess the merits of aggressive medical resuscitation and blood pressure management. J Neurosurg 1997; 87:239–246.
31. Kirschblum SC, O'Connor KC. Predicting neurologic recovery in traumatic cervical spinal cord injury. Arch Phys Med Rehabil 1998;79:1456–1466.
32. Waters RL, Adkins RH, Yakura JS, Sie I. Effect of surgery on motor recovery following traumatic spinal cord injury. Spinal Cord 1996;34:188–192.
33. Waters RL, Adkins RH, Yakura JS, Sie I. Motor and sensory recovery following incomplete paraplegia. Arch Phys Med Rehabil 1994;75:67–72.

34. American Spinal Injury Association. American Spinal Injury Association: Standard for Neurological Classification of Spinal Injury Patients. Chicago, IL: American Spinal Injury Association, 1982.

35. Bracken MB, Shepard MJ, Collins WF, et al. A randomized, controlled trial of methylprednisolone or naloxone in the treatment of acute spinal-cord injury. Results of the Second National Acute Spinal Cord Injury Study. N Engl J Med 1990;322:1405–1411.

36. Bracken MB, Shepard MJ, Holford TR, et al. Administration of methylprednisolone for 24 or 48 hours or tirilazad mesylate for 48 hours in the treatment of acute spinal cord injury. Results of the Third National Acute Spinal Cord Injury Randomized Controlled Trial. National Acute Spinal Cord Injury Study. JAMA 1997;277:1597–1604.

37. Geisler FH, Dorsey FC, Coleman WP. Recovery of motor function after spinal-cord injury—a randomized, placebo-controlled trial with GM-1 ganglioside. N Engl J Med 1991;324:1659–1660.

38. Guttmann L. The conservative management of closed injuries of the vertebral column resulting in damage to the spinal cord and spinal roots. In: Vinken PJ, Brwyn GW, eds. Handbook of Clinical Neurology. New York: American Elsevier, 1976:285–306.

39. Young JS, Dexter WR. Neurological recovery distal to the zone of injury in 172 cases of closed, traumatic spinal cord injury. Paraplegia 1978;16:39–49.

40. Burke DC, Murray DD. The management of thoracic and thoraco-lumbar injuries of the spine with neurological involvement. J Bone Joint Surg Br 1976;58:72–78.

41. Leidholt JD, Young JJ, Hahn HR, Jackson RE, Gamble WE, Miles JS. Evaluation of late spinal deformities with fracture-dislocations of the dorsal and lumbar spine in paraplegics. Paraplegia 1969;7:16–28.

42. Nash CL, Schatzinger LH, Brown RH, Brodkey J. The unstable thoracic compression fracture. Spine 1977;2:261–265.

43. Schaefer DM, Flanders AE, Osterholm JL, Northrup BE. Prognostic significance of magnetic resonance imaging in the acute phase of cervical spine injury. J Neurosurg 1992;76:218–223.

44. Alander DH, Parker J, Stauffer ES. Intermediate-term outcome of cervical spinal cord-injured patients older than 50 years of age. Spine 1997;22:1189–1192.

45. Carlson GD, Minato Y, Okada A, et al. Early time-dependent decompression for spinal cord injury: Vascular mechanisms of recovery. J Neurotrauma 1997;14:951–962.

46. Delamarter RB, Sherman J, Carr JB. Pathophysiology of spinal cord injury. Recovery after immediate and delayed decompression. J Bone Joint Surg Am 1995;77:1042–1049.

47. Guha A, Tator CH, Endrenyi L, Piper I. Decompression of the spinal cord improves recovery after acute experimental spinal cord compression injury. Paraplegia 1987;25:324–339.

48. Aebi M, Mohler J, Zach GA, Morscher E. Indication, surgical technique, and results of 100 surgically-treated fractures and fracture-dislocations of the cervical spine. Clin Orthop 1986;203:244–257.

49. Benzel EC, Larson SJ. Clinical observation and notes: Functional recovery after decompressive operations for thoracic and lumbar spine fractures. Neurosurgery 1986;19:722–728.

50. Wilberger JE. Diagnosis and management of spinal cord trauma. J Neurotrauma 1991; Suppl 1:S21–S30.

51. Levi L, Wolf A, Rigamonti D, Ragheb J, Mirvis S, Robinson WL. Anterior decompression in cervical spine trauma: Does the timing of surgery affect the outcome? Neurosurgery 1991;29:216–222.

52. Tator CH, Duncan EG, Edmonds VE, Lapczak LI, Andrews DF. Comparison of surgical and conservative management in 208 patients with acute spinal cord injury. Can J Neurol Sci 1987;14:60–69.

53. Vaccaro AR, Daughtery RJ, Sheehan TP, et al. Neurologic outcome of early versus late surgery for cervical spinal cord injury. Spine 1997;22:2609–2613.
54. Farmer J, Vaccaro A, Albert TJ, Malone S, Balderston RA, Cotler JM. Neurologic deterioration after cervical spinal cord injury. J Spinal Disord 1998;11:192–196.
55. Heiden JS, Weiss MH, Rosenberg AW, Apuzzo ML, Kurz T. Management of cervical spinal cord trauma in Southern California. J Neurosurg 1975;43:732–736.
56. Marshall LF, Knowlton S, Garfin SR, et al. Deterioration following spinal cord injury. A multicenter study. J Neurosurg 1987;66:400–404.
57. Gertzbein SD. Scoliosis Research Society. Multicenter spine fracture study. Spine 1992; 17:528–540.
58. Bradford DS, Akbarnia BA, Winter RB, Seljeskog EL. Surgical stabilization of fracture and fracture dislocation of the thoracic spine. Spine 1977;2:185–196.
59. Cantor JB, Lebwohl NH, Garvey T, Eismont FJ. Nonoperative management of stable thoracolumbar burst fractures with early ambulation and bracing. Spine 1993;18:971–976.
60. Chakera TM, Bedbrook G, Bradley CM. Spontaneous resolution of spinal canal deformity after burst-dispersion fracture. Am J Neuroradiol 1988;9:779–785.
61. Fidler MW. Remodeling of the spinal canal after burst fracture. A prospective study of two cases. J Bone Joint Surg Br 1988;70:730–732.
62. Mumford J, Weinstein JN, Spratt KF, Goel VK. Thoracolumbar burst fractures. The clinical efficacy and outcome of nonoperative management. Spine 1993;18:955–970.
63. Brown CW, Gorup JM, Chow GH. Thoracic burst fractures; nonsurgical treatment. In: Zdbelick TA, Benzel EC, Anderson PA, Stillerman CB, eds. Controversy in Spine Surgery. St. Louis, MO: Quality Medical, 1999:86–96.
64. Denis F, Armstrong GW, Searls K, Matta L. Acute thoracolumbar burst fractures in the absence of neurologic deficit. A comparison between operative and nonoperative treatment. Clin Orthop 1984;189:142–149.
65. Kostuik JP. Anterior fixation for burst fractures of the thoracic and lumbar spine with or without neurological involvement. Spine 1988;13:286–293.
66. Bradford DS, McBride GG. Surgical management of thoracolumbar spine fractures with incomplete neurologic deficits. Clin Orthop 1987;218:201–216.
67. Harrington RM, Budorick T, Hoyt J, Anderson PA, Tencer AF. Biomechanics of indirect reduction of bone retropulsed into the spinal canal in vertebral fracture. Spine 1993;18: 692–699.
68. Esses SI, Botsford DJ, Kostuik JP. Evaluation of surgical treatment for burst fractures. Spine 1990;15:667–673.
69. Shono Y, McAfee PC, Cunningham BW. Experimental study of thoracolumbar burst fractures. A radiographic and biomechanical analysis of anterior and posterior instrumentation systems. Spine 1994;19:1711–1722.
70. Triantafyllou SJ, Gertzbein SD. Flexion distraction injuries of the thoracolumbar spine: A review. Orthopedics 1992;15:357–364.
71. Willen J. Unstable thoracolumbar injuries. Orthopedics 1992;15:329–335.
72. Bohlman HH, Freehafer A, Dejak J. The results of treatment of acute injuries of the upper thoracic spine with paralysis. J Bone Joint Surg Am 1985;67:360–369.
73. Larson SJ, Holst RA, Hemmy DC, Sances A, Jr. Lateral extracavitary approach to traumatic lesions of the thoracic and lumbar spine. J Neurosurg 1976;45:628–637.
74. Fessler RG, Dietze DD, Jr., Millan MM, Peace D. Lateral parascapular extrapleural approach to the upper thoracic spine. J Neurosurg 1991;75:349–355.
75. Kostuik JP. Anterior fixation for fractures of the thoracic and lumbar spine with or without neurologic involvement. Clin Orthop 1984;189:103–115.
76. Sharan AD, Przybylski GJ, Tartaglino L. Approaching the upper thoracic vertebrae without sternotomy or thoracotomy: A radiographic analysis with clinical application. Spine 2000;25:910–916.

77. Lesoin F, Thomas CE III, Autricque A, Villette L, Jomin M. A transsternal biclavicular approach to the upper anterior thoracic spine. Surg Neurol 1986;26:253–256.
78. Birch R, Bonney G, Marshall RW. A surgical approach to the cervicothoracic spine. J Bone Joint Surg Br 1990;72:904–907.
79. McCullen G, Vaccaro AR, Garfin SR. Thoracic and lumbar trauma: Rationale for selecting the appropriate fusion technique. Orthop Clin North Am 1998;29:813–828.
80. Luque ER. The anatomic basis for the development of segmental spinal instrumentation. Spine 1982;7:256–259.
81. Cotrel Y, Dubousset J, Guillaumat M. New universal instrumentation in spinal surgery. Clin Orthop 1988;227:10–23.
82. McCormack T, Karaikovic E, Gaines RW. The load sharing classification of spine fractures. Spine 1994;19:1741–1744.
83. McLain RF, Sparling E, Benson DR. Early failure of short segment pedicle instrumentation for thoracolumbar fractures. J Bone Joint Surg Am 1993;75:162–187.
84. Waters RL, Adkins RH, Yakura JS, Sie I. Motor and sensory recovery following complete tetraplegia. Arch Phys Med Rehabil 1993;74:242–247.

32

Thoracolumbar Trauma

GLENN R. RECHTINE

University of Florida, Gainesville, Florida, U.S.A.

MICHAEL J. BOLESTA

University of Texas Southwestern Medical Center, Dallas, Texas, U.S.A.

I INTRODUCTION

Fractures and other injuries at the thoracolumbar region are the most common spinal injuries. The rigid thoracic segment and the mobile lumbar spine create a junction with a concentration of stresses that account for higher likelihood of injury between T10 and L2 than in other areas of the spine. Not only are these injuries the most common, but also they provide some of the greatest controversy as to the appropriate treatment.

II NONCONTIGUOUS INJURIES

Once a spinal fracture has been identified, the search is not over. Approximately 20 to 25% of patients will have more than one spinal injury. Half of these will be at the adjoining segment. The other half will be at other levels of the spine. Junctional injuries (cervicothoracic, occipital thoracolumbar, and lumbosacral fractures) are commonly associated noncontiguous injuries (1–5). Each injury must be evaluated and an appropriate treatment plan developed. The clinician must also take any other nonspinal injuries into account and synthesizes a comprehensive care plan.

III REMODELING

The development of computed tomography (CT) technology demonstrated the canal compromise associated with burst fractures (Fig. 1C). As a result, there was a huge increase in spinal canal decompressions, using a variety of approaches and tech-

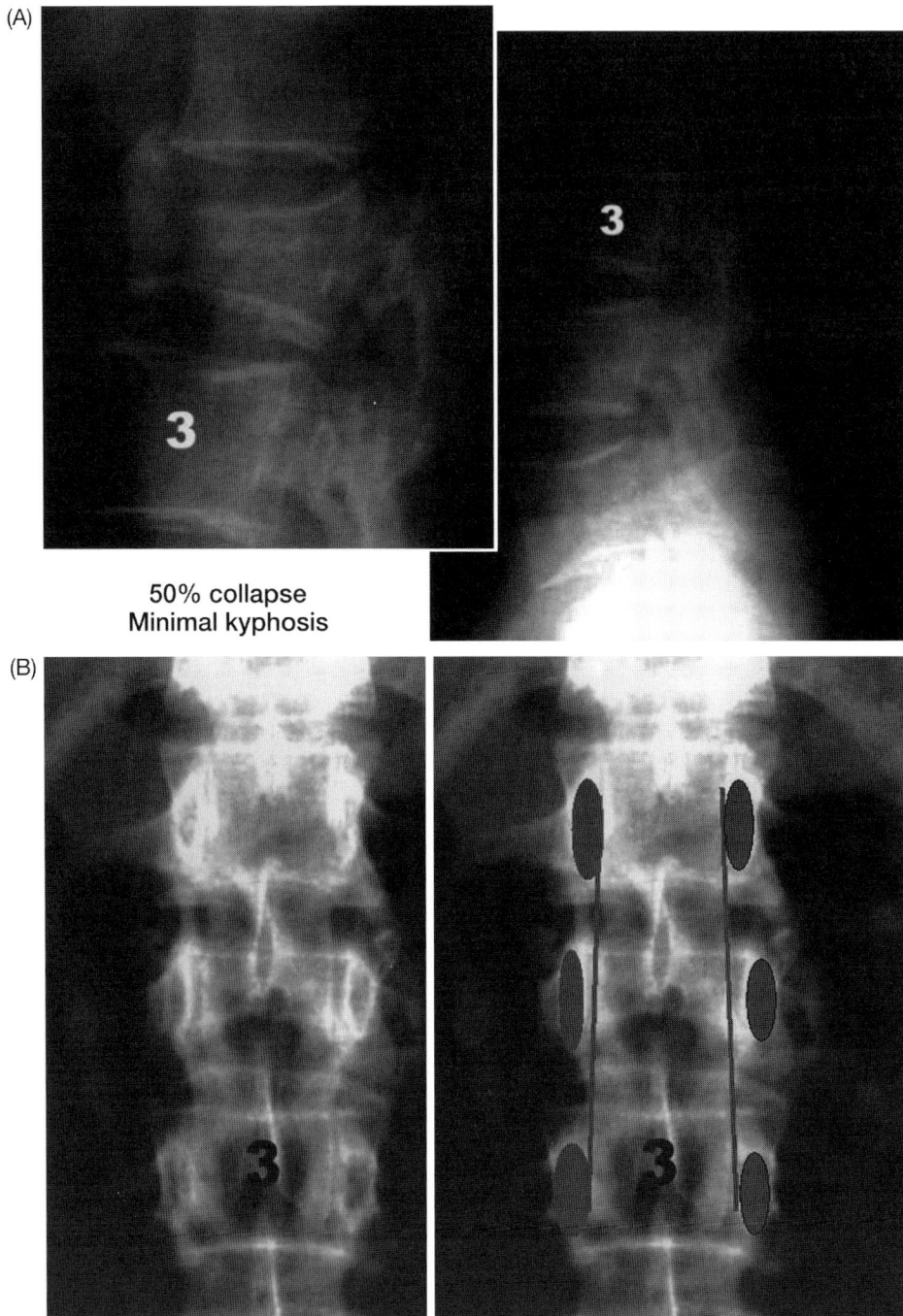

(A)

50% collapse
Minimal kyphosis

(B)

Figure 1 (A) Lateral x-ray showing L2 fracture. (B) AP x-ray showing interpedicular widening. (C) Axial CT image showing burst component.

(C)

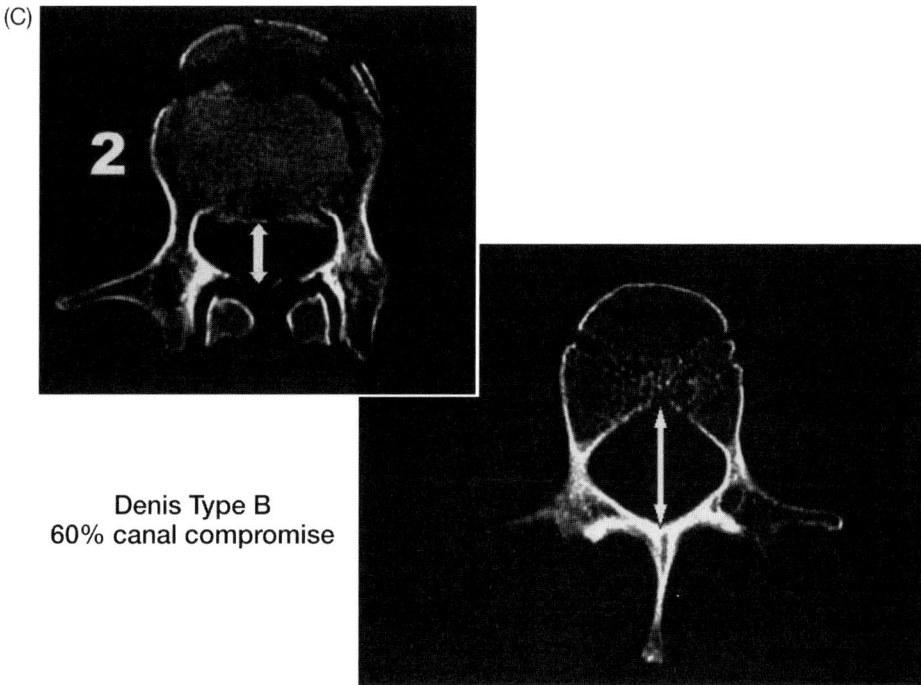

Denis Type B
60% canal compromise

Figure 1 Continued

niques. With long-term follow-up, there was also the realization that the spinal canal will commonly remodel, with or without surgical intervention (6–13). Furthermore, the degree of neurological dysfunction, if any, correlated poorly with the degree of residual canal stenosis. The mere presence of bony canal stenosis does not justify surgical intervention in the absence of other signs or symptoms (14).

IV CLASSIFICATION

The classification of thoracolumbar injuries is a major debate. Originally, Holdsworth had a two-column theory. Plain radiographs are used to differentiate various thoracolumbar injuries. In the 1980s, the Denis classification, based on a three-column concept, emerged as the standard. McAfee modified this scheme (15). The most recent comprehensive classification system is that of the Association for the Study of Internal Fixation (AO/ASIF). Magerl and his team developed this mechanistic classification through analysis of 1200 fractures (16).

A Holdsworth Classification

In the Holdsworth classification, the vertebral body, disks, and longitudinal ligaments constitute the anterior column. The posterior bony elements and ligaments make up the posterior column. The anterior column is loaded in compression; the poster elements are loaded in tension. In this classification system, the instability patterns are associated with posterior column failure.

B Denis Classification

In 1983, Denis introduced the notion of the middle column, which is the posterior half of the vertebral body, the disk, and the posterior longitudinal ligament. This arose from the development of the CT scan. The burst fracture that Holdsworth described is better delineated by the Denis classification. He described five variations of the burst fracture. The Denis B involves only the superior and endplate alone and was by far the most common (Fig. 1A,B). Axial loading typically produces this type of burst fracture. For many years surgery was carried out to decompress the spinal canal for fear of late spinal stenosis symptoms. With the observation of spontaneous spinal canal remodeling, it became apparent why delayed neurogenic claudication was quite rare. The development of the CT scanner engendered a fallacious indication for surgery. The stenosis of the burst fracture had occurred throughout human history, but resolved without intervention. McAfee's addition to the Denis classification was the so-called "unstable burst fracture," which had ligamentous instability as well as bony disruption. The Denis classification includes the slice fracture. The presence of a rotational component in the Denis type D burst fracture actually makes it a fracture dislocation. All three columns are injured and the spine is globally unstable.

C Magerl Classification

Magerl spent years evaluating the fracture patterns in 1200 injuries. He then developed an AO/ASIF classification that consists of an ABC system. The A patterns are axial loading injuries. The B injuries are the result of distraction. The C lesions are characterized by rotation. Obviously, many injuries are produced by combinations of these forces. Magerl accommodated this by subdividing each section of the classification into several levels. In this mechanistic classification, severity of injury tends to progress from A to B to C, and there is an associated increase in concomitant neurological injury. In its most basic form, ABC is a very good classification. In its full form, it is difficult to use. Consider an injury with an axial load anteriorly and a distraction component posteriorly. Some clinicians would class this as an A injury because of the axial portion; others would call it a type of the B injury.

Perhaps the original Holdsworth classification of anterior and posterior columns is adequate and most appropriate. It is posterior ligamentous disruption that significantly changes the overall stability of the fracture. The middle-column concept does not assist patient management. In general, everyone should be familiar with all the different classification systems listed above. It is unlikely that one will be universally accepted, although that would facilitate outcomes research. Each individual physician will have to decide which classification system best facilitates patient care.

V NONOPERATIVE TREATMENT

At the present time, one of the most controversial aspects of thoracolumbar fracture care revolves around the indications for surgical intervention. This can be considered by addressing the indications for nonsurgical treatment. The original treatment of all thoracolumbar injuries was nonoperative. Laminectomy for trauma was described at least as early as the seventh century A.D., but rarely decompresses the neural elements, often worsens any neurological deficit, destabilizes the spinal column, and leads to painful deformity. It is of historical significance, but should almost never be performed in isolation. Bedrest, casting, and bracing have been the mainstays of nonsurgical treatment in the modern era. A recent clinical series by Rechtine et al. showed that acute hospitalization complications were less in patients with nonoperative treatment consisting of 6 weeks of Roto-Rest bed treatment as compared to surgical intervention (17). Pulmonary problems, mortality, skin (decubitus ulceration), and other medical complications were the same in both populations. There was a significant risk of infection with surgical intervention that could not occur in those treated nonoperatively. Two studies demonstrated that patients who are neurologically intact have less than 20 degrees of kyphosis, less than 50% canal compromise, and less than 50% compression are best managed with recumbency. The cost of such treatment can be half of that of surgical intervention (18–20). Cantor demonstrated the effective use of a thoraco-lumbo-sacro-orthosis (TLSO) and short-term hospitalization for thoracolumbar injuries (21). They were adamant that posterior ligamentous injury is a contraindication for this type of fracture management.

Not every patient requires 6 weeks of bedrest. The vast majority of thoracolumbar injuries can be managed with early mobilization and no surgery. Currently we use the Roto-Rest bed until the injury site is nontender. Then the patient is fit with an orthosis.

Ligamentous instability is not an injury that is amenable to nonsurgical management. This will most likely result in a progressive painful deformity. Even if the original studies do not suggest a ligamentous injury, every patient should be evaluated for radiographic evidence of instability. Usually this is accomplished with upright (standing or sitting) anteroposterior and lateral radiographs in the cast or orthosis. If the posterior ligaments are incompetent, a progressive kyphosis can result. The upright radiographs should be repeated at regular intervals to assess for progressive deformity. A series from Colorado showed that, even in the face of interspinous widening, the injury could be managed with a hyperextension cast with no deleterious long-term effects (22). The degree of ligamentous disruption that mandates surgical stabilization is unknown. With a minimum of 2-year follow-up, Kraemer showed no difference in the functional outcome of patients treated operatively or nonoperatively. Singer and Knight reported similar findings (23–25).

VI BRACES AND ORTHOSES

Braces are commonly used after surgery or nonoperative treatment. There is no good scientific evidence that they are effective at preventing deformity or hardware failure. One in vivo study suggested that braces and harnesses were ineffective at reducing the loads on the spinal instrumentation. In fact, some of the loads were even higher in the orthoses (26). Braces are probably best used as a reminder for the patient and family members to restrict activities.

VII TIMING OF SURGERY

There is no consensus as to the best timing of surgery. The arguments range from immediate to late decompressions. Bohlman et al. demonstrated that pain relief and neurological function could be improved even if surgery was delayed an average of 4.5 years after injury (27). If the surgery is done within the first 2 years after injury, the results as measured by neurological improvement are better (28). Clohisy suggests that the results are better if done within the first 48 h as compared to a group that underwent surgery an average of 61 days postinjury (29).

Yazici compared patients who underwent indirect canal reduction within 24 h of injury to those operated outside that period (13). This retrospective study involved 18 patients (10 early, 8 late). The indirect canal clearance and restoration of sagittal correction was better with surgery performed within 24 h of injury. A larger series of cases from Syracuse indicated that the first 72 h were optimal for surgery in patients with multiple injuries (ISS equal or greater than 18) and in those with concomitant cervical injuries with a neurological deficit (30).

VIII SPINAL CORD MONITORING

Spinal cord monitoring in surgery for intact or incomplete injuries is a way to reduce the risk of iatrogenic injuries. Robinson has shown that femoral nerve monitoring can be used to assess the midlumbar roots in the face of thoracolumbar injuries (14).

IX POSTERIOR SURGERY

The oldest and simplest surgical intervention for spinal trauma is the laminectomy. Described as early as the seventh century A.D., this surgery actually predated the development of general anesthesia. At the thoracolumbar junction, it is rare that a laminectomy would be performed in isolation. Paul Harrington's deformity instrumentation was adapted to trauma in the late 1970s. This was extremely controversial at the time and began a history of operative treatment with reasonably successful results. The hope was the surgical procedure would decrease the time of hospitalization as well as the cost, and increase the likelihood of neurological recovery. Over the years, many studies have attempted to document this, but unsuccessfully to date. Studies have shown that surgical treatment will decrease the hospital time over a period of long-term bed rest, but otherwise the complications and neurological recovery appear to be the same.

The original Harrington instrumentation required long segment fusions extending two to three segments proximal and distal to the injury to achieve mechanical stability. For the thoracolumbar junction, this involved fusion of much of the lumbar spine. In the mid-1980s, Rae Jacobs suggested the rod-long–fuse-short technique. The rods spanned the five or more segments required by the Harrington technique, but only the injured levels were grafted with bone. This necessitated rod removal at 9 months to 1 year after the injury. There have been several studies documenting an excellent return of motion of the segments that had been up immobilized but not fused.

About the same time, short segment fixation was developed in Europe. This technique involves placing pedicle screws at the level above and below the level of the injury. This allowed for short segment fixation, short segment fusion, and, theoretically, the avoidance of problems with injuring noninjured segments. Initial problems were loss of reduction and failure of fixation. The construct did not restore the integrity of the anterior structure, loading the device in a cantilever mode. Nonetheless, the results for this technique were comparable to other methods. There was a high incidence of screw fracture from fatigue, but the clinical results were good. Bone grafting through the pedicle was performed in an attempt to reconstitute the anterior column. These techniques were fraught with infrequent, but sometimes catastrophic, complications. One may adopt the strengths of long and short segment fixation by placing a claw construct above and a pedicle screw fixation two levels below the injury. There is sufficient leverage to reduce and hold most fractures. If there is a globally unstable fracture dislocation, more segments may be included. Some sort of cross-linkage between the rods will improve rotational stability.

X   ANTERIOR SURGERY

The addition of anterior surgery for thoracolumbar trauma is relatively recent. The spinal canal compression is usually anterior. The anterior or lateral approach allows for a direct spinal canal decompression and visualization of the decompression. The requirement for thoracotomy or retroperitoneal approach demands greater surgical skill and increases the risks of complications as compared to the posterior approach (31). Anteriorly, allograft has been used with good success as opposed to the dismal results from the use of allograft for posterior or posterolateral fusion in adults (32).

Anterior structures are manipulated, but the approach, decompression, and instrumentation are really lateral. All instrumentation must be placed so that there is no contact with any pulsating vessel to avoid catastrophic complications. A safe location for the instrumentation must be determined from the preoperative CT scan or MRI. Patient anatomy dictates whether a left- or right-sided approach will be used for the surgery. Selecting the incorrect side may preclude instrumentation, limit the instrumentation to intervertebral cages, or risk late vessel erosion. The angle of approach can vary from a transpedicular approach to a costotransversectomy to a transthoracic or retroperitoneal approach. The more anterior, the better the visualization of the spinal canal. Selection will vary with the experiences and preferences of the surgeon. A possible variation is to perform a transthoracic extrapleural dissection. This may reduce the need for a thoracostomy tube.

XI   ANTERIOR INSTRUMENTATION

The recent popularity of anterior surgery is in part the result of advances in anterior instrumentation. Without instrumentation, anterior decompressions and fusions required either bedrest or posterior stabilization as well. With rigid instrumentation, it is possible to achieve decompression and stabilization with one surgery.

A   Biomechanics

Currently there are over 15 different varieties of anterior instrumentation. Almost every manufacturer of spinal implants has at least one anterior thoracolumbar implant. The differences include unicortical versus bicortical screw purchase, ability to compress and distract, strength, rigidity of the implant, and fatigue life (33–36). None of them will adequately stabilize a fracture dislocation as a stand-alone device.

B   Clinical Results

Professor Kaneda has extensive experience with anterior decompression and instrumentation. His series of 140 patients with thoracolumbar injuries and neurological deficits with 5 to 12 years follow-up is a landmark publication (37). There was a 93% successful fusion. He noted nine broken implants; 95% of the patients improved neurological function by one Frankel grade. Smaller series with shorter follow-up and other implants have shown similar results (38–47).

XII   360 FUSION

Several authors have advocated the use of a combined anterior and posterior procedure (48–50). There are no good controlled studies to indicate that the results are superior to either anterior or posterior surgery alone. Defino's series of 43 patients included four deaths (9%) and three infections (7%).

XIII   COMPARISON OF METHODS OF TREATMENT

Grace surveyed the need for anterior decompression after vertebral burst fractures (51). In this survey, 56% of neurosurgeons and 81% of orthopedic surgeons treated a neurologically intact patient with stabilization alone. Patients with partial, stable, or improving neurological injuries were managed with anterior direct decompression by 84% of the neurosurgeons and 77% of the orthopedic surgeons.

In a comparison of anterior, posterior, and combined surgery for thoracolumbar burst fractures, there was no significant difference as measured by kyphosis correction, neurological function, pain, or return to work. The cost, operative time, and blood loss was less with isolated posterior surgery (52).

In a retrospective analysis of 24 patients with greater than 2-year follow-up after thoracolumbar spine fracture without neurological deficit, the SF-36 and Roland scales were found to be comparable to patients with diabetes and low back pain. The scores did not demonstrate any functional difference between those patients treated operatively and those managed nonoperatively. There was poor correlation between residual kyphosis and outcome (23). What constitutes appropriate indications for surgical intervention of thoracolumbar fractures is an ongoing debate. The recommendation from Iowa is that patients who are neurologically intact, with angular deformity less than 20 degrees, residual spinal canal area greater than 50%, and preservation of greater than 50% anterior vertebral height should be treated nonoperatively (19,20). The outcomes of such patients were good. Complications noted in the literature with nonoperative treatment and specific operative approaches for thoracolumbar spine trauma are detailed in Table 1.

XIV   PEDIATRICS

In the pediatric population, there are concerns that differ from adult injuries. In the adolescent population, fractures of the apophyseal ring will present with disklike symptoms (i.e., radiculopathy). These are usually not diagnosed without CT and can be missed with MRI (65,66).

Table 1 Complications of Thoracolumbar Spine Trauma Intervention

Approach	Complication
Anterior	Pseudomeningocele, infection, meningitis (53), vessel injury, viscus injury, chylothorax (54,55), iatrogenic neurological deficit
Posterior	Transdural screw placement (56), infection, instrumentation migration (57), iatrogenic neurological deficit
Nonsurgical	Main bronchus laceration by thoracic fracture fragments (58), rupture of descending aorta with T11 compression fracture (59), thoracic spine fracture with esophageal rupture (60,61), traumatic pseudomeningocele through spina bifida occulta deformity (62,63) subarachnoid hematoma 4/100 (64)

In children, the possibility of further growth provides different options. In a child with remaining growth and a post-traumatic kyphosis, one alternative is a short segment posterior fusion. Continued anterior growth will reduce the kyphosis (67).

Flexion distraction injuries are most commonly associated with seat-belt usage. In contrast, Sturm and coworkers reported seven cases of compression fractures in children with seat-belt usage. They presumed that the posterior ligamentous complex was sufficient to withstand the applied load. This would concentrate the forces on the anterior column, which fails in compression (68).

One of the concerns after any significant pediatric injury is the long-term effect. Even in young patients, the injury could have lasting consequences. In a series of patients who were 8 to 20 years of age at the time of injury, half of them had disk degeneration and endplate changes adjacent to a compression fracture (69).

XV HIGH-TECH FUTURE POSSIBILITIES

Minimally invasive techniques are being used for fracture stabilization. The theoretical advantages of less tissue damage, quicker recovery, and fewer complications have not yet been realized. Small series of endoscopically assisted surgery have been reported (70–73). As more and more experience is obtained, the role of such technology will be defined. Verheyden reported 16 patients who had surgery with the assistance of real-time intraoperative MRI monitoring. The artifact from the instrumentation did not seem to be insurmountable (74).

REFERENCES

1. Albertsen AM, Jurik AG. Posttraumatic spinal osteolysis in ankylosing spondylitis as part of pseudoarthrosis. A case report. Acta Radiol 1996; 37(1):98–100.
2. Arthornthurasook A, Thongmag P. Thoracolumbar burst fracture with another spinal fracture. J Med Assoc Thai 1990; 73(5):279–282, 1990.
3. Pouilles JM, Tremollieres F, Roux C, Sebert JL, Alexandre C, Goldberg D, Treves R, Khalifa P, et al. Effects of cyclical etidronate therapy on bone loss in early postmenopausal women who are not undergoing hormonal replacement therapy. Osteoporos Int 1997; 7(3):213–218.

4. Rechtine GR, Sutterlin CE, Wood GW, Boyd RJ, Mansfield FL. The efficacy of pedicle screw/plate fixation on lumbar/lumbosacral autogenous bone graft fusion in adult patients with degenerative spondylolisthesis. J Spinal Disord 1996; 9(5):382–391.

5. Vedantam R, Crawford AH. Multiple noncontiguous injuries of the spine in a child: atlantooccipital dislocation and seat-belt injury of the lumbar spine. Acta Orthop Belg 1997; 63(1):23–27.

6. de Klerk LW, Fontijne WP, Stijnen T, Braakman R, Tanghe HL, van Linge B. Spontaneous remodeling of the spinal canal after conservative management of thoracolumbar burst fractures. Spine 1998; 23(9):1057–1060.

7. Ha KI, Han SH, Chung M, Yang BK, Youn GH. A clinical study of the natural remodeling of burst fractures of the lumbar spine. Clin Orthop 1996; (323):210–214.

8. Karlsson MK, Hasserius R, Sundgren P, Redlund-Johnell I, Ohlin A. Remodeling of the spinal canal deformed by trauma. J Spinal Disord 1997; 10(2):157–161.

9. Kuner EH, Schlickewei W, Kuner A, Hauser U. Restoration of the spinal canal by the internal fixator and remodeling. Eur Spine J 1997; 6(6):417–422.

10. Johnsson R, Herrlin K, Hagglund G, Stromqvist B. Spinal canal remodeling after thoracolumbar fractures with intraspinal bone fragments. 17 cases followed 1–4 years. Acta Orthop Scand 1991; 62(2):125–127.

11. Scapinelli R, Candiotto, S. Spontaneous remodeling of the spinal canal after burst fractures of the low thoracic and lumbar region. J Spinal Disord 1995; 8(6):486–493.

12. Sjostrom L, Jacobsson O, Karlstrom G, Pech P, Rauschning W. Spinal canal remodelling after stabilization of thoracolumbar burst fractures. Eur Spine J 1994; 3(6):312–317.

13. Yazici M, Atilla B, Tepe S, Calisir A. Spinal canal remodeling in burst fractures of the thoracolumbar spine: a computerized tomographic comparison between operative and nonoperative treatment. J Spinal Disord 1996; 9(5):409–413.

14. Robinson L, Slimp J, Anderson P, Stolov W. The efficacy of femoral nerve intraoperative somatosensory evoked potentials during surgical treatment of thoracolumbar fractures. Spine 1993; 18(13):1793–1797.

15. McAfee P, Yuan H, Lasda N. The unstable burst fracture. Spine 1982; 7(4):365–373.

16. Magerl F, Aebi M, Gertzbein SD, Harms J, Nazarian S. A comprehensive classification of thoracic and lumbar injuries. Eur Spine J 1994; 3(4):184–201.

17. Rechtine G, Cahill D, Chrin A. Treatment of thoracolumbar trauma: comparison of complications of operative versus nonoperative treatment. J Spinal Disord 1999; 12(5): 406–409.

18. Domenicucci M, Preite R, Ramieri A, Ciappetta P, Delfini R, Romanini L. Thoracolumbar fractures without neurosurgical involvement: surgical or conservative treatment? J Neurosurg Sci 1996; 40(1):1–10.

19. Hitchon PW, Torner JC, Haddad SF, Follett KA. Management options in thoracolumbar burst fractures. Surg Neurol 1998; 49(6):619–626.

20. Mumford J, Weinstein J, Spratt K, Goel V. Thoracolumbar burst fractures. The clinical efficacy and outcome of nonoperative management. Spine 1993; 18(8):955–970.

21. Cantor J, Lebwohl N, Garvey T, Eismont F. Nonoperative management of stable thoracolumbar burst fractures with early ambulation and bracing. Spine 1993; 18(8):971–976.

22. Chow GH, Nelson BJ, Gebhard JS, Brugman JL, Brown CW, Donaldson DH. Functional outcome of thoracolumbar burst fractures managed with hyperextension casting or bracing and early mobilization. Spine 1996; 21(18):2170–2175.

23. Kraemer WJ, Schemitsch EH, Lever J, McBroom RJ, McKee MD, Waddell JP. Functional outcome of thoracolumbar burst fractures without neurological deficit. J Orthop Trauma 1996; 10(8):541–544.

24. Singer BR. The functional prognosis of thoracolumbar vertebrae fractures without neurological deficit: a long-term follow-up study of British Army personnel. Injury 1995; 26(8):519–521.

25. Knight R, Stornelli D, Chan D, Devanny J, Jackson K. Comparison of operative versus nonoperative treatment of lumbar burst fractures. Clin Orthop 1993; (293):112–121.
26. Rohlmann A, Riley LH, 3rd, Bergmann G, Graichen F. In vitro load measurement using an instrumented spinal fixation device. Med Eng Phys 1996; 18(6):485–488.
27. Bohlman H, Kirkpatrick J, Delamarter R, Leventhal M. Anterior decompression for late pain and paralysis after fractures of the thoracolumbar spine. Clin Orthop 1994; (300): 24–29.
28. Transfeldt EE, White D, Bradford DS, Roche B. Delayed anterior decompression in patients with spinal cord and cauda equina injuries of the thoracolumbar spine. Spine 1990; 15(9):953–957.
29. Clohisy J, Akbarnia B, Bucholz R, Burkus J, Backer R. Neurologic recovery associated with anterior decompression of spine fractures at the thoracolumbar junction (T12-L1). Spine 1992; 17(8 Suppl):S325–330.
30. Schlegel J, Bayley J, Yuan H, Fredricksen B. Timing of surgical decompression and fixation of acute spinal fractures. J Orthop Trauma 1996; 10(5):323–330.
31. Peel NF, Moore DJ, Barrington NA, Bax DE, Eastell R. Risk of vertebral fracture and relationship to bone mineral density in steroid treated rheumatoid arthritis. Ann Rheum Dis 1995; 54(10):801–806.
32. Finkelstein JA, Hu RW, al-Harby T. Open posterior dislocation of the lumbosacral junction. A case report. Spine 1996; 21(3):378–380.
33. Chen WJ, Niu CC, Chen LH, Chen JY, Shih CH, Chu LY. Back pain after thoracolumbar fracture treated with long instrumentation and short fusion. J Spinal Disord 1995; 8(6): 474–478.
34. Dick JC, Brodke DS, Zdeblick TA, Bartel BD, Kunz DN, Rapoff, AJ. Anterior instrumentation of the thoracolumbar spine. A biomechanical comparison. Spine 1997; 22(7): 744–750.
35. An HS, Lim TH, You JW, Hong JH, Eck J, McGrady L. Biomechanical evaluation of anterior thoracolumbar spinal instrumentation. Spine 1995; 20(18):1979–1983.
36. van Loon JL, Slot GH, Pavlov PW. Anterior instrumentation of the spine in thoracic and thoracolumbar fractures: the single rod versus the double rod Slot-Zielke device. Spine 1996; 21(6):734–740.
37. Kaneda K, Taneichi H, Abumi K, Hashimoto T, Satoh S, Fujiya, M. Anterior decompression and stabilization with the Kaneda device for thoracolumbar burst fractures associated with neurological deficits. J Bone Joint Surg Am 1997; 79(1):69–83.
38. Aydin E, Solak A, Tuzuner M, Benli I, Kis, M. Z-plate instrumentation in thoracolumbar spinal fractures. Bull Hosp Joint Dis 1999; 58(2):92–97.
39. Bayley JC, Yuan HA, Fredrickson BE. The Syracuse I-plate. Spine 1991; 16(3 Suppl): S120–124.
40. Been HD. Anterior decompression and stabilization of thoracolumbar burst fractures using the Slot-Zielke-device. Acta Orthop Belg 1991; 57(Suppl 1):144–161.
41. Carl AL, Tranmer BI, Sachs BL. Anterolateral dynamized instrumentation and fusion for unstable thoracolumbar and lumbar burst fractures. Spine 1997; 22(6):686–690.
42. Ghanayem AJ, Zdeblick TA. Anterior instrumentation in the management of thoracolumbar burst fractures. Clin Orthop 1997; (335):89–100.
43. Kirkpatrick JS, Wilber RG, Likavec M, Emery SE, Ghanayem A. Anterior stabilization of thoracolumbar burst fractures using the Kaneda device: a preliminary report. Orthopedics 1995; 18(7):673–678.
44. Haas N, Blauth M, Tscherne H. Anterior plating in thoracolumbar spine injuries. Indication, technique, and results. Spine 1991; 16(3 Suppl):S100–111.
45. Matsuzaki H, Tokuhashi Y, Wakabayashi K, Ishihara K, Shirasaki Y, Tateishi T. Rigix plate system for anterior fixation of thoracolumbar vertebrae. J Spinal Disord 1997; 10(4):339–347.

46. Okuyama K, Abe E, Chiba M, Ishikawa N, Sato K. Outcome of anterior decompression and stabilization for thoracolumbar unstable burst fractures in the absence of neurologic deficits. Spine 1996; 21(5):620–625.

47. Rao SC, Mou ZS, Hu YZ, Shen HX. The IVBF dual-blade plate and its applications. Spine 1991; 16(3 Suppl):S112–119.

48. Dimar JR, 2nd, Wilde, PH, Glassman SD, Puno RM, Johnson JR. Thoracolumbar burst fractures treated with combined anterior and posterior surgery. Am J Orthop 1996; 25(2): 159–165.

49. Defino HL, Rodriguez-Fuentes AE. Treatment of fractures of the thoracolumbar spine by combined anteroposterior fixation using the Harms method. Eur Spine J 1998; 7(3): 187–194.

50. Shiba K, Katsuki M, Ueta T, Shirasawa K, Ohta H, Mori E, Rikimaru, S. Transpedicular fixation with Zielke instrumentation in the treatment of thoracolumbar and lumbar injuries. Spine 1994; 19(17):1940–1949.

51. Findlay J, Grace M, Saboe L, Davis L. A survey of vertebral burst-fracture management in Canada. Can J Surg 1992; 35(4):407–413.

52. Danisa OA, Shaffrey CI, Jane JA, Whitehill R, Wang GJ, Szabo TA, Hansen CA, Shaffrey ME, et al. Surgical approaches for the correction of unstable thoracolumbar burst fractures: a retrospective analysis of treatment outcomes. J Neurosurg 1995; 83(6):977–983.

53. Nairus JG, Richman JD, Douglas RA. Retroperitoneal pseudomeningocele complicated by meningitis following a lumbar burst fracture. A case report. Spine 1996; 21(9):1090–1093.

54. Nagai H, Shimizu K, Shikata, J, Iida H, Matsushita M, Ido K, Nakamura, T. Chylous leakage after circumferential thoracolumbar fusion for correction of kyphosis resulting from fracture. Report of three cases. Spine 1997; 22(23):2766–2769.

55. Silen ML, Weber TR. Management of thoracic duct injury associated with fracture-dislocation of the spine following blunt trauma. J Trauma 1995; 39(6):1185–1187.

56. Donovan DJ, Polly DW, Jr, Ondra SL. The removal of a transdural pedicle screw placed for thoracolumbar spine fracture. Spine 1996; 21(21):2495–2498.

57. Vanichkachorn JS, Vaccaro AR, Cohen MJ, Cotler JM. Potential large vessel injury during thoracolumbar pedicle screw removal. A case report. Spine 1997; 22(1):110–113.

58. Korovessis PG, Stamatakis M, Baikousis A. Unrecognized laceration of main bronchus caused by fracture of the T6 vertebra. Eur Spine J 1998; 7(1):72–75.

59. Murakami R, Tajima H, Ichikawa K, Kobayashi Y, Sugizaki K, Yamamoto K, Kurokawa A, Kumazaki T. Acute traumatic injury of the distal descending aorta associated with thoracic spine injury. Eur Radiol 1998; 8(1):60–62.

60. Lee J, Harris JH, Jr, Duke JH, Jr, Williams JS. Noncorrelation between thoracic skeletal injuries and acute traumatic aortic tear. J Trauma 1997; 43(3):400–404.

61. Brouwers MA, Veldhuis EF, Zimmerman KW. Fracture of the thoracic spine with paralysis and esophageal perforation. Eur Spine J 1997; 6(3):211–213.

62. Johnson JP, Lane, JM. Traumatic lumbar pseudomeningocele occurring with spina bifida occulta. J Spinal Disord 1998; 11(1):80–83.

63. Cook DA, Heiner JP, Breed AL. Pseudomeningocele following spinal fracture. A case report and review of the literature. Clin Orthop 1989; (247):74–79.

64. Deeb ZL, Rothfus WE, Goldberg AL, Daffner RH. Absent cord sign in acute spinal trauma. Clin Imag 1990; 14(2):138–142.

65. Beggs I, Addison J. Posterior vertebral rim fractures. Br J Radiol 1998; 71(845):567–572.

66. Peh WC, Griffith JF, Yip DK, Leong JC. Magnetic resonance imaging of lumbar vertebral apophyseal ring fractures. Australas Radiol 1998; 42(1):34–37.

67. Horsley MW, Taylor TK. Spontaneous correction of a traumatic kyphosis after posterior spinal fusion in an infant. J. Spinal Disord 1997; 10(3):256–259.
68. Sturm PF, Glass RB, Sivit CJ, Eichelberger MR. Lumbar compression fractures secondary to lap-belt use in children. J Pediatr Orthop 1995; 15(4):521–523.
69. Kerttula L, Serlo W, Tervonen O, Paakko E, Vanharanta H. Post-traumatic findings of the spine after earlier vertebral fracture in young patients: clinical and MRI study. Spine 2000; 25(9):1104–1108.
70. Hertlein H, Hartl WH, Dienemann H, Schurmann M, Lob G. Thoracoscopic repair of thoracic spine trauma. Eur Spine J 1995; 4(5):302–307.
71. Karahalios DG, Apostolides PJ, Vishteh AG, Dickman CA. Thoracoscopic spinal surgery. Treatment of thoracic instability. Neurosurg Clin North Am 1997; 8(4):555–573.
72. McAfee PC, Regan JR, Fedder IL, Mack MJ, Geis WP. Anterior thoracic corpectomy for spinal cord decompression performed endoscopically. Surg Laparosc Endosc 1995; 5(5):339–348.
73. Olinger A, Hildebrandt U, Mutschler W, Menger M. First clinical experience with an endoscopic retroperitoneal approach for anterior fusion of lumbar spine fractures from levels T12 to L5. Surg Endosc 1999; 13(12):1215–1219.
74. Verheyden P, Katscher S, Schulz T, Schmidt F, Josten C. Open MR imaging in spine surgery: experimental investigations and first clinical experiences. Eur Spine J 1999; 8(5):346–353.

33

Lower Lumbar Fractures

STANLEY D. GERTZBEIN

Baylor College of Medicine, Houston, Texas, U.S.A.

I LOWER LUMBAR FRACTURES [L3–L5]

Because fractures of the lower lumbar spine are uncommon, the most frequent injuries being burst fractures (1), the management of these injuries is somewhat controversial (2–4). Unique anatomical features of the lower lumbar spine and their biomechanical characteristics create fracture patterns which differ from those at the thoracolumbar junction (5). The location of the vertebral bodies below the pelvic rim as well as the iliolumbar ligaments stabilize the L4 and L5 vertebrae resulting in less post-traumatic instability than injuries elsewhere, with implications for management.

A Classification of Lower Lumbar Fractures

Previous classifications of thoracolumbar fractures have been based on morphology (6–9), mechanisms of injury (10,11) or both (4,12,13). Most classifications, however, fail to take into account the severity of the injury relative to the fracture categories or fail to predict the prognosis. Instability, which is an indicator of severity, should be identified in any classification along with a spectrum of increasing involvement of the spinal structures. Furthermore, the classification should take into account the involvement of both the bony elements and the soft tissues. One such classification (14–16) does address these issues and provides additional information regarding the planes of disruption.

The main categories of this classification include type A, compression injuries, primarily involving the vertebral bodies; type B, distraction injuries, affecting both the anterior and posterior elements; and type C, rotational injuries that also affect the anterior and posterior elements of the spine secondary to multidirectional injuries, one of which is rotation (Fig. 1) (Table 1).

455

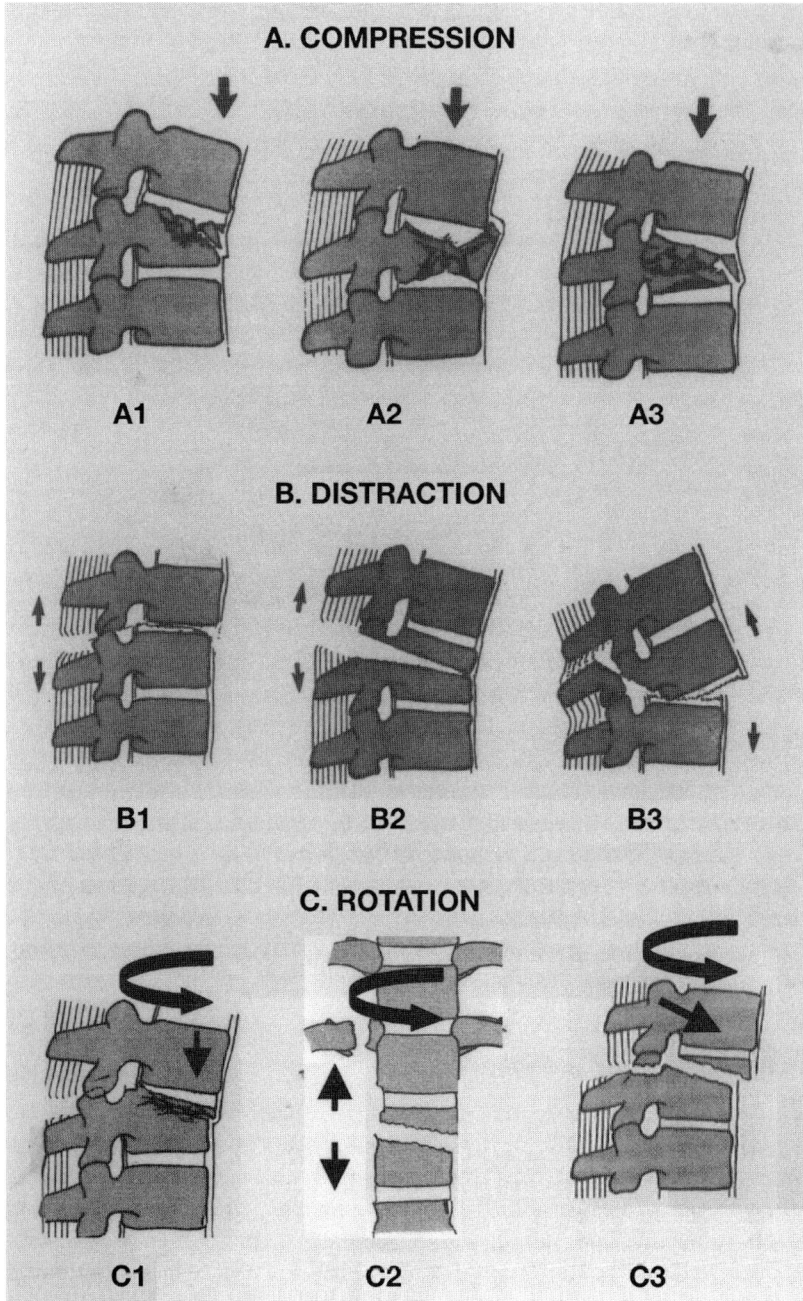

Figure 1   Comprehensive classification. Diagrammatic representation of three types (A, B, and C) and nine groups (A1–A3, B1–B3, C1–C3).

Table 1 Comprehensive Classification of Thoracic Lumbar Fractures

Type	Group
A. Compression	A_1 Impaction (e.g., wedge)
	A_2 Split (e.g., coronal)
	A_3 Burst (e.g., complete burst)
B. Distraction	B_1 Through the soft tissues posteriorly (e.g., subluxation)
	B_2 Through the arch posteriorly (e.g., chance fracture)
	B_3 Through the disk anteriorly (e.g., extension spondylosis)
C. Rotation	C_1 With compression
	C_2 With distraction
	C_3 With shear

Type A, compression injuries, involve the vertebral body and are caused by an axial load with or without flexion. Vertebral height is lost. If a fracture of the posterior arch is present it is often a vertical split injury and does not substantially affect the stability of the injury. Posterior soft tissues are not disrupted nor is one vertebral body translated on the other. Examples of this type include impaction injuries (group A1), of which the wedge compression fracture is a typical fracture; split fractures (group A2), in which a sagittal or coronal split occurs in the vertebral body; and burst fractures (group A3), which present in varying degrees of comminution and displacement. This is the most common type of fracture in the low lumbar region (Fig. 1).

Type B injuries involve the posterior and anterior elements with distraction. The distraction occurs in the transverse plane, posteriorly through the soft tissues (group B1) or the bony arch (group B2) or distraction anteriorly through the disk (group B3) with minimal, if any, translation (Fig. 1). As the forces are carried anteriorly in groups B1 and B2, the injury may occur through the disk (subluxation) or, if an axial load occurs anteriorly, a compression injury is seen in the vertebral body similar to the above-mentioned type A compression injuries. Group B3 injuries occur with distraction anteriorly usually associated with extension forces. The anterior injury passes posteriorly from the disk and may create a fracture of the arch (extension spondylolysis) or a disruption through the soft tissues (posterior subluxation).

Type C injuries also affect the posterior and anterior elements of the spine with significant translation. These are the most unstable of all spinal injuries (Fig. 1). In group C1, there is rotation with axial loading causing compression of the vertebral bodies, producing vertebral body injuries comparable to those noted in type A vertebral body fractures. In group C2, translation is in the anteroposterior direction and is associated with rotation, as well as flexion. In group C3, there is axial loading causing a shearing effect in combination with rotation. This pattern reveals an oblique fracture with marked disruption of all of the posterior and anterior elements (e.g., Holdsworth slice fracture) (1).

The classification is set up in an order of increasing severity of bony and soft tissue disruption. Comminution and displacement, as well as number of planes of disruption, also increase from group 1 through group 3. Fractures are more unstable as one progresses through the classification and the neurological deficit also increases from type A to type C (16).

Because of progressive instability, fractures are more likely to be treated surgically the further down one moves in the classification. The principles of management are established by understanding both the forces causing the injury and the planes of disruption. For example, in type A injuries caused by axial load with compression, reversal of the forces (i.e., distraction) leads to restoration of alignment and vertebral height. In type B injuries, distraction is the primary mechanism, so corrective forces of compression are required. And, finally, for type C injuries with rotation and multidirectional forces, there is significant instability requiring additional stabilizing techniques, such as fixation of the vertebral bodies two or more levels above and/or below (instead of only at one level above and below) or a combination of anterior and posterior stabilization may be necessary.

Minor isolated injuries such as fractures of the transverse (Fig. 2) or spinous processes are secondary to avulsions and do not have instability implications. Fractures of the pars interarticularis are usually a result of an anterior distraction injury with disruption of the disk anteriorly, resulting in significant instability requiring surgical stabilization (Fig. 2).

B Clinical Assessment

The clinical features are related to both the back itself and to the nervous system. A history of violent trauma should alert the clinician to the possibility of a spinal injury. Pain is the most common symptom and is aggravated by the slightest movement of the spine. Neurological symptoms such as loss of sensation, strength, and bladder function are lower motor neuron injuries related to the cauda equina.

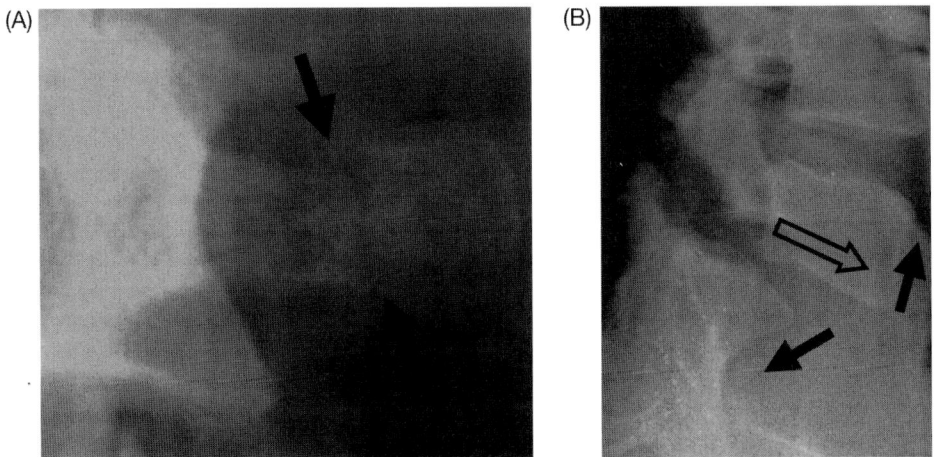

Figure 2 (A) Transverse process fracture. Isolated fracture of the transverse process of L3. This is an avulsion of the psoas muscle and is a stable injury. (B) Pars interarticularis fracture. This fracture is often secondary to an extension-distraction injury (black arrows) and may be combined with a disk disruption with forward slip (open arrows) resulting in significant instability, even though only a minimal amount of bony disruption has occurred.

Typical signs of spinal injury include acute tenderness at the fracture site, widening or gap between the spinous processes, a fullness or swelling of the tissues secondary to hematoma, and muscle spasm. Contusions or abrasions should arouse suspicion particularly if they are unilateral since they may reflect a torsional component to the forces applied to the spine. Malalignment of the spinous processes may be seen or felt. A gibbus may be seen or felt as well. Anterior contusions and abrasions over the abdominal wall often indicate a significant seatbelt injury of the lower lumbar spine (Fig. 3). A rectal examination may indicate a lax sphincter with no perianal sensation or voluntary contraction.

A careful neurological assessment must be performed at regular intervals whether or not a deficit was originally present since the neurological status may change with movement of the patient or local disturbances at the fracture site.

C Imaging Studies

An accurate assessment of injuries of the spinal column and neural tissues will facilitate the management of patients with injuries to the lower lumbar spine. Routine radiological investigations are essential but newer techniques are now available to determine the extent of injury in exquisite detail, providing a better understanding of not only the bony injuries, but also the soft tissue lesions, including the nervous system. It is important to evaluate the entire spine so that lesions at other sites can be identified. Up to 20% of all major spinal fractures will be associated with additional spinal injuries at distant levels (17).

D Plain Radiographs

When assessing the spine radiographically, it is just as important to identify lesions associated with spinal injury as it is to define the precise pattern of the lesion itself. For example, fractures of the ribs may indicate a violent trauma associated with

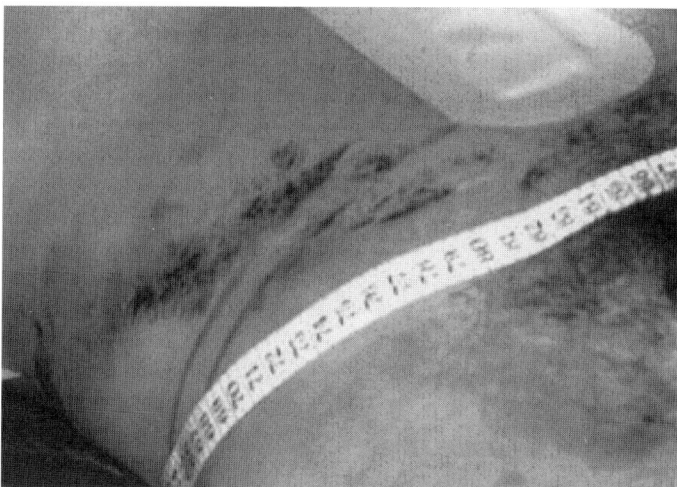

Figure 3 Seatbelt injury. Note the contusion across the lower abdomen resulting from the impact of the seatbelt following a flexion distraction injury.

rotation. A transverse process fracture or fractures at the same or another level may reflect a rotational component in combination with other forces resulting in a more severe fracture of lumbar spine. Both anteroposterior and lateral x-rays of the suspected region of injury should be performed. Cone-down views may be of further assistance in defining the injury more precisely. Using plain radiographs, the fracture pattern, the deformity (kyphosis or scoliosis) and the loss of vertebral height can be determined. Accurate measurements of the deformity, particularly the kyphosis, is recommended. The loss of vertebral height can be determined by averaging the vertebral height of the radiograph of the normal vertebrae bodies above and below the fracture (Fig. 4).

Evaluation of all three columns as described by Denis (6) should be performed. The extent of the vertebral body fracture should be determined not only from the standpoint of involvement of the anterior and middle columns (type A injuries), but also with respect to identifying fragments of the bone in the spinal canal (Fig. 4). This is determined best on the lateral projection. The posterior elements should be assessed to identify vertical fractures of the lamina or transverse lesions through the posterior bony arch (Fig. 4). An increased distance between the bony elements posteriorly and/or anteriorly is indicative of injuries caused by distraction (i.e., type B injuries) (Fig. 5).

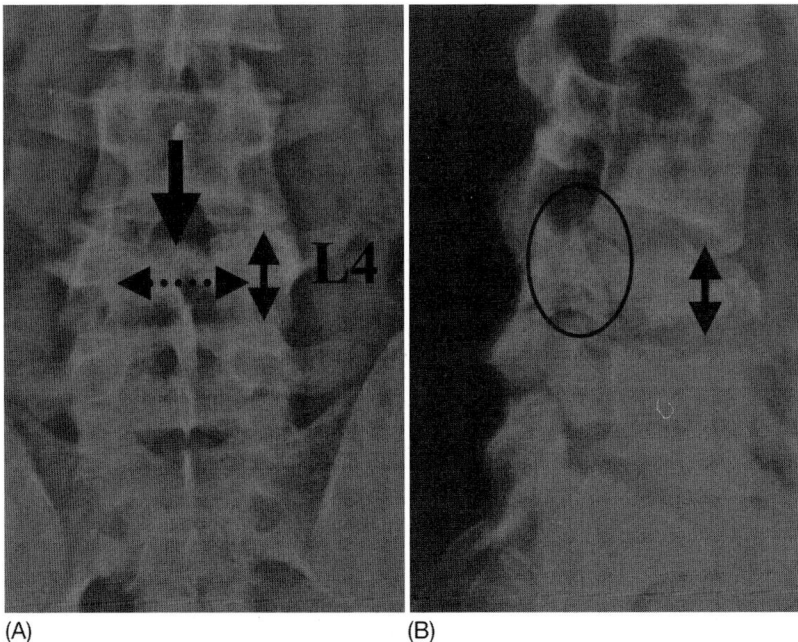

(A)   (B)

Figure 4   (A,B) Type A injury: burst fracture of L4. This axially loaded injury with severe reduction of the vertebral height (2-headed arrow) is associated with significant instability of the anterior and middle columns. In addition, there is a vertical fracture of the laminae (arrow), which often does not produce further instability but may entrap the neural elements. The transpedicular distance is increased (dotted double arrow). Note the lack of translation or rotation, which is in keeping with a type A injury. A fragment of bone from the vertebral body is retropulsed in the spinal canal (circle).

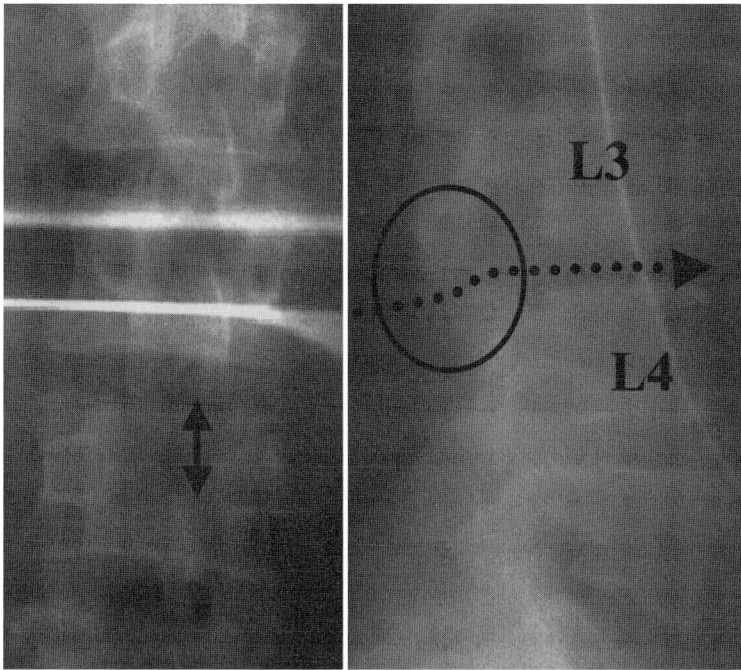

(A) (B)

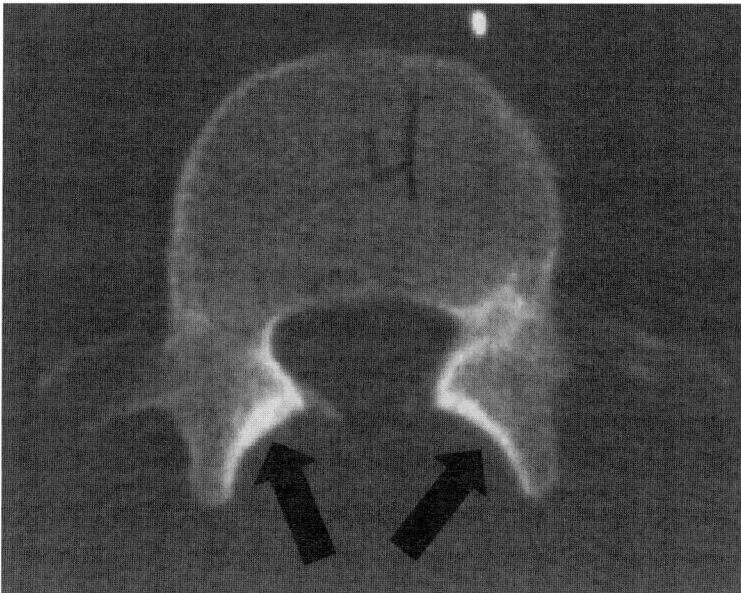

(C)

Figure 5 Type B injury. (A) Note the widening of the intraspinous distance and the subluxation of the facets of L3–L4 (double arrow). (B) This distraction injury through the L3–L4 motion segment is a result of a soft-tissue injury (subluxation) through the facets (circle), posterior ligaments, and disk (dotted arrow). (C) A CT scan at the C3–C4 level. Note the lack of articulation of the facet joints of L3 resulting in a "naked facet" appearance (arrow). (D), (E) Postoperative repair of this type B1 injury with simple interspinous wiring and facet screw fixation along with posterolateral fusion.

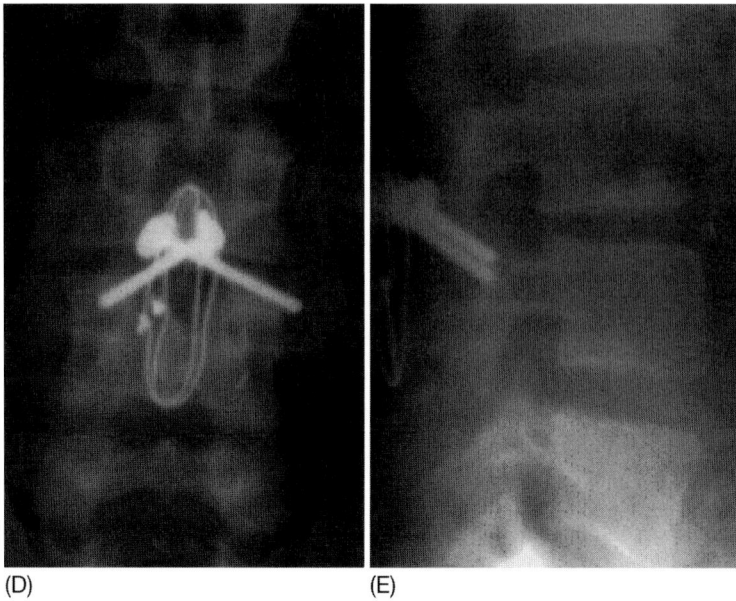

(D)   (E)

Figure 5 Continued

Of paramount importance is the identification of signs of rotation (type C injuries). These include unilateral fractures of the transverse processes, offset of the spinous processes, and/or bodies of the vertebrae, asymmetrical pedicle diameter, and "lateral" subluxation of one vertebral body on the other (Fig. 6). A fracture of the lateral corner of the vertebral body is a little known but important finding suggestive of rotation.

E CT Scan

The CT scan provides excellent images for determining the extent of encroachment of the spinal canal by bony and/or soft tissue fragments (Fig. 7). The amount of canal intrusion can be estimated by determining the sagittal diameter of the bony fragment in the midline as a percentage of normal (calculated by averaging the diameters of the vertebrae immediately above and below the fracture). The cross-sectional surface area of the fragment can also be determined and compared to the normal cross-sectional area. Subluxation or dislocations of facet joints are readily seen on cuts through these joints by the appearance of the so-called "naked facets" appearance (Fig. 5C). The presence of disk material in the spinal canal may also be detected.

F Magnetic Resonance Imaging

The use of MRI in the investigation of spinal injuries is very helpful (18). Not only can the bony elements be easily assessed but the soft tissues, namely the disk and ligamentous structures may also be visualized (Fig. 8). Of even greater relevance, compression of the cauda equina can be readily identified. The relationship between

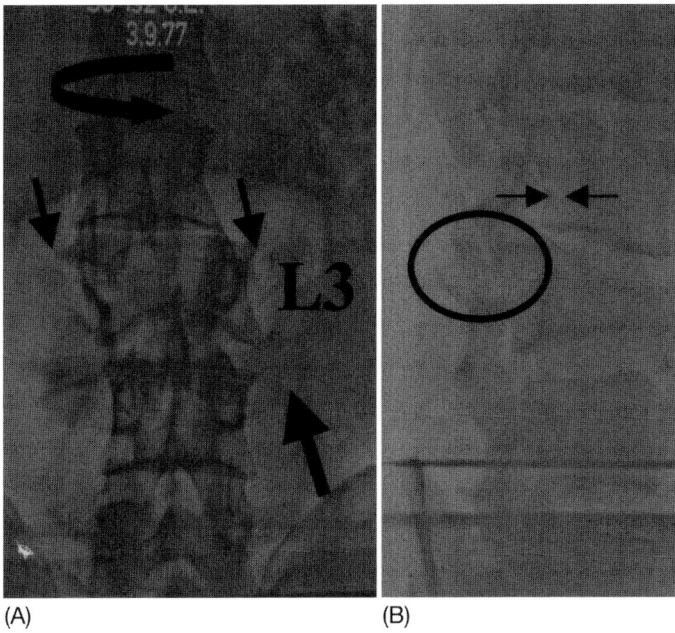

Figure 6 Type C injury: rotational burst fracture of L3. (A) Malalignment of the spinous process and off-set of the vertebral bodies along with asymmetrical pedicle diameter are indications of rotation in this axially loaded fracture. In combination with transverse process fractures (arrows), this rotational injury is very unstable. (B) Note the double shadow of the posterior body wall indicative of rotation (arrows). The retropulsed fragment (circle) is consistent with the burst component.

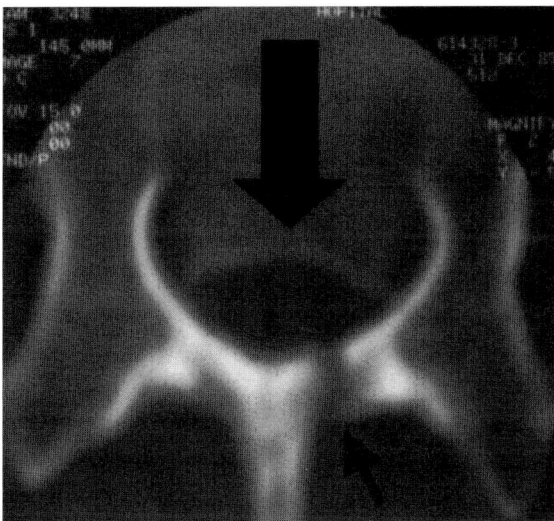

Figure 7 CT scan of burst fracture of L4. The propulsion of the bony fragment posteriorly from the vertebral body has resulted in more than 50% compromise of the spinal canal (heavy arrow). A vertical laminar fracture is seen (small arrow).

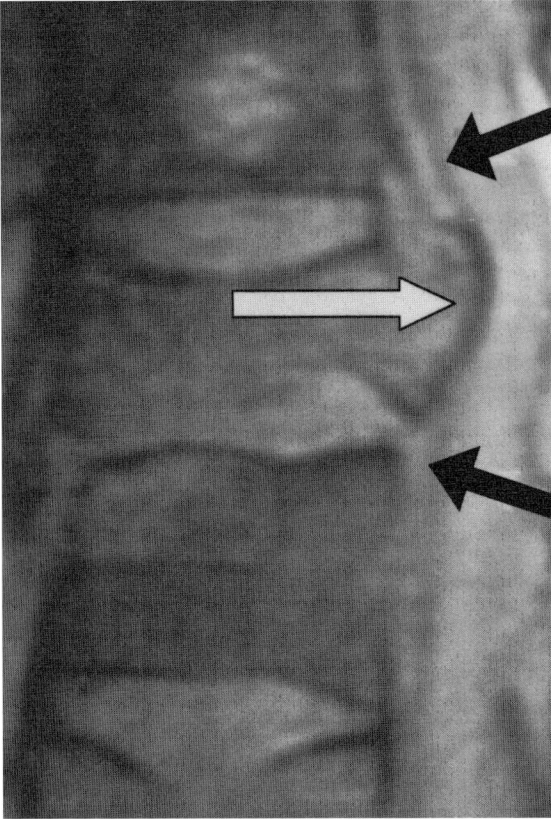

Figure 8 MRI. This burst fracture demonstrates intrusion of the bony fragment into the spinal canal with significant compromise (white arrow). In addition, it demonstrates the intactness of the posterior longitudinal ligament (black arrows).

the bony trauma and neurological deficit may be understood better using this investigative tool.

G Other Imaging Studies

Myelography, conventional tomography, and three-dimensional CT scans have all been used in the past to delineate traumatic lesions. Currently, these are not as effective as the imaging studies described above but can be used in special situations.

II ALGORITHM FOR IMAGING SELECTION

An algorithm is suggested that provides a logical approach to the use of imaging techniques (Fig. 9). A careful clinical assessment along with the appropriate radiological investigations will not only lead to an accurate diagnosis but should result in effective management of patients with these injuries.

Suspected Fracture

```
Suspected Fracture
        │
        ▼
AP & Lateral   ────────────►  Fracture not
Radiographs                   Identified
        │                          │
        ▼                          ▼
Fracture Identified ◄──────── Repeat Films
        │
        ▼
Cone-down Views                              Suspect Soft Tissue Injury
        │
        ▼
1. Posterior Complex          Neurological
2. Canal Fragments            Deficit
3. Disc
        │                          │
        ▼                          ▼
       CT                         MRI  ◄────
```

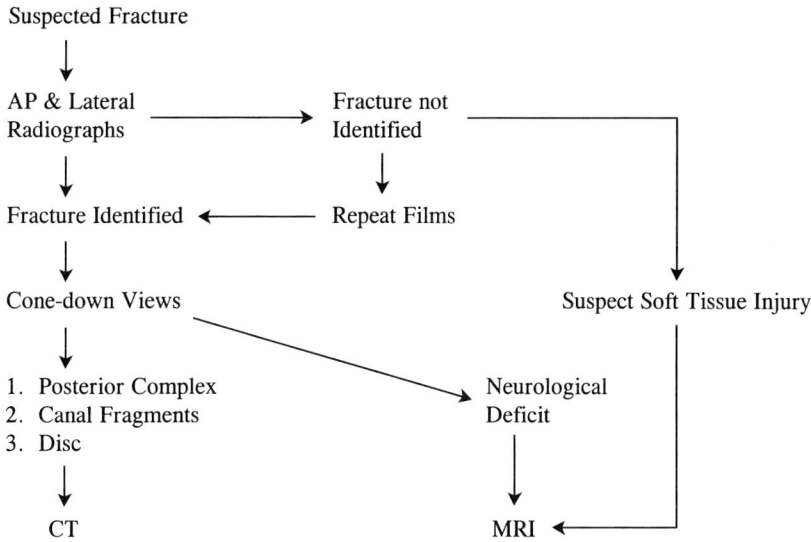

Figure 9   Algorithm for the use of imaging techniques in spinal fractures.

A   Management

Many fractures of the lumbar spine can be treated nonoperatively (1,4,20–22). In most simple burst fractures without neurological deficit and mild deformity, simple measures such as early bed rest, analgesics, and bracing are appropriate (Fig. 10).

Isolated transverse and spinous process fractures require only symptomatic treatment since they are avulsions and are unassociated with instability or neural deficits. Pars interarticularis fractures, however, are more unstable and often require a stabilizing procedure.

The primary indications for surgical intervention are injuries affecting both the posterior and anterior elements (i.e., the three columns of Denis) (3). Such injuries include some type A (burst fractures) (Fig. 11), many type B injuries (Fig. 12), and most type C fractures (Fig. 13). The indications for surgery of the lower lumbar region include (1) instability; (2) neurological deficit; and (3) deformity. When the lesion is mainly a soft tissue injury, as in the case of many type B injuries, inadequate healing of the soft tissues may result in late deformity accompanied by pain. With neurological deficits, a posterior decompression may be necessary to release en-trapped neural elements within the vertical laminar fracture, not an uncommon se-quelae of burst fractures in this region (2,9,19). Posterior decompression of the canal by pushing the body fragments forward through a laminectomy exposure is often effective (Fig. 12). Fusion is usually recommended following decompression surgery. Anterior decompression of the spinal canal at L5 also necessitates an arthrodesis to the sacrum because of the lack of anterior vertebral support following the decom-pression.

To stabilize an unstable segment affecting L5 and occasionally L4, posterior instrumentation down to the sacrum is required, particularly in type C injuries in which all of the posterior and anterior elements have been disrupted and instability is a significant concern (Fig. 13).

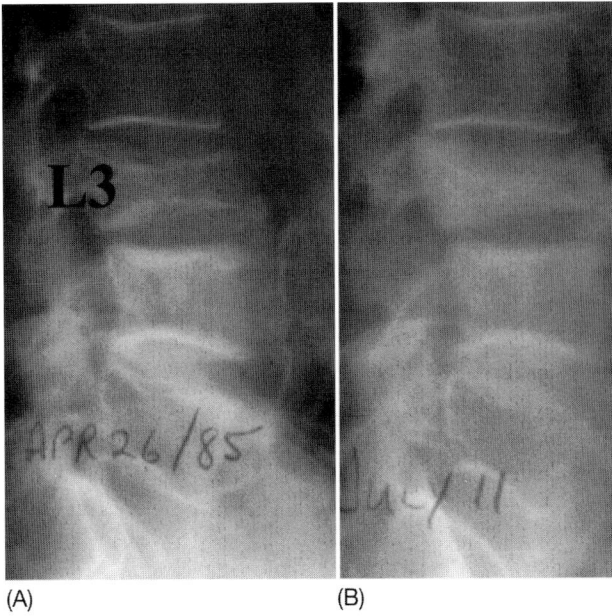

(A)   (B)

Figure 10   Burst fracture of L3. (A) This type A injury is in acceptable alignment of the spinal column with no neurological associated deficit. (B) Three months post-injury on conservative treatment, the fracture is healed in satisfactory alignment and the patient has no significant pain.

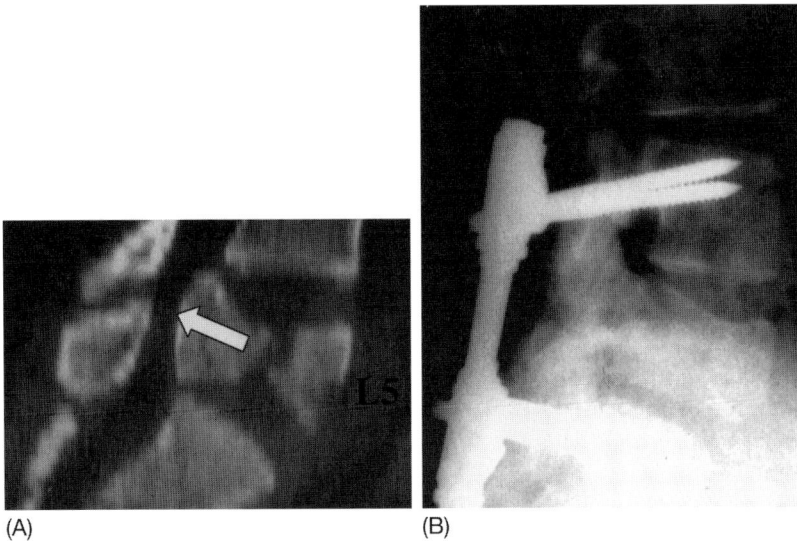

(A)   (B)

Figure 11   (A) Burst fracture of L5 with intrusion into the spinal canal (white arrow) associated with neurological deficit. (B) Postoperative radiograph following decompression laminectomy, reduction of the posterior fragment by direct forward impaction and stabilization with pedicle screw fixation and posterolateral fusion.

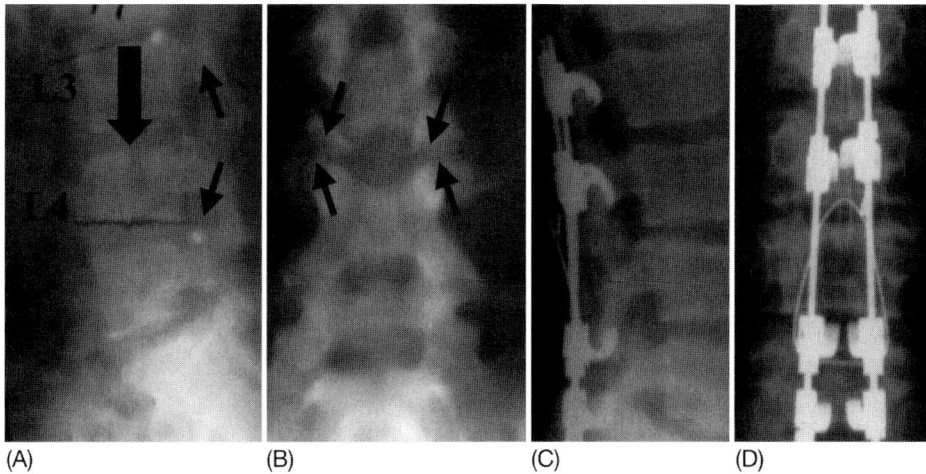

(A)   (B)   (C)   (D)

Figure 12 Type B injury. (A, B) AP and lateral projections with distraction in a transverse plane posteriorly (smaller arrows) through the bony elements and anterior compression of the vertebral body (heavy arrow). (C, D) Posterior compression of this L3–L4 motion segment injury using interspinous wiring and compression instrumentation resulted in good alignment and a stable construct.

Any kyphosis of the lumbar spine is significant since the normal contour is that of lordosis. A kyphosis of 30° at the lower lumbar region is equivalent to a 40° deformity. A kyphosis of this magnitude would require instrumentation to achieve and maintain the normal lumbosacral lordosis (10).

B   Posterior Versus Anterior Surgery

Burst fractures and many type B and type C injuries can be adequately treated with a posterior approach, both by decompression of the entrapped neural elements in the vertical split fracture of the lamina (Fig. 4) with laminectomy, and by anterior impaction of the vertebral body fragments located within the spinal canal. The anterior approach should be reserved for decompression of the vertebral body of L5 in cases of severe crush injuries of the vertebral body (greater than 50 to 60% of the vertebral height) because posterior surgery alone to correct lost vertebral height may result in loss of the reduction and implant failure.

C   Surgical Technique

Most fractures requiring a fusion can be performed by a posterolateral arthrodesis. Instrumentation to the sacrum is required for L5 fractures to ensure the restoration of alignment, the stability of the lesion, and enhancement of the fusion rate. For posterior instrumentation, pedicle screws and rods are the instrumentation of choice since the number of levels required for stabilization compared to nonpedicle devices are minimized. In most cases fractures of the fifth lumbar vertebra can be stabilized by means of screws in the pedicles of L4 and S1 (Fig. 11). For L4 fractures, in most cases, it is sufficient to fuse from L3 to L5. Occasionally, with severe disruptions,

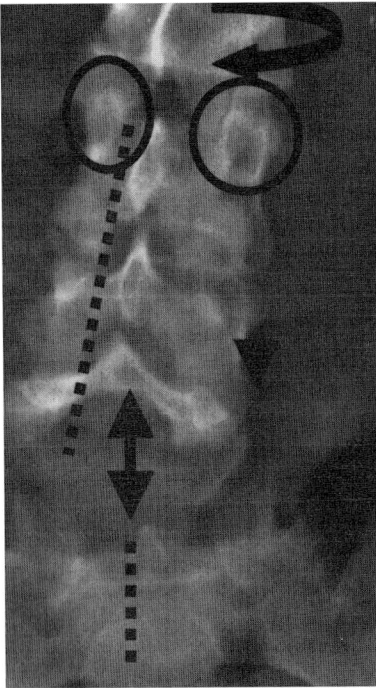
(A)

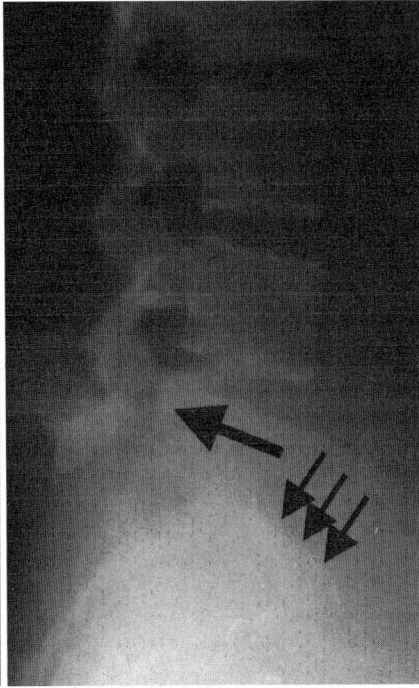
(B)

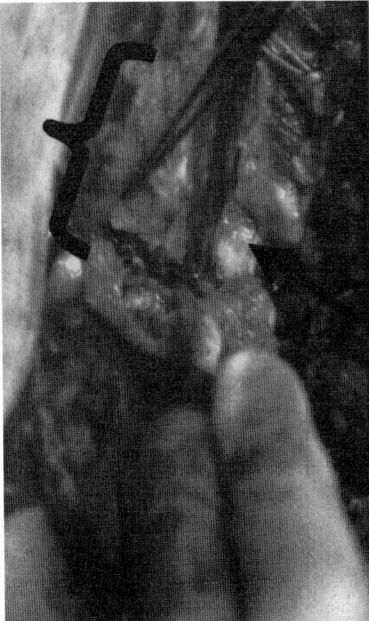
(C)

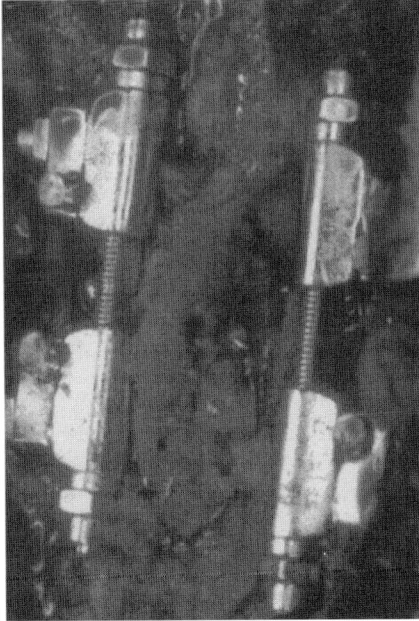
(D)

Figure 13 Type C Injury. (A, B) AP and lateral radiographs of a posterior dislocation at L5–S1. Note the translation of L5 posteriorly on the sacrum (arrows) with rotation and angulation of the spine on the AP projections. There is distraction of L5 on S1 (double arrow) and asymmetry of the pedicle diameter (circles) and a fracture of the L5 transverse process (arrowhead) indicative of rotation. (C) This injury resulted in avulsion of the cauda equina (arrow). (Reprinted with permission from Ref. 23.)

468

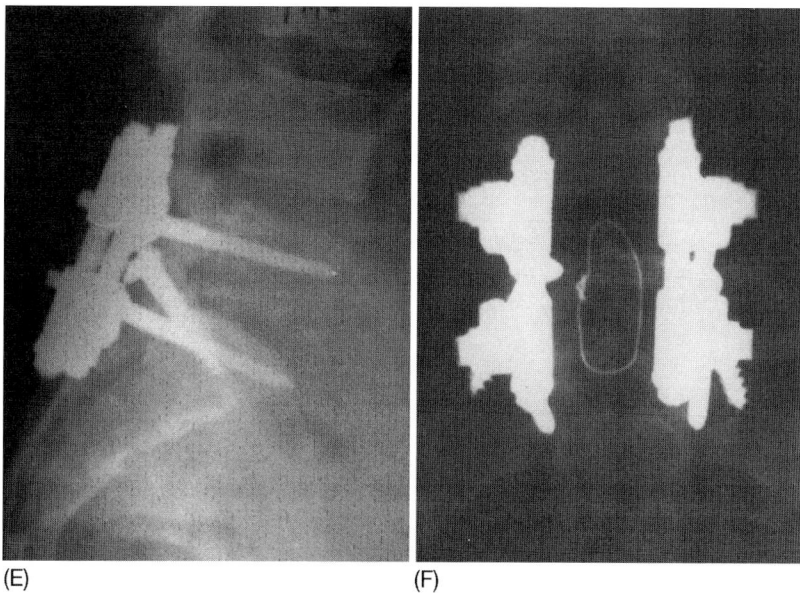

(E) (F)

Figure 13 Continued. Intraoperative view of the severely distracted lumbosacral junction posteriorly (bracket) is noted. (D) Post-intraoperative view of the gap closed by posterior pedicle screw fixation. (E, F) Lateral and AP projection postoperatively demonstrating intraspinous wiring and pedicle screw fixation L5 and S1 with reduction of the gap and normal alignment.

in which additional levels are required to maintain stability, extension of the instrumentation down to the sacrum and up to L2 may be necessary.

Insertion of screws along the ala of the sacrum is just as effective in obtaining satisfactory purchase as inserting into the pedicles and may be used in cases in which there is some difficulty in converging the screws through the pedicles (i.e., a narrow pelvis with overriding iliac crest posteriorly). Anterior decompression of the L5 vertebral body results in a large anterior defect that must be corrected. Restoration of stability and the formation of a solid anterior bridge can be achieved by an anterior bone strut extending from L4 to the sacrum. An autologous tricortical iliac crest graft is recommended followed by posterior pedicle screw fixation to compress the graft from posteriorly.

The approach for decompression is difficult at the lumbosacral level and is best achieved by a direct anterior approach either transperitoneally or retroperitoneally (22). A lateral oblique or transverse incision retroperitoneally is not effective in gaining clear access to the posterior L5 vertebral body. Unfortunately, anterior instrumentation at this level is extremely difficult by any approach. Once the anterior strut graft has been inserted, posterior instrumentation using pedicle screw fixation from L4 to the sacrum can stabilize and maintain alignment (23).

The use of a lumbosacral brace is recommended to prevent undue activity that might interfere with the fusion. A hip spica with leg extension is rarely required.

III CONCLUSIONS

Fractures of the lower lumbar spine (L4 and L5) is uncommon. Conservative measures are effective in dealing with some of these injuries particularly the type A injuries; however, arthrodesis with instrumentation is required for the following indications: (1) stabilization of unstable injuries (some type A injuries, many type B injuries, and most type C injuries); (2) neurological decompression resulting in further instability; and (3) correction of deformity particularly if associated with soft tissue disruption. Pedicle screw fixation appears to offer the best form of fixation, immobilizing the minimum number of motion segments.

REFERENCES

1. Gertzbein SD, Triantafyllou SJ. The management of low lumbar burst fractures (L4 and L5). Orthopaed Proc J Bone Joint Surg 1992;74:255.
2. Garfin S, Gertzbein SD, Eismont FJ. Fractures of the lumbar spine: evaluation, classification and treatment. In: Weinstein J, ed. The Lumbar Spine. Philadelphia: Saunders, 1989:822–873.
3. Levine AM. The surgical treatment of low lumbar burst fractures. Sem Sine Surg 1990; 2:41–53.
4. Seybold EA, Sweeney CA, Fredrickson BE, Warhold LG, Bernini PM. Functional outcome of low lumbar burst fractures. A Multicenter Review of Operative and Nonoperative Treatment. Spine 1999;24:2154–2161.
5. Panjabi MM, Oxland TR, Lin RM, McGowen TW. Thoracolumbar burst fractures: a biomechanical investigation of its multidirectional flexibility. Spine 1994;19:578–585.
6. Denis F. The three column spine and its significance in the classification of acute thoracolumbar spinal injuries. Spine 1983;3:817–831.
7. Kelly RP, Whitesides TE Jr. Treatment of lumbosacral fracture dislocation. Ann Surg 1968;167:705–717.
8. Nicoll EA. Fractures of the dorso-lumbar spine. J Bone Joint Surg 1949;31B:376–394.
9. Pickett J, Blumenkoopf B. Dural lacerations and thoracolumbar fractures. J Spine Disord 1989;2:99–103.
10. Bohler L. The Treatment of Fractures, ed 4 English. Baltimore: W Wood & Co, 1935.
11. Ferguson RL, Allen BL Jr. A mechanistic classification of thoracolumbar spine fractures. Clin Orthop 1984;189:77–78.
12. Gertzbein SD, Court-Brown C. Decompression and circumferential stabilization of unstable spinal fractures. Spine 1988;13:892–895.
13. Holdsworth F. Fractures, dislocations and fracture-dislocations of the spine. J Bone Joint Surg 1970;52A:1534–1551.
14. Gertzbein SD. Fractures of the Thoracic and Lumbar Spine. Baltimore: Williams and Wilkins, 1992.
15. Magerl F, Harms J, Gertzbein SD, et al. A new classification of spinal fractures. Presented at the Societe Internationale Orthipedie et Traumatologie Meeting. Montreal, Canada, September 9, 1990.
16. Magerl F, Harms J, Gertzbein SD, et al. A new classification of thoracic and lumbar fractures. Eur Spine J 1994;3:184–200.
17. Korres DS, Katasara A, Pontazopoulos T, Hartofilakeidis-Garofalidis G. Double or multiple level fractures of the spine. Injury. 13(2):147–152, 1981.
18. Gertzbein SD, et al. Thoraco-lumbar spinal injuries: Injury. Curr Orthoped 1988;2:218–226.

19. Denis F, Burkus JK. Diagnosis and treatment of cauda equina entrapment in the vertebral lamina fracture of lumbar burst fractures. Spine 1991;16(8):S433–S439.

20. An HS, Simpson JM, Ebraheim NA, et al. Low lumbar burst fractures: comparison between conservative and surgical treatments. Orthoped 1992;15(3):367–373.

21. An HS, Vaccar A, Cotler JM, et al. Low lumbar burst fractures: comparison among body cast, Harrington rod, Lugue rod and Steffee plate. Spine 1990;16(8):S440–S444.

22. Court-Brown, CM, Gertzbein SD. The management of burst fractures of the fifth vertebrae. Spine 1987;12:308–312.

23. Gertzbein SD. Posterior dislocation of the lumbosacral joint: a case report. J Spinal Disord 1990;3:174–178.

34

Fractures of the Sacrum and Coccyx

KIRKHAM B. WOOD

University of Minnesota, Minneapolis, Minnesota, U.S.A.

FRANCIS DENIS

Twin Cities Spine Center, Minneapolis, Minnesota, U.S.A.

I   INTRODUCTION

The sacrum is the distal spinal segment, less commonly injured than the more cephalad spinal segments. However, injury to the sacrum may be a source of significant and complex disability. In this chapter we will present the spectrum of sacral and coccygeal trauma, classification schemes, radiological diagnoses, treatment, both operative and nonoperative, and any associated complications. The first section deals with higher intensity sacral trauma resulting in fracture; the second reviews sacral insufficiency fractures—a frequent cause of acute low back pain in the elderly—and sacral stress fractures wherein normal sacral bone fails under repetitive elevated stresses; finally, fractures of the distal coccyx are described.

II   TRAUMATIC SACRAL FRACTURES

The stability of the sacrum is largely determined by its anatomical shape with the more caudal aspect shaped like a wedge, and the anterior surface wider than the posterior aspect. The weight of the body imposes a vertical load that passes through the hips, such that the sacrum is the principal keystone transferring loads for the spine to the pelvis (1). When any deforming force is applied to the head or shoulders, the thoracolumbar spine typically sees the greatest impact, but when applied more distally, the lumbosacral region is affected especially if the knees are extended. Nicoll has suggested that transverse fractures of the sacrum are thought to occur typically with the individual in a hip-flexed, knee-extended sitting position (2).

In 1937, Medelman (3) was the first to classify sacral trauma into three groups according to the direction of the fracture—longitudinal, horizontal, or oblique. In 1945, Bonnin (4) subsequently divided fractures into six different types: (1) juxtailiac marginal fractures; (2) fractures through the first or second sacral foramina; (3) compressed and comminuted body fractures; (4) traction fractures at the site of connecting ligaments; (5) transverse body fractures at the level of S2 or S3; or (6) fissure fractures separating the lateral masses from the most proximal sacral foramina.

Denis et al. (5) provided us with one of the most readable and usable fracture schemes based on the medial or lateral location of the fracture relative to the sacral foramina (Fig. 1). They studied 236 sacral fractures in 776 pelvic injuries over a 10-year period and classified them into three principal zones. Zone I (alar) involves fractures through the lateral ala which tend to be most commonly associated with lateral compression pelvic injuries (e.g., pedestrians hit by motor vehicles). There is no damage to either the foramina or the central sacral canal. Superiorly displaced zone I fractures can be associated with trauma to the exiting L5 nerve root (5,6) (Fig. 2). Zone II (foraminal) involves a fracture line through one or more of the sacral foramina. These commonly extend over multiple levels (Fig. 3). Fractures here may also include the lateral ala, but do not extend into the central canal. Zone III (central canal) fractures involve the central nerve root canal, but frequently also include zones I and II. Burst fractures of the sacrum or fracture dislocations—commonly seen in high-energy falls—are examples of zone III injuries (Fig. 4).

Transverse fractures of the sacrum are another type of zone III fracture. Rare in isolation and typically seen with other pelvic ring fractures, they are frequently associated with neurological embarrassment (5–7). They usually occur at S2–S3 as this represents the apical kyphotic angulation between the upper and lower aspect of the sacrum (Fig. 4B). Additionally, the superior aspect of the sacrum is stabilized by the sacroiliac joint while the distal sacrum, the distal coccyx, and their ligamentous support may act as a lever arm on the superior body (8).

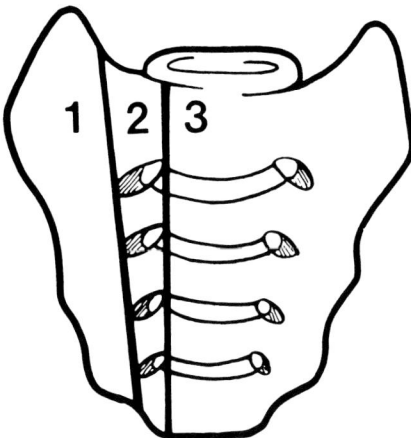

Figure 1   Schematic view of the sacrum divided into the three zones as described by Denis et al. (5): (1) alar, (2) foraminal, and (3) central.

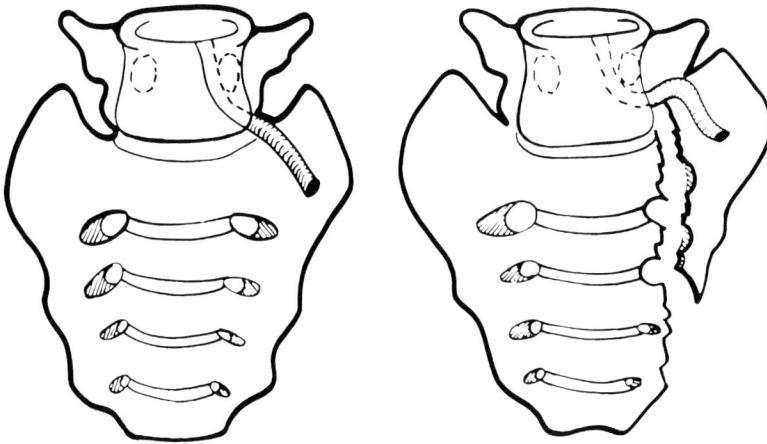

Figure 2 A/P view of the sacrum wherein a displaced alar fracture impinges on the exiting L5 nerve root (right).

Approximately one-fourth of sacral fractures are complicated by neurological injury (4–10). These deficits can be either cauda equina-type radiculopathies of the sacral or lumbar nerve roots or whole plexopathies. They can occur either intra-durally, extradurally within the canal, within the neural foramina, extraforaminally (plexus), or within the nerves beyond the sacrum itself. Injury to the L5 nerve root induces changes in sensation in the dorsum of the foot and lateral calf as well as weakness of dorsiflexors of the foot. The S1 and S2 nerve roots are responsible mainly for hip extension, knee flexion, and plantar flexion with corresponding sensory dermatomes in the posterior aspect of the thigh, leg, the sole and lateral foot, and the genitalia (S2). The ankle jerk will typically be diminished in lesions involving the S1 nerve root.

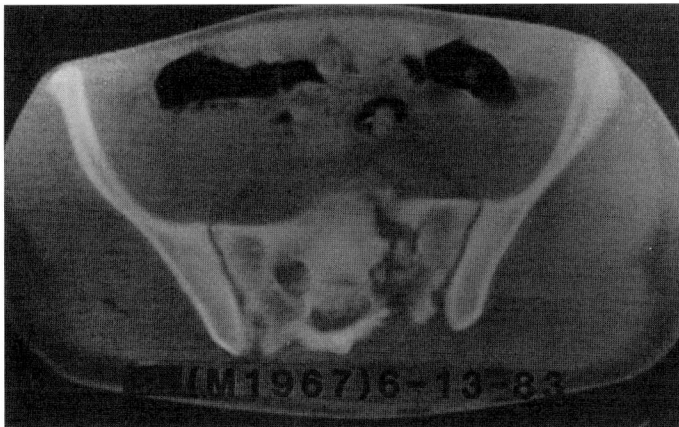

Figure 3 Foraminal fracture with impingement of left S1 nerve root. (Reprinted with permission from Ref. 5.)

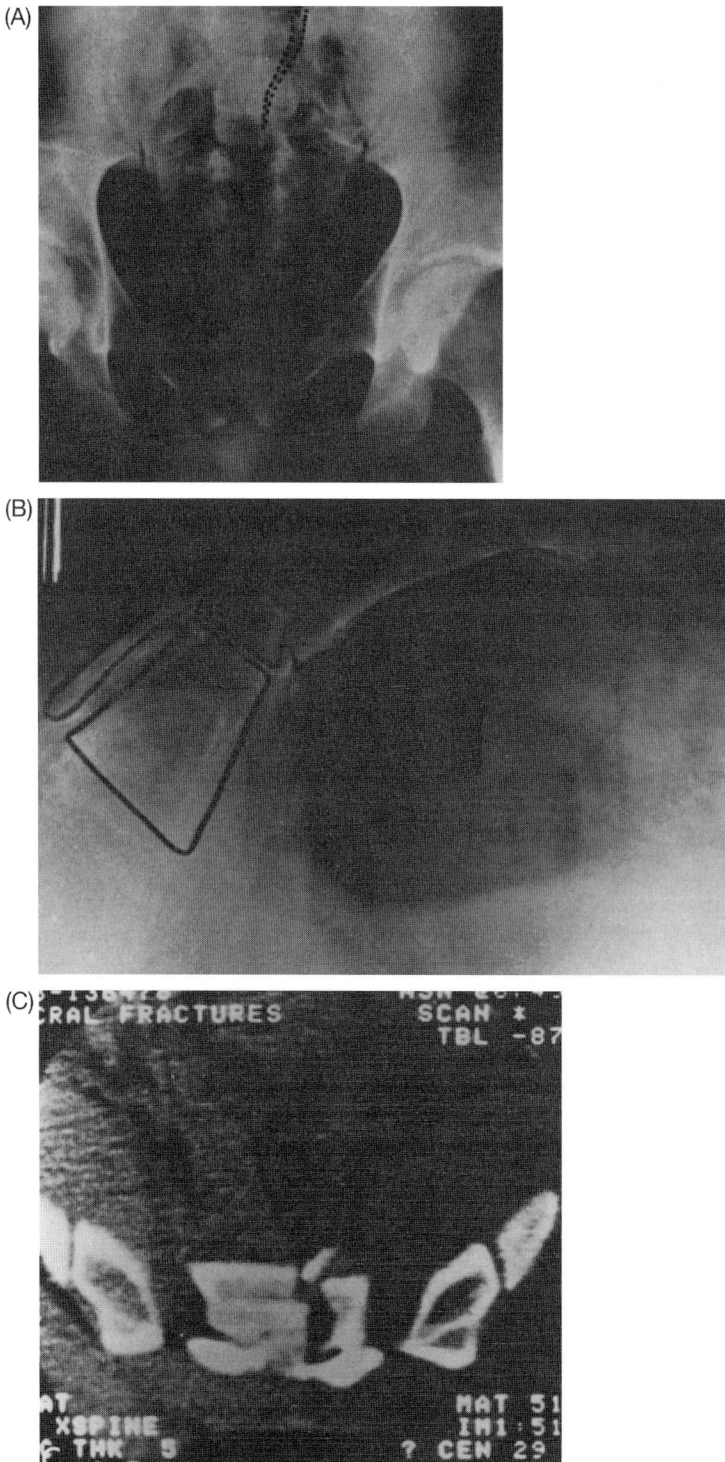

Figure 4   (A) AP view of pelvis with sacral burst fracture difficult to detect. (B) Lateral view shows sagittal angulation. (C) CT scan demonstrating central canal occlusion from retropulsed bone. (Reprinted with permission from Ref. 5.)

Injuries to the nerve roots S2 through S5 are commonly overlooked in trauma settings in large part due to the lack of obvious motor or sensory involvement in the lower extremities. The principal function of the S2 root is its role as a main contributor to the pudendal nerve. S2 innervates the musculature forming the external urethral and anal sphincters while S4 and S5 give sensation to the penis, labia, urethra, posterior scrotum, and anal canal (8,9). S3 provides sensation to the uppermost medial thigh.

Coordinated voluntary control of the bladder and rectum is governed principally by the pelvic splanchnic autonomic nerves from S2 to S4. They are parasympathetic rami distributed to the bladder and rectum as the inferior hypogastric plexus. Their afferent fibers carry awareness of vesicle filling while the efferent fibers initiate detrusor and rectal contraction. Sympathetic splanchnic nerves derive from the S2 and S3 ganglia. Their afferent fibers are responsible for pain and thermal information while the efferent transmissions provide contraction of the urethral and anal sphincters and inhibit contraction of the muscular walls within their respected organ.

Neural injury to the roots S2 to S5 manifests principally by impairment of bowel and bladder continence and disturbances of sexual function. Often this aspect of the neurological examination is overlooked or incomplete in the setting or urgent or multiple trauma (8). The first indication of lower sacral neuropathology sometimes comes days or weeks later when the first complaints of perineal numbness or voiding difficulties are noted.

Neurological injuries were seen in 51 of Denis' 236 patients (5). They were much more common in zones III (56.7%) and II (28.4%) than zone I (5.9%). Within the central sacral canal, neurological damage involved bowel, bladder, and sexual function in 16 of 21 patients. Ebraheim, et al. (6) described eight zone III fractures over a 7-year period of time, seven of whom had complete loss of bowel and bladder function; five also with sexual dysfunction.

The geometry and orientation of the sacral fracture plays a strong role in the development of any neurological sequelae. Foraminal fractures, when comminuted, can have a high association with segment radiculopathy, especially at the more cephalad levels of the sacrum (S1–S2). Transverse fractures of the sacrum are nearly always associated with some degree of neural injury (6,8,9) usually cauda equina, occasionally plexopathy. Most all patients complain of disturbance of bladder function consistent with the bilateral deficit within the canal. Vertical sacral fractures, on the other hand, are much less commonly associated with neurological injury, probably due in part to their proclivity for the lateral alar zone I. However, when a neuropathy is found, it tends to be either radicular (L5) or plexopathic (L5–S1) in nature (e.g., "far-out syndrome") (5,9).

It has been noted that sacral fractures occur in conjunction with some form of pelvis fracture in 80 to 90% of cases. Other injuries associated with sacral fractures include thoracolumbar fractures, varying degrees of pelvic disruption, bladder damage and bladder neck tearing, presacral hematoma from laceration of the middle sacral artery or presacral venous plexus, rectal lacerations, and cerebrospinal fluid leakage (8).

III RADIOLOGY

Conventional radiographs of the pelvis can fail to adequately demonstrate trauma to the sacrum for a number of reasons: Anteroposterior radiographs are often obscured by overlying intestinal gas, and because the sacrum is curved, the upper segments may be superimposed on one another making fracture identification difficult. Adequate lateral images also may be difficult to obtain in the acute trauma setting and can also be obscured in the obese patient by the overlying pelvis (6,9). Often because of these radiological difficulties, as well as the aforementioned lack of obvious neuropathology during the acute trauma admission, sacral fractures can experience a significant delay in diagnosis (7).

There are, however, certain radiographic signs that should heighten suspicion of a sacral injury (4,11): (1) patterns of pelvic ring fractures known to be associated with a sacral fracture (e.g., bilateral rami fractures); (2) fracture of the transverse process of L5 (6,12) (e.g., detection of an apparently isolated lower lumbar transverse process fracture may actually be a warning signal for a sacral fracture, and additional imaging is recommended. A sacral fracture should also be suspected in cases of significant anterior disruption of the pelvic ring even if the sacroiliac joint appears intact (6).

The diagnostic yield using plain radiography in more subtle cases can be increased by angling the A-P x-ray beam 50 degrees cephalad to the pelvis to show the sacrum en face (Fig. 5). This image not only gives adequate view of the body of the sacrum, but will also demonstrate clearly the ventral foramina of zone II. Such fractures are commonly comminuted and careful inspection allows identification of subtle fracture lines (9) (Fig. 6).

Lateral radiography is most useful in demonstrating the sagittal angulation seen in cases of transverse fractures or sacrolisthesis (1,6,7) (Fig. 4B).

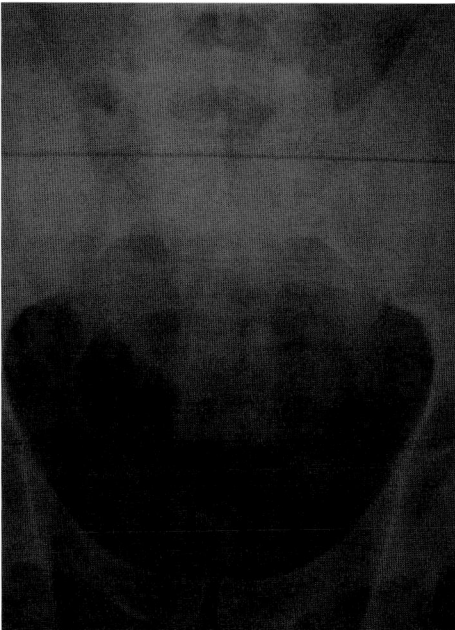

Figure 5 A/P view of the sacrum with the beam angled 50° cephalad shows the foramina en face.

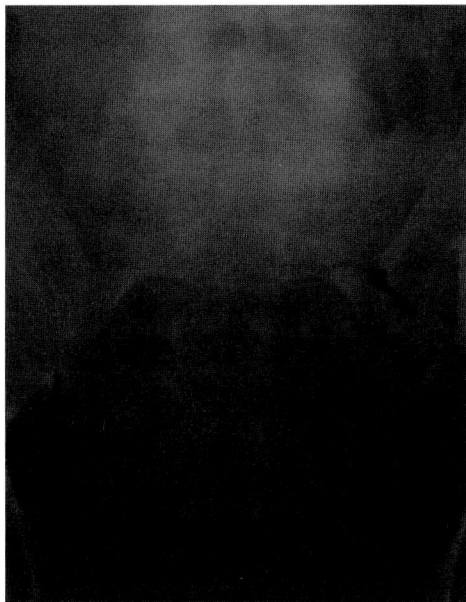

Figure 6 Zone II foraminal fractures seen with the x-ray beam angled at 50° cephalad (arrows).

CT scanning offers superior resolution and is probably the radiographic procedure of choice in evaluating complex sacral fractures especially those within zone III, or any fracture associated with a neurological deficit. Sagittal reconstruction is also advised so as to detect subtle transverse fractures (6).

MR imaging is becoming more and more useful, primarily because of its ability to describe the nerve roots within the canal and foramina. It is also useful in highlighting areas of bony edema surrounding subtle fractures that may be missed on conventional radiography. Finally, MR provides excellent sagittal images that can include the lumbar and sacral spine all on one view (Fig. 7).

IV   PHYSIOLOGICAL TESTING

Electromyography (EMG) can be useful at times in helping to localize an area of a sacral injury and even suggest prognosis (9). For example, injuries within the lumbar or sacral plexuses will yield diffuse patchy electromyelographic changes: As the paraspinal muscles derive their innervation proximally from the dorsal rami, plexus injuries therefore spare these muscles, whereas neuropathology from within the canal includes them in the injury pattern. The principal drawback to EMG is that several weeks are needed to pass for real abnormalities to appear. It is also useful for only the lumbar and uppermost sacral roots as more caudal levels below S2 have no real myotomal distribution.

A simple test in the clinical evaluation of bladder function is measuring post-void residuals. Additionally, cystometrography (CMG) can be used to elicit detrusor contraction through the active instillation of liquid into the bladder, as part of the examination of the mid- to lower sacral roots. Structural lesions of the sacrum will

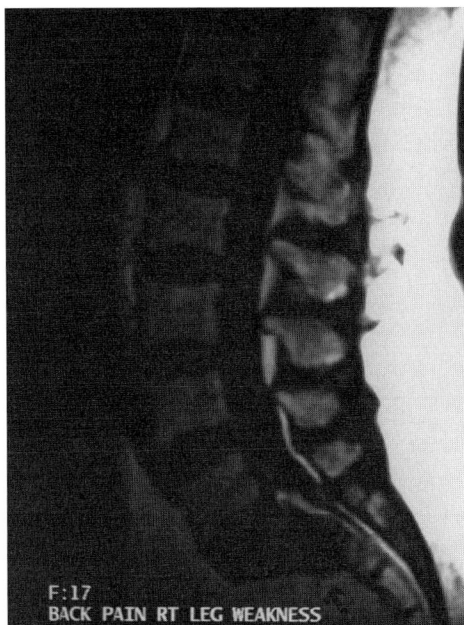

Figure 7 Sagittal MRI allows imaging of the lumbar spine and sacrum in one view. This 17-year-old female presents with a transverse fracture of the upper sacrum (arrows).

usually affect both sympathetic and parasympathetic control of the urinary system and manifest as detrusor areflexia and uninhibited sphincter relaxation. CMG is most useful in confirming clinical impressions, but it can also be of some value in excluding a neurological etiology for bowel or bladder dysfunction in the setting of local trauma to the lower urinary tract (8,9).

V TREATMENT

Because so many reports of sacral fractures have been anecdotal case reports or retrospective reviews describing multiple treatment techniques, there actually has been very little experience compiling a large series of similar injuries treated with various methods, operative or nonoperative (5,9,10). Denis et al.'s (5) experience remains the most comprehensive to date and is probably the most useful in planning treatment.

The majority of adequately reduced and neurologically stable sacral fractures such as in zones I and II can be easily managed by initial bedrest followed by progressive mobilization as comfort allows. If closed reduction is necessary, such as in vertically displaced alar fractures with L5 nerve root impingement, correction and maintenance of alignment can be maintained through rest, skeletal traction, if necessary, and/or hip spica casts.

Gunterberg's biomechanical data (13) suggests that actually much of the sacrum distal to the S1–S2 level can be disrupted—including the lower half of the sacroiliac joint—without significantly weakening the pelvic ring. He concluded that in instances of subtotal destruction of the sacrum below S1 (e.g., transverse fractures, gunshot wounds, etc.), it was probably safe to allow full-weight-bearing at a relatively early stage. Higher transverse fractures (above S1–S2) have been treated with bedrest and traction with moderate success (7,9).

As the majority of sacral fractures are associated with other pelvic ring fractures, anterior external fixation of the injured ring actually indirectly stabilizes the fractured sacrum (6,9). It is important to remember, however, that while external fixation is a means of stabilizing the injured and bleeding pelvis, none of the "anterior" frames adequately stabilizes a major posterior injury so as to permit early weight bearing.

When surgery is considered, anterior approaches to the injured sacrum are rare and ill-advised, for many of these injuries can have large presacral hematomas and surgical violation may precipitate massive hemorrhage. Diastases of the pubic symphysis may render some alar fractures unstable, but may be stabilized with anterior pubic plating.

Most neurological deficits will improve with time, although commonly it is not complete. Sacral laminectomy is the most common procedure, but a comparison of results with those of nonoperative management does not exist (5,6). Posterior laminectomy and decompression of affected sacral neural structures provide the best chance of nerve root recovery. Especially with transverse fractures that show varying degrees of angulation and fragment displacement, often with kinking, tethering, or even occasional transection of nerve roots (6,8,14,15).

On the other hand, Phelan et al. (7), described four patients with transverse fractures of the sacrum and neurological deficits of bowel and bladder, who recovered complete function with conservative treatment of bedrest and progressive ambulation. Even in instances of surgical decompression, perioperative bedrest with or without traction is indicated to effect osseous union.

In instances of displaced and unstable longitudinal or vertical fractures, direct stabilization of the fractured sacrum is occasionally possible (6,14,16). A distinct advantage to this approach is that it can in many instances allow immediate mobilization of the patient out of bed (10,16). While the indications for internal fixation of isolated sacral fractures is variable, Templeman et al. (10) writes that most authorities agree that the pelvis is unstable if more than 1 cm of posterior displacement exists.

Transforaminal zone II fractures with displacement should be realigned with open reduction, decompression, and internal fixation. If the sacroiliac joint is disrupted posteriorly and the alar region is intact or with minimal comminution, direct internal fixation such as iliosacral screws or trans-sacral plating is possible (and can be supplemented with an anterior external frame) (6,16). Care should be exercised when fixing longitudinal or foraminal fractures with screws by not overcompressing the fragments and risk trapping nerve roots. Lag screw fixation alone should not be performed in instances of significant foraminal fracture (i.e., one should probably consider using posterior plating instead). Somatosensory-evoked potential monitoring may be useful in avoiding this complication (6,16).

Closed reduction of displaced fractures with percutaneous fixation has been advocated by some for several reasons: it simplifies the treatment and extensile exposure and the attendent wound problems can be avoided (10,16). Blood loss is minimized and potential infectious contamination in the polytrauma setting is lessened. Concomitant anterior reduction and fixation can be accomplished without turning the patient prone. Their technique is dependent on adequate fluoroscopic visualization, however, and the surgeon must have a thorough understanding of the complex anatomical variations of the pelvis. Also, closed reductions are rarely perfectly anatomical. Many authors actually prefer open reduction of sacral fractures associated with foraminal debris and associated neurological injuries or with documented instability (5,14,16).

VI INSUFFICIENCY FRACTURES

Insufficiency fractures of the sacrum can be an unsuspected cause of acute low back pain in the elderly, especially women, who have sustained unknown or relatively minimal trauma. They occur in abnormally fragile bone with reduced elastic resistance secondary to structural alterations as seen in osteopenia, involutional osteoporosis, or other metabolic bone disorders, including corticosteroid- or radiation-induced osteoporosis (17–20).

The frequency of insufficiency fractures of the sacrum within the general population is not well known. A prospective study by Gaucher et al. (21) in a health clinic in Europe, found an annual incidence of approximately 2% in women over 60. Weber et al. (20) found 20 sacral insufficiency fractures out of 2366 patients (0.9%) presenting with low back pain to the Department of Rheumatology at Stadtspital Triemli Zuerich during a 20-year period.

The demographics of sacral insufficiency fracture heavily favor postmenopausal women in their seventh, eighth, or ninth decade (20). Most patients complain of dull low back pain, many of whom will report exacerbation of the pain with direct pressure. Because the etiology is unclear, many patients will complain of chronic pain for weeks and the diagnosis may frequently be quite delayed (22). Although insufficiency fractures of the sacrum almost universally have a normal neurological exam (19,20,23), neurological findings have occasionally been reported, including paresthesias and urinary or bowel incontinence (18,24–26). Finiels et al. (27) reviewed almost 500 cases of sacral insufficiency fractures and found an approximately 2% rate of neurological compromise, sphincter dysfunction being the most common. The true incidence may be somewhat underestimated, however, for many elderly individuals will report "sphincter dysfunction" and concomitant symptoms of distal paresthesias and leg weaknesses may be overlooked (26).

Imaging insufficiency fractures of the sacrum can be difficult because, in the elderly, the sacrum is frequently irregularly structured and osteolytic, and osteosclerotic areas can be seen as well. Plain radiography can be relatively insensitive and often the fracture can be missed completely, especially longitudinal fractures within the cancellous body of the lateral ala (19,20,22,24). Bone scans, on the other hand, are remarkably adept at pinpointing the diagnosis (19,22,25). The most common anatomical presentation in insufficiency fractures is a longitudinal break parallel with the sacroiliac joint and can be seen as H- or butterfly-shaped when the fractures are bilateral (Fig. 8). Commonly, due both to the patient's age and the rather insidious onset of the pain, many patients with insufficiency fractures have been presumed initially to have metastatic disease (23). The increased uptake on bone scans confounded by the patchy osteoporosis has on many occasions caused such a diagnosis and unnecessary biopsies to be made (25).

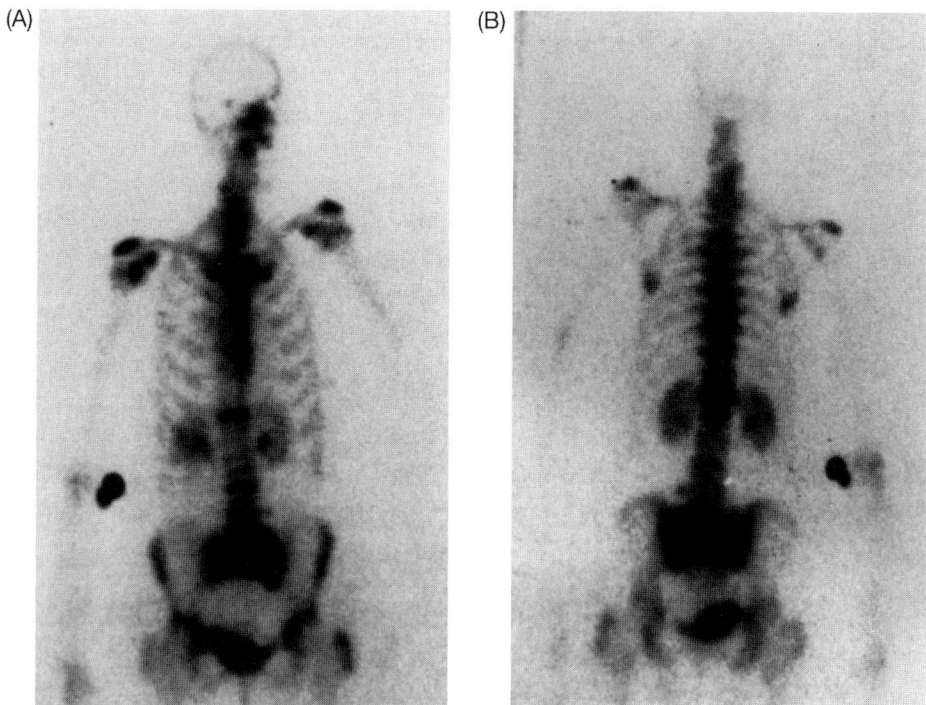

Figure 8 (A) Anterior and (B) posterior bone scan demonstrating typical "H" pattern of bilateral sacral insufficiency fractures.

Computerized tomography is the definitive study (22,25) and will reliably show fracture lines within the anterior margin of the sacrum. Vacuum-like phenomena can be sometimes be seen within the fractures yet without the destructive processes or soft tissue masses seen in metastatic disease. CT is best when combined with scintigraphy as longitudinal fractures can on occasion be misinterpreted as sacroilitis on radionuclide imaging.

MR is playing an increasing role in the examination and diagnosis of patients with subclinical insufficiency fractures due to its ability to image the reactive edema within the surrounding bone and also rule out metastatic pathology and sagittal images of the entire spinal axis on one film is possible (25).

Fortunately, instability is not a problem with most sacral insufficiency fractures and surgical intervention is almost never required. Bed rest with pain control, followed by gradual mobilization, is all that is typically needed. Even those patients with clinical neuropathy or cauda equina-type syndromes will often respond well this way (26). Most patients become pain-free and fully independent within 6 to 12 months.

VII STRESS FRACTURES

Stress fractures differ from insufficiency fractures in that they occur when the mechanical or elastic resistance of bone is normal, but stressed beyond normal capacity.

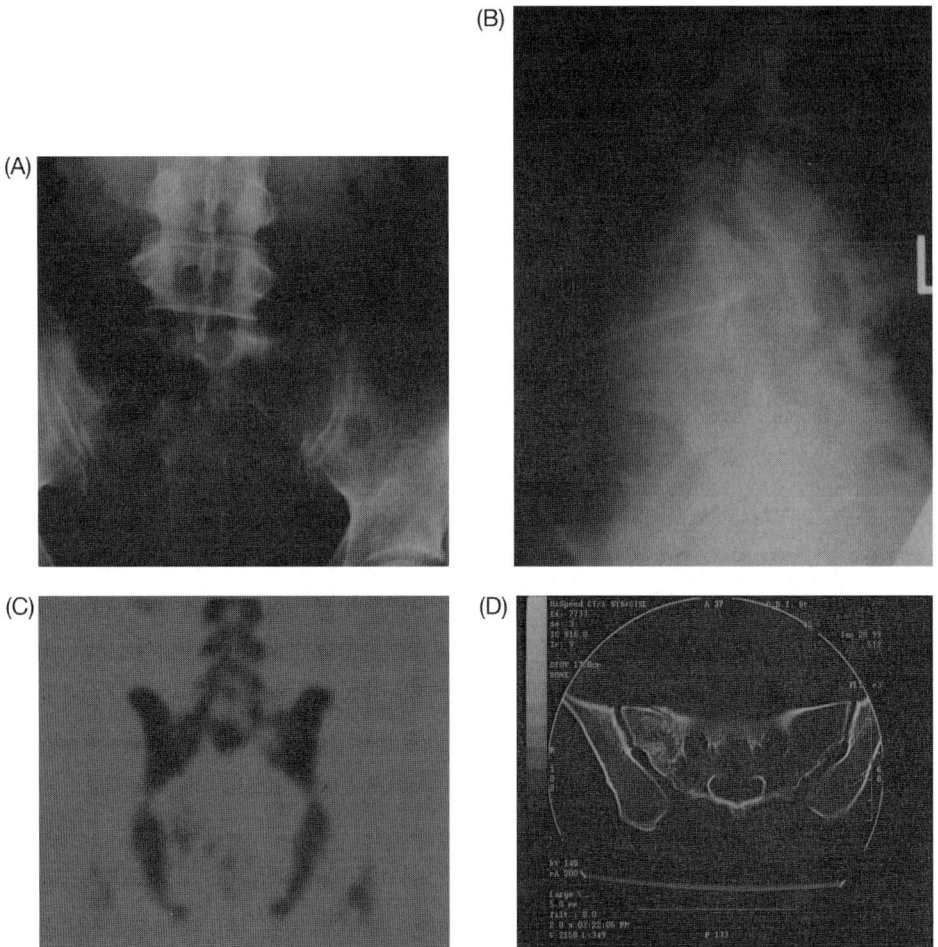

Figure 9   (A) A/P and (B) lateral views of the sacrum of a 29-year-old female long-distance runner. (C) Bone scan shows increased uptake in the right sacral alar. (D) CT scan demonstrating a subtle break in the anterior alar cortex. (E) Repeat CT scan 4 months later shows healing after 4 months of rest and reduced running. (F) Axial MRI on presentation with (R) sacral alar stem fracture. Note mild increase in T2W signal (R) alar. (G) Three months later, the increased T2W signal is evident. (H) Seven months following treatment fracture appears healed, yet increased T2W signal persists.

Stress fractures of the lower extremities are a common finding in certain patient populations, including military recruits, athletes, and long-distance runners (28,29) and, to a lesser degree, the lower lumbar spine and pelvis including the sacrum can be affected as well (28,30). Stress fractures may also be nutritionally based: in the female long-distance runner, amenorrhea is common, which can lead to a general weakening of bone in the sacrum (29).

The diagnosis of a sacral stem fracture is entertained when low back and buttock or groin pain is found in susceptible individuals, such as long-distance runners,

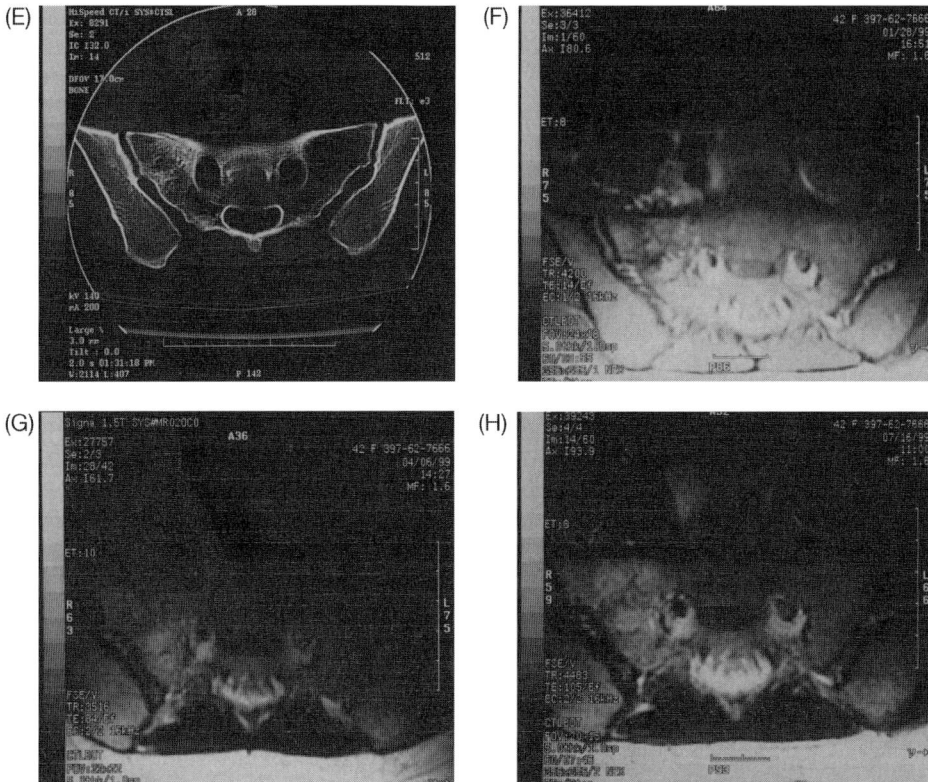

Figure 9 Continued

in whom osteoporosis and malignancy have been ruled out and there is no history of previous pelvic radiation. Many will have localized tenderness over the sacrum and sacroiliac joint.

As in insufficiency fractures, stress fractures of the sacrum are extremely difficult to visualize with plain radiography and bone scintigraphy will remain the initial screening image of choice. CT scanning provides great bony detail, typically showing a sclerotic zone in the cancellous bone of the anterior aspect of the sacrum surrounding a faint linear lesion within the cortical bone (Fig. 9).

Most individuals recover well with 4 to 6 weeks of rest and should be able to return to their normal activities by 2 months. The resumption of activities should be gradual, regulated by pain, however, so as to prevent recurrent injury.

VIII   COCCYGEAL FRACTURES

Coccygeal fractures can be a source of coccygodynia—tail bone pain—and are most commonly due to direct trauma to the coccyx (31–34) or fracture associated with child birth (35).

Plain radiography can often show an angulated sacrococcygeal or intercoccygeal segment; however, some interpretive difficulty persists in that normal variations of the angulation of the distal sacrococcyx have been described in asymptomatic populations (31,32). Bone scan imaging may help confirm the diagnosis.

Treatment includes symptomatic maneuvers such as cushions and supports, injection therapy, and in cases resistant to nonoperative care, coccygectomy. Wood et al., in unpublished data (36), studied 21 patients at a minimum of 2 years follow-up for total coccygectomy following painful traumatic coccygodynia, and found 86% good or excellent results as reported by patient questionnaire.

REFERENCES

1. Rodriguez-Fuentes AE. Traumatic sacrolisthesis S1-S2. Spine 1993;18:768–771.
2. Nicoll EA. Fractures of the dorsolumbar spine. J Bone Joint Surg [Br] 1949;31:376.
3. Medelman JP. Fractures of the sacrum. Their incidence in fractures of the pelvis. Am J Roentgenol 1937;42:100–105.
4. Bonnin JG. Sacral fractures and injuries of the cauda equina. J Bone Joint Surg [Am] 1945;27:113–127.
5. Denis F, Davis S, Comfort T. Sacral fractures: an important problem. A retrospective analysis of 236 cases. Clin Orthop Rel Res 1988;227:67–81.
6. Ebraheim NA, Biyani A. Zone III fractures of the sacrum. A case report. Spine 1996; 21:2390–2396.
7. Phelan ST, Jones DA, Bishay M. Conservative management of transverse fractures of the sacrum with neurological features. A report of four cases. J Bone Joint Surg [Br] 1991;73:969–971.
8. Fountain SS, Hamilton RD, Jameson RM. Transverse fractures of the sacrum. J Bone Joint Surg [Am] 1977;59:486–489.
9. Scmidek HH, Smith D, Kristiansen TK. Sacral fractures: issues of neural injury, spinal stability, and surgical management. In: Dunsker SB, Schmidek HH, Frymoyer J, Kahn A, editors. The Unstable Spine. New York: Harcourt, 1986.
10. Templeman D, Goulet J, Duwelius PJ, Olson S, Davidson M. Internal fixation of displaced fractures of the sacrum. Clin Orthop Rel Res 1996;329:180–185.
11. Laasonen EM. Missed sacral fractures. Ann Clin Res 1977;9:84–87.
12. Fardon DF. Displaced fracture of the lumbosacral spine with delayed cauda equina deficit. Report of a case and review of literature. Clin Orthop 1976;120:155–158.
13. Gunterberg B. Effects of major resection of the sacrum. Acta Orthop Scand (Suppl 2) 1976;162:1–38.
14. Taguchi T, Kawai S, Kaneko K, Yugue D. Operative management of displaced fractures of the sacrum. J Orthop Sci 1999;4:347–352.
15. Rao SH, Laheri MR. Traumatic transverse fracture of sacrum with cauda equina injury —a case report and review of literature. J Postgrad Med 1998;44:14–15.
16. Routt ML, Simionian PT. Closed reduction and percutaneous skeletal fixation of sacral fractures. Clin Orthop Rel Res 1996;329:121–128.
17. Saraux A, Valls I, Guedes C, Baron D, Le Goff P. Insufficiency fractures of the sacrum in elderly subjects. Revue Du Rhumatisme [EE] 1995;62:582–586.
18. Lien HH, Blomlie V, Talle K, Tveit K. Radiation-induced fracture of the sacrum: Findings on MR. Am J Roentgenol 1992;159:227.
19. Schulman LL, Addesso V, Starton RB, McGregor CC, Shane E. Insufficiency fractures of the sacrum: A cause of low back pain after lung transplantation. J Heart Lung Trans 1997;16:1081–1085.
20. Weber M, Hasler P, Gerber H. Insufficiency fractures of the sacrum: twenty cases and review of the literature. Spine 1993;18:2507–2512.

21. Gaucher A, Pere P, Regent D, Bannwarth B. Les fractures de contrainte de la ceinture pelvienne des sujets ages: fractures de insuffisance osseuse. Semin Hop Paris 1986;62: 2157–2161.

22. Leroux JL, Denat B, Thomas E, Blotman F, Bonnel F. Sacral insufficiency fractures presenting as acute low-back pain: Biomechanical aspects. Spine 1993;18:2502–2506.

23. Gotis-Graham I, McGuigan L, Diamond T, Portek I, Quinn R, Sturgess A, Tulloch R. Sacral insufficiency fractures in the elderly. J Bone Joint Surg [Br] 1994;76:882–886.

24. Lock SH. Osteoporotic sacral fracture causing neurological deficit. Br J Hosp Med 1993; 49:210.

25. Stabler A, Beck R, Bartl R, Schmidt D, Reiser M. Vacuum phenomena in insufficiency fractures of the sacrum. Skeletal Radiol 1995;24:31–35.

26. Jacquot JM, Finiels H, Fardjad S, Belhassen S, Leroux JL, Pelissier J. Neurological complications in insufficiency fractures of the sacrum. Three case reports. Rev Rhumatisme [EE] 1999;66:109–113.

27. Finiels H, Finiels PJ, Jacquot JM, Strubel D. Fractures du sacrum par insuffisance osseuse: meta-analyse de 508 cas. Presse Med 1997;26:1568–1573.

28. Schils J, Hauzeur JP. Stress fracture of the sacrum. Am J Sports Med 1992;20:769–770.

29. Major NM, Helms CA. Sacral stress fractures in long-distance runners. Am J Roentgenol 2000;174:727–729.

30. Belkin SC. Stress fractures in athletes. Orthop Clin North Am 1980;11:735–742.

31. Postacchini F, Massobrio M. Idiopathic coccygodynia. J Bone Joint Surg [Am] 1983; 65:1116–1124.

32. Grosso NP, van Dam BE. Total coccygectomy for the relief of coccygodynia: A retrospective review. J Spinal Disord 1995;8:328–330.

33. Gutierrez PR, Mas-Martinez JJ, Arenas J. Salter-Harris type I fracture of the sacrococcygeal joint. Pediatr Radiol 1998;28:734.

34. Raissaki MT, Williamson JB. Fracture dislocation of the sacro-coccygeal joint: MRI evaluation [letter]. Pediatr Radiol 1999;29:642–643.

35. Jones ME, Shoaib A, Bircher MD. A case of coccygodynia due to coccygeal fracture secondary to parturition. Injury 1997;28:549–550.

36. Wood KB, Mehbod A, Goldsmith M. Coccygectomy for treatment of painful coccygodynia. In progress.

35

Nonoperative Treatment of Thoracolumbar Fractures

MITCHEL B. HARRIS

Wake Forest University, Bowman Gray School of Medicine, Winston-Salem, North Carolina, U.S.A.

I INTRODUCTION

The management of thoracolumbar fractures remains controversial. The controversy continues primarily due to the lack of a significant functional difference noted when comparing the results of operative and nonoperative treatment methods. Advanced imaging techniques such as computed axial tomography (CAT scan) and magnetic resonance imaging (MRI) have facilitated a better appreciation of fracture pattern morphology and the implied injury mechanism, the status of the neural elements, and our understanding of the ill-defined concept of spinal stability. However, these advances have not enabled us to identify the specific factors that determine whether surgery will lead to a better functional outcome than nonoperative treatment techniques.

Advocates of surgical intervention for thoracolumbar fractures cite the potential for decompression of the spinal cord and conus, restoration of spinal alignment, and earlier mobilization with unencumbered (braceless) rehabilitation as compelling reasons for their approach. Advocates of the nonoperative approach counter with clinical evidence of similar neurological recovery while avoiding the potential complications inherent in spinal surgery. These complications include postoperative infection, iatrogenic neurological injury, pseudarthrosis, hardware failure, and anesthetic complications. Contemporary studies highlight the lack of difference in functional outcomes between operatively and nonoperatively treated thoracolumbar spine fractures with the submission that chronic spinal pain seems to be more common in the operatively managed group (1–8).

Regardless of the treatment method chosen, the goals of thoracolumbar spine fracture management remain the same. The primary emphasis should be to prevent or limit neurological injury. Secondary issues include restoring spinal stability, re-aligning the spine to a balanced sagittal and coronal alignment, minimizing the number of functional spinal units rendered immobile by fusion, and facilitating the earliest possible rehabilitation. The treatment plan should provide an environment conducive to healing bony and soft tissue and eventually to achieving a stable pain-free spinal column. This should be done without accepting a high risk for complications. By these generally accepted criteria, it would seem that surgical treatment should be reserved either for patients with a progressive or incomplete neurological deficit or for those felt to have an unstable spine. Further narrowing the scope of the problem allows us to focus on the true basis of this persistent controversy: what are the identifiable and reversible factors that predict spinal cord recovery and the determination of the degree of mechanical instability that can be safely and effectively treated nonoperatively?

II NEUROLOGY

Although the majority of the clinical literature addressing thoracolumbar fractures does not statistically support the commonly held belief that surgery leads to greater improvement in the neurological condition compared to nonoperative treatment (1,9–12), surgery is generally recommended for patients with incomplete or progressive spinal cord injuries. This is primarily because it proposes an action that can potentially lead to some neurological recovery, even in a delayed fashion (13). More precisely, successful surgical treatment of a thoracolumbar burst fracture with neural injury should result in the neural elements being freed of compression from the retropulsed bone/disk material, and should eliminate the pathological motion (instability) present until fusion occurs across the operated segments. This combination of decompressed neural elements and the absence of pathological motion is felt to improve the likelihood of neural recovery. These principles have been clearly and consistently demonstrated in animal models (14–19), but not in humans. Fehlings and Tator (11) succinctly summarize the current literature regarding the impact of surgical decompression and stabilization on the recovery of spinal cord function in their recent article:

> There is biological evidence from experimental studies in animals that early decompressive surgery may improve neurological recovery after SCI, although the relevant interventional timing in humans remains unclear. To date, the role of surgical decompression in patients with SCI is only supported by Class III and limited Class II evidence (Class III = retrospective study, Class II = well-designed comparative clinical studies). Accordingly, decompressive surgery for SCI can only be considered a practice option.

Therefore, with respect to the role of the neurological condition of the patient with a thoracolumbar fracture, there is little hard clinical evidence (statistics) to support the notion that surgical intervention will alter the natural history of neurological improvement. Despite that, we advocate surgical decompression and stabilization for the incomplete or neurologically progressive injury.

III SPINAL STABILITY

The concept of spinal stability remains undefined. Despite numerous classification systems and proposed treatment algorithms, there is no uniform agreement as to the definition of spinal stability. The range of these proposed definitions spans nearly 60 years, starting with Watson-Jones in 1938, reporting on his experience with 250 fractures of the spine (20). Fifteen years later, Holdsworth and Hardy (21) furthered the work of Nicoll (22) and established a classification system that has withstood the "test of time." One of the more recently proposed definitions of spinal stability belongs to Panjabi et al. (23), with their "neutral zone theory."

Holdsworth's classification (21) allows a clinician to evaluate the injury, define its presumed mechanism, and determine its stability based on intact or structurally compromised anatomical structures. This classification strongly emphasizes the integrity of the posterior ligamentous complex. Despite its relative simplicity and its lack of dependence on modern imaging techniques (CT scan, MRI), recent studies have further supported its merits. James et al. (24), utilizing cadaveric specimens, biomechanically evaluated the relative contributions of the anterior, middle, and posterior columns [of Denis (25)] with respect to their role in maintaining spinal stability. The authors concluded the following:

1. The integrity of the posterior column is crucial to spinal stability and resistance to kyphotic progression in a thoracolumbar burst fracture.
2. There is little additive contribution to spinal stability from the middle column (Denis) in a burst fracture, and thus its role in spinal stability may be overemphasized.
3. The experimental data support the relevance of the two-column theory of spinal stability.

The two columns consist of the anterior column (anterior longitudinal ligament, vertebral body, intervertebral disk, annulus, and posterior longitudinal ligament) and the posterior column (osteoligamentous complex including facets, ligamentum flavum, inter- and supraspinous ligaments).

In contrast to Holdsworth, Panjabi's neutral zone theory (23,26) emphasizes the continuum between stability (with physiological motion), hypermobility (associated with normal degenerative changes), and eventually the painful and dangerous consequences of instability. This latter end-stage condition can also occur as a direct result of spinal trauma. This concept has been nicely applied to illustrate the varying degrees of instability in the laboratory setting, but has yet to be applied in the clinical setting to determine the stability of specific injury patterns.

Despite the 50-year period of discussion and the numerous proposed definitions of stability, there remains no consensus opinion. In this confused setting, it is helpful to remember and ponder the definition provided by White and Panjabi (12):

> Clinical instability is the inability of the spine to maintain its pattern of displacement under physiological loads so there is no neurological deficit, pain, nor deformity.

Unfortunately, this exquisitely practical and succinct guideline has neither been defined nor substantiated by clinical or radiographic measurements/parameters. In fact, the range of definitions currently purported to imply instability still parallel the extreme positions advocated by Watson-Jones (20) and Nicoll. (22) Therefore, despite the fact that spinal stabilization procedures (fusions) are performed daily for instability, whether it be posttraumatic, postoperative (postlaminectomy syndrome), or for restoring stability to the spine that has been rendered unstable secondary to the naturally occurring degenerative process, the definition of instability still remains largely within the context of the surgeon who is describing it.

Thus far, we have reviewed the issues of neurological improvement and restoration of stability with respect to operative versus nonoperative intervention. With close scrutiny of the available data, it is clear that neither of these primary treatment pathways has sufficient data to support strict guidelines. Although we, as treating surgeons, want to improve the potential for neurological recovery by decompression and stabilization, this has not proved to be a consistent result. Likewise, due to our ill-defined understanding of instability, there is documentation of excellent functional results from nonoperatively treated "unstable" fracture patterns and, conversely, there are multiple reports of residual impairment despite the "appropriate" surgical treatment of unstable fracture patterns. The final treatment objective concerns the need to intervene early to avoid latent back pain.

IV POST-TRAUMATIC KYPHOSIS

Unfortunately, the topic of post-traumatic kyphosis and its relationship to latent back pain is similarly clouded. It is impossible to ignore the results reported by Mumford et al. (5) with respect to the absence of clinical correlation of final x-rays and pain/impairment. These data lend further credibility to Nicoll's classic article (22), which reported full return to mining activities in 7/10 miners with "unstable injuries" when they healed. No attempt at reduction was performed. Additional support to the notion that deformity does not necessarily cause pain and impairment is noted upon closer review of articles by Weinstein et al. (7,8), Cantor et al. (2), and, more recently, Kraemer et al. (4).

Chow et al. (27) emphatically demonstrated the potential efficacy of nonoperative treatment by including thoracolumbar fractures with evidence of posterior ligament injury in their patient cohort. Thus, by all criteria, these injuries are classified as "unstable." This subset of patients fared no worse with respect to radiographic collapse or clinical outcome compared to the remainder of the treatment group, following the completion of their bracing.

Soreff (28) is generally credited with scientifically documenting a relationship between residual deformity and back pain. In his treatise, he identified "... a connection between radiological changes originating from the injury and the severity of the residual symptoms." Furthermore, his results revealed that "... severe compression fractures at levels Th11–L1 give rise to the most pronounced residual symptoms." His study group consisted of 147 patients with a minimum follow-up period of 8 years. Fifty percent of the study cohort were evaluated at least 15 years after their spinal injury.

Why the clinical picture varies so much despite similar-appearing radiographs remains puzzling. However, Baab (29) and later Young (30) brought attention to the possibility that it is *not* the bony injury but rather the associated soft-tissue injury that leads to the long-term sequelae of back pain. Baab wrote:

> A compression fracture of the spine should be considered as a joint injury and not as an injury to the bone (alone). The fracture always heals regardless of the treatment, but the damaged soft tissue produces the residual symptoms.

In a similar vein, Savastano and Pierik (31) suggest that it is the injured and subsequently fibrosed soft-tissue component of the spinal injury that leads to the long-term painful sequelae. Thus, if the fibrosis and increased stiffness that generally occur as a result of the injury are avoided by earlier mobilization, the facet joints and the associated soft tissues can more readily adapt to the bony injury and thus minimize the development of pain.

V TREATMENT GUIDELINES

Nonoperative treatment of thoracolumbar fractures should remain the primary treatment option. It should be initially entertained with most injury patterns. A comprehensive physical examination including a thorough neurological exam and direct palpation of the injured segment is essential. In addition, appropriate x-rays are necessary before any treatment option can be determined.

In the neurologically intact patient, the first step in our evaluation is the status of the posterior ligamentous complex. Evaluation of the posterior ligamentous complex is the key determinant of fracture stability. Integrity of these structures provides significant resistance to the deforming forces of kyphosis and translation. Direct evaluation of its structural integrity can be difficult because of patient size or inability to provide useful feedback during the examination (closed head injury, alcohol, drugs, distracting injuries). Supine radiographs also may mask an occult injury to these tissues. However, it is the authors' belief that the integrity of these tissues is the major determinant of stability and thus a high priority. Therefore, if the patient cannot assist the evaluating surgeon during the physical examination and the plain radiographs are not diagnostic of a posterior injury, an MRI is suggested to evaluate the integrity of these soft tissues. If the patient's body habitus does not allow MRI evaluation, the patient should be assumed to have an "unstable" spine until a better clinical examination can be obtained. This management includes strict log-rolling with bedrest precautions. Ultimately, once the patient is more able to cooperate, in addition to direct palpation of the area, a functional examination can be performed with progressive upright lateral films obtained to evaluate the presence or absence of a progressive kyphosis. Once the posterior structures are accurately assessed, the anterior column can be similarly evaluated.

In the neurologically intact patient, the presence of canal compromise is irrelevant. Latent neurological compromise is exceedingly rare and is generally associated with an occult injury to the posterior column (32). In the neurologically compromised patient, a CAT scan will allow accurate assessment of the canal compromise and facilitate a surgical plan. Despite the lack of clinical evidence, we recommend surgical decompression and stabilization for thoracolumbar fractures with incomplete neurological injuries. It is our bias to approach the majority of these injuries anteriorly and to both decompress and stabilize through a singular approach. The one exception is the fracture dislocation, which generally requires both anterior decompression and reconstruction followed by posterior stabilization for optimal stability.

In the neurologically "complete" spinal cord injury patient, our treatment plan is directed by the stability issues rather than the neurological picture. Generally, if we operate on the neurologically "complete" injury, it is through a posterior approach with the surgical goals of realignment and restoration of stability. We also attempt to obtain sufficient stability to obviate the need for a brace. Technically, we limit the number of levels stabilized/fused in order to maximize the number of free lumbar segments to optimize wheelchair mobility.

Finally, the most common scenario—the neurologically intact thoracolumbar spine fracture with intact posterior ligaments and an initial local kyphosis of 25 to 35 degrees. Our treatment algorithm is very individualized in this setting. When discussing the treatment options with the patient, several factors are taken into consideration. These include the patient's body habitus, their general health condition, lifestyle, and expectations, as well as their motivation. A young, thin, active individual with a labor-intensive profession would initially be offered nonoperative treatment. However, if the local gibbus proved bothersome or the post-traumatic pain sequelae interfered with necessary daily activities, surgical reconstruction would be offered. Similarly, an individual with multiple comorbidities such as osteoporosis, diabetes mellitus, or obesity would be given the option of nonoperative treatment due to the potential for less than optimal results. In the neurologically intact patient with intact posterior ligaments, it is difficult to encourage acute surgical treatment when the likelihood of successful nonoperative treatment is similar to that reported with surgery. If necessary, secondary reconstructive surgery can provide a favorable result.

In general, when nonoperative treatment is provided, bracing and ambulation are initiated when the acute traumatic pain has diminished. This is rarely much more than 7 to 10 days. Slow and progressive ambulation is then encouraged, and repeat upright x-rays are obtained during the acute hospital phase. If there is a significant increase in kyphosis or the patient is experiencing long tract signs, surgery is again entertained. Once ambulation is initiated, and repeat films are checked, the patient is discharged and followed closely in the outpatient setting. Bracing is generally continued for 8 to 12 weeks, depending on fracture configuration and patient comfort. Once the brace is discontinued, active flexion–extension x-rays are obtained to evaluate for pathological motion. If motion continues in association with pain, the brace is continued or surgical intervention is suggested. If the films show no residual motion, the brace is weaned and strengthening exercises are initiated under the supervision of a therapist.

REFERENCES

1. Burke DC, Murray DD. The management of thoracic and thoraco-lumbar injuries of the spine with neurological involvement. J Bone Joint Surg 1976;58B:72–78.
2. Cantor JB, Lebwohl NH, Garvey T, Eismont FJ. Nonoperative management of stable thoracolumbar burst fractures with early ambulation and bracing. Spine 1993;18:971–976.
3. Fredrickson N, Yuan HA, Bayley JC. The nonoperative treatment of thoracolumbar injuries. Sem Spine Surg 1990;2:70–78.
4. Kraemer WJ, Schemitsch EH, Lever J, McBroom RJ, McKee MD, Waddell JP. Functional outcome of thoracolumbar burst fractures without neurological deficit. J Orthoped Trauma 1996;10:541–544.
5. Mumford J, Weinstein JN, Spratt KF, Goel, VK. Thoracolumbar burst fractures. The clinical efficacy and outcome of nonoperative management. Spine 1993;18:955–970.

6. Rechtine GR, Cahill D, Chrin AM. Treatment of thoracolumbar trauma: comparison of complications of operative versus nonoperative treatment. J Spin Disord 1999;12:406–409.

7. Weinstein JN, Collalto P, Lehmann TR. Long-term follow-up of nonoperatively treated thoracolumbar spine fractures. J Orthop Trau. 1987;1:152–159.

8. Weinstein JN, Collalto P, Lehmann TR. Thoracolumbar "burst" fractures treated conservatively: a long-term follow-up. Spine 1988;13:33–38.

9. Davies WE, Morris JH, Hill V. An analysis of conservative (non-surgical) management of thoracolumbar fractures and fracture-dislocations with neural damage. J Bone Joint Surg 1980;62A:1324–1328.

10. Dickson JH, Harrington PR, Erwin WD. Results of reduction and stabilization of the severely fractured thoracic and lumbar spine. J Bone Joint Surg 1978;60A:799–805.

11. Fehlings MG, Tator CH. An evidence-based review of decompressive surgery in acute spinal cord injury: rationale, indications, and timing based on experimental and clinical studies. J Neurosurg 1999;91:1–11.

12. White AA, Panjabi MM. Clinical Biomechanics of the Spine. 2nd ed. Philadelphia: JB Lippincott, 1990.

13. Bohlman HH. Treatment of fractures and dislocations of the thoracic and lumbar spine. J Bone Joint Surg 1985;67A:165–169.

14. Carlson GD, Minato Y, Okada A, et al. Early time-dependent decompression for spinal cord injury: Vascular mechanisms of recovery. J Neurotrauma 1997;14:951–962.

15. Delamarter RB, Sherman J, Carr JB. Pathophysiology of spinal cord injury. Recovery after immediate and delayed decompression. J Bone Joint Surg 1995;77A:1042–1049.

16. Dolan EJ, Tator CH, Endrenyi L. The value of decompression for acute experimental spinal cord compression injury. J Neurosurg 1980;53:749–755.

17. Guha A, Tator CH, Endrenyi L, Piper I. Decompression of the spinal cord improves recovery after acute experimental spinal cord compression injury. Paraplegia 1987;25:324–339.

18. Rivlin AS, Tator CH. Objective clinical assessment of motor function after experimental spinal cord injury in the rat. J Neurosurg 1977;47:577–581.

19. Rivlin AS, Tator CH. Effect of duration of acute spinal cord compression in a new acute cord injury model in the rat. Surg Neurol 1978;10:38–43.

20. Watson-Jones R. The results of postural reduction of fractures of the spine. J Bone Joint Surg 1938;20:567–586.

21. Holdsworth FW, Hardy A. Early treatment of paraplegia from fractures of the thoracolumbar spine. J Bone Joint Surg 1953;35B:540–550.

22. Nicoll EA. Fractures of the dorso-lumbar spine. J Bone Joint Surg [Br] 2000;376.

23. Panjabi MM, Oxland TR, Lin RM, McGowen TW. Thoracolumbar burst fracture. A biomechanical investigation of its multidirectional flexibility. Spine 1994;19:578–585.

24. James KS, Wenger KH, Schlegel JD, Dunn HK. Biomechanical evaluation of the stability of thoracolumbar burst fractures. Spine 1994;19:1731–1740.

25. Denis F. The three column spine and its significance in the classification of acute thoracolumbar spinal injuries. Spine 1983;8:817–831.

26. Panjabi MM, Goel VK, Takata K. Physiologic strains in the lumbar spinal ligaments. An in vitro biomechanical study—1981 Volvo Award in Biomechanics. Spine 1982;7:192–203.

27. Chow GH, Nelson BJ, Gebhard JS, Brugman JL, Brown CW, Donaldson DH. Functional outcome of thoracolumbar burst fractures managed with hyperextension casting or bracing and early mobilization. Spine 1996;21:2170–2175.

28. Soreff J. Assessment of the late results of traumatic compression fractures of the thoracolumbar vertebral bodies. 1–95. 1977.

29. Baab OD. Fractures of the dorsal and lumbar spine. Clin Orthop Rel Res 1966;49:195–200.
30. Young MH. Long-term consequences of stable fractures of the thoracic and lumbar vertebral bodies. J Bone Joint Surg 1973;55:295–300.
31. Savastano AA, Perik J. Traumatic compression fractures of the dorsolumbar portion of the spine. J Int Coll Surg 1960;34:93–101.
32. Gertzbein SD. Neurologic deterioration in patients with thoracic and lumbar fractures after admission to the hospital. Spine 1994;19:1723–1725.

36

Operative Techniques: Posterior Thoracolumbar Techniques and Surgical Approaches

JAMES S. HARROP

Jefferson Medical College, Philadelphia, Pennsylvania, U.S.A.

GREGORY J. PRZYBYLSKI

Northwestern University, Chicago, Illinois, U.S.A.

I INTRODUCTION

Many surgical approaches have been developed to treat a variety of pathological lesions of the thoracolumbar spine. The route for exposure of the spine is often chosen to facilitate a direct line of sight to the pathology while minimizing the risk of injury to surrounding tissue.

Although an anterior exposure typically offers the most direct route to vertebral body lesions, this approach has some anatomical constraints. The heart and great vessels limit access to the rostral thoracic spine, whereas the diaphragm limits the exposure of the thoracolumbar junction. In contrast, the middle thoracic region can be exposed easily, allowing access for extensive decompression, arthrodesis, and instrumentation. The anterior approach is particularly useful for correcting severe thoracic kyphosis, midline thoracic disk protrusions, and anterior lumbar diskectomy and arthrodesis (1). One concern regarding anterior exposures involves transgression of pleural or peritoneal cavities, which may place patients at greater operative risks than either posterior or posterolateral approaches. The postoperative pulmonary and gastrointestinal complications may be debilitating, particularly in the elderly. Despite growing utilization of anterior approaches, many spinal surgeons require the assistance of a thoracic or general surgeon for access to the anterior thoracolumbar spine.

In contrast, spinal surgeons are most familiar with the dorsal thoracolumbar spinal exposure through a translaminar or transpedicular approach. Both are performed through a midline incision and represent the most common approaches for spinal pathology. Although a laminectomy limits visualization to the dorsal thecal sac, a unilateral transpedicular approach can offer exposure to eccentric disk or vertebral pathology, whereas a bilateral transpedicular approach can provide circumferential access for decompression of the anterior and posterior spinal canal. However, direct visualization of the anterior dura cannot be achieved using these midline dorsal approaches.

Consequently, posterolateral approaches were developed to achieve more direct visualization of the vertebral body or disk from a dorsal incision. These approaches include the costotransversectomy and lateral extracavitary approach. Although the costotransversectomy allows a limited thoracic exposure, this extrapleural approach is particularly useful for the treatment of thoracic disk disease. In contrast, the lateral extracavitary approach allows circumferential exposure of the vertebra. The purpose of this chapter is to illustrate the techniques, advantages, and limitations of posterior and posterolateral thoracolumbar surgical approaches.

II ANATOMY

In order to appreciate the line of vision provided by these approaches, it is important to understand the anatomical relationships among vertebrae, ribs, muscles, and diskoligamentous structures. This will facilitate choosing the approach that allows appropriate visualization of the pathological target and adequate space within the exposed tissue planes.

The superficial muscles of the thoracic and lumbar regions are dorsal to the thoracolumbar fascia and consist of the latissimus dorsi, trapezius, rhomboid, and serratus posterior inferior muscles. The latissimus dorsi muscle arises from the spinous processes of T6–T12 and forms the posterior wall of the axillae prior to inserting on the proximal humerus. The serratus posterior inferior muscle arises from the last two thoracic and first two lumbar vertebrae and inserts onto the thoracic ribs. The trapezius also arises from the thoracic spinous processes T1–T12 and inserts onto the scapula. Deep to the superficial muscles and the thoracolumbar fascia are the erector spinalis muscles. These muscles, which are important for maintaining posture and motion of the vertebral column, are located between the spinous and transverse process and are termed the paraspinal muscles (2).

After dissection of muscular attachments to the vertebrae, a variety of ligamentous structures can be identified which limit visualization of the underlying bone. In the thoracic region, the rib tubercle articulates with the transverse process of the vertebral body, supported by the large superior costotransverse ligament that bridges the superior rib segment to the inferior portion of transverse process. The rib head attaches to the vertebral body with support from the costovertebral ligaments, articulating over the disk space of the superior vertebral body along with the transverse process to which it is attached. Since the transverse process is perpendicular and dorsal to the pedicle, removal of the rib head and transverse process allows visualization of the lateral pedicle. By exposing the pedicle, the neurovascular bundle can be identified and preserved.

Each vertebral segment has a segmental nerve that leaves the spinal canal through the neural foramen to join with others to become peripheral nerves. The foramen is bounded rostrally and caudally by adjacent pedicles, anteriorly by the vertebral body, and posteriorly by the pars interarticularis. In the thoracic region, the segmental nerve joins the thoracic segmental vein and artery to form the neurovascular bundle located along the inferior surface of the rib. The spinal cord ends as the conus medullaris, which modulates bowel and bladder function. The actual anatomical location of the conus varies, but is typically near the L1–L2 level. Perfusion of the distal spinal cord is somewhat restricted by the limited vascular supply. Often, the thoracic cord receives prominent blood supply from a single dominant vessel termed the artery of Adamkiewicz. This artery is usually observed on the left side between T10 and L2. Some surgeons recommend spinal angiography to identify this vessel for resections between the T6 and L2 level (3). However, division of a limited number of segmental vessels close to the aorta may allow preservation of sufficient collateral vessels to allow inadvertent sacrifice of this important vessel, particularly in left-sided approaches.

III PREPARATION

The preparation of a patient is an integral portion of any spinal procedure. Proper attention to positioning provides maximal unobstructed visualization of the pathology, allowing the surgeon to realize the approach to its full advantage, while concurrently protecting pressure points on the body. Prior to induction of anesthesia, the patient's range of cervical motion is assessed so that a comfortable position can be maintained. In addition, pneumatic compression stockings are placed and, if appropriate, neurophysiological monitoring equipment is utilized and baseline parameters are determined. One should ensure that the operating table has radiolucent parts to facilitate intraoperative radiographs.

Within a half hour prior to skin incision, the patient should receive preoperative antibiotics. In addition, intravenous steroids and H2 blockers may be given, if indicated, and an indwelling bladder catheter may be inserted. The types and quantity of intravenous access should be considered so that any blood loss may be replaced efficiently. If significant blood loss is anticipated, a central venous catheter and arterial line can be placed to monitor the patient's hemodynamic status during surgery. The operating table may include laminectomy rolls or other devices to reduce venous outflow obstruction from abdominal pressure, thereby theoretically reducing venous bleeding while allowing normal respiration. The head and neck are maintained in a neutral position and excessive manipulation is avoided. If the patient has an unstable spine, supine transfer to a rotating operating table (e.g., Stryker or Jackson tables) facilitates subsequent placement in a prone position.

If the operative site is above the sixth thoracic level or a lengthy operative duration is expected, then the patient's head is placed in three-point fixation with the Mayfield frame. This allows support of the head and neck without external pressure on the face or neck. Particular attention should be given to the ocular and nasal regions to avoid compression of the eyes that may result in permanent visual loss. After prone positioning, the patient is secured to the table with wide tape. Typically the arms are abducted at the shoulder and flexed at the elbow to prevent compression or entrapment of neurovascular structures. Padding to these areas may be helpful. If the operative site is in the rostral to midthoracic region, the arms are padded and positioned at the patient's side to allow the surgeon to stand closer to the operative field. Proper padding, taping, and head positioning allow the surgeon to more safely rotate the operating table to further improve visualization.

The planned incision is marked on the back and the thoracolumbar regions are prepped. The iliac crest region and/or chest wall should be prepped and draped in the field to allow access to harvest sites for autologous bone, if needed. The preparation, including positioning, is similar for each of the four approaches.

A Posterior Laminectomy

In 1911, Hibbs and Albee first described the use of this approach for fusions of spinal deformities resulting from tuberculosis. The posterior midline approach is the most common spinal exposure used. Laminectomies are performed for disk excision, canal decompression, intradural tumor resection, posterior spinal fusion, deformity correction, and stabilization. This approach exposes the dorsal spinal elements including the spinous processes, laminae, superior and inferior facets, pars interarticularis, and transverse processes.

A midline incision is carried down through the thoracolumbar fascia. The spinous processes are identified and a subperiosteal dissection is performed to expose the dorsal spine. Retractors on the paraspinal muscles are positioned to maintain exposure of the dorsal spine. The extent of exposure of the facet capsule is predicated upon the lateral extent of the intraspinal target. Exposure of central structures can end at the junction of the lamina and medial aspect of the facet. In contrast, exposing a portion of the medial facet capsule may be helpful in accessing the lateral recess. Finally, subperiosteal dissection beyond the lateral facet to the transverse processes provides the necessary exposure for a posterolateral fusion. An intraoperative radiograph may be taken to identify the level of exposure. Since interpreting radiographs with markers on the spinous process may be misleading, a radio-opaque marker is placed under the inferior lamina, thereby identifying the plane of the interspace below. Alternatively, a marker on the transverse process identifies the level of the pedicle and may allow more accurate identification of spinal level. A surgical table that allows posteroanterior radiographs may help in identifying thoracic levels. The interspinous ligaments at the rostral and caudal limits of the planned laminectomy are divided. A Horsley bone cutter facilitates rapid removal of the spinous processes at the spinolaminar junction. Several methods may be utilized to perform a laminectomy. The lamina may be thinned with a rongeur or drill. A curved curette can be used to develop a plane between the lamina and yellow ligament. Preservation of the flaval ligament initially facilitates protection of the underlying dura to the upper portion of the lamina. The laminectomy is typically performed in a caudal to cranial direction. Alternatively, a drill can be used to remove a trough of bone bilaterally at the junction of the medial facet and lamina, thereby creating a "floating" lamina. This can be dissected from the flaval ligament attachments with a curette so that the lamina is removed in one piece. Occasionally, a rapid laminectomy may be required for spinal cord decompression (Fig. 1). If a dorsal epidural process is present that displaces the dura anteriorly, a high-speed drill with footplate may be cautiously used to divide the lateral lamina at its junction with the facet joints. Since the thoracic spinal canal is narrower than the lumbar canal and is also occupied by the spinal

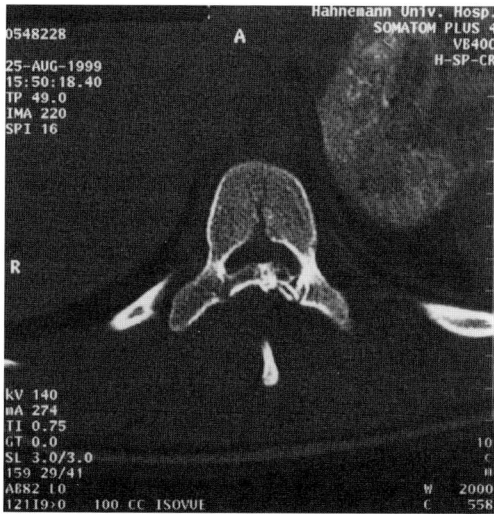

Figure 1   Axial CT image of an impacted laminar fracture sustained by a young man who fell onto a fence, sustaining a severe spinal cord injury. He underwent a posterior laminectomy alone and subsequently regained ambulatory function.

cord, a thoracic laminectomy performed with bilateral troughs may reduce manipulation of the spinal cord by sublaminar placement of a rongeur footplate. It is important to drill perpendicularly to the lamina, which requires medial angulation, to avoid inadvertent removal of a portion of the medial facet. Drilling may be carried down through both cortices of the lamina until the flaval ligament caudally and dura rostrally are seen at each laminar level. Alternatively, the cortex closest to the dura may be preserved and removed with a narrow rongeur. If the lamina appears to be unusually thick, one should reassess the angle of drilling to be certain that one is not drilling into the facet complex. Subsequently, the laminectomy may be widened laterally with a rongeur. If the decompression is performed too far laterally, then excessive bleeding may be encountered from the epidural venous plexus. This can be controlled with bipolar cautery and packing. The laminae are set aside and can be replaced in the form of a laminoplasty at the end of the procedure with small plates or wire fixation.

B   Posterior Transpedicular Approach

The transpedicular approach was described by Patterson et al. as an alternative method to excise extruded thoracic disk fragments (4), given the high frequency of neurological morbidity after a laminectomy alone (5). Although Patterson performed a complete facetectomy, others have shown that complete diskectomies and vertebrectomies can be done through a bilateral transpedicular approach (6,7). A unilateral procedure may be preferred if only a limited exposure of the posterolateral vertebral body is necessary (Fig. 2), whereas a bilateral approach allows complete circumferential decompression of the dural sac, including the ability to perform a vertebrectomy (Fig. 3). As a result, a vertebrectomy can be performed along with placement of posterior instrumentation through a single exposure.

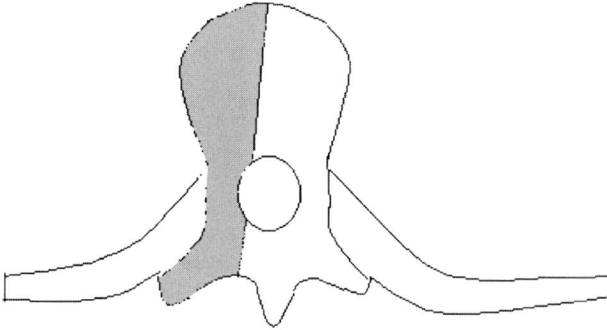

Figure 2 A schematic estimating the amount of bone removal achieved in a unilateral transpedicular approach.

If a bilateral transpedicular approach is planned, the dissection is carried laterally to expose the facets and transverse processes bilaterally. A complete laminectomy may be performed over the involved vertebral body, but is not necessary for a unilateral approach. However, removal of the lateral lamina allows identification of the exiting nerve root before removing the pedicle.

Significant excision of the facets overlying the targeted pedicle is accomplished with rongeurs or a high-speed drill. Subsequently, the drill is used to remove the pedicle down to the vertebral body, protecting the exiting nerve root below. This allows visualization of the rostral intervertebral disk and rostral lateral part of the vertebral body (Fig. 4). Placement of an interbody graft requires complete excision of the facets and pars unilaterally, as well as the costovertebral joint. Excision of the caudal pars interarticularis allows visualization of the caudal lateral portion of the vertebral body. Lateral exposure from the rostral to the caudal disk allows a trajectory for the vertebrectomy. In the thoracic region, the exiting nerve root can be sacrificed by suture ligation at its take-off from the dural sac. Patients do not typically describe sensory loss, even if a pair of adjacent thoracic intercostal nerves are sacrificed. However, the lumbar roots typically cannot be sacrificed without sustaining a neurological injury. The disk is removed in a piecemeal fashion with curettes and pi-

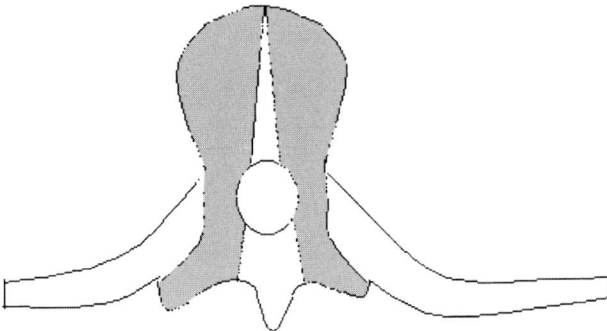

Figure 3 A schematic estimating the amount of bone removal achieved in a bilateral transpedicular approach.

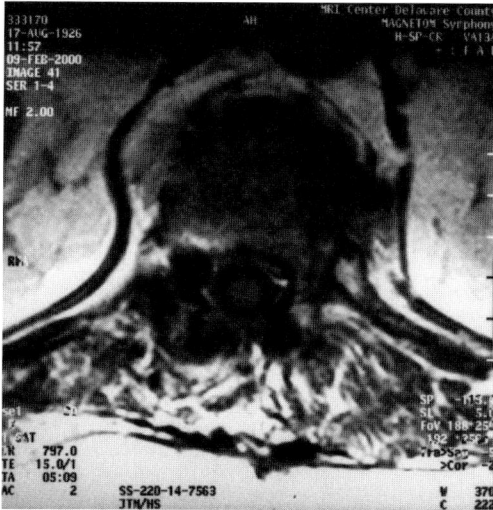

Figure 4 Axial T1-weighted MR image demonstrates a laminectomy and right pedicle removal after a unilateral transpedicular approach to a lateral thoracic disk displacement.

tuitary rongeurs. The high-speed drill is used to remove portions of the vertebral body alongside and tangential to the dural sac. The procedure is repeated contralaterally, isolating a midline remnant of posterior vertebral body adjacent to the dura. Once a corpectomy defect is created, a plane is developed between the dura and the posterior cortical remnant, which is then pushed into the defect. The dura can be visualized anteriorly with a dental mirror.

Once decompression is completed, a structural graft the width of the iliac crest can be placed lateral to the dural sac. With a laminar distractor, a slightly oversized graft can be placed in compression after distraction is released. The posterior instrumentation can be fashioned and placed (Fig. 5). This allows the surgeon the ability to adjust the spinal alignment.

C Posterolateral Costotransversectomy

In 1894, Menard first described this approach through a midline incision for drainage of tuberculous paraspinal abscesses in patients with Pott's disease (8). Decades later, Alexander and Capener modified this approach into the lateral rhachotomy for treatment of thoracic spinal deformities (9,10). Although the costotransversectomy approach is similar to the lateral extracavitary exposure in principle, a lesser exposure is necessary. In fact, a comparatively smaller paramedian incision is made such that the posterior spinal elements are not even exposed. Several modifications to this procedure have been proposed (11–13).

Although the patient is typically positioned prone as previously described for midline dorsal approaches, others prefer to position patients laterally (13). The side approach should be predicated on the laterality of the pathology. The inferior rib head articulates over the desired disk space. The thoracic ribs should be counted in a caudal direction on all imaging since a small proportion of patients have fewer

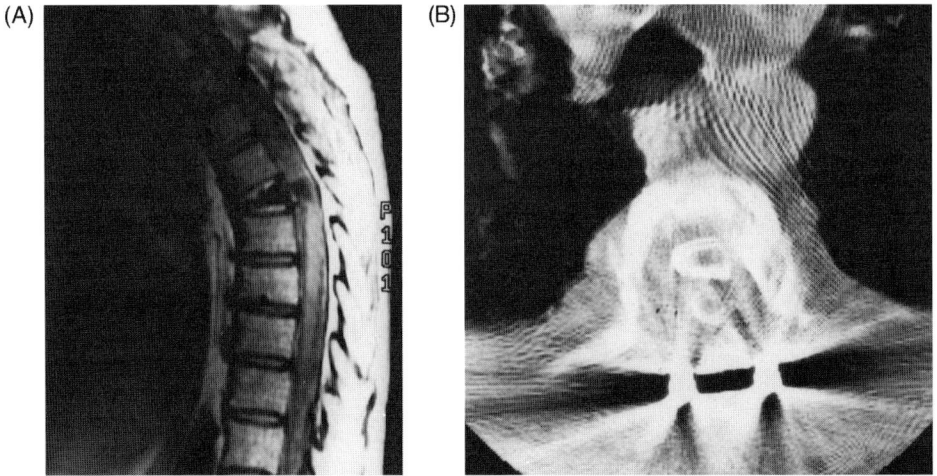

Figure 5   (A) A sagittal MR shows a midthoracic metastasis in a patient with acute paraplegia. (B) After resection and reconstruction using a bilateral transpedicular approach, a postmyelographic CT demonstrates canal decompression and anterior graft placement.

than 12 ribs. A paramedian incision is made laterally on the border of the paraspinal muscles, approximately 12 to 15 cm in length.

The thoracolumbar fascia and superficial muscles are incised and the dorsal aspect of the ribs is exposed. A blunt dissection is then carried medially along the rib cage, anterior to the paraspinal muscles. A Doyen is used to circumferentially dissect the periosteum off the ribs toward the vertebral attachment. Subsequently, cautery is used to dissect the costotransverse and costovertebral ligaments from the transverse process and vertebral body at the rib head. The rib is cut laterally and disarticulated from the vertebral body. Rongeurs or a high-speed drill may be required to remove the remaining rib head. The neurovascular bundle, which was identified during the subperiosteal dissection, is dissected and traced to its origin at the neural foramen. The superior and inferior pedicle borders are defined with a curved curette, which facilitates development of an epidural plane behind the pedicle. Subsequently, the pedicle is removed in a piecemeal fashion with the rongeur and high-speed drill, allowing visualization of the lateral thecal sac. The disk is incised and a posterior diskectomy is performed using curettes and pituitary rongeurs. The retropulsed disk in the central canal may be removed by pushing the remaining disk into the empty intervertebral space (Fig. 6). An anterior arthrodesis is typically not required since this approach spares nearly all of the dorsal spinal elements.

D   Posterolateral Lateral Extracavitary Approach

Alexander and Capener first reported the posterolateral approach to the thoracic and lumbar spine for the treatment of tuberculous spondylitis. Subsequently, Larson further refined the procedure (14) and described the advantages for treating thoracolumbar fractures (15) and thoracic disk disease (16). The approach provides excellent exposure of the lateral thoracolumbar vertebrae, allowing performance of a verte-

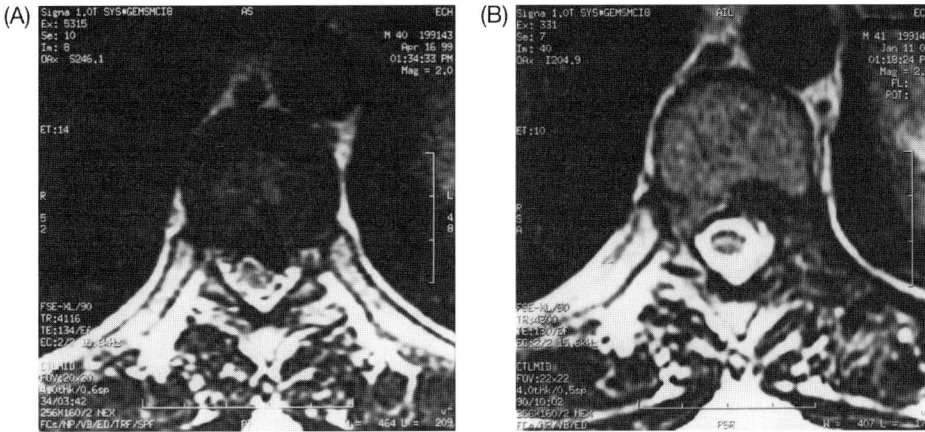

Figure 6 (A) An axial T2-weighted MR shows a left posterolateral disk displacement. (B) Postoperative axial T2-weighted MR shows excision of the disk by a costovertebral approach.

brectomy from a unilateral approach without sacrifice of the nerve root, interbody reconstruction, and a posteriorly instrumented fusion through a single incision. This approach allows the surgeon to expose the lamina, facets, transverse processes, and lateral vertebral body of the exposed side (Fig. 7). Moreover, the iliac crest may be exposed in the same incision for lumbar approaches. Although the procedure may be performed across the entire thoracolumbar spine, the scapula can limit exposure of the rostral-most thoracic vertebra, whereas the iliac crest may interfere with exposure of the caudal-most lumbar vertebra. In addition, circumferential access to the vertebral body can be attained if the approach is performed bilaterally. Although blood loss may be substantial, this dissection allows vertebrectomy without transgressing the pleural or peritoneal cavities. In traumatic injuries, cell saver salvage may limit the need for blood transfusion.

Although the patient may be positioned as described previously, the approach has also been performed in a three-quarter (17) or full lateral position (18). Typically,

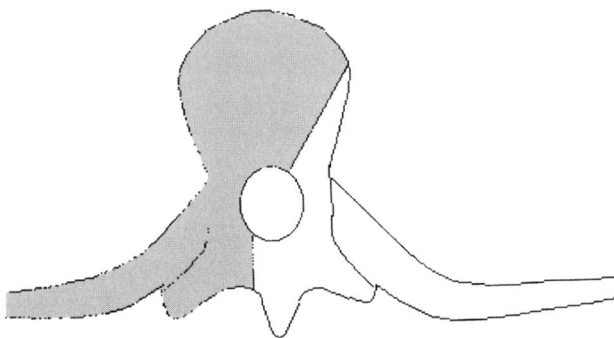

Figure 7 A schematic estimating the amount of bone removal achieved in a lateral extracavitary approach.

the midline incision is performed three vertebral segments rostral and caudal to the targeted vertebra. The incision is then carried laterally at least 8 cm to either the right or left side. The laterality of approach is based upon asymmetry of pathology and location of the artery of Adamkiewicz. A subperiosteal dissection of the posterior bony elements may be performed first in preparation for subsequent instrumentation and posterolateral fusion. Packing for hemostasis is then placed dorsally.

Subsequently, a plane is developed between the layers of the thoracodorsal fascia to expose the paraspinal muscles out to their lateral extent. Several bridging vessels between the subcutaneous layer and the muscles are coagulated and divided. In the thoracic region, the ribs are encountered lateral to the paraspinal muscles. Blunt dissection from the lateral border taken anteromedially allows circumferential mobilization of the paraspinal muscles on one side. The muscle bundle can then be brought across midline to the opposite side, allowing visualization of the dorsolateral spine. The subcutaneous flap is retracted downward and laterally. In the thoracic spine, the rib of the targeted vertebra and the next inferior one are exposed subperiosteally with a combination of Adson and Doyen periosteal elevators. A rib cutter is then used to resect the rib laterally. Then, the medial portion of the costovertebral attachment, including the costovertebral and costotransverse ligaments, is dissected free with cautery so that the rib can be disarticulated in a similar fashion as described in the costotransversectomy. Although care should be taken to avoid entry into the pleural or peritoneal cavities, small defects may be closed primarily. However, larger lacerations may need to be treated with a chest tube postoperatively. Typically, a single rib is removed to expose an interspace, whereas two ribs are removed for each vertebral body that needs to be resected. In addition, the transverse process is resected in order to facilitate visualization of the lateral pedicle.

The neurovascular bundle that was freed from the inferior border of the rib is marked with a vessel loop and dissected medially to identify the neural foramen. A subperiosteal dissection is carried down over the lateral vertebral body from interspace to interspace. The segmental vessels at the midportion of the vertebral body should be coagulated and divided. Although one may ligate and divide thoracic nerve roots to prevent traction on the spinal cord, these can often be preserved. After identifying the pedicle, a curette is used to dissect the superior and inferior borders of the pedicle, developing an epidural plane behind the pedicle. The pedicle is then removed with rongeurs or a high-speed drill, allowing identification of the lateral thecal sac. If a retropulsed bone fragment (e.g., burst fracture) is present, only the more caudal portion of the lateral dura may be seen initially. The pedicle is then removed with rongeurs or a high-speed drill. Identification of the dural sac before visualizing the pathology is one great advantage of this exposure.

Once exposure of the lateral vertebra from rostral to caudal disk space is achieved and the pedicle has been excised, the annulus of each intervertebral disk is incised and a diskectomy performed. Then, the corpectomy is performed with either rongeurs or a high-speed drill. A thin rim of posterior cortical bone is left in place to protect the dural contents. This also helps maintain compression of the epidural veins to reduce bleeding until the final fragment is removed. One must be careful to maintain a lateral trajectory, as there is a tendency to perform the corpectomy more anteriorly as one crosses to the contralateral side. Operating in a seated position and rotating the patient away from the surgeon may facilitate a more directed lateral bony removal. Once the dissection has crossed to the opposite pedicle, the annular ligament attachments to the posterior vertebral body cortex are excised, thereby creating a "free-floating" posterior cortical remnant. Finally, this cortical rim can be pushed into the corpectomy defect with a reverse angle curette away from the spinal cord and dura. In contrast, the anterior vertebral body cortex can be preserved, since it provides no benefit in decompressing the canal, increases blood loss, and increases the risk of aortic or vena caval injury. However, sufficient bone must be removed anteriorly to allow adequate space for an interbody graft. A dental mirror can be placed in the corpectomy defect to confirm decompression across midline. Finally, an interbody graft is positioned into the corpectomy defect after preparation of the endplates (Fig. 8).

In the lumbar region, the iliac crest can impede visualization of the lateral L5 vertebral body. By bringing the lateral limb of the incision over the iliac crest, one can resect a larger border of the ilium to improve caudal exposure. The exposure of the lumbar region is similar, except that the neurovascular bundle is not superficially associated with the undersurface of the rib. Instead, dissection through the transverse ligament allows identification of the exiting nerve root. One dissects proximally and distally along the root, marking it with a vessel loop. This allows mobilization of the lumbar nerves, which usually cannot be sacrificed without significant neurological deficit. The roots can be held on slight traction to maintain the exposure of the lateral vertebral body. The nerve root is followed proximally into the foramen, and the procedure continues as previously described in the thoracic spine.

Another advantage of this exposure is the ability to reposition the anterior graft while adjusting the posterior instrumentation. Once the spinal cord is decompressed, attention can then be directed to midline posterior instrumentation, reduction of deformity, and interbody reconstruction. Although this approach allows concurrent anterior and posterior exposure through a single skin incision, there are associated

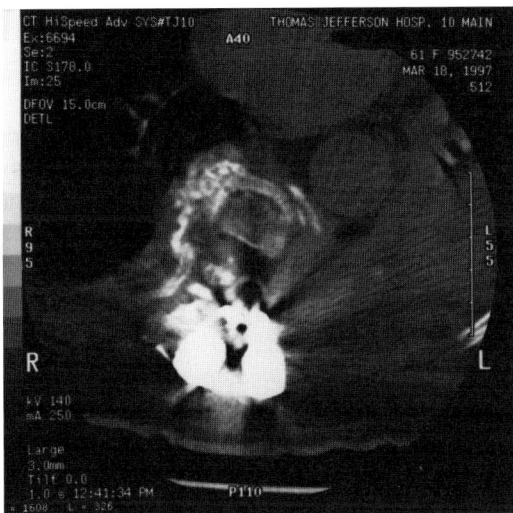

Figure 8 A postmyelographic axial CT demonstrates a vertebrectomy with anterior graft placement and posterior instrumentation through a left lateral extracavitary approach.

morbidities including increased blood loss and operative time in comparison to transpedicular and staged anteroposterior approaches (19). While this procedure allows significant advantages, it is technically demanding and tedious. An experienced assistant may help facilitate the exposure.

In conclusion, posterior and posterolateral approaches represent a series of progressively more lateral views of the spine from an initial dorsal spinal incision. Although several of these approaches allow anterior vertebrectomy and interbody reconstruction, these are technically more difficult since one is working around and deep to the thecal sac. However, the ability to perform concurrent posterolateral arthrodesis and instrumentation through the same incision without entering the pleural cavity offers significant advantages as well. Ultimately, the unique pathology of the patient should be carefully evaluated in order to choose the most appropriate approach for the given condition.

REFERENCES

1. Perot PL, Munro DD. Transthoracic removal of midline thoracic disc protrusions causing spinal cord compression. J Neurosurg 1969;31:452–458.
2. Moore KL. Clinically Oriented Anatomy, 2nd ed. Baltimore: Williams & Wilkins, 1985.
3. Maiman DJ, Larson SJ. Lateral extracavitary approach to the thoracic and lumbar spine. In: Rengachary, SS, Wilkins, RH, eds. Neurosurgical Operative Atlas, AANS. Baltimore: Williams & Wilkins, 1992:153–161.
4. Patterson RH, Arbit E. A surgical approach through the pedicle to protrude thoracic discs. J Neurosurg 1978;48:768–772.
5. Arseni C, Nash F. Thoracic intervertebral disc protrusion: a clinical study. J Neurosurg 1960;17:418–430.
6. Akeyson EW, McCutcheon IE. Single-stage posterior vertebrectomy and replacement combined with posterior instrumentation for spinal metastasis. J Neurosurg 1996;85: 211–220.
7. Le Roux PD, Haglund MM, Basil HA. Thoracic disc disease: experience with the transpedicular approach in twenty consecutive patients. Neurosurgery 1993;33(1):58–66.
8. Menard V. Causes de la paraplegic dans la mal de pott. Rev Orthop 1894;5:47–64.
9. Alexander GL. Neurological complications of spinal tuberculosis. Proc R Soc Med 1946; 39:730–734.
10. Capener N. The evolution of lateral rhachotomy. J Bone Joint Surg 1954;36B:173–179.
11. Ahlgren BD, Herkowitz HN. A modified posterolateral approach to the thoracic spine. J Spinal Disord 1995;8:69–75.
12. Hulme A. The surgical approach to thoracic intervertebral disc protrusions. J Neurol Neurosurg Psychiatry 1960;23:133–137.
13. Simpson MJ, Silveri CP, Simeone FA, Balderson RA, An HS. Thoracic disc herniation re-evaluation of the posterior approach using a modified costotransversectomy. Spine 1993;18(13):1872–1877.
14. Larson SJ, Holst RA, Hemmy DC, Sances A Jr. Lateral extracavitary approach to traumatic lesions of the thoracic and lumbar spine. J Neurosurg 1976;45:628–637.
15. Larson SJ. The lateral extrapleural and extraperitoneal approaches to the thoracic and lumbar spine. In: D Ruge, L Wiltse, eds. Spinal Disorders: Diagnosis and Treatment. Philadelphia: Lea and Febiger, 1977:137–141.
16. Maiman DJ, Larson SJ, Luck E, El-Ghatit A. Lateral extracavitary approach to the spine for thoracic disc herniation: report of 23 cases. Neurosurgery 1984;14:178–182.

17. Benzel EC. The lateral extracavitary approach to the spine using the three-quarter prone position. J Neurosurg 1989;71:837–841.
18. McCormick PC. Retropleural approach to the thoracic and thoracolumbar spine. Technique and application. Neurosurgery 1995;37(5):908–914.
19. Resnick DK, Benzel EC. Lateral extracavitary approach for thoracic and thoracolumbar spine trauma: operative complications. Neurosurgery 1998;43:796–803.

37

Posterior Thoracolumbar Spine Surgical Techniques

GLENN M. AMUNDSON

University of Kansas Medical Center, Kansas City, Kansas, U.S.A.

I INTRODUCTION

Before the use of spinal instrumentation, most paraplegic patients died as a result of large bedsores and urinary tract infections. Poor nonoperative treatment results and a host of complications, including gross angulation of the spine, stiffness of joints, contractures and deformities, seriously delayed or even prevented rehabilitation. Denis et al. documented a 25% incidence of late pain in patients with burst fractures treated nonsurgically (1). Internal fixation of the lumbar spine was first described in 1897 when Wilkins reported tying a carbolized silver suture around the pedicles of the T12 and L1 vertebrae in an infant who was born with a fracture dislocation (2). Early fixation devices, including Weiss springs, the Wilson plate, wire loops, and the Meurig-Williams plate, did not allow early mobilization due to inadequate fixation resulting from metal failure, wire cut-out, or bone fracture (3–6) (Fig. 1).

A thoracolumbar spine rendered unstable by traumatic injury requires safe reduction and stabilization techniques to (1) allow early mobilization of the patient to prevent pulmonary, vascular, urological, and psychological complications; (2) relieve pain; (3) reduce and maintain alignment of the spine and spinal canal; (4) decompress directly or indirectly the neural elements; (5) restore stability to promote healing and prevent increased neurological loss; and (6) attain solid fusion (7–10). Early operative stabilization and mobilization reduces morbidity and shortens rehabilitation time and hospital stay, thereby curtailing cost (11–13). The ideal instrumentation system should demonstrate the following characteristics: (1) low morbidity; (2) secure fixation with a low failure rate; (3) minimize external immobilization; (4) cost-effectiveness; and (5) high success rate measured by a low pseudarthrosis rate and

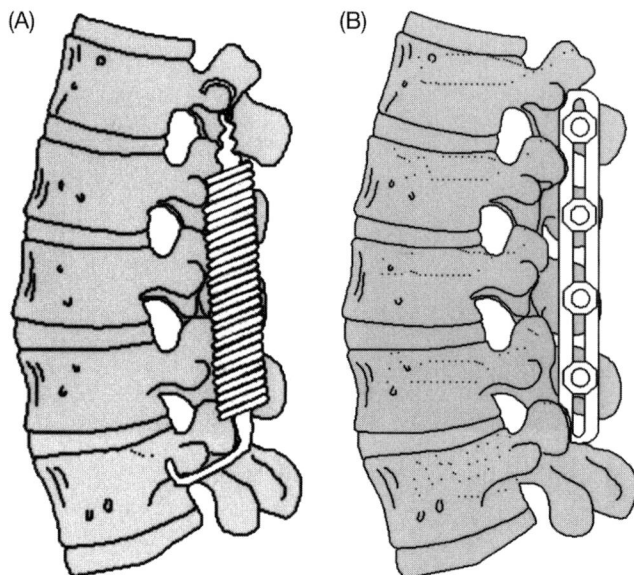

Figure 1 Early posterior spinal instrumentation. (A) Weiss springs. (B) Meurig-Williams plate.

absence of pain and deformity after surgery (12). Injured spinal column structures should be protected from load, or their function replaced by an appropriate surgical implant (14). Modern posterior spinal instrumentation for thoracolumbar trauma meets much of these expectations (1,15).

Historically, posterior spinal instrumentation for thoracolumbar trauma has grown from efforts to correct and stabilize chronic, progressive, spinal deformities. A natural extension of these techniques has been to apply the principles of scoliosis posterior spinal fixation to the more acute spinal deformities related to trauma. Since its contemporary introduction by Harrington, in 1959, posterior spinal instrumentation for unstable thoracolumbar spine fractures has been the most often applied method of stabilization and fusion. Patients treated with early posterior spinal instrumentation techniques required the addition of rigid external bracing for the postoperative protection of the hook–lamina interface until solid arthrodesis was achieved (10). In the hopes of improving correction and construct stability, the Harrington system underwent various modifications. These Harrington "variants" included square-ended "Moe" rods and hooks, Edwards' hooks and sleeves, Jacob's locking hook-rod, and the addition of compression rods and sacral bars.

In the 1970s, Edwardo Luque of Mexico City, Mexico, developed a segmental spinal fixation system for the treatment of severe progressive scoliotic deformities that often decreased the need for rigid external bracing. His system allowed purchase and application of force to multiple levels of the deformed spine and began the era of segmental spinal fixation. Subsequently, the combination of the Harrington system with the Luque segmental wiring technique and square-ended hooks allowed anatomical sagittal contouring and resulted in better control of axial, translational, and rotational forces over shorter spinal segments.

In the early 1980s, Cotrel and Dubousset of France developed a universal posterior segmental spinal fixation system that allowed for multiple variable hook fixations on a knurled rod as a device to aid in the correction and fusion of spinal deformities. The past decade has witnessed a dramatic increase in the availability of spinal instrumentation devices, enabling surgeons to treat a variety of spinal disorders with improved results and lower morbidity. The use of transpedicular screw fixation of the thoracolumbar spine allows for excellent segmental fixation over shortened constructs, even in the absence of posterior elements, and has significantly improved the fusion rate.

Harrington and Tullos were the first to report use of a transpedicular screw. They attempted the reduction of a spondylolisthesis in conjunction with a Harrington rod (16). In France, Roy-Camille et al. developed the first spinal fixation system that truly utilizes the pedicle (17). Steffee et al. improved upon the Roy-Camille plate by rigidly anchoring the screw to the plate independent of the plate–bone contact (18). Current trends in posterior spinal instrumentation are noted: (1) the application of implants over shorter distances, therefore immobilization and/or fusing the least number of normal spinal segments; (2) more rigid implants and stiffer segmental spinal fixation techniques; and (3) a better understanding of the ability of posterior spinal implants to provide immediate stability to the unstable thoracolumbar spine (10).

II POSTERIOR APPROACH

Posterior spinal instrumentation has the primary advantage of using the familiar technique of posterior midline exposure. In 1995, Danisa et al. retrospectively studied 49 nonparaplegic patients who sustained acute unstable thoracolumbar burst fractures (19). Three treatment groups were reviewed: one group of 16 patients underwent anterior decompression and fusion with instrumentation; a second group of 27 patients underwent posterolateral decompression and fusion; and a third group of six patients had combined anterior–posterior surgery. These groups were composed of patients of similar age, gender, level of injury, percentage of canal compromise, neurological function, and degree of kyphosis. Patients treated with posterior surgery had a statistically significant diminution in operative time, blood loss, and number of units transfused. There were no significant intergroup differences when considering postoperative kyphotic correction, neurological function, pain assessment, or the ability to return to work. This study is representative of more recent work documenting posterior surgery to be as effective as anterior or anterior–posterior surgery when treating unstable thoracolumbar burst fractures. Posterior surgery, however, required the least time and resulted in the least blood loss and expense of the three techniques (19).

III CANAL DECOMPRESSION

Hashimoto et al. evaluated CT scans of 112 consecutive patients with thoracolumbar burst fractures to investigate the relationship between traumatic canal stenosis and neurological deficits. They found burst fractures associated with the following ratios of canal occlusion to be at significant risk of neurological involvement: at T11 to T12 with 35% or more; at L1 with 45% or more; and at L2 and below with 55%

or more (20,21). Lemons et al. confirmed that the greater the initial spinal canal compromise, the more severe the neurological deficit. With injuries involving L1 and above, this relationship increased. They thought the relationship between initial spinal canal encroachment and neurological deficit reflects the kinetic energy transferred at the time of impact. The major determinant of neurological loss and ultimate outcome is the severity of the initial injury (22). Several clinical reviews have documented a lack of correlation between the extent of spinal canal reconstruction (decompression) and neurological recovery, suggesting that ongoing neural compression is not the sole cause of persistent neurological deficits (22–25).

IV INDIRECT DECOMPRESSION

The anatomical reduction of thoracolumbar burst fractures should include correction of multiplane spinal deformity. The optimal reconstruction of vertebral burst fractures is dependent on successful application of distractive forces in combination with the restoration of normal spinal lordosis. Distraction, whether it is applied before or after kyphosis correction, is the major corrective force required to reduce retropulsed fragments in the spinal canal. However, intracanal fragments are best reduced when the anatomical lordosis is restored, in addition to correction of the vertebral height. Zou et al. suggested the reduction of fragments in the canal may not be due to the ligamentotaxis of the posterior ligament alone, but also to the symmetrical tightening of all bony attachments along the vertebral body, including the anterior longitudinal ligament and annulus fibrosis (26). The reduction and stabilization provided by a variety of posterior instrumentation systems have shown excellent restoration of sagittal alignment. However, the reduction capability of the intracanal bone fragments is variable, distinctly limited, and associated with fracture pattern and instrumentation technique (23–29)

Shono et al. have experimentally shown that it is not possible to produce an anteriorly directed force in the posterior longitudinal ligament at less than 35% canal occlusion (23,29,30). Pedicle screw fixation systems can apply multiple corrective forces while allowing three-dimensional adjustments. These systems permit direct reduction-force transmission to both the anterior and middle columns of the spine. Symmetric three-column lordotic distraction obtains the best possible reduction of intracanal fragments. Short-segment pedicle screw fixation systems allow force transmission while minimizing the number of immobilized segments, particularly in comparison to Harrington, Luque, and CD rod systems. Shiba et al. showed that canal clearance was most effective when carried out in the first 4 days after injury in their patients with an initial canal compromise of 34 to 66% (31).

V POSTERIOR DECOMPRESSION

Historically, the posterior approach for decompression of neural elements has been associated with a low success rate. Many investigators attest to poor results of laminectomy in addressing neurological deficits resulting from anterior compression. With more than 35% ventral canal occlusion from vertebral body retropulsion, laminectomy demonstrates no decompressive effect for the neural elements (32). Extensive laminectomy compounds the problem by further destabilizing the spine (4,10,33). Specific indications for laminectomy include the need to (1) facilitate ultrasonography of the spinal canal; (2) decompress epidural hematoma associated with ankylosing spondylitic spinal fractures; (3) perform a posterolateral decompression; and (4) repair a dural leak identified at the time of surgery, usually associated with burst and concomitant laminar fractures (10). Approximately one-third of patients with an incomplete neurological deficit and a laminar fracture seen on computed tomography (CT) scan have an associated dural tear, with 13% having neural elements entrapped within the fracture (34,35).

VI   POSTEROLATERAL DECOMPRESSION

The posterolateral approach includes a laminotomy, transpedicular approach, or resection (partial or complete), and direct reduction or resection of the compromising anterior fracture (Fig. 2). The efficacy of this approach in relieving anterior fracture fragment impingement has been documented by Cigliano et al., Hu et al., Garfin et al., Shaw et al., and Silvestro et al. (27,33,36–38). Shaw et al. described a one-stage posterolateral decompression-stabilization procedure for nine patients with thoracolumbar spine tumors and pathological fractures. Marked lasting improvement was observed in all patients with preoperative neurological deficits and in four patients with severe back pain and/or radiculopathy. Three nonambulators and two marginal ambulators could walk postoperatively without assistance. No patient deteriorated neurologically due to the procedure. The investigators concluded that adequate one-stage decompression-stabilization of spinal epidural lesions is possible via the posterolateral approach and should be considered in certain cases as an alternative to the anterior (33). Hu et al. compared the efficacy of anterior and posterolateral decompression and found no difference in neurological outcome results in 69 patients

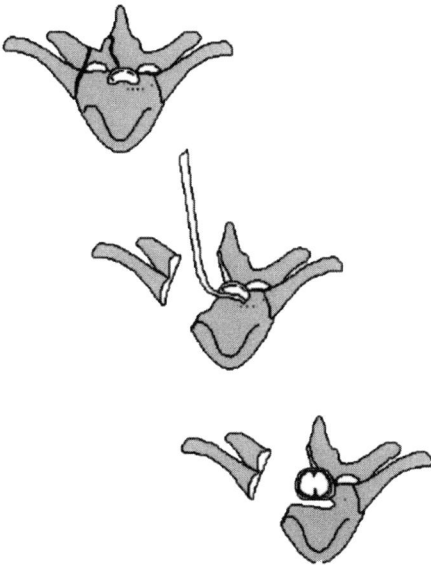

Figure 2   Posterolateral decompression.

(37). These studies support the recent trend of reporting posterolateral and anterior decompression approaches as equally effective (39).

VII ANTERIOR DECOMPRESSION

Bradford and McBride documented the results of surgical decompression in 59 patients with neurological deficits secondary to thoracic or lumbar fractures and represents of the findings of earlier series. They documented greater neurological improvement in anterior compared with posterior or posterolateral spinal decompression groups (88% vs. 64 %). The return of normal bowel and bladder control also occurred more frequently in the anterior spinal decompression group (69% vs. 33%) (40). However, anterior incisions tend to be more painful and debilitating than posterior incisions, and may result in longer hospital stays and more perioperative morbidity such as hemothorax, pneumothorax, chylothorax, or ileus. Additionally, mediastinal, pulmonary, or retroperitoneal disease may make the anterior approach unacceptably risky or even impossible. Finally, supplemental posterior stabilization is often required, necessitating another incision and stage of surgery (41). Although the decompressive efficacy of the anterior approach is well established, its associated morbidity potential must be weighed against the recently reported, equally efficacious, less morbid posterolateral decompression-stabilization procedures (33,37,38,40,42).

VIII POSTERIOR SPINAL IMPLANTS

A Harrington Instrumentation

In 1958, Harrington first applied his method of instrumentation and fusion of the spine, originally devised for scoliosis, to a patient with a spinal fracture dislocation (Fig. 3). Dickson et al. described the use of dual Harrington distraction rods as the "classic" for posterior fixation of the unstable thoracolumbar fracture or fracture dislocation. Ninety-five patients were treated and followed up for an average of 21 months between 1962 and 1976 for thoracolumbar spine fracture dislocations, with noncontoured Harrington distraction rods. A modified body cast was applied 1 week postoperatively to protect the hook–lamina interface. Hooks were placed two interspaces above and two below the fracture level. The rods were removed between the nineth and twelfth postoperative months. They documented a 93% union rate and only a 4° loss of reduction at follow-up (10,43).

Harrington rod fixation depends on hook–laminar bone contact and deformity correction is achieved by rod position and axial distraction. The recommended hook placement for optimal spinal realignment, strength, and stability, while minimizing hook dislodgement, was "three spinal levels above and two to three levels below" the injury interspace (5,44,45). The advantages of the early Harrington instrumentation series as compared to nonsurgical treatment were: (1) improved stability; (2) earlier mobilization; (3) shortened hospital stay; (4) neurological function maintenance/improvement; (5) prevention of late deformity (kyphosis); (6) less pain; and (7) higher fusion rates (14,43,44,46–53). Disadvantages of the procedure included the requirement for postoperative external immobilization for 4 to 6 months to protect the hook–lamina interface.

The concept of "rodding long and fusing short," popularized by Jacobs, offered advantages of a more accurate reduction and secure fixation while minimizing the

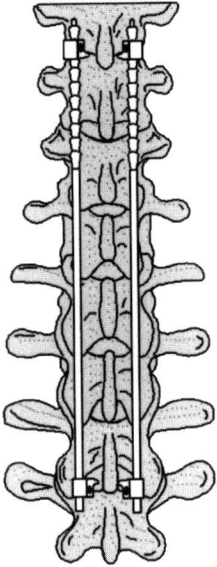

Figure 3 Harrington distraction rods.

length of the arthrodesis, resulting in a more normal spine (14,44). Optimal alignment was achieved by this technique when five or more spinal segments were instrumented (51). Jacobs et al. reduced the number of levels fused from 4.8 to 1.4. The postoperative vertebral height was 92% and 88% at final follow-up. Kyphosis immediately postoperatively measured 0° and 9° at last follow-up (54). Proposed timing of rod removal ranged from 6 to 19 months, reflecting the uncertainty of time needed for fusion maturity (44,45,54–56).

The disadvantages of Harrington posterior distraction rodding are excessive length of spinal segment immobilization and inability to sagittally contour, resulting in kyphosis or iatrogenic "flat back." Two-point fixation predisposed to hook dislodgement in 6% and showed particularly poor ability to resist torsional loads (12,57,58). Metal fatigue fractures occurred at the rod/ratchet interface (59). Overdistraction with subsequent neural and vascular injury was possible if the anterior longitudinal ligament was disrupted (48,59,60). Other disadvantages and complications included the potential for instrumentation-spanned facet arthritis and disk degeneration, instrument failure, and the late occurrence of kyphosis (10,48,49,54–56,59,61–63). Despite these shortcomings, the Harrington instrumentation system is still used worldwide, offering a viable alternative for the management of most unstable thoracolumbar spinal fractures.

B   Harrington Variants

The Harrington posterior spinal instrumentation system has been modified to improve the fixation, versatility, and ability to correct and maintain sagittal contours. These refinements include: (1) the addition of a posterior midline interspinous process wire or compression rod to prevent overdistraction; (2) square-ended (Moe) hooks and rods (64); Edward's anatomical hooks, universal rods, and polyethylene rod sleeves; and (4) the Jacob's threaded-rod locking-hook system (Fig. 4) (61,64–66).

The midline posterior interspinous compression rod or wire and Harrington rod construct act in concert, allowing correction of kyphosis and restoration of vertebral and diskal height while preventing overdistraction of the spinal cord (61). The dual Harrington rod system delivers the distractive (kyphosing) reduction force via a two-point hook–lamina bone interface. The round-ended Harrington rods rotate within the hooks explaining their inability to maintain the orientation of a sagittally contoured rod. The square-ended (Moe) hook-rod and Jacob's threaded-rod locking-hook systems solved this problem by preventing rod rotation at the hook rod interface (61,64,65). Edward's polyethylene sleeves provide a third point of fixation with an anteriorly directed (lordosing) force application to restore sagittal plane alignment (64).

C Segmental Dual Rod Instrumentation

The prototype of segmental dual rod constructs is the Luque rod segmental wire instrumentation system. The rods are smooth-surfaced 316-L stainless steel in $\frac{3}{16}$- and $\frac{1}{4}$-in. diameters. Surgical technique includes the addition of a transverse bend in the rod to fabricate an "L." Later, continuous loops or "Luque" rectangles were introduced. The solid cross-link feature of the rectangular constructs improved rotational stability. The rods are attached to the spine by single- or double-stranded 16- or 18-gauge sublaminar stainless steel wires. The Luque constructs are low profile, affording considerable stability to all but axial loads, and were particularly popular in the fracture-dislocation cord-injured patient. The segmental purchase and stability allowed early rehabilitation without cumbersome external immobilization, a significant advantage in the neurologically impaired or unreliable patient (10,12,67–69). However, clinical and laboratory studies have documented neurological injuries due to cord, or conus-level passage of sublaminar wires (70,71).

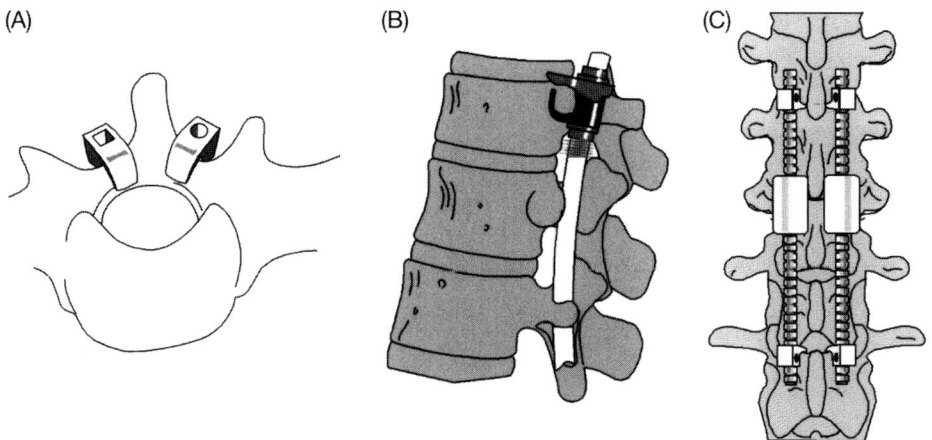

Figure 4 Harrington instrumentation variants. (A) Moe hooks with square rod hold. (B) Jacob's threaded rod-locking hook system. (C) Edward's universal rod, anatomical hook, polypropylene sleeve system.

   The lack of an axial distraction mechanism is a shortcoming of the Luque system. Without distraction, Luque instrumentation is less efficient in obtaining reduction and unable to prevent axial load-related deformation. Other methods of fixation are necessary for injuries that rendered the middle spinal column incompetent to resist axial load, potentiating further progression of deformity and canal compromise. An answer to Luque's axial loading weakness was found in the Harrington–Luque hybrid. Dual square-ended Harrington sagittally contoured rods provided three-point fixation, axial distraction force, and sagittal plane realignment. Luque sublaminar wires provided segmental stability and resistance to pullout. The fracture constructs and fusion typically extend at least two levels above and below the injury (11,60,67,72–75).

   A segmental spinous process wire (Wisconsin) system was introduced as an alternative to sublaminar wire passage. Dual wires are passed through the base of the spinous process, through a "button" that reduces wire cut-out. The segmental purchase of this system is inferior to sublaminar wires and more significantly affected by bone quality (Fig. 5).

D   Multiple Hook Rod Instrumentation

The Cotrel-Dubousset instrumentation (CDI) system is the prototype of the multiple hook rod constructs (Fig. 6). The system consists of a variety of open and closed hooks applied to a $\frac{1}{4}$-in. knurled, stainless steel rod. The transverse process, lamina, and pedicle provide varying points of purchase for the hooks. Multiple hooks can

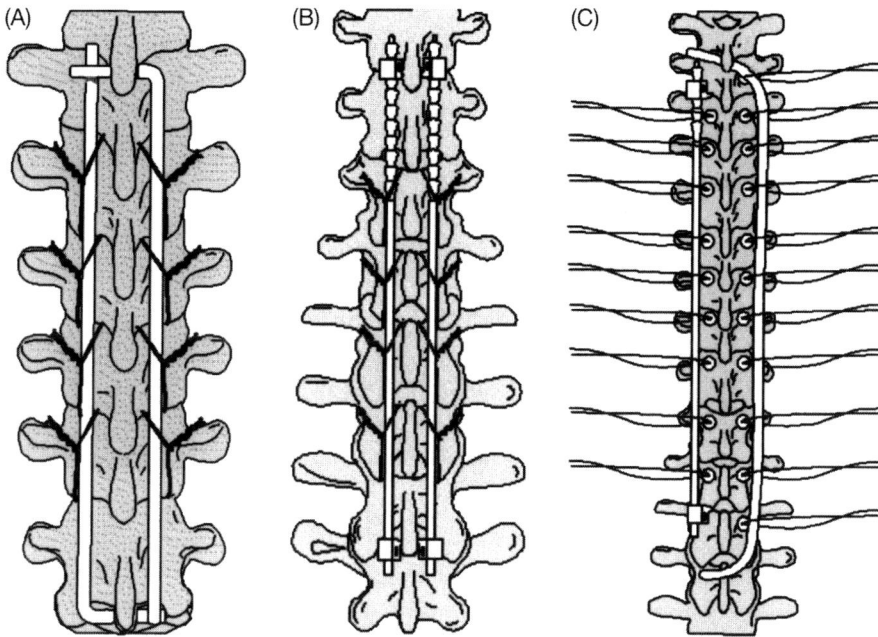

Figure 5   Segmental dual rod constructs. (A) Luque segmental wiring system-"L" rods. (B) "Hari-Luque" hybrid instrumentation. (C) Wisconsin spinous process "button" wires.

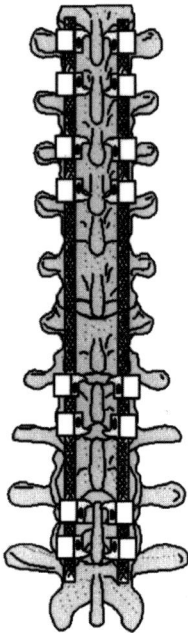

Figure 6 Multiple hook constructs with Cotrel-Dubousset instrumentation (CDI). "Claw" hook pattern is shown.

be applied to the rod and their orientation determines whether they provide distraction or compression corrective forces. The application of multiple hooks on a single rod allows the benefits of segmental fixation and load sharing, facilitating sagittal plane contouring, stability, and shortened constructs. Opposing-hook orientation creates a "claw" to rigidly fix the instrument to spinal segments. Once the rod is "locked" to the spine, the sagittal plane reconstruction is determined by the contour of the rod. A variety of hook applications allows multiple points of purchase and force application resulting in load sharing. At the completion of rod seating, the rods can be cross-connected, affording greater rigidity and construct stability.

A variety of other multiple hook rod constructs have evolved: Texas Scottish Rite Hospital, Isola, Moss-Miami, and Synthes to name a few. The primary advantages of these systems are that they are rigid, low profile, allow for a variety of fixation methods to be applied to a single rod, and decrease the need for external immobilization. These systems have been shown to provide and maintain excellent correction of deformity and stability, resulting in a fusion rate of more than 95% (10). One of the disadvantages of these systems is related to their versatility: The fabrication of these constructs requires a fairly steep, time-dependent learning curve.

Stambough and Nayak reviewed 17 patients treated with CD or Luque instrumentation for unstable thoracolumbar fracture dislocations and complete paraplegia. Both instrumentation systems provided long-term posterior spinal stabilization with no clear advantage of one system over the other (76). Graziano reviewed 14 fracture patients whose CD construct included a transverse-pedicular "claw" hybrid. They found the CDI multiple hook constructs with claw patterns lessened the chance of

hook dislodgement. The two-hook transverse-pedicle and laminar-laminar claw configurations greatly improved fixation to the spine. The use of thoracic claw patterns
allowed for safe instrumentation into the thoracic spine where pedicle screw placement may be hazardous or even impossible, due to small pedicle diameter (77). Benli
et al. reviewed 20 unstable thoracic or lumbar fractures treated with CDI. They found
the Cotrel-Dubousset instrumentation established vertebral stability by forming a
rigid frame and allowed restoration of physiological thoracic and lumbar postural
contours due to its powerful corrective effect in the sagittal plane. One vertebra above
and one below the fractured level were instrumented in six patients; two above and
one below in eight patients; and two above and two below in five patients. One
patient required the inclusion of six mobile levels within the instrumentation. All
patients were instrumented with laminar or transverse-pedicular claws at the top and
laminar claws at the caudal end of the construct. The thoracolumbar sagittal plane
alignment was normalized and maintained in 65% of the cases (78). Stambough
reported on 55 patients treated with Cotrel-Dubousset instrumentation for unstable
thoracolumbar spine fractures. Sixty percent of patients were braced with a custom-
molded thoracolumbosacral orthosis (TLSO) after surgical stabilization. Radiographic analysis showed significant correction in fracture angle, vertebral body compression, and fracture displacement. At follow-up, there was little to no deterioration.
Two levels above and two levels below the injury level were instrumented, with the
exception of the fracture-dislocation group where three levels above and two levels
below injury were often used. There was no significant loss of fixation, instrumentation dislodgement, instrument fatigue failure, or nonunion (9).

Stambough outlined the principles of hook placement, construct formulation,
and implantation as follows: (1) the shoe of each hook should fully contact bone
(lamina are the preferred site of attachment); (2) each hook should fit snugly, preventing canal encroachment by the hook; (3) closed hooks should be used at the
ends of a construct; (4) multiple fixation points on a single rod should be obtained;
(5) bone graft posteriorly should be placed over the decorticated bone before final
rod insertion; (6) sagittal contouring of the rod should closely match the anatomy of
the fracture level (kyphosis and/or lordosis); (7) hooks are placed in a construct to
reverse the injury mechanism (e.g., compression for chance type or flexion distraction
injuries); (8) cross-link both rods whenever possible; and (9) avoid dissimilar metals
(either stainless steel or titanium alloy) (10).

E   Transpedicle Screw Instrumentation

Michele and Krueger originally described transpedicular fixation in 1949 (79). Since
1963, Roy-Camille of France has used pedicle screw plates (PSP) as his routine
method of spine fixation (80). In the United States, Steffee was one of the first to
introduce the transpedicular fixation technique and developed the variable screw
placement (VSP) plate system. Many studies document advantages and efficacy of
transpedicular fixation systems (6,10,29,31–36,60,80–99). There are multiple effective versatile transpedicular instrumentation systems available (Fig. 7). Most investigators think that choosing the proper surgical approach and techniques is more
important than the selection of a particular transpedicular fixation system in achieving
an excellent surgical result (31,83).

The insertion of a screw or Schanz pin in the pedicle of the involved vertebra
allows three-column spinal purchase. Three-column spinal purchase allows excellent

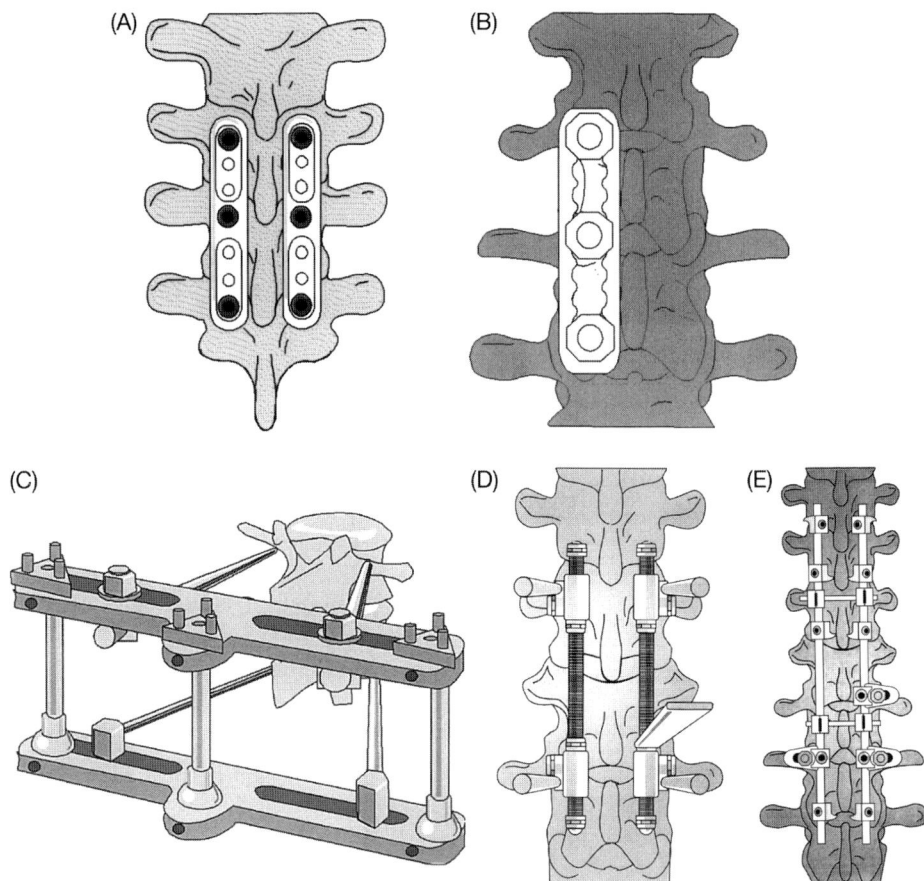

Figure 7 Transpedicular screw instrumentation. (A) Roy-Camille's pedicle screw plate (PSP). (B) Steffee's VSP instrumentation system. (C) Magrel's external fixator. (D) Dick's internal fixator. (E) Isola instrumentation system.

stable, reliable, fixation and three-dimensional correction of deformity. Transpedicular instrumentation systems include screws attached to plates, rods, and external fixation devices. One of the main concerns with pedicle screw systems is placement of the screw within the pedicle. Screw placement deviations can subject the nerve root and spinal contents immediately medial and the nerve root inferior to the pedicle to injury.

Many technological advances have occurred over the past decade, which have facilitated the placement of thoracolumbar pedicle screws. When first marketed, most pedicle screw systems were produced from stainless steel. Today, the surgeon may choose to utilize titanium screws and rods, which are more compatible with postoperative MRI imaging. In addition, "top-loading" and "top-tightening" systems have now considerably simplified the placement of pedicle screws. Modern systems are now considered "low profile" to limit the occurrence of postoperative hardware prominence. More recently developed systems offer screws with a multiaxial design.

This feature facilitates placement of the rod if the pedicles are not symmetrically aligned as seen in many disease processes (2).

New systems have been designed to aid surgeons in the placement of pedicle screws. These systems are based on the concept of frameless stereotaxy and require a preoperative CT scan. A reference base is fixed to a standard immobile anatomical landmark, usually the spinous process of the vertebral body that is being instrumented. A locator tool is then used to match the actual anatomical landmarks of the patient's vertebrae to preoperatively chosen ones on the reformatted CT scan. Locator tools can work using either magnetic, ultrasound, or light-emitting sensors to record their position. Accuracy of placement has been recorded in the 95.7 to 100% range (100,101). Reported neurological complications associated with pedicle screw placement are low to nonexistent in most series (24,80,92,99).

Currently available transpedicular fixation systems offer the following advantages: (1) true three-dimensional fixation; (2) shortened instrumentation, even with posterior element fractures; (3) elimination of deliberate fixation encroachment of the spinal canal; (4) improved power, quality, and maintenance of spinal realignment; and (5) a high rate of fusion (31,57,96). Fixation is often not affected, nor does it need to be extended due to laminar absence or fracture. Fixation is obtained using the strongest part of the vertebrae, the pedicle (94). Restoration of lumbar lordosis and previous lumbosacral junction fixation "problem areas" is more effectively treated than with any previous fixation methods.

These transpedicular devices, similar to all other spinal implants, require obtaining a solid arthrodesis to prevent fixation failure and ensure clinical success. Failure of fusion will result in instrumentation deformation, loosening, or breakage (80,86,91,92,97–99,102,103). Some degree of recurrent deformity usually accompanies instrumentation failure due to failed arthrodesis. Failure of short-segment (one level above and below injury) constructs has been a recurrent problem when incompetent anterior and middle columns are not reconstructed at the time of instrumentation or three-point fixation is not obtained (10,88,91,103,104). Most hardware failures have been noted at the first or second lumbar levels, which reflect the increased mechanical stresses at the thoracolumbar junction. Constructs that do not support or load share across the anterior column of the spine have a powerful bending movement acting on the screws at the point where it enters the pedicle (105). Spines with burst fractures showed a bilinear load displacement behavior with significant instability at low loads in flexion, lateral bending, and, particularly, axial rotation (106–108). Stresses measured in the roots of pedicle screws were found to exceed the endurance limit of the stainless steel in those systems in which the pedicle screws were attached rigidly to the plates (83). Without three-point contact, bending moments are resisted only by the intrinsic stiffness of the screw and rod. McCormack et al. published a point assignment system—the Load Sharing Classification of Spine Fractures—which they found predictive of hardware failure (102). When the anterior column remains incompetent after posterior fracture instrumentation, additional external orthotic support should be considered (88,107).

The basic transpedicular system fixation technique involves screw placement in the pedicles of the vertebrae adjacent to the injured level. Whenever possible, an additional fixation point should be obtained at the injured vertebral level. If a posterolateral canal decompression is anticipated, the side opposite the intended decompression is instrumented. Plate or rod contour corrects kyphosis and distraction restores loss of vertebrae and disk height. If the anterior column is severely deficient, transpedicular vertebral and intradiskal grafting can be performed. Posterolateral grafting should be performed, and the remainder of the instrumentation implanted. Final contouring and tensioning of the instrumentation are assessed and adjustments performed in situ, if necessary/possible. Once the instrumentation is "set," the canal is inspected on one final occasion. Transpedicular decompression combined with vertebral and intradiskal grafting, when indicated, provides excellent clinical results, decreasing the need for a formal anterior decompression (Fig. 8).

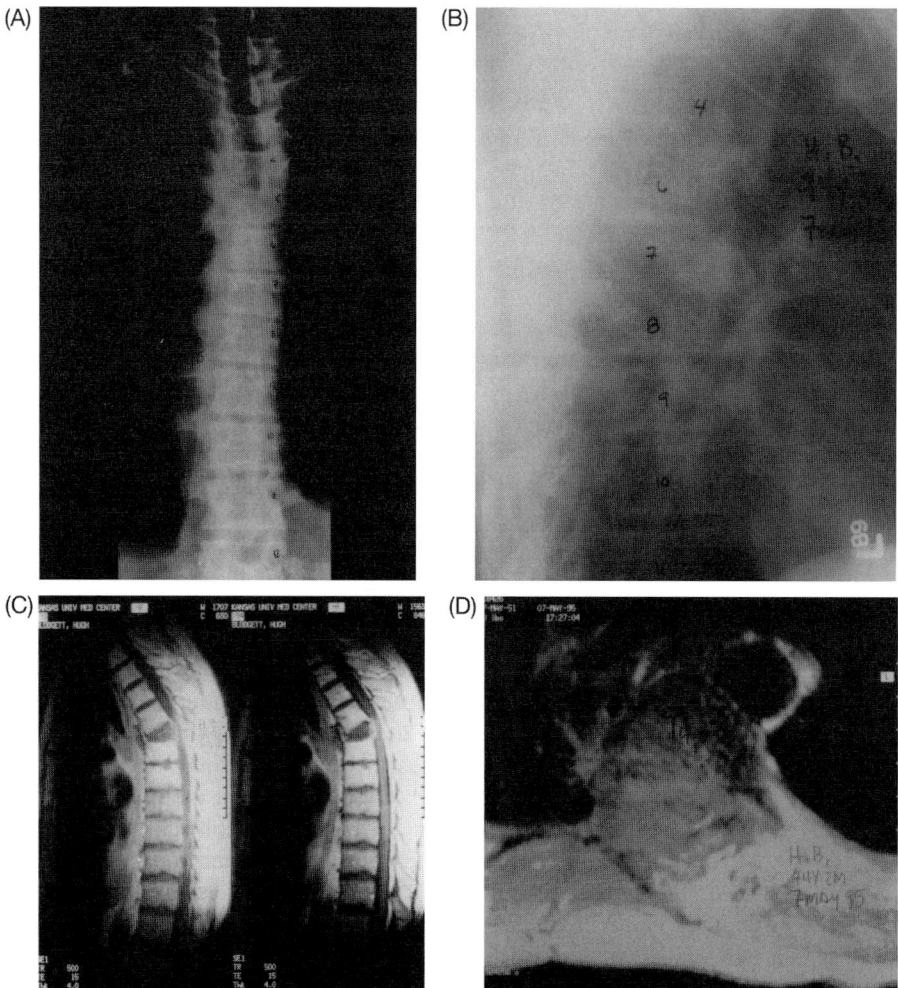

Figure 8 H.B., 44-year-old male with a pathological fracture of T5 and paraparesis due to metastatic lung cancer. (A) AP radiograph of injured T5. (B) Lateral. (C) MRI demonstrates T5 destruction and canal compromise. (D) MRI axial view at T4,5. Post-operative (E) AP and (F) lateral spine after Isola instrumentation and posterolateral decompression.

(E)   (F)

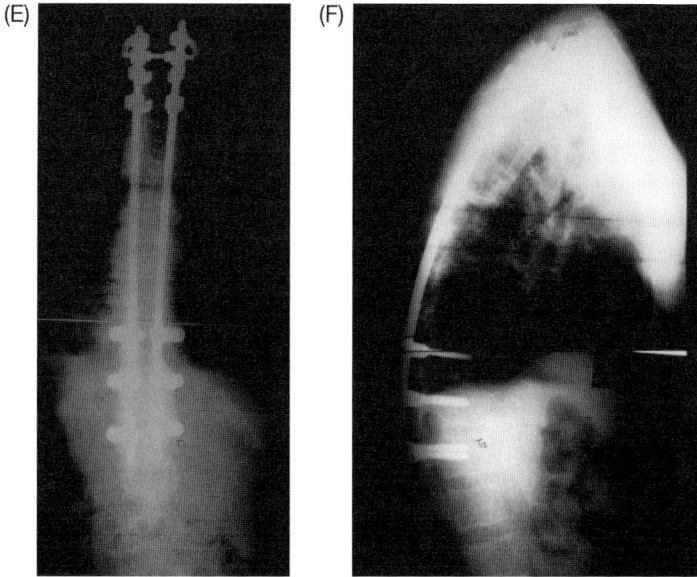

Figure 8   Continued

IX   SUMMARY

The nonsurgical treatment result for a patient's spine rendered unstable by tumor or traumatic destruction is often fair to poor. Posterior thoracolumbar spinal instrumentation has evolved from the early fixation techniques with wire loops and spinous process plates. The Harrington instrumentation system subsequently provided two-point hook fixation and a distraction corrective force. Shortcomings noted were the inclusion of too many normal spinal motion segments in the construct, lack of anatomical reduction, and the requirement of rigid protective postoperative external immobilization devices. Segmental rod-wire and hook systems provided greater stability, multiple points of fixation, and corrective force application, thereby shortening constructs and decreasing the need for rigid external protective immobilization. Current posterior instrumentation systems provide strong, secure, multiple-point, transpedicular, three-column fixation. Spinal purchase is not affected by laminar incompetence or absence. Due to the strength of the fixation and corrective forces supplied by the instrumentation, the constructs involve the least number of spinal segments possible. Arthrodesis spans the instrumentation length, eliminating the need for later instrumentation removal. A limitation of current systems includes a high rate of failure if the anterior and middle columns remain chronically insufficient. If disk injury, osteopenia, or severe comminution results in expected long-term spinal column insufficiency, anterior reconstruction should be considered to accompany posterior reduction and instrumentation procedures.

The posterior approach to the spine is the most familiar and is associated with the least surgical time, blood loss, and expense of approaches used to treat destructive processes of the spine. Early studies touted the anterior decompression as the most efficacious. Anterior instrumentation has improved and, particularly at the thoracolumbar junction, often eliminates the need for second-stage posterior instrumentation procedure. However, most anterior decompressive and reconstructive techniques at upper thoracic and lower lumbar levels require stabilization by a second-stage posterior spinal instrumentation procedure. More recent literature supports the effectiveness of the posterolateral decompression and reconstructive approach.

Posterolateral and anterior decompressions are reported as equally effective. Posterolateral decompression allows the familiar posterior approach and instrumentation and eliminates the need for a second-stage stabilization procedure. Optimal timing of the procedure with regard to intracanal fragment reduction is within the first 4 days of injury. In the multiply traumatized patient, complications are markedly reduced if the procedure can be performed within 72 h of injury.

Present transpedicular instrumentation systems provide strong versatile fixation and, as might be expected, longer learning curves than the original systems. Many excellent transpedicular posterior spinal instrumentation systems exist, but most investigators believe it is now the choice of surgical approach and technique that is more important in determining a successful outcome than the specific transpedicular device.

REFERENCES

1. Denis F, Armstrong GW, Searls K, Matta L. Acute thoracolumbar burst fractures in the absence of neurologic deficit. a comparison between operative and nonoperative treatment. Clin Orthop 1984; (189):142–149.
2. Bennett CR, Bendo JA. Lumbar pedicular fixation: An update. In: Errico TJ, ed. Spine: State of the Art Reviews. 1999; 13:313–327.
3. Aho AJ, Savunen TJ, Makela PJ. Operative fixation of fractures of the thoracic and lumbar vertebrae by williams plates with reference to late kyphosis. Injury 1988; 19(3): 153–158.
4. Kaufer H, Hayes JT. Lumbar fracture dislocation. J Bone Joint Surg [Am] 1966; 48(4): 712–730.
5. Purcell GA, Markolf KL, Dawson EG. Twelfth thoracic-first lumbar vertebral mechanical stability of fractures after harrington-rod instrumentation. J Bone Joint Surg [Am] 1981; 63(1):71–78.
6. Stauffer ES, Neil JL. Biomechanical analysis of structural stability of internal fixation in fractures of the thoracolumbar spine. Clin Orthop 1975; (112):159–164.
7. Babu ML, Wani MA. Management of thoraco-lumbar fractures. Acta Neurochir (Wien) 1990; 102(1–2):54–57.
8. Dunn HK. Spinal instrumentation. Part I. Principles of posterior and anterior instrumentation. Instr Course Lect 1983; 32:192–202.
9. Stambough JL. Cotrel-dubousset instrumentation and thoracolumbar spine trauma: a review of 55 cases. J Spinal Disord 1994; 7(6):461–469.
10. Stambough JL. Posterior instrumentation for thoracolumbar trauma. Clin Orthop 1997; 335:73–88.
11. Gaines RW, Breedlove RF, Munson G. Stabilization of thoracic and thoracolumbar fracture-dislocations with harrington rods and sublaminar wires. Clin Orthop 1984; (189):195–203.
12. Sullivan JA. Sublaminar wiring of harrington distraction rods for unstable thoracolumbar spine fractures. Clin Orthop 1984; (189):178–185.
13. Schlegel J, Bayley J, Yuan H, Fredricksen B. Timing of surgical decompression and fixation of acute spinal fractures. J Orthop Trauma 1966; 10(5):323–330.

14. Jacobs RR, Casey MP. Surgical management of thoracolumbar spinal injuries. General principles and controversial considerations. Clin Orthop 1984; (189):22–35.

15. Holdsworth FW, Hardy A. Early treatment of paraplegia from fractures of the thoraco-lumbar spine. J Bone Joint Surg [Br] 1953; 35(4):540–550.

16. Harrington PR, Tullos HS. Reduction of severe spondylolisthesis in children. South Med J 1969; 62(1):1–7.

17. Roy-Camille R, Saillant G, Berteaux D, Salgado V. Osteosynthesis of thoraco-lumbar spine fractures with metal plates screwed through the vertebral pedicles. Reconst Surg Traumatol 1976; 15:2–16.

18. Steffee AD, Biscup RS, Sitkowski DJ. Segmental spine plates with pedicle screw fix-ation: a new internal fixation device for disorders of lumbar and thoracolumbar spine. Clin Orthop Rel Res 1986; 203:45–53.

19. Danisa OA, Shaffrey CI, Jane JA, Whitehill R, Wang GJ, Szabo TA, Hansen CA, Shaffrey ME, Chan DP. Surgical approaches for the correction of unstable thoraco-lumbar burst fractures: a retrospective analysis of treatment outcomes. J Neurosurg 1995; 83(6):977–983.

20. Hashimoto T, Kaneda K, Abumi K. Relationship between traumatic spinal canal ste-nosis and neurologic deficits in thoracolumbar burst fractures. Spine 1988; 13(11):1268–1272.

21. Sapkas G, Efstathiou P, Makris A, Kyratzoulis J. Thoracolumbar burst fractures: cor-relation between post-traumatic spinal canal stenosis and initial neurological deficit. Bull Hosp Jt Dis 1996; 55(1):36–39.

22. Lemons VR, Wagner FC Jr., Montesano PX. Management of thoracolumbar fractures with accompanying neurological injury. Neurosurgery 1992; 30(5):667–671.

23. Crutcher JP Jr., Anderson PA, King HA, Montesano PX. Indirect spinal canal decom-pression in patients with thoracolumbar burst fractures treated by posterior distraction rods. J Spinal Disord 1991; 4(1):39–48.

24. Doerr TE, Montesano PX, Burkus JK, Benson DR. Spinal canal decompression in traumatic thoracolumbar burst fractures: posterior distraction rods versus transpedicular screw fixation [see comments]. J Orthop Trauma 1991; 5(4):403–411.

25. Esses SI, Botsford DJ, Kostuik JP. Evaluation of surgical treatment for burst fractures. Spine 1990; 15(7):667–673.

26. Zou D, Yoo, JU, Edwards WT, Donovan DM, Chang KW, Bayley JC, Fredrickson BE, Yuan HA. Mechanics of anatomic reduction of thoracolumbar burst fractures. compar-ison of distraction versus distraction plus lordosis, in the anatomic reduction of the thoracolumbar burst fracture. Spine 1993; 18(2):195–203.

27. Garfin SR, Mowery CA, Guerra J Jr., Marshall LF. Confirmation of the posterolateral technique to decompress and fuse thoracolumbar spine burst fractures. Spine 1985; 10(3):218–223.

28. Greenwald TA, Keene JS. Results of Harrington instrumentation in type a and type b burst fractures. J Spinal Disord 1991; 4(2):149–156.

29. Shono Y, McAfee PC, Cunningham BW. Experimental study of thoracolumbar burst fractures. a radiographic and biomechanical analysis of anterior and posterior instru-mentation systems. Spine 1994; 19(15):1711–1722.

30. Harrington RM, Budorick T, Hoyt J, Anderson PA, Tencer AF. Biomechanics of indirect reduction of bone retropulsed into the spinal canal in vertebral fracture. Spine 1993; 18(6):692–699.

31. Shiba K, Katsuki M, Ueta T, Shirasawa K, Ohta H, Mori E, Rikimaru S. Transpedicular fixation with zielke instrumentation in the treatment of thoracolumbar and lumbar in-juries. Spine 1994; 19(17):1940–1949.

32. Tencer AF, Allen BL, Ferguson RL. A biomechanical study of thoracolumbar spinal fractures with bone in the canal: I. The effect of laminectomy. Spine 1985; 10:580–585.

33. Shaw B, Mansfield FL, Borges L. One-stage posterolateral decompression and stabilization for primary and metastatic vertebral tumors in the thoracic and lumbar spine [see comments]. J Neurosurg 1989; 70(3):405–410.

34. Cammisa FP, Eismont FJ, Green BA. Dural laceration occurring with burst fractures and associated laminar fractures. J Bone Joint Surg (Am) 1989; 71:1044–1052.

35. Hardaker WT, Cook WA, Friedman AH, et al. Bilateral transpedicular decompression and Harrington Rod stabilization in the management of severe thoracolumbar burst fractures. Spine 1992; 17:162–171.

36. Cigliano A, de Falco R, Scarano E, Russo G, Profeta G. A new instrumentation system for the reduction and posterior stabilization of unstable thoracolumbar fractures. Neurosurgery 1992; 30(2):208–216.

37. Hu SS, Capen DA, Rimoldi RL, Zigler JE. The effect of surgical decompression on neurologic outcome after lumbar fractures. Clin Orthop 1993; (288):166–173.

38. Silvestro C, Francaviglia N, Bragazzi R, Viale GL. Near-anatomical reduction and stabilization of burst fractures of the lower thoracic or lumbar spine. Acta Neurochir (Wien) 1992; 116(1):53–59.

39. Heller M, Perrin I, Macnab I, McBroom JR. Treatment of metastatic disease of the spine with posterolateral decompression and Luque instrumentation. J Bone Joint Surg [Br] 1986; 68(5):852–853.

40. Bradford DS, McBride GG. Surgical management of thoracolumbar spine fractures with incomplete neurologic deficits. Clin Orthop 1987; (218):201–216.

41. Gertzbein SD, Court-Brown CM, Jacobs RR, Marks P, Martin C, Stoll J, Fazl M, Schwartz M, Rowed D. Decompression and circumferential stabilization of unstable spinal fractures. Spine 1988; 13(8):892–895.

42. Kostuik JP, Errico TJ, Gleason TF. Spinal stabilisation of vertebral column tumours. J Bone Joint Surg [Br] 1986; 68(5):853.

43. Dickson JH, Harrington PR, Erwin WD. Results of reduction and stabilization of the severely fractured thoracic and lumbar spine. J Bone Joint Surg [Am] 1978; 60(6):799–805.

44. Dekutoski MB, Conlan ES, Salciccioli GG. Spinal mobility and deformity after Harrington rod stabilization and limited arthrodesis of thoracolumbar fractures. J Bone Joint Surg Am 1993; 75(2):168–176.

45. Myllynen P, Bostman O, Riska E. Recurrence of deformity after removal of Harrington's fixation of spine fracture. seventy-six cases followed for 2 years. Acta Orthop Scand 1988; 59(5):497–502.

46. Aebi M, Mohler J, Zach G, Morscher E. Analysis of 75 operated thoracolumbar fractures and fracture dislocations with and without neurological deficit. Arch Orthop Trauma Surg 1986; 105(2):100–112.

47. Convery FR, Minteer MA, Smith RW, Emerson SM. Fracture-dislocation of the dorsal-lumbar spine. acute operative stabilization by Harrington instrumentation. Spine 1978; 3(2):160–166.

48. Devilee R, Sanders R, de Lange S. Treatment of fractures and dislocations of the thoracic and lumbar spine by fusion and Harrington instrumentation. Arch Orthop Trauma Surg 1995; 114(2):100–102.

49. Fang D, Leong JC, Cheung HC. The treatment of thoracolumbar spinal injuries with paresis by conservative versus surgical methods. Ann Acad Med Singapore 1982; 11(2):203–206.

50. Flesch JR, Leider LL, Erickson DL, Chou SN, Bradford DS. Harrington instrumentation and spine fusion for unstable fractures and fracture-dislocations of the thoracic and lumbar spine. J Bone Joint Surg [Am] 1977; 59(2):143–153.

51. Jodoin A, Dupuis P, Fraser M, Beaumont P. Unstable fractures of the thoracolumbar spine: a 10-year experience at sacre-coeur hospital. J Trauma 1985; 25(3):197–202.

52. Kornberg M, Rechtine GR, Herndon WA, Reinert CM, Dupuy TE. Surgical stabilization of thoracic and lumbar spine fractures: a retrospective study in a military population. J Trauma 1984; 24(2):140–146.
53. McEvoy RD, Bradford DS. The management of burst fractures of the thoracic and lumbar spine. experience in 53 patients. Spine 1985; 10(7):631–637.
54. Gardner VO, Armstrong GW. Long-term lumbar facet joint changes in spinal fracture patients treated with Harrington rods. Spine 1990; 15(6):479–484.
55. Akbarnia BA, Crandall DG, Burkus K, Matthews T. Use of long rods and a short arthrodesis for burst fractures of the thoracolumbar spine. a long-term follow-up study. J Bone Joint Surg Am 1994; 76(11):1629–1635.
56. Karjalainen M, Aho AJ, Katevuo K. Operative treatment of unstable thoracolumbar fractures by the posterior approach with the use of williams plates or Harrington rods. Int Orthop 1992; 16(3):219–222.
57. Dickman CA, Yahiro MA, Lu HT, Melkerson MN. Surgical treatment alternatives for fixation of unstable fractures of the thoracic and lumbar spine. a meta-analysis. Spine 1994; 19(20 Suppl):S2266–2273.
58. Gaines RW Jr., Carson WL, Satterlee CC, Groh GI. Experimental evaluation of seven different spinal fracture internal fixation devices using nonfailure stability testing. the load-sharing and unstable-mechanism concepts. Spine 1991; 16(8):902–909.
59. Meyer PR Jr. Posterior stabilization of thoracic, lumbar, and sacral injuries. Instr Course Lect 1986; 35:401–419.
60. Wenger DR, Carollo JJ. The mechanics of thoracolumbar fractures stabilized by segmental fixation. Clin Orthop 1984; (189):89–96.
61. Floman Y, Fast A, Pollack D, Yosipovitch Z, Robin GC. The simultaneous application of an interspinous compressive wire and Harrington distraction rods in the treatment of fracture-dislocation of the thoracic and lumbar spine. Clin Orthop 1986; (205):207–215.
62. Kahanovitz N, Bullough P, Jacobs RR. The effect of internal fixation without arthrodesis on human facet joint cartilage. Clin Orthop 1984; (189):204–208.
63. Svensson O, Aaro S, Ohlen G. Harrington instrumentation for thoracic and lumbar vertebral fractures. Acta Orthop Scand 1984; 55(1):38–47.
64. Denis F, Ruiz H, Searls K. Comparison between square-ended distraction rods and standard round-ended distraction rods in the treatment of thoracolumbar spinal injuries. a statistical analysis. Clin Orthop 1984; (189):162–167.
65. Gertzbein SD, Jacobs RR, Stoll J, Martin C, Marks P, Fazl M, Rowed D, Schwartz M. Results of a locking-hook spinal rod for fractures of the thoracic and lumbar spine. Spine 1990; 15(4):275–280.
66. Jacobs RR, Schlaepfer F, Mathys R Jr., Nachemson A, Perren SM. A locking hook spinal rod system for stabilization of fracture-dislocations and correction of deformities of the dorsolumbar spine. a biomechanic evaluation. Clin Orthop 1984; (189):168–177.
67. Akbarnia BA, Fogarty JP, Tayob AA. Contoured Harrington instrumentation in the treatment of unstable spinal fractures. the effect of supplementary sublaminar wires. Clin Orthop. 1984; (189):186–194.
68. Bernard TN Jr., Whitecloud TS 3d, Rodriguez RP, Haddad RJ Jr. Segmental spinal instrumentation in the management of fractures of the thoracic and lumbar spine. South Med J 1983; 76(10):1232–1236
69. Fidler MW. Posterior instrumentation of the spine. an experimental comparison of various possible techniques. Spine 1986; 11(4):367–372.
70. Cervellati S, Bettini N, Bianco T, Parisini P. Neurological complications in segmental spinal instrumentation: analysis of 750 patients. Eur Spine J 1966; 5(3):161–166.

71. Coe JD, Becker PS, McAfee PC, Gurr KR. Neuropathology with spinal instrumentation. J Orthop Res 1989; 7(3):359–370.

72. Akbarnia BA, Fogarty JP, Smith KR Jr. New trends in surgical stabilization of thoracolumbar spinal fractures with emphasis for sublaminar wiring. Paraplegia 1985; 23(1): 27–33.

73. Hardaker WT Jr., Cook WA Jr., Friedman AH, Fitch RD. Bilateral transpedicular decompression and harrington rod stabilization in the management of severe thoracolumbar burst fractures. Spine 1992; 17(2):162–171.

74. Louw JA. Unstable fractures of the thoracic and lumbar spine treated with harrington distraction instrumentation and sublaminar wires. S Afr Med J 1987; 71(12):759–762.

75. Munson G, Satterlee C, Hammond S, Betten R, Gaines, RW. Experimental evaluation of harrington rod fixation supplemented with sublaminar wires in stabilizing thoracolumbar fracture-dislocations. Clin Orthop 1984; (189):97–102.

76. Stambough JL, Nayak S. Frankel a paraplegia: a comparison of two spinal instrumentation systems. South Med J 1996; 89(6):597–602.

77. Graziano GP. Cotrel-dubousset hook and screw combination for spine fractures. J Spinal Disord 1993; 6(5):380–385.

78. Benli IT, Tandogan NR, Kis M, Tuzuner M, Mumcu EF, Akalin S, Citak M. Cotrel-dubousset instrumentation in the treatment of unstable thoracic and lumbar spine fractures. Arch Orthop Trauma Surg 1994; 113(2):86–92.

79. Michele AA, Krueger FJ. Surgical approach to the vertebral body. J Bone Joint Surg Am 1949; 31:873–878.

80. Roy-Camille R, Saillant G, Mazel C. Internal fixation of the lumbar spine with pedicle screw plating. Clin Orthop 1986; (203):7–17.

81. Aebi M, Etter C, Kehl T, Thalgott J. Stabilization of the lower thoracic and lumbar spine with the internal spinal skeletal fixation system. indications, techniques, and first results of treatment. Spine 1987; 12(6):544–551.

82. Akeyson EW, McCutcheon IE. Single-stage posterior vertebrectomy and replacement combined with posterior instrumentation for spinal metastasis. J Neurosurg 1996; 85(2): 211–220.

83. Ashman RB, Galpin RD, Corin JD, Johnston CE II. Biomechanical analysis of pedicle screw instrumentation systems in a corpectomy model. Spine 1989; 14(12):1398–1405.

84. Bridwell KH, Jenny AB, Saul T, Rich KM, Grubb RL. Posterior segmental spinal instrumentation (pssi) with posterolateral decompression and debulking for metastatic thoracic and lumbar spine disease. limitations of the technique. Spine 1988; 13(12): 1383–1394.

85. Dick W, Kluger P, Magerl F, Woersdorfer O, Zach G. A new device for internal fixation of thoracolumbar and lumbar spine fractures: the 'fixateur interne.' Paraplegia 1985; 23(4):225–232.

86. Ebelke DK, Asher, MA, Neff JR, Kraker DP. Survivorship analysis of vsp spine instrumentation in the treatment of thoracolumbar and lumbar burst fractures. Spine 1991; 16(8 Suppl):S428–432.

87. Esses SI, Botsford DJ, Wright T, Bednar D, Bailey S. Operative treatment of spinal fractures with the ao internal fixator. Spine 1991; 16(3 Suppl):S146–150.

88. Gurwitz GS, Dawson JM, McNamara MJ, Federspiel CF, Spengler DM. Biomechanical analysis of three surgical approaches for lumbar burst fractures using short-segment instrumentation. Spine 1993; 18(8):977–982.

89. Heller JG, Zdeblick TA, Kunz, DA, McCabe R, Cooke ME. Spinal instrumentation for metastatic disease: in vitro biomechanical analysis. J Spinal Disord 1993; 6(1):17–22.

90. Hirabayashi S, Kumano K, Kuroki T. Cotrel-dubousset pedicle screw system for various spinal disorders. merits and problems. Spine 1991; 16(11):1298–1304.

91. Kramer DL, Rodgers WB, Mansfield FL. Transpedicular instrumentation and short-segment fusion of thoracolumbar fractures: a prospective study using a single instrumentation system. J Orthop Trauma 1995; 9(6):499–506.
92. Lindsey RW, Dick W. The fixateur interne in the reduction and stabilization of thoracolumbar spine fractures in patients with neurologic deficit. Spine 1991; 16(3 Suppl): S140–145.
93. Magerl FP. Stabilization of the lower thoracic and lumbar spine with external skeletal fixation. Clin Orthop 1984; 189:125–141.
94. Markel DC, Graziano GP. A comparison study of treatment of thoracolumbar fractures using the ace posterior segmental fixator and cotrel-dubousset instrumentation A comparison study of treatment of thoracolumbar fractures using the ace posterior segmental fixator and cotrel-dubousset instrumentation. Orthopedics 1995; 18(7):679–686.
95. Olerud S, Karlstrom G, Sjostrom L. Transpedicular fixation of thoracolumbar vertebral fractures. Clin Orthop 1988; 227:44–51.
96. Sasso RC, Cotler HB. Posterior instrumentation and fusion for unstable fractures and fracture-dislocations of the thoracic and lumbar spine. a comparative study of three fixation devices in 70 patients. Spine 1993; 18(4):450–460.
97. Sasso RC, Cotler HB, Reuben JD. Posterior fixation of thoracic and lumbar spine fractures using dc plates and pedicle screws. Spine 1991; 16(3 Suppl):S134–139.
98. Sim E, Stergar PM. The fixateur interne for stabilising fractures of the thoracolumbar and lumbar spine. Int Orthop 1992; 16(4):322–329.
99. Simpson JM, Ebraheim NA, Jackson WT, Chung S. Internal fixation of the thoracic and lumbar spine using roy-camille plates. Orthopedics 1993; 16(6):663–672.
100. Carl AL, Khanuja HS, Sachs BL, et al. In vitro simulation: Early results of stereotaxy for pedicle screw placement. Spine 1997; 22:1160–1164.
101. Laine T, Schlenzka D, Makitalo K, et al. Improved accuracy of pedicle screw insertion with computer-assisted surgery: A prospective clinical trial of 30 patients. Spine 1997; 22:1254–1258.
102. McCormack T, Karaikovic E, Gaines RW. The load sharing classification of spine fractures. Spine 1994; 19(15):1741–1744.
103. McLain RF, Sparling E, Benson DR. Early failure of short-segment pedicle instrumentation for thoracolumbar fractures. a preliminary report [see comments]. J Bone Joint Surg Am 1993; 75(2):162–167.
104. Gurr KR, McAfee PC, Shih CM. Biomechanical analysis of posterior instrumentation systems after decompressive laminectomy. an unstable calf-spine model. J Bone Joint Surg [Am] 1988; 70(5):680–691.
105. Ferguson RL, Tencer AF, Woodard P, Allen BL Jr. Biomechanical comparisons of spinal fracture models and the stabilizing effects of posterior instrumentations. Spine 1988; 13(5):453–460.
106. Gurr KR, McAfee PC, Shih CM. Biomechanical analysis of anterior and posterior instrumentation systems after corpectomy. a calf-spine model. J Bone Joint Surg [Am] 1988; 70(8):1182–1191.
107. Mann KA, McGowan DP, Fredrickson BE, Falahee M, Yuan HA. A biomechanical investigation of short segment spinal fixation for burst fractures with varying degrees of posterior disruption. Spine 1990; 15(6):470–478.
108. Slosar PJ Jr., Patwardhan AG, Lorenz M, Havey R, Sartori M. Instability of the lumbar burst fracture and limitations of transpedicular instrumentation. Spine 1995; 20(13): 1452–1461.

38

Spinopelvic Fixation Techniques

LOUIS G. QUARTARARO, ALEXANDER R. VACCARO, and JUSTIN P. KUBECK

Thomas Jefferson University Hospital and the Rothman Institute, Philadelphia, Pennsylvania, U.S.A.

JOHN J. CARBONE

Johns Hopkins Bayview Hospital, Baltimore, Maryland, U.S.A.

JENS CHAPMAN

Harborview Medical Center, Seattle, Washington, U.S.A.

I INTRODUCTION

The successful fusion of the lumbrosacral articulation is often a challenge to the spinal surgeon. The proximity of important neurovascular structures makes operative accesses to, and placement of, stable spinal hardware across this region extremely challenging (Fig. 1). More importantly, the high stresses in this area create a biomechanical environment hostile to a stable bony fusion. Thus, even the most experienced of spinal fusion surgeons have had difficulty in achieving a successful lumbrosacral arthrodesis, with reported pseudoarthrosis rates ranging from 8 to 41% (1–5).

In light of these fusion difficulties, it is not unexpected that several different lumbrosacral fixation techniques have been described. The different techniques can be divided into two major groups: sacral and iliosacral.

II SACRAL TECHNIQUES

Several techniques of sacral fixation have been described. These include S1 pedicle screws, S2 pedicle screws, sacral alar screws, and the Jackson technique.

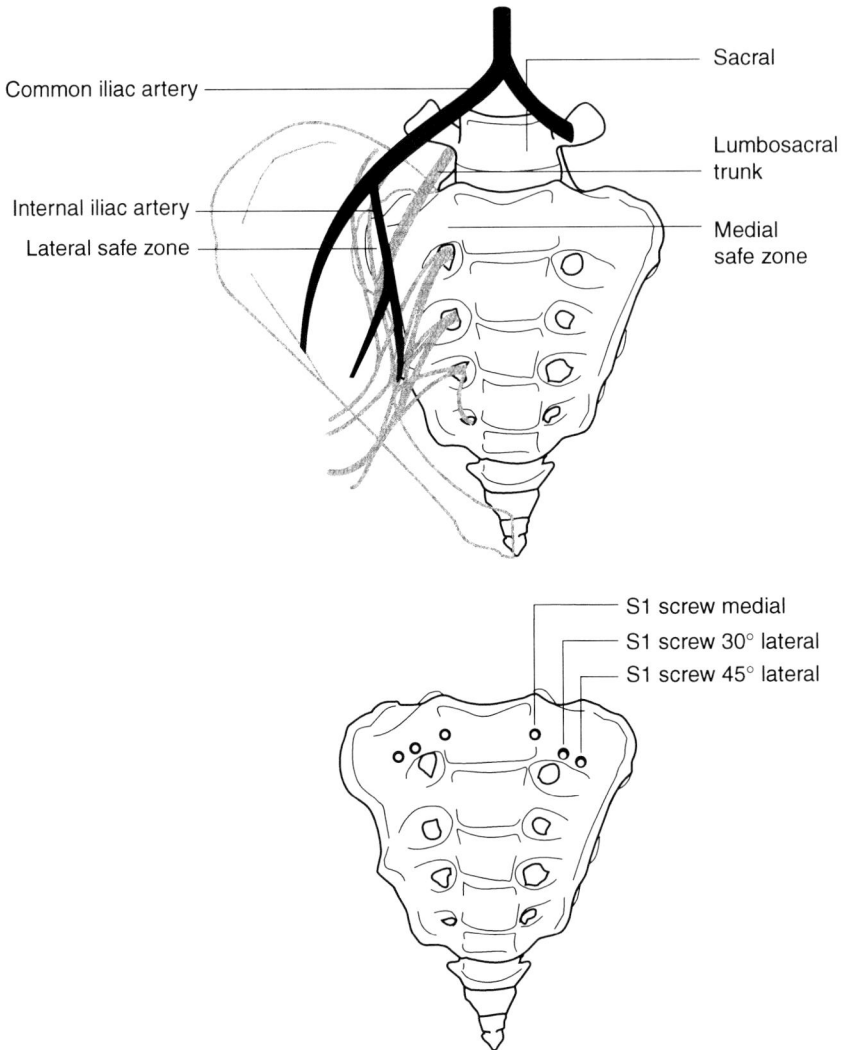

Figure 1 Anterior sacral anatomy demonstrating important vascular structures as well as areas for safe screw placement.

A S1 Pedicle Screws

S1 pedicle screws are the most commonly used mode of spinal fixation to the pelvis. Placement involves using standard instruments and techniques that are used for insertion of lumbar pedicle screws. The starting point is just cephalad to the S1 foramen, below the lumbrosacral facet joint, in line with L5 pedicle. An awl or burr is used to penetrate the outer bony cortex. The pedicle seeker is angled medially 10 to 20 degrees. Bicortical purchase through the sacral promontory is preferable, enhancing fixation. A drill may be required to perforate the thick bone of the promontory.

B   S2 Pedicle Screws

S2 pedicle screws are inserted using a technique similar to S1 screws. The starting point in the transverse plane is the midpoint between the S1 and S2 foramen, and in the vertical plane, halfway between the midline and the line between the sacral foramen. S2 screws should be considered an adjunct to sacral fixation, and should not be used alone as the sole source of terminal sacral stability (6).

C   Sacral Alar Screws

Sacral alar screws are inserted by creating a starting hole just cephalad to the S1 foramen. The pedicle seeker or drill is directed 45 degrees laterally. Bicortical purchase enhances fixation. Care must be taken, however, to avoid aggressive anterior cortical penetration, as the iliac vessels are directly anterior to this point. The anterior cortex should not be penetrated more than 1 to 2 mm.

There is some debate as to whether sacral alar or pedicle screws are stronger. Several good scientific studies argue both sides (7–9). Whichever technique you choose, it is generally felt that bicortical purchase enhances fixation. Once again, neurovascular structures are at risk and care must be taken to avoid overpenetration of the anterior cortex. Some surgeons prefer to use both S1 pedicle and alar screws in the same construct. Several devices have been developed to allow this, including the Chopin block and Tacoma plate. These require more extensive exposure, but afford more points of fixation (Fig. 2).

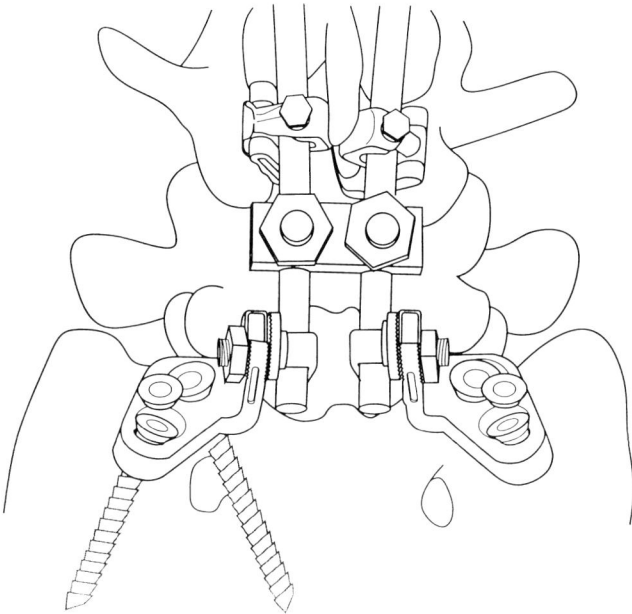

Figure 2   Schematic representation of the Tacoma sacral plate system. This particular sytem allows for both S1 pedicle and alar screw placement. This affords more points of fixation at the expense of a more extensive exposure procedure.

D   Jackson Intrasacral Technique

Jackson has described a technique that involves termination of the caudal end of the rod in the sacrum. S1 screws are placed in the manner mentioned above. The slot in the screw head is oriented obliquely, aiming lateral to the sacral neuroforamen, but medial to the SI joint. The sacrum is drilled in this direction, exiting at the level of the S2 foramen intrapelvically. The contoured terminal portion of the rod is inserted, as in Figure 3 (10,11). Jackson showed that the morphometry of the posterior portion of the ilium provided additional external buttressing of the sacrum in approximatly 92% of the population enhancing rod stability (11).

The above method offers protection of the S1 screws from pullout, added sacral fixation, and avoids crossing the SI joints. Biomechanical studies comparing different AP fusion techniques have found the Jackson technique to be the strongest posterior construct when used in conjunction with an anterior interbody fusion (10).

III   ILIOSACRAL TECHNIQUES

Common to all the iliosacral techniques is the extension of the terminal fixation points into the ilium. This results in a longer lever arm, and thus, in theory, more effectively counterbalances the cantilever forces experienced at the lumbrosacral junction. Drawbacks include increased dissection, more extensive rod contouring, and the crossing of the sacroiliac joint, which may cause postoperative SI joint degenerative changes and pain.

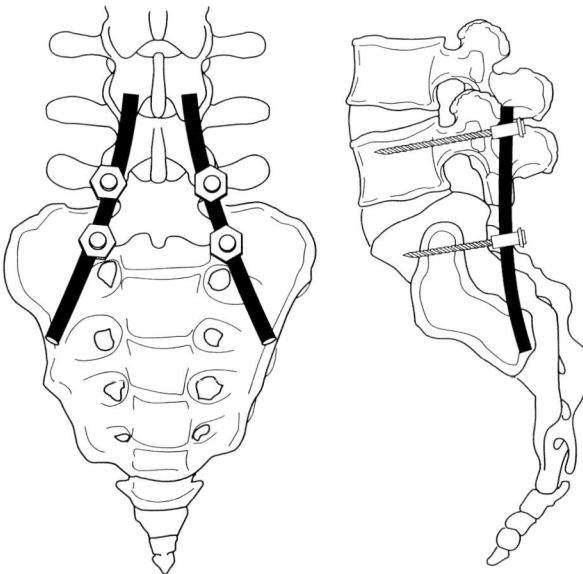

Figure 3   Schematic representation of the Jackson intrasacral technique (AP and lateral views).

A Galveston Technique

The original Galveston technique, as described by Allen and Ferguson, has inherent limitations (12). These include limited biomechanical stiffness, implant loosening within the ilium, and technical difficulties of implantation in conjunction with multilevel lumbar segmental screw or hook fixation. Moreover, its application in patients with iliac defects, such as caused by posterior crest bone graft harvesting or tumor, is technically challenging and frequently not achievable to a satisfactory degree. Placement of iliac screws in projection angles similar to the Galveston technique have been proposed by Letournel, Roy-Camille, Asher, Abumi, and Schildhauer in a variety of technical refinements and for different clinical indications (13,14).

1 Indications

Potential clinical indications for iliolumbar instrumentation are patients with either complex spinal deformity or patients with pathological conditions of the posterior pelvic ring. Patients who need correction of thoracolumbar deformities, such as neuromuscular scoliosis or severe kyphosis, or who require fusion to the S1 segment, may benefit from an improved caudal instrumentation purchase gained from the ileum (15). Tumor disease affecting the lumbosacral junction, such as found in patients with sacral chordoma or chondrosacroma makes solid iliac fixation a necessity. Patients with traumatic disruption of the posterior pelvic ring, such as found with vertically displaced zone II or zone III sacral fractures may similarly benefit from this instrumentation technique (Table 1).

2 Decision Making

Basic requirements for iliolumbar screw fixation remain the same as originally proposed for the Galveston modification for lumbopelvic fixation: to provide biome-

Table 1 Potential Indications for Lumbopelvic Instrumentation

---

Deformity
   Neuromuscular scoliosis
   Correction of decompensated lumbar idiopathic scoliosis
   Sagittal balance correction necessitating sacral fixation
   Revision surgery for high-grade spondylolisthesis
Trauma
   Displaced sacral insufficiency fracture
   Vertically displaced zone 2 sacral fracture
   Displaced zone 3 sacral fracture
     "H" patterns
     "U" patterns
   Corrective osteotomy for malunion
Neoplasia
   Sacrectomy for
     Sacral chordoma
     Sacral chondrosarcoma
     Other indications for sacrectomy

---

chanically strong, yet low-profile fixation to the ilium as an anchor for stabilization of long thoracolumbar deformity corrections or for patients with an unstable posterior pelvic ring. Unavailability of a low-profile construct assembly and limitations in the ability to individually manipulate the various iliolumbar fixation points has traditionally hampered the clinical usefulness of iliolumbar fixation systems.

The most common type of failure of a traditional Galveston type iliolumbar instrumentation technique has been toggle loosening of the iliac part of the rod, leading to a typical windshield wiper appearance on radiographs. The goal of any iliolumbar screw fixation, therefore, is to optimize screw purchase by placing iliac screws of maximum length and diameter (16). If need be, more than one screw should be placed in order to accommodate a patient's specific needs. Placement of transilial screws, however, has to be intraosseous within the ilium to minimize intraoperative complications. Extraosseous screw placement could result in injury of the superior gluteal vessels in the area below the greater sciatic notch with subsequent bleeding, superior gluteal nerve injury, injury of intrapelvic structures, as well as fractures of the iliac wing. Excessively caudal screw angulation might result in intraarticular acetabular screw positioning. Therefore, the surgeon should be well familiar with the pelvic anatomy of the ilium before placement of such screws and needs to be knowledgeable of the screw size to avoid extraosseous placement.

To date, the scientific validation of iliolumbar screw fixation in aspects of biomechanical performance and clinical outcomes remains in a state of evolution (17). Iliolumbar screw and rod fixation was shown to be biomechanically superior to sacroiliac screw fixation and Galveston rod technique in a cadaveric model with a unilateral, vertically destabilized lumbosacral junction (14). Using a trajectory between the posterior superior iliac spine and the anterior inferior iliac spine, a maximum potential iliac screw length of an average of 140 mm with an 8- to 9-mm diameter was found for male patients, as compared to 130 mm in female patients (14).

IV   SUGGESTED SURGICAL TECHNIQUE

The patient is positioned prone on a suitable radiolucent spinal operating table, such as a Jackson table or a Wilson frame. A posterior midline exposure is performed. The multifidus is stripped from its posterior alar attachment to reveal the medial cortex of the iliac crest (18). The posterior superior iliac crest is now exposed and the outer iliac table developed in subperiosteal fashion. A periosteal elevator, such as a Cobb, is then used as guide to determine the inclination angle of the iliac wing. The cortical condensation above the sciatic notch can be bluntly probed to confirm a drill trajectory above the sciatic notch (15). Depending upon the specific indications, the posterior aspect of the superior iliac crest can also be exposed. This superior posterior pelvic crest can later be used as a bone graft harvest site without compromising iliac screw placement. The intended decompression and thoracolumbar instrumentation surgery can now be completed as necessary. The caudal end of any rod should be contoured to lie in the groove formed by the posterior iliac crest and the sacral ala. The distal rod end should reach to the level of the caudal end of the posterior superior iliac spine.

Using a side opening screw system, such as the Universal Spine System (USS, Synthes, Paoli, PN), allows for a simple and direct iliac screw to rod attachment without connector pieces after the main instrumentation rods have been placed. Other systems require placement of the iliac screws first and then utilize a number of connector components to achieve rod attachment. The following description pertains to use of a side-opening screw system such as the USS.

A C-arm is positioned in a true lateral projection to the patient's pelvis as shown by exact superimposition of the left and right sciatic notches. It is not used until iliac instrumentation is performed. A starting point on the ilium is selected immediately lateral to the already placed fixation rod on the inferior end of the posterior iliac spine. Since the widest iliac cancellous passage space is located in the area above the sciatic notch, this area is usually preferred for initial screw placement. For patients with an unstable hemipelvis, reduction of the pelvis is performed with one or more iliac Schanz pins. The drill direction should be perpendicular to the longitudinal rod axis. The inclination of the drill should parallel the ilium. Use of a clinical alignment guide, such as a periosteal elevator held parallel to the outer iliac cortical table, is helpful in determining this angle. Drilling is then performed with a "high speed–slow advance" technique, using a long 3.2-mm drill and a drill guide. Some surgeons prefer the use of a "bounce" drill technique, others an oscillating drill to minimize the risk of premature cortical penetration. The C-arm is used to assure correct drill passage above the sciatic notch and toward the anterior inferior iliac spine. Correct maintenance of this trajectory avoids penetration of the acetabulum. Screw length is ultimately dictated by a patient's anatomy and clinical needs. If needed, bicortical screw lengths of 130 mm or more using a 8-mm diameter screw are possible. After probing of the drill tract with a suitably long depth gauge, an appropriately measured screw is then inserted. Patients with very dense cancellous bone may require overdrilling or tapping of the drill hole to facilitate screw placement. The starting hole is then widened with a rongeur to accommodate the screw head. A screw is then manually advanced into the hole, recessed into the posterior iliac crest, and locked against the rod using conventional coupling devices. The USS screw head configuration is of a narrow profile and thus allows for screw placement in close proximity of an already placed rod. Larger screw head designs are prone to create a cavity around the insertion site due to eccentric screw deviation during insertion. The use of polyaxial screws has not been necessary and may lead to undesirable hardware prominence. If needed, a second screw can now be placed midway between the S1 screw and the previously placed iliac screw. It should be noted that the more cranial iliac screws usually require a more lateral screw trajectory than the screw placed above the sciatic notch. This, again, can be clinically confirmed by placing a periosteal elevator alongside the outer iliac table at the level of the intended screw placement.

Radiographic confirmation of intraosseous screw placement is then performed with the C-arm in an anteroposterior oblique pathway, in which the C-arm beam is coaxially centered over the trajectory of the iliac screw. The screw should remain confined within the iliac tables, preferably in the triangular supra-acetabular cancellous bone.

Arthrodesis is now carried out by decorticating the posterolateral bony elements of the instrumented segments of the lumbar spine and the superior shoulder of the sacral ala. If desired, the posterior iliosacral ligaments can be removed as well and decortication of the posterior aspect of the iliosacral joint can be performed. Iliac crest bone graft is now harvested by resecting flakes of corticocancellous bone from the superior posterior iliac crest.

A   Iliac Screws

Another modification of Galveston fixation to the pelvis involves the use of an iliac screw, described by Asher et al. (Fig. 4) (19). Essentially, a long pedicle screw is placed between the tables of the ilium, along the same path as the Galveston rod. This screw is linked to an eyebolt rod or slotted connector which then mates with a longitudinal rod member (Fig. 5 a,b).

B   Iliosacral Screws

Iliosacral screws, described by Duboisset (20) are inserted from lateral to medial, through the ilium's outer table, then inner table, then finally through the sacrum, for "tri-cortical" purchase. The screw does not directly cross the sacroiliac joint, but is inserted cephalad to this anatomical articulation. Thus, it has an "in-out-in" orientation. From the starting point on the outer table of the ilium, the drill is directed 30 degrees caudal and 30 degrees anterior. The drill is then visualized as it exits the inner table of the ilium. The entry point on the sacrum is 1 cm caudal and 1 cm lateral to the lumbrosacral facet joint. The lumbar longitudinal member (rod) is then connected to the screw, not at the screw head but at the screw shaft between the sacral ala and the posterior ilium. Thus, pullout forces are perpendicular to the direction of screw placement, making the stability of the connection highly efficient. Drawbacks include the very extensive dissection required to place this screw, and the indirect crossing of the SI joint.

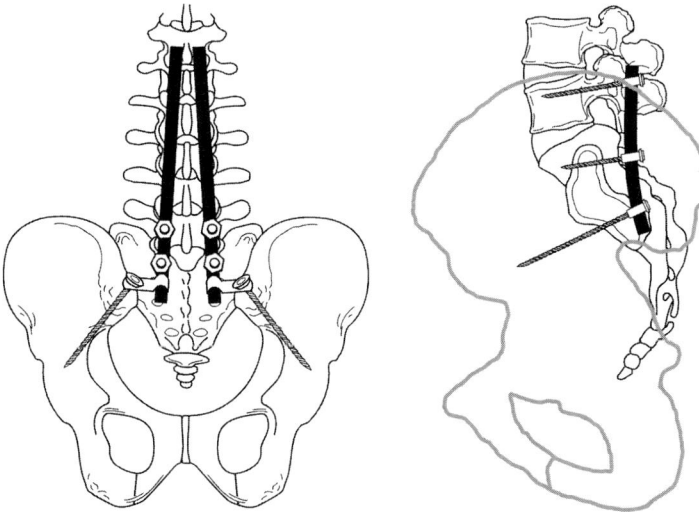

Figure 4   Schematic representation of iliac screw placement. This particular system uses transpedicular screws in the lumbar area, an S1 pedicle screw into the sacral promontory, iliac fixation via intrailiac screws and cross connectors.

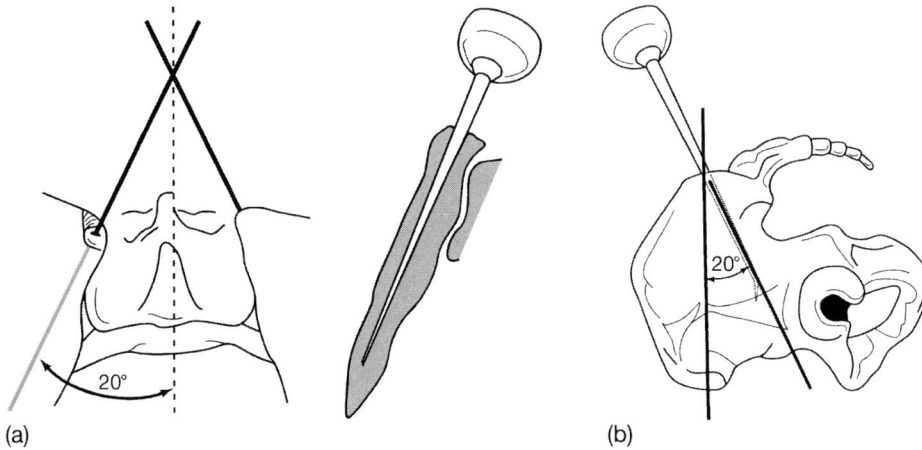

Figure 5 (a) Schematic representations of intrailiac post/screw anchor placement. (b) In the normal adult pelvis, the axial plane passage line is approximately 20 degrees lateral from the midsagittal plane and 20 degrees caudal to a transverse plane.

C   Kostuik Transsacral Bar Technique

The transsacral bar technique was used by Harrington for long posterior spine fusions. With the advancement of fixation techniques, Kostuik has introduced a newer version of the transsacral bar. In essence, it consists of a horizontal bar embedded in both posterior ilium and connected to two S1 pedicle screws, and then connected to a standard longitudinal lumbar rod construct. To place the bar construct, S1 pedicle screws are placed initially. The screw heads are oriented horizontally, so as to receive a horizontal, transsacral bar. An ''L''-shaped awl is then used to punch a hole in the ilium, using the screw head as a guide. The distance between both ilium posteriorly is measured and 6 cm is added to this measurement, for the appropriate rod length. The rod is then contoured to the curve of the sacrum, and driven into the aforementioned holes in the ilium. This is then attached to the S1 pedicle screws in the standard fashion. A rod called a ''sacral connector rod'' is then used, which allows for a perpendicular, rod-to-rod, connection to the transsacral bar. Lumbar pedicle screws can now be connected in standard fashion to the sacral connector rod. Alternatively, this rod can be connected to an existing lumbar pedicle screw, rod construct with a side-to-side, bar-to-bar connector. This technique provides increased stability, without the need for extensive additional dissection, as in the Galveston techniques. It does, however, cross the SI joints, and may cause late degenerative changes and pain.

Each of the above techniques has its good features and its pitfalls. The authors prefer the sacral techniques, because of the debatable belief that crossing the SI joint may cause late problems. Their placement also avoids more extensive dissection. The concominant use of anterior arthrodesis at L5–S1, whether by anterior lumbar interbody fusion (ALIF), transforaminal lumbar interbody fusion (TLIF), or posterior lateral interbody fusion (PLIF), has been shown to enhance fusion rates, and thus is also recommended (21).

REFERENCES

1. Boachic-Adjei O, Dendrinos GK, Ogilvie JW, Bradford DS. Management of adult spinal deformity with combined anterior-posterior arthrodesis and Luque-Galveston instrumentation. J Spinal Disord 1991;4:131–141.
2. Devlin VJ, Boachic-Adjei O, Bradford DS, et al. Treatment of adult spinal deformity with fusion to the sacrum using C-D instrumentation. J Spinal Disord 1991;4:1–14.
3. Kostuik JP, Errico TJ, Gleason TF. Techniques of internal fixations for degenerative conditions of the lumbar spine. Clin Orthop 1986; 203:212–231.
4. Kostuik JP, Musha Y. Fusion to the sacrum in adult idiopathic scoliosis using C-D instrumentation (1986–1990). Presented at the SRS Annual Meeting, Portland Oregon, September 1994.
5. Saer E, Winter RB, Lonstein J. Long scoliosis fusion to the sacrum in adults with nonparalytic scoliosis: An improved method. Spine 1990; 15:650–653.
6. McCord DH, Cunningham BW, Shonto S, et al. Biomechanical analysis of lumbrosacral fixation. Spine 1992; 17(85):235–243.
7. Asher MA, Strippgen WE. Anthropometric studies of the human sacrum relating to dorals trans-sacral implant designs. Clin Orthop 1986; 203:58–62.
8. Smith SA, Abitbol JJ, Carlson GD, et al. The effects of depth penetration, screw orientation, and bone density on sacral screw fixation. Spine 1993; 18:1006–1010.
9. Zindrick MR, Wiltse LL, Widell EH, et al. A biomechanical study of intrapedicular screw fixation in the lumbrosacral spine. Clin Orthop 1986; 203:99–112.
10. Glazer PA, Collins O, Lotz, Bradford DS. Biomechanical analysis of lumbar fixation. Spine 1996; 21:1211–1222.
11. Jackson RP, McManus AC. The iliac buttress. A computed tomographic study of sacral anatomy. Spine 1993; 18:1318–1328.
12. Allen BL, Ferguson RL. A 1988 perspective of the Galveston technique of pelvic fixation. Orthop Clin North Am 1988; 19:409–418.
13. Letournel E, Judet R. Fractures of the acetabulum, 2nd ed. Berlin: Springer-Verlag, 1993.
14. Schildhauer TA, Josten C, Muhr G. Triangular osteosynthesis of vertically unstable sacrum fractures: a new concept allowing early weight-bearing. J Orthop Trauma 1998; 12(5):307–314.
15. Berry, JL, Stahurski T, Asher MA. Morphometry of the supra sciatic notch intrailiac implant anchor passage. Spine 2001; 26:E143–148.
16. Chapman JR, Harrington RM, Lee K, et al. The influence of screw design and insertion technique on the pull-out strength of screws in porous materials. Trans Orthop Res Soc 1992; 17:406.
17. Glazer PA, Colliou O, Lotz JC, et al. Biomechanical analysis of lumbosacral fixation. Spine 1996; 21:1211–1222.
18. Miller F, Moseley C, Koreska J. Pelvic anatomy relative to lumbosacral instrumentation. J Spinal Disord 1990; 3:169–173.
19. Asher MA. Lumbropelvic fixation with the ISOLA spinal implant system. In: Marguiles JY, Floman Y, Farcy J-PC, Neuwirth MG, eds. Lumbrosacral and Spinopelvic Fixation. Philadelphia: Lippincott-Raven, 1996.
20. Dubousset J. Pelvic obliquity correction. In: Marguiles JY, Floman Y, Farcy J-PC, Neuwirth MG, eds. Lumbrosacral and Spinopelvic Fixation. Philadelphia: Lippincott-Raven, 1996.
21. Wetzel FT, Larocca H. The failed posterior lumbar interbody fusion. Spine 1991; 16: 839.

39

Anterior Thoracolumbar Techniques: Surgical Approaches

ROCCO R. CALDERONE

St. John's Regional Medical Center, Oxnard, California, U.S.A.

I TRANSTHORACIC EXPOSURE

Access to the anterior thoracic spine is achieved through a transthoracic exposure (Table 1). The limits of the exposure include the second thoracic vertebra through the twelfth thoracic vertebra, depending on the placement of the incision and the level of the diaphragm. Exposure and intervention to the anterior thoracic spine is undertaken through the pleural cavity.

A Positioning and Incision Placement

The transthoracic exposure requires an incision parallel to the course of the ribs. The left-sided approach is favored by most for several anatomical reasons. On the left side, the aorta can be mobilized and manipulated with more retraction pressure than the thin-walled vena cava. The thicker-walled aorta also serves to protect the thinner-walled vena cava, azygos vein system, and thoracic duct. The heart is handled with more mobility on the left, with anterior displacement in contrast to right side of the heart with superior and inferior vena caval attachments. In addition, on the right side, the liver raises the diaphragm to a higher level, allowing less caudal access of the thoracic spine without incision of the diaphragm and entry into the retroperitoneal space.

Surgeons advocating a right-sided approach argue for safer internal fixation placement on the left side. There are few cited cases of pseudoaneurysm formation from internal fixation devices adjacent to the aorta. Also deformity cases involving a right-sided convexity may necessitate a right-sided approach. A bifurcated endotracheal tube is required for selective lung deflation during thoracotomy exposure.

Table 1   Transthoracic Exposure of the Thoracic Spine

In lateral position left-side approach.
Incision placed along left side following the rib two levels above vertebra.
Latissimus and serratus anterior muscles are divided.
Rib periosteum is elevated and stripped.
Intercostal nerve and vessels below rib protected.
Pleura is incised, ribs spread, lung deflated, packed with sponge.
Parietal pleura reflected from vertebra.
Intercostal vessels ligated and divided, aorta retracted.
Vertebral body, disks and pedicle exposed.

For a left-sided approach, the patient is positioned in the lateral decubitus position with the right side appropriately padded against the table with an axillary roll. The right side of the waist is also supported with padding. Flexure of the table allows the ribs on the left side to spread for maximum exposure. This position also curves the spine toward the right. This may serve to correct spinal deformity. A convex deformity to the right would be exacerbated in this position. Table flexion must be eliminated prior to final spinal fixation in order to avoid deformity.

Placement of the incision depends on the exposure desired. For isolated exposure of one segment, the incision can be centered over the rib at that vertebral level. A more extensive exposure requires an incision one or two rib levels above the central vertebra of the range involved in the procedure or at the rib corresponding to the cephalic vertebra of the range. It is much easier to work and expose levels caudal to the incision than it is to expose cephalad levels. Since the ribs slope distally as they are followed around the chest wall it is better to begin at a rib level above the main vertebral level. Horizontally oriented ribs are the exception, allowing incision placement centered over the spinal levels.

For the upper thoracic levels cephalad to T-5, a periscapular incision is required. The scapula and periscapular muscles overlie the ribs of the upper thoracic spine. Retraction of the overlying scapula is required to expose the appropriate rib level.

B   Superficial Dissection

The incision at the chosen level begins about four fingerbreadths lateral to the spinous process and follows the selected rib level around anteriorly to the costochondral junction. The incision is deepened through the skin and subcutaneous tissue encountering the first muscle layers: trapezius, latissimus dorsi, and serratus anterior. The trapezius attaches to the spinous processes as far down as T6 and usually remains posterior and superior to the field dissection. The latissimus requires division transverse to its muscle fibers as caudal as possible to avoid its innervation, which originates proximally. The serratus anterior is similarly divided in the anterior region of the exposure. Cautery muscle division aids in hemostasis.

The periosteum of the selected rib can now be identified. The periosteum of the rib is incised and elevated. Subperiosteal dissection proceeds toward the upper border of the rib, detaching the intercostal muscles from over the top of the rib. The intercostal nerve, artery, and vein course underneath each rib. Access over the superior edge of the rib avoids injury to the neurovascular bundle.

The intercostal muscles are composed of three adjacent layers: external, internal, and innermost intercostal muscles. The neurovascular bundle lies between the internal and innermost intercostal muscle layers. Subperiosteal exposure is required for rib removal. Alternatively, incision through the intercostal muscles close to the superior rib margin can be used for limited exposures not requiring rib removal.

For rib removal, subperiosteal dissection is advanced over the top of the rib and around to the inner and under surface. Gaining access to the under surface requires close adherence to the bone to dissect above the neurovascular bundle. Once access to the undersurface of the rib is achieved, a rib stripper is inserted and used to carry the subperiosteal plane around to the remainder of the rib. This section of rib is then excised from about two fingerbreadths lateral to the transverse process anteriorly to the costochondral junction using a rib cutter. Occasionally, an extended exposure is required with removal of an additional adjacent rib or a separate, more caudal, incision. Excised ribs serve as an additional source of bone graft.

The parietal pleura lies in the bed of the excised rib. It is divided while protecting the underlying lung. Rib-spreading retractors are inserted and the anterior thoracic spine is visualized underneath the mediastinal parietal pleura.

Alternatively, a retropleural approach can be used. This requires careful, blunt dissection of the parietal pleura away from the intercostal muscle layer. Complete resection of the rib helps in continuing this plane of dissection posteriorly.

C   Deep Dissection

For a deep dissection, a Finochietto rib-spreading retractor should be inserted (Fig. 1). Protect the adjacent lung. Pack it away from the field of dissection. Deflation of the left lung is achieved with a bifurcated endotracheal tube through which the anesthesiologist may selectively deflate the left side. Spinal level localization can be confirmed by inserting a marker needle into the disk space followed a radiograph or fluoroscopic image confirming the position.

Anterior spinal exposure is accomplished with incision through and reflection of the parietal pleura. The segmental intercostal artery and veins cross the mid aspect of the vertebral body. These are controlled with clipping and ligation. Paralysis as a result of impeding the blood supply to the spinal cord with vessel ligation is rare. Winter et al. have documented 1197 cases involving anterior vessel ligation without resultant paralysis (1). Collateral circulations from the opposite side, as well as from vessels proximal and distal to the area of dissection, are abundant. To preserve this collateral circulation through branches adjacent to the spinal canal, segmental arteries should be ligated as far anteriorly as possible adjacent to the aorta, away from the neural foramen.

Rib disarticulation from its transverse process and hemifacet vertebral body articulations allows better visualization of the neuroforamen. The rib articulates with the transverse costal facet at the anterior lateral aspect of the tip of the transverse process. It is also anchored to the posterior lateral corner of the vertebral body above and below through superior and inferior costal facets. Locate and protect the intercostal neurovascular bundle during excision of these articulations. Once the rib attachments have been removed, the intercostal nerve can be traced back to the intervertebral foramen.

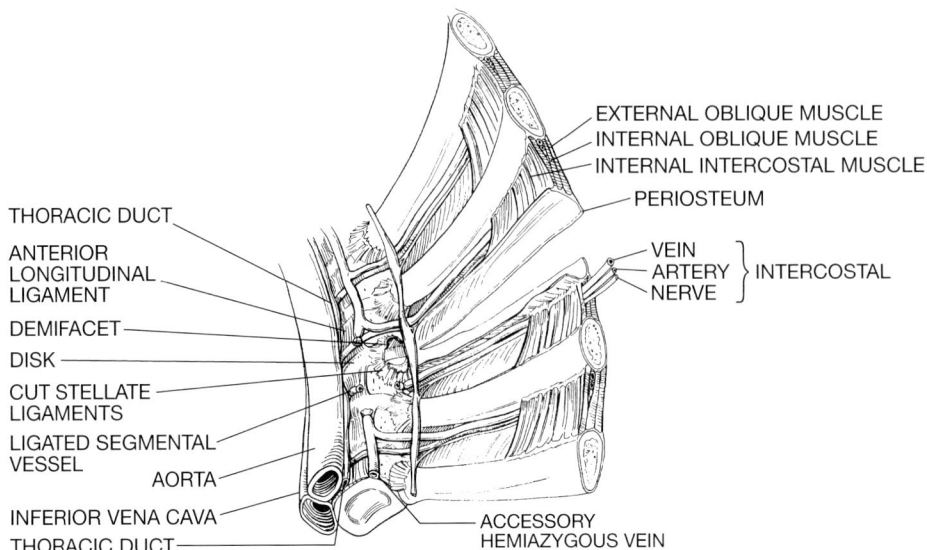

Figure 1 Transthoracic exposure: deep dissection with division of intercostal vessels and exposure of the thoracic spine.

The sympathetic trunk and greater splanchnic nerve lie along the lateral aspect of the vertebral bodies adjacent to the head of the ribs. Injury to the sympathetic chain in the upper thoracic spine may result in Horner's syndrome.

Posterior mediastinal structures to be avoided include the thoracic duct, azygos and hemiazygos veins. The thoracic duct and azygos vein generally lie to the right side of the aorta. The hemiazygos vein lies along the left side and has a more varied pattern. Anatomical variations exist and attention to these structures avoid complications of profuse venous bleeding or chylothorax from thoracic duct injury. Segmental vessel ligation and division above and below the spinal segment on the left side allows the aorta to move away to the right and protect the azygos, thoracic duct, and vena cava.

Subperiosteal dissection can then expose the vertebral body, disks, and pedicle. The aorta generally lies over the anterior lateral aspect of the vertebral body on the left with some anatomical variation on its exact course. The border of the anterior longitudinal ligament begins under the aorta. The periosteum is adherent to the annulus at each disk level. Intervertebral disk excision can be undertaken using a scalpel or cautery with Cobb elevators and ring curettes. The exposure also allows corpectomy. The pedicle will identify the limit of the posterior vertebral body. Anterolateral placement of internal fixation rather than anterior placement avoids hardware impingement against the aorta. Deformity correction and arthrodesis with spinal fixation can be accomplished. Correct the table position, as needed, prior to final fixation.

D   Wound Closure

Stability of a bone graft and fixation is achieved. The periosteal layer usually is not intact enough for closure in adults. The pleura of the posterior mediastinum usually cannot be reapproximated. Hemostasis is required for all transsected vessels. Avoid any absorbable hemostatic sponges or other space-occupying substance in the vicinity of the spinal cord.

A chest tube is inserted to drain postoperative fluid accumulation and oozing. The chest tube will evacuate and prevent any pleural effusion. Also, initial continuous suction eliminates a pneumothorax as the pleural lining reforms. The chest tube is sutured into the skin. A purse string suture is often used in the skin for site closure when the tubes are pulled.

Sponges and packing are removed and counted. The lung is reinflated. The lung is inflated intermittently with slight positive pressure to eliminate areas of atelectasis. The ribs above and below the area of dissection are reapproximated with the rib approximator. The table can be flexed toward the side of closure to aid in bringing the ribs together. The pleura layer and intercostal muscle layer are brought together in a watertight fashion with a running suture. Chest wall closure is reinforced, as needed, with absorbable sutures around the upper rib and below the lower rib, taking care to avoid injury to the neurovascular bundle. Serratus anterior, latissimus, and trapezius muscle layers are repaired. Subcutaneous and skin layers are closed in routine fashion.

The chest tube is maintained to suction for the first few days. The tubes are removed when drainage sufficiently decreases to 100 cc or less per 24 h and risk of pneumothorax and effusion decreases. Purse-string sutures are tightened closing off the chest tube site and an occlusive dressing is placed. Frequent incentive spirometry, coughing, and deep breathing are essential to the patient.

II THORACOABDOMINAL EXPOSURE

Exposure of the thoracolumbar spine requires a thoracoabdominal approach (Table 2). Exposure through the pleural space allows access of the spine through to about the T12 vertebra. Through the retroperitoneal space the upper lumbar spine can be exposed. Taking down the diaphragm reveals a continuous segment of the thoracolumbar junction. This allows a wide and safer region of exposure for access above T12 and below L1. The approach is a combined transthoracic and retroperitoneal

Table 2 Transthoracic Retroperitoneal Exposure of the Thoracolumbar Spine

---

In semilateral position, incision placed along tenth rib and curving distally toward umbilicus.
Periosteum elevated and tenth rib excised.
External, internal oblique, and transversus abdominus muscles is divided.
Transversalis fascia is divided peritoneum exposed.
Parietal pleura incised, lung deflated, and packed with sponge.
Peritoneum bluntly dissected away exposing the retroperitoneal space.
Diaphragm is incised 2 cm from periphery around to aorta.
Pleura, peritoneum, and periosteum reflected from spine.
Intercostal and lumbar artery and veins ligated and divided.
Aorta retracted, vertebrae and disks exposed.

---

exposure as detailed in two other sections of this chapter. In addition to these two exposures, dissection of the diaphragm is required as described below.

A   Positioning and Incision Placement

A left-sided approach is preferred. The right side requires exposure under and behind the liver as well as dissection of the inferior vena cava. The right-sided approach may present significantly more difficulty. The patient is thus positioned with the right side padded against the table in a semilateral position. A beanbag positioner may be used to hold the patient lateral angled slightly toward supine. Flexing the table down or padding under the waist will allow the left side to bend away or open for easier exposure. This sideways positioning may need to be corrected toward the end of the case for proper spinal alignment or fixation. Lung deflation on the left side will be performed with a bifurcated endotracheal tube, which can be placed in preparation for this.

The incision begins posteriorly about four fingerbreadths from the spinous process and proceeds along the course of the chosen rib. Generally, the tenth rib serves for exposure distal to T10 vertebra. For easier access to the superior aspect of T10, the ninth rib is chosen for incision placement. This varies according to the obliquity of the ribs. Generally one or two ribs above the desired vertebral access level are required.

A curvilinear incision is made extending distally at the costochondral junction just past the midaxillary line. The obliquity of the incision continues around to the lateral border of the rectus muscle. The distal extent of the incision depends on the desired access of the lumbar spine. An incision to the level of the umbilicus would allow access to the L2–L3 region.

B   Superficial Dissection

The superficial dissection approach (Fig. 2) has been advocated both as proceeding first with a retroperitoneal exposure followed by a transthoracic exposure, as well as vice versa, by various sources. It is best to familiarize oneself with both retroperitoneal and transthoracic dissection individually, and then to proceed according to preference. Also a retropleural retroperitoneal approach has been described and differs only in dissecting the pleural away after rib resection rather than entering the pleural cavity. This description will focus on the more common transpleural technique.

Incision through the subcutaneous tissues requires hemostasis of multiple venous branches, including the lateral thoracic vein in the midaxillary line. Division of the muscle layer proceeds through the latissimus dorsi and serratus anterior muscles along the chest and the external abdominal oblique, internal abdominal oblique, and transverses abdominis muscles along the abdominal aspect of the incision. The incision is carried distally to the edge of the rectus abdominus sheath. Ascending branches of the deep circumflex iliac artery are encountered along the abdominal musculature.

The periosteum is incised over the rib. The rib is stripped subperiosteally, carefully avoiding the intercostal neurovascular bundle riding along the inferior margin. The rib is removed, cutting it posteriorly adjacent to the paraspinal muscles and anteriorly close to the costochondral junction. A small section of internal oblique

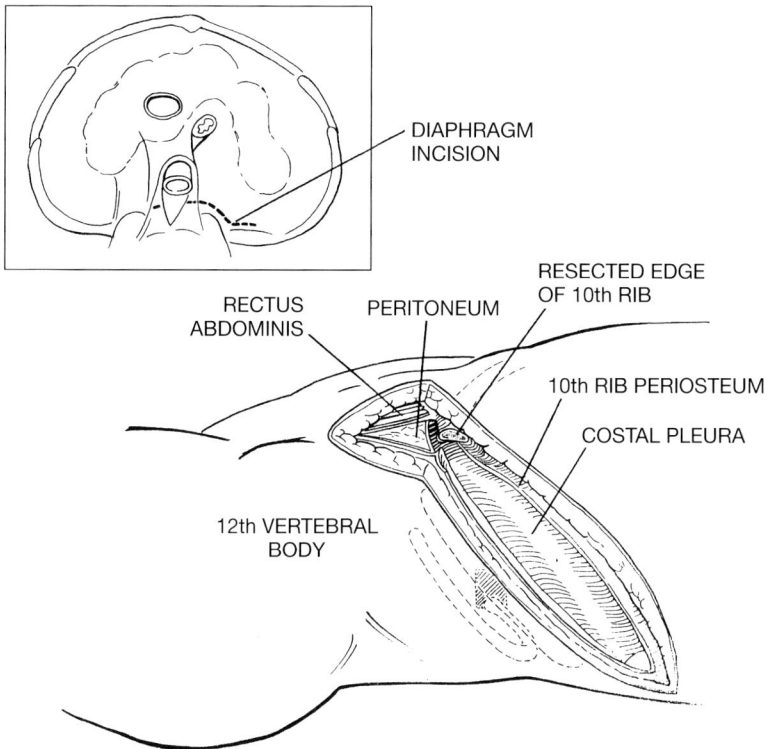

Figure 2 Thoracoabdominal exposure: superficial dissection with division of latissimus, serratus anterior, intercostal, external oblique, internal oblique, and transversus abdominus muscles followed by rib resection, pleural incision, retroperitoneal dissection, and diaphragm incision.

muscle can be left attached to the costochondral junction. After rib removal, the costal cartilage can be split leaving a small piece of cartilage on the internal oblique muscle as a landmark to facilitate reattachment of the abdominal musculature at this junction. The pleura are visible in the bed of the rib. The pleura are divided with protection of the underlying lung and caudally arching diaphragm. The pleural cavity is now accessible. The lung is deflated and protected and packed away from the field of dissection. Chest-spreading retractors are inserted.

Along the abdominal region, the transversalis fascia is exposed under the muscle layer. The peritoneal layer is now visible. The peritoneum is bluntly dissected away from the abdominal wall, developing the retroperitoneal space. The peritoneum is packed away with protecting sponges and self-retaining retractors inserted. Access to both the pleural cavity and retroperitoneal space has now been achieved. The diaphragm is now visible separating the two cavities. The deep dissection of this exposure describes the access to the spine in this region.

C   Deep Dissection

Access to the thoracolumbar region of the spine requires taking down the diaphragm (Fig. 3). The peritoneum is bluntly dissected away from the inferior surface of the

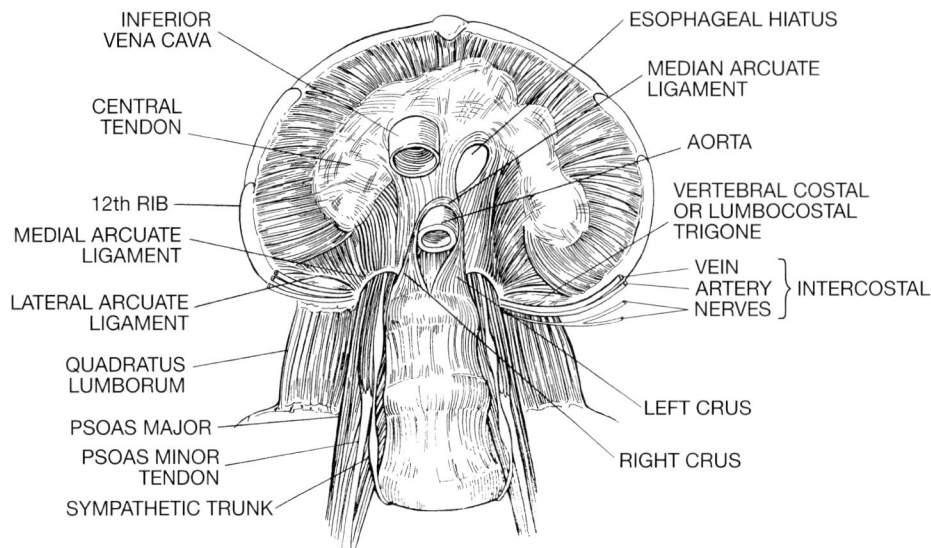

Figure 3 Thoracoabdominal exposure: deep dissection, diaphragmatic anatomy.

diaphragm. The superior and inferior surfaces of the diaphragm are now visible. The phrenic nerves course down through the mediastinum on either side of the heart, which rests on the central portion of the diaphragm. The phrenic nerves course through the central tendinous portion of the diaphragm, branching out toward the periphery along the superior and inferior surfaces. The inferior phrenic arteries arise from the aorta along the undersurface of the diaphragm, branching out toward the periphery. Incisions in the diaphragm are placed in the periphery because the innervation and circulation originates in the central tendinous portion.

The esophagus courses through the central portion of the diaphragm. The esophageal hiatus is formed by the fibers from the right crus of the diaphragm passing around the right and left sides of the esophagus and branches of the vagus nerves. The aorta passes posterior to the esophagus and anterior to the spine between the right and left crura under the median arcuate ligament of the diaphragm. The vena cava passes through the central tendenous portion of the diaphragm to the right through the vena caval foramen. The right lobe of the liver is adherent to the right subphrenic space separated from a narrow area of diaphragm behind the right triangular ligament of the liver close to the rib. A right-sided approach requires the incision to pass through this narrow area of diaphragm to mobilize the liver with the diaphragm and allow retraction to the left for exposure of the spine. A right-sided approach also requires control and ligation of the right lumbar veins to mobilize the diaphragm and vena cava out to the left of the path of the anterior spinal dissection.

The dome-shaped diaphragm is attached anteriorly to the xiphoid process of the sternum and anterolaterally along the costochondral region of the lower six ribs, anchoring posterolaterally on the twelfth rib and posteriorly on the transverse process of L1 vertebra. The posterior attachments form three arcuate ligaments or lumbocostal arches. The region between the twelfth rib to L1 transverse process forms the lateral arcuate ligament under which passes the quadratus lumborum muscle and twelfth costal nerve. This region includes a triangular tendinous extension referred to as the lumbocostal trigone. The diaphragmatic attachments from the L1 transverse process to anterior L1 vertebral body form the medial arcuate ligament under which passes the psoas muscle, ilioinguinal and iliohypogastric nerves, as well as the sympathetic trunk. The right and left crura of the diaphragm continue in the midline posteriorly descending and inserting into the prevertebral fascia of L1, L2, and L3. This forms the median arcuate ligament in the midline under which passes the aorta. Other important structures pass through the diaphragm in this region between the medial and intermediate crura, including the thoracic duct, azygos vein, and hemiazygos or ascending lumbar vein as well as the greater, lesser, and least splanchnic nerves.

Continuing with the approach, the diaphragmatic incision remains along the periphery to prevent denervation of a large portion of the diaphragm, which is innervated from the central region and outward. The incision lies along the periphery approximately 1 to 2 cm from the chest wall, allowing a rim for later repair. Sutures may be used to mark corresponding points for later reattachment. The curved incision passes anterior to the lateral arcuate ligament, medial arcuate ligament to the left crus of the diaphragm. The left medial crus is the final portion of diaphragm attaching to the left side of the anterior spine. The left crus extends down the lumbar region, attaching to L2 and L3 anterior vertebral bodies adjacent to the anterior longitudinal ligament and aorta. The proximal medial aspect of left crus ascends proximally, joining into the median arcuate ligament over the top of the aorta. The incision continues through the medial left crus of the diaphragm 1 to 2 cm above the lateral and medial arcuate ligaments, but behind the greater, lesser, and least thoracic splanchnic nerves and hemiazygos or ascending lumbar vein. Branches of the hemiazygos vein are ligated and divided, as needed, for mobilization of the diaphragm. The sympathetic trunk lies posterior to the field of dissection passing through the diaphragm in the region of the intermediate and lateral crura near the medial arcuate ligament. The aorta is protected with a curved clamp inserted in front of the vessel wall and behind the median arcuate ligament as the incision is completed through the medial crus to the aortic hiatus.

The anterior spine can now be exposed. Parietal pleura and retroperitoneal tissue are carefully dissected away. The aorta is mobilized with ligation of segmental lumbar and intercostal vessels. These vessels are ligated and divided toward the aorta side to preserve collateral circulation to the spinal cord near the neuroforamen. Subperiosteal dissection is undertaken overlying the intervertebral disks proceeding along to the midvertebral bodies, where the segmental vessels are found, exposed, and ligated, as needed. The sympathetic trunk is retracted laterally and protected during exposure of the spine toward the transverse process. The psoas muscle is detached from vertebra and retracted to expose laterally along the vertebral body and toward the neuroforamen.

D   Wound Closure

The area of dissection overlying the anterior thoracolumbar spine is inspected. Adequate hemostasis is maintained. Internal fixation and bone graft are positioned without pressure on the aorta. Insertion of absorbable hemostatic sponges or other hemostatic agents near the spinal canal is avoided, as swelling and expansion can cause pressure and injury to the spinal cord. In general, the anterior spinal and retroperitoneal areas lack adequate tissues or periosteum for any closure.

The diaphragm is repaired. The medial left crus is repaired back to its insertion on the anterior L1, L2, and L3 vertebral bodies. The diaphragm is then sutured back to its peripheral rim anterior to the medial and lateral arcuate ligaments. Previously placed marking sutures aid in anatomical alignment. The peritoneum is repaired of any breeches in this layer and laid back into position with removal of packing sponges and retractors. Sponges are counted as the retroperitoneal space is allowed to close. A retroperitoneal drain is placed, if desired.

Retractors are removed from the chest portion as well. The small section of costal cartilage remaining from the twelfth rib can serve as a marker for reattachment of the external oblique to the costal chondral junction. A pleural drain or chest tube is required for the transthoracic segment of the incision. This is placed out through the skin for suction and drainage postoperatively to avoid hemothorax, pneumothorax, or pleural effusion as the wound is healing. Purse-string sutures may be placed through the skin around the exiting chest tubes for later closure. The chest tubes are also secured to the skin. Packing sponges are removed and counted. The lung is reinflated with three or four forced inspirations to eliminate areas of atelectasis.

The pleural layer and intercostal muscle layers are repaired with watertight closure. Table positioning angled toward the incision can aid in closing the wound. The neurovascular bundle of the excised rib is avoided during suturing. The muscle layer along the chest region includes closure of the serratus anterior and latissimus muscles.

The abdominal region is closed with a repair of the transversalis fascia. The muscle layers of the transverses abdominus, internal abdominal oblique, external abdominal oblique, and latissimus are repaired. The subcutaneous tissue and skin are closed in routine fashion.

Chest tube management is performed in routine fashion with suction for several days until clamping of suction confirms adequate seal of the pleural incision and drainage has decreased to 100 cc or less per 24 h. Pleural drains are removed with tying of previously placed purse-string sutures and placement of an airtight occlusive dressing. Postoperative incentive spirometry, coughing, and deep breathing is required of the patient.

III   RETROPERITONEAL EXPOSURE

The anterior retroperitoneal approach exposes the lumbar spine through to the first sacral vertebra (Table 3A, B). This approach uses the potential space anterior to the quadratus lumborum and psoas muscles and behind the peritoneum and renal fascia.

A   Positioning and Incision Placement

A left-sided approach is generally used (Fig. 4). This avoids retroperitoneal dissection around the overlying liver on the right side as well as dissection in proximity to the thin-walled inferior vena cava. The patient may be positioned supine for limited exposure and anterior interbody fixation or semilateral position lying on the right side midway between lateral and supine. Flexing the table in the semilateral position allows the body to flex away opening the space between the twelfth rib and the iliac

Table 3A Lateral Retroperitoneal Exposure of the Lumbar Spine

In lateral position, incision placed along left side in transverse fashion toward
  umbilicus.
Incision lies between twelfth rib and iliac crest, depending on level of desired
  exposure.
Latissimus, external, and internal obliques and transversus abdominus muscles are
  divided.
Transversalis fascia is divided, peritoneal layer exposed.
Peritoneum bluntly dissected away exposing the retroperitoneal space.
Lumbar arteries and veins ligated and divided, aorta retracted.
Psoas muscle elevated laterally, vertebral body exposed.

Table 3B Anterior Retroperitoneal Exposure of the Lumbosacral Spine

In a supine position, longitudinal incision is placed in midline of abdomen.
Anterior rectus sheath is incised, rectus muscle retracted toward midline.
Posterior rectus sheath and transversalis fascia is incised longitudinally.
Peritoneal layer bluntly dissected toward the midline and patient's right side.
Retroperitoneal space is developed laterally and posteriorly around the patient's left side.
Lumbar vessels are ligated and divided, aorta is retracted to right.
Vertebrae exposed and psoas muscle elevated away.

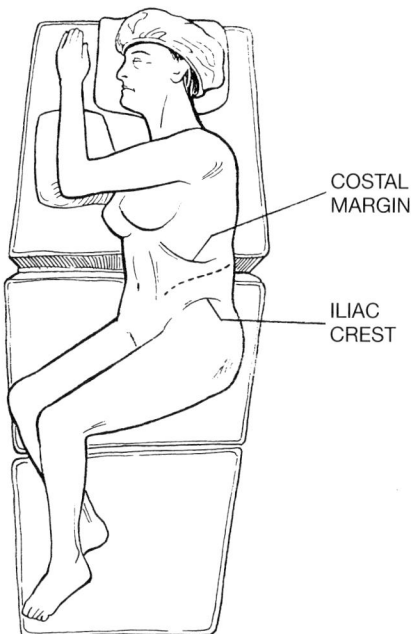

Figure 4 Retroperitoneal exposure: supine positioning with longitudinal incision or,
as shown, lateral position with incision along left side.

crest. Unbend the table when correcting spinal deformity. Flexing the hips will relax the psoas muscle for retraction away from the spine.

Incision placement depends on the level of access desired. For a direct anterior approach, the incision is orientated in a longitudinal fashion slightly to the left of the midline. L1 exposure generally involves an incision above the umbilicus. L2 and L3 are at the level of the umbilicus and slightly below. Exposure of levels L4 and L5 generally lie below the umbilicus. An incision for exposure to S1 extends close to the pubis. A variation of this approach includes a cosmetic Pfannenstiel incision, transversely above the pubic symphysis, which affords a limited exposure to L5–S1 exposure.

The classic incision lies transversely from the left side toward the midline. It begins at or below the twelfth rib on the patient's left side and proceeds transversely or obliquely to the anterior abdomen. The obliquity of the incision depends on the level of the spine requiring exposure. Incisions for the upper lumbar spine begin at or just below the twelfth rib and proceed transversely around to the anterior abdomen above the level of the umbilicus. Exposure of the lower lumbar spine is suited by an incision beginning below the costal margin or midway between the twelfth rib and the iliac crest on the left and sloping obliquely and anteriorly below the umbilicus. An extended exposure of the entire lumbar spine should begin over the twelfth rib on the left and course obliquely over the abdomen below the umbilicus.

B   Superficial Dissection

For the anterior midline approach, a longitudinal incision is made through the skin and subcutaneous tissues. Control bleeding and coagulate as needed branches of the paraumbilical veins and superficial epigastric artery and veins. Small anterior cutaneous branches of the intercostal nerve are also encountered. Divide the anterior layer of the rectus sheath, which is the first fascial layer, encountered. Bluntly dissect around the lateral border of the rectus abdominus muscle. The inferior epigastric artery and vein arises laterally deep and inferior to the arcuate line and runs longitudinally behind and within the rectus muscle. It may be necessary to proceed medial to the rectus muscle if the exposure involves a more caudal incision to avoid the inferior epigastric vessels.

Behind the rectus muscle, a second fascial layer is encountered which is the posterior rectus sheath. The posterior rectus sheath extends down to the arcuate line. Beneath the posterior rectus sheath is a layer of transversalis fascia. Below the arcuate line, the transversalis fascia is encountered without an overlying posterior rectus sheath layer of fascia. Below this layer is the peritoneum. The delicate peritoneal layer is bluntly dissected away from the fascial layer above. Proceed around to the left exposing the potential retroperitoneal space.

A classic incision begins on the left side. The oblique incision crosses through the thoracoepigastric vein and branches of the deep circumflex iliac artery in the region of midaxillary line. Small lateral cutaneous branches of the intercostal nerve are encountered. The muscle layer is divided through the lateral edge of the latissimus muscle and transversely through the external abdominal oblique, internal abdominal oblique, and transverses abdominis muscles. Anteriorly the field of dissection extends to the lateral border of the rectus muscle. Below the muscle layer, divide the transversalis fascia. The next layer is the peritoneum and extraperitoneal areolar tissue. Bluntly develop the retroperitoneal space around posteriorly. Repair any violations of the peritoneum. Pack away the peritoneum protecting it with a lap pad. Insert a rib-spreading or Finochietto retractor and Deaver retractors.

C Deep Dissection

The retroperitoneal space is developed bluntly by dissecting the peritoneum around exposing the psoas muscle and anterior lumbar spine (Figs. 5 and 6). The ureter traverses the field of dissection lying atop the psoas muscle. The ureter is occasionally confirmed with gentle pressure producing peristaltic contraction. Other important structures include the genitofemoral nerve coming through and overlying the psoas muscle and the sympathetic trunk lateral to the vertebral body.

The lumbar arteries branch out from the aorta at each vertebral level transversely crossing the middle of the vertebral body at each level. These are ligated and divided at each level necessary for mobilization of the aorta. This may require division of lumbar arteries one or two levels above and below the instrumented vertebral levels. These vessels are best divided closer to the aorta to preserve col-

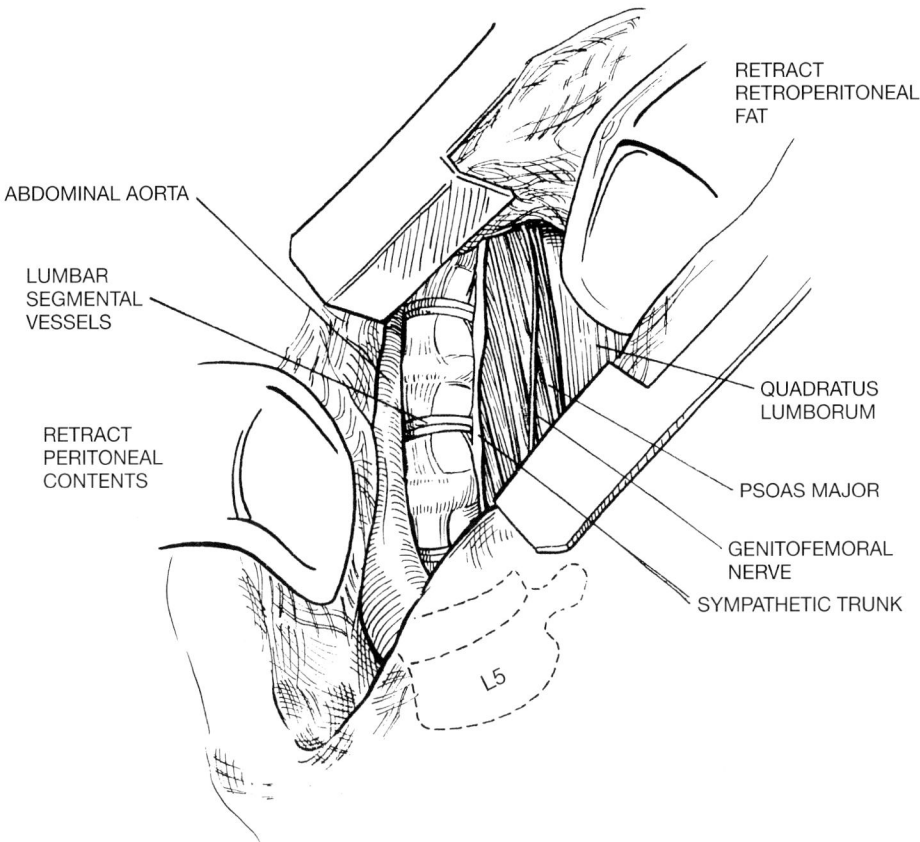

Figure 5 Retroperitoneal exposure: deep dissection with division of lumbar arteries and veins, aorta, and psoas muscle retracted, lumbar spine exposed.

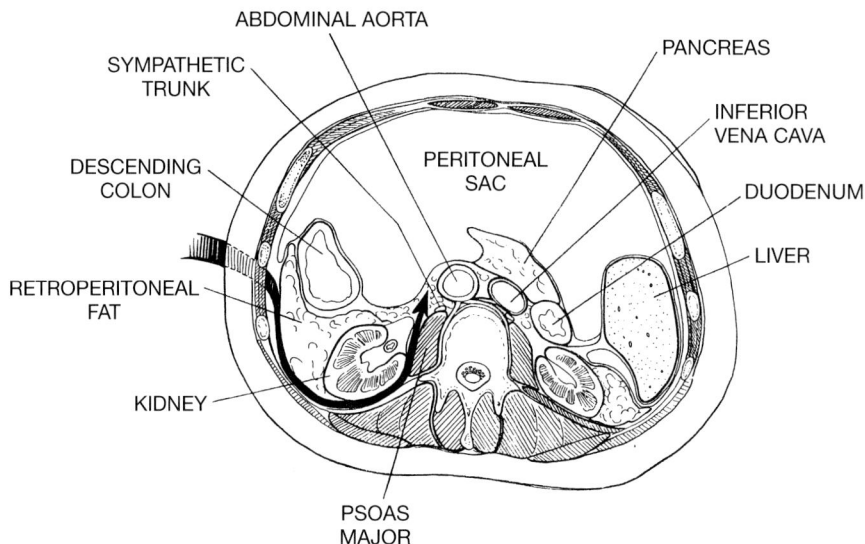

Figure 6 Retroperitoneal exposure: cross-sectional view of retroperitoneal path of dissection.

lateral sources of circulation among branches closer to the neuroforamen. Corresponding lumbar veins are similarly divided. Note that there is also an ascending lumbar vein running longitudinally and parallel to the aorta and vena cava interconnecting the lumbar veins at each level. Branches of the aorta in the region of the lumbar spine from proximal to distal include the inferior phrenic arteries below the diaphragm, the celiac trunk, superior mesenteric artery, superior, middle, inferior suprarenal arteries, bilateral renal arteries, bilateral testicular or ovarian arteries, inferior mesenteric artery. Lumbar arteries arise posteriorly at each vertebral level from level 1 through 4 of the lumbar spine. The aorta bifurcates into the common iliac arteries in the vicinity of the L4 vertebra. The middle sacral artery arises within the bifurcation traversing distally along the L5 vertebra and sacrum. The exact level of bifurcation varies, as does the fifth lumbar artery, which may arise from the middle sacral artery. Further anatomical description of this region is noted in the transperitoneal approach in this chapter.

Exposure of the spine is accomplished after mobilization and protection of the aorta and inferior vena cava. Subperiosteal dissection and elevation of the psoas muscle exposes the lateral aspect of the vertebra and the neuroforamen. This region requires attention to and protection of the sympathetic trunk, lumbar nerve roots, and lumbosacral trunks. The lumbar spine is now exposed for appropriate spinal procedures.

D   Wound Closure

Wound closure is accomplished with adequate hemostasis. Internal fixation is positioned such that excessive pressure against arterial or venous structures is prevented. Avoid pressure that may impede circulation or cause cumulative trauma with arterial pulsations with possible bleeding or pseudoaneurysm formation. Allow the vessels to gently lie back in their anatomical position. Deep posterior structures and peri-osteum generally do not require any suturing. The peritoneum is allowed to fall back into place with removal of packing. Account for all sponges and lap pads placed within the wound at this point. A retroperitoneal drain may be placed, if desired. Allow the drain to be brought through the skin adjacent to the incision. Violations of the peritoneum in any area are repaired with suture.

Fascial layers are now repaired. The transversalis fascia and rectus sheath are closed with running suture for midline approaches. The layers of the transversus abdominis, internal abdominal oblique, external abdominal oblique, and latissimus muscles are repaired for the classic oblique incision. The subcutaneous layer and skin are closed in routine fashion.

IV TRANSPERITONEAL EXPOSURE

An alternate exposure to the anterior lumbar spine involves a transperitoneal ap-proach (Table 4). The transperitoneal exposure is essentially a laparotomy. This ap-proach offers a direct anterior exposure to the lumbar spine.

A Positioning and Incision Placement

The patient is positioned supine. Slight flexion of the hips removes tension from the psoas muscle, which may aid in exposure during spinal dissection. A towel roll below the lumbar spine may be used to place the lumbar spine in a lordotic position for arthrodesis, if needed.

A midline incision as in a laparotomy is used. The umbilicus corresponds with approximately the L3 vertebra. The length of the incision above and below the umbilicus varies according to the lumbar levels needed to expose. Alternatively, a cosmetic low transverse or Pfannenstiel incision can be used for exposure below the L4 level.

B Superficial Dissection

A longitudinal incision is made through the skin and subcutaneous tissue around the umbilicus down to the fascial layer of the anterior rectus sheath. The subcutaneous layer contains a rich supply of venous branches from the paraumbilical and super-

Table 4 Transperitoneal Exposure of the Lumbar Spine

In a supine position, longitudinal incision is placed in midline of abdomen.
Alternatively low transverse incision is placed above the pubis.
Anterior and posterior rectus sheath are incised through midline linea alba.
Transversalis fascia and peritoneum are incised.
Greater omentum and bowels are packed to the right side of abdomen.
Posterior peritoneum is incised and prevertebral tissues spread.
For L5–S1, nerve plexus is bluntly spread in the aortic bifurcation.
Middle sacral artery and veins are ligated in area of bifurcation.
Left common iliac vein is retracted and L5–S1 vertebrae and disk
    exposed.

ficial epigastric veins. A low transverse incision through the skin and subcutaneous tissue also proceeds to the fascial layer at which time the fascial layer can be divided in a longitudinal direction along the midline. Continuing in a transverse direction with a Pfannenstiel incision would require entering the rectus sheath and dividing the rectus muscle transversely. The transverse fascial approach would also encounter the inferior epigastric vessels along the right and left sides of the incision. A transverse fascial incision would avoid this and is further described.

The fascial incision is placed in the midline through the linea alba. The anterior and posterior rectus sheath is confluent in one layer here. Below this layer lies the transversalis fascia and peritoneum. A longitudinal incision is made through these layers, allowing entry into the peritoneal cavity. Care is taken to protect underlying bowel and abdominal contents during incision.

The greater omentum and underlying small intestines are encountered within the abdomen. The peritoneal contents are carefully packed away to the right side of the abdomen protecting the intestines with sponges. The field is now prepared for deep dissection into the retroperitoneal space.

C   Deep Dissection

The posterior peritoneum layer overlying the aorta and aortic bifurcation is identified (Fig. 7). Exposure of the upper lumbar spine through this approach can be difficult because of the retroperitoneal nature of the pancreas and duodenum crossing the field transversely. The posterior peritoneal layer is carefully incised to enter the retroperitoneal area.

Exposure of the anterior lumbar spine is performed meticulously and carefully with ligation of small vessels, including lumbar arteries and veins as described above in the retroperitoneal approach. The arterial branches from the aorta are also noted

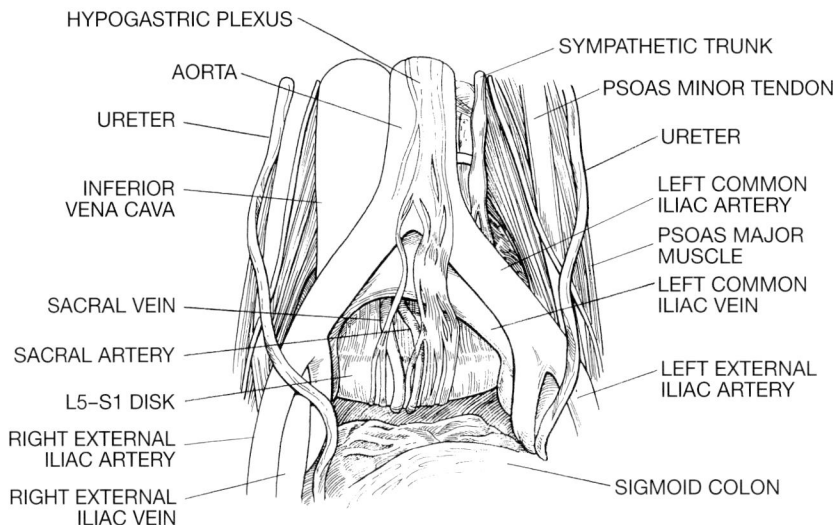

Figure 7   Transperitoneal exposure: deep dissection with lumbosacral spine exposure within common iliac bifurcation of aorta and vena cava.

above. The transperitoneal exposure generally proceeds toward the left side of the spinal column. Approaching the spine to the left side allows dissection around the aorta. This avoids dissection around the thin-walled inferior vena cava, which may bleed more easily and is more difficult to repair than the aorta. The area within the aortic bifurcation is described in further detail.

The area between the bifurcation of the great vessels is commonly used to approach the L5 vertebral body, L5–S1 intervertebral disk, and sacrum. The aorta and inferior vena cava bifurcate in the vicinity of the fourth lumbar vertebra. Recent studies have documented anatomical variations in this region. Reviews of series of angiograms and venograms have shown that approximately 14% of patients have a bifurcation of the aorta at the L3 level, 48% at the L4 level, and 38% at the L5 level. The inferior vena cava was shown to bifurcate with the left iliac vein overlying L5 in 86% of patients and overlying L4 in the remainder (2). Anatomical studies of magnetic resonance images have shown that iliac vein is overlying the L5–S1 intervertebral disk in approximately 18% of patients studied (3). Within the tissues of the retroperitoneum overlying this region is the superior hypogastric nerve plexus. This plexus supplies sympathetic function to the urogenital region. Blunt dissection of this area is recommended. In males, retrograde ejaculation has been reported and attributed to injury of this plexus of fine nerves (4).

Lateral to the bifurcation, the ureter and superior rectal vessels cross the field atop the iliac vessels closer to the bifurcation of the internal and external iliac vessels. Bluntly dissect through the prevertebral tissue. The middle sacral artery and vein lie between the common iliac vessels. There may be multiple vessels in common, particularly veins. Ligate or coagulate these vessels. The anterior spine at the lumbosacral junction may now be exposed. Further vessel mobilization and retraction may be necessary, according to the anatomical variation as noted above.

D Wound Closure

The main aspect of wound closure of the deep area of dissection is hemostasis. In most instances, there is no remaining posterior peritoneal layer to close. In addition, suturing the perivascular tissues together may risk further bleeding. The retroperitoneal space can be sutured closed if there is an easily identifiable peritoneal layer that can be closed without excessive tension. Otherwise, the deep posterior peritoneal layer will reform along with wound healing. Again, inspect any internal fixation or structural bone grafts to assure that there is no pressure on surrounding structures.

Sponges used for packing are removed and counted. Intra-abdominal contents are allowed to fall loosely back into their anatomical position with the greater omentum over the top. The anterior peritoneal layer is closed. The transversalis fascia and rectus abdominus sheath are closed in the midline. Subcutaneous tissue and skin are closed in routine fashion.

V ANTERIOR CERVICOTHORACIC EXPOSURE

The great vessels and the heart overlie the anterior cervicothoracic spine (Table 5A, B). At this junction, the lordotic cervical spine transitions into a kyphotic thoracic spine. This creates an anterior-to-posterior depth of dissection well beyond that of the lower cervical spine approach. Because of these challenges, several variations

Table 5A   Anterior Exposure of the Cervicothoracic Spine

In supine position, incision placed longitudinally on the left side.
It begins along border of sternomastoid and is continued over the sternum.
Platysma is divided, plane developed lateral to trachea, medial to sternomastoid.
Carotid sheath protected laterally, esophagus medially.
Partial or complete sternotomy performed.
Sternohyoid and sternothyroid muscles detached and sternum retracted.
Inferior and middle thyroid vessels ligated and divided.
Vertebral levels confirmed on radiograph with needle marker.
Longus colli muscle elevated and retractors placed.
Left brachiocephalic vein ligated and divided for caudal exposure beyond T2.
Vertebrae and disks exposed.

exist to the approach and exposure of the anterior cervicothoracic spine. These variations in technique can be divided into two major approaches. The cervicothoracic junction can be approached from an anterior direction above the clavicle, through the clavicle, or through the sternum via an anterior thoracotomy. This region can also be approached from an anterolateral direction through a high lateral transthoracic dissection or lateral thoracotomy. The surgical approach to this region will be discussed from these two perspectives.

A   Positioning and Incision Placement

1   Direct Anterior

Positioning for exposure of the cervicothoracic junction depends on the approach chosen. For a direct anterior approach through the clavicle or sternum, the patient is positioned supine (Fig. 8). A left-sided dissection allows greater access around the great vessels and avoidance of the recurrent laryngeal nerve. The recurrent laryngeal nerves pass under the arch of the aorta on the left side but under the subclavian artery on the right side. This allows the left recurrent laryngeal nerve to ascend in the tracheal esophageal groove at a more caudal level away from the field of dissection. The head is thus turned slightly to the right with the neck positioned in moderate extension, if not contraindicated. A soft bump or towel roll between the

Table 5B   Transthoracic Exposure of the
Cervicothoracic Spine

In lateral position, periscapular incision placed on left side.
Latissimus and trapezius muscles are divided, scapula is elevated.
Periosteum of second or third rib is incised and stripped.
Rib is removed, pleura incised, and ribs spread.
Lung is deflated and packed with sponge.
Segmental intercostal vessels are ligated.
Great vessels, esophagus, and trachea retracted toward midline.
Vertebrae of cervicothoracic spine exposed.

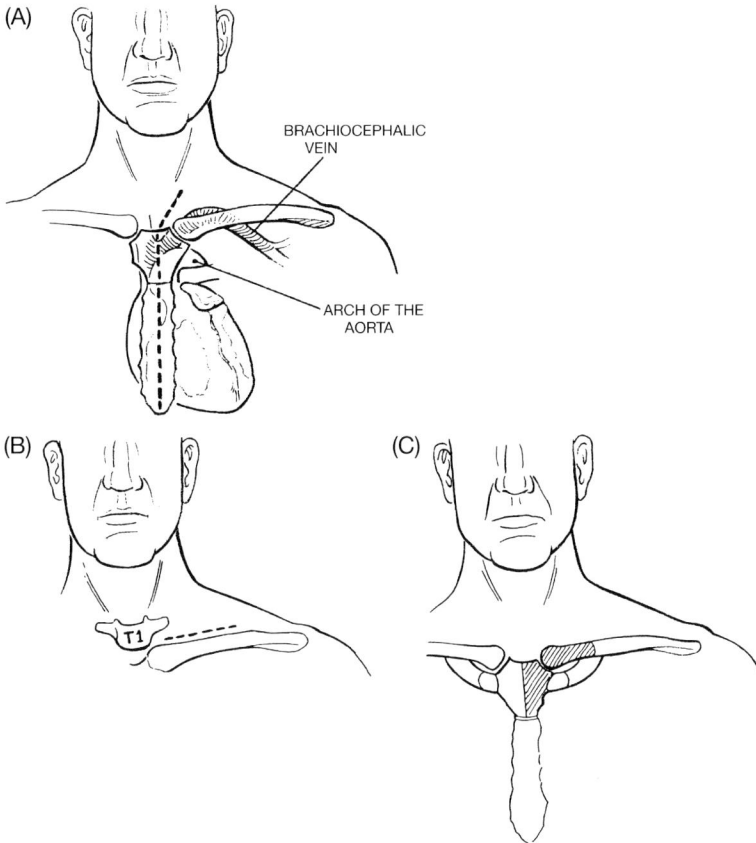

Figure 8 Anterior cervicothoracic exposure: supine positioning with anterior incision for (A) transsternal approach. (B) Low anterior cervical approach to the cervicothoracic junction-supraclavicular. (C) Low anterior cervical approach to the cervicothoracic junction via partial claviculotomy and sternotomy allowing access to T1 to T3.

shoulder blades under the thoracic spine aids in positioning the cervical spine in the desired amount of extension.

The anterior cervical incision is placed longitudinally along the medial border of the left sternocleidomastoid muscle for a low anterior cervical approach. In most patients, this will allow adequate exposure through to the cephalad aspects of the T1 vertebra. Beyond this region, it may be necessary to extend the incision over the clavicle, sternoclavicular joint, or curved down along the midline over the top of the sternum. This will depend on the chosen access route for the upper thoracic spine. An esophageal tube can be placed for later palpation and identification of landmarks intraoperatively.

2 Lateral Thoracotomy

The transthoracic approach requires a lateral position with the patient's arm extended forward at the shoulder, supported under the forearm (Fig. 9). The head needs to be

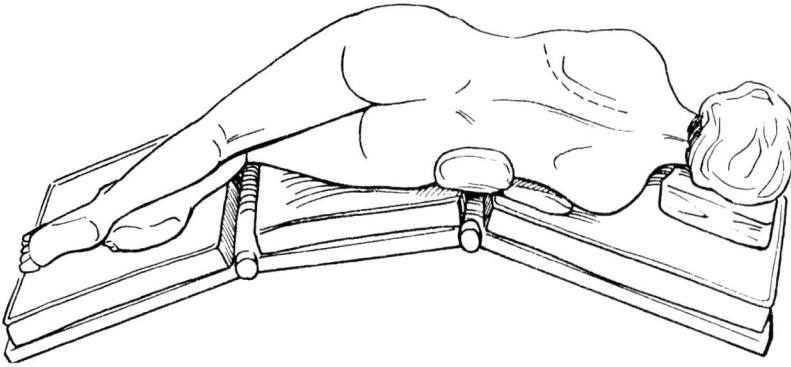

Figure 9 Lateral cervicothoracic exposure: positioning with left lateral periscapular incision for high transthoracic approach.

supported with padding and avoidance of tilt causing stretch to the nerve roots of the left side of the cervical spine. Axillary padding is placed under the right side. Flexing the table away from the side of the incision will open the rib cage on the side of dissection. The undersurface of the right waist and iliac crest is also appropriately padded. A bifurcated endotracheal tube is used for selective left lung deflation later in the procedure.

The transthoracic incision begins posteriorly behind the scapula and runs parallel to the medial border of the scapula. It continues around the tip of the scapula and curves anteriorly toward the anterior chest approximately at the level of the nipple. This will allow access under the scapula to the upper ribs. A left-sided approach is preferred as the mobilization and retraction of the aorta are easier and safer than a right-sided approach involving dissection in the region of the thinner-walled superior vena cava. Also, the left side of the heart is more mobile and can be displaced anteriorly in contrast to right side of the heart with superior and inferior vena caval attachments.

B Superficial Dissection

1 Direct Anterior

The incision for the anterior approach to the cervicothoracic spine is carried through the skin and subcutaneous tissues. Small sensory branches of the transverse cervical nerves and supraclavicular nerves may be found overlying the platysma and underneath overlying the cervical fascia. The incision is deepened dividing the platysma muscle and proceeding distally toward the jugular notch of the sternum. Small venous branches lying underneath the platysma are coagulated. The incision is deepened to the periosteum and extended distally as far as the planned incision. For access caudally to T1, the incision may not require incising the manubrium. For access to T3 and cephalad T4, the incision will require osteotomy of the manubrium and sternum.

The anterior border of the sternocleidomastoid muscle is identified. The external jugular vein lies lateral to the field of dissection; however, branches including the communicating vein and anterior jugular vein lie parallel to the sternocleidomastoid muscle and sternohyoid muscle, respectively. The interval between the sternocleidomastoid muscle and the trachea is identified. The cervical fascia is divided longitudinally in this area. A plane of dissection is developed in this interval with blunt instrument or fingertip spreading. The carotid sheath containing the vagus nerve, internal jugular vein, and carotid artery is protected behind the sternocleidomastoid muscle. The pulse can be palpated for identification. The trachea, larynx, and underlying esophagus are retracted toward the midline. Palpation of the nasogastric tube helps identify the esophagus. The interval is developed medial to the muscle bellies of the omohyoid. The strap muscles beneath the sternocleidomastoid include the sternohyoid and sternothyroid. Exposure with sternotomy requires release of the strap muscles from the manubrium; this allows retraction of the bone as the strap muscles are generally left to the medial side while the trachea and esophagus, the sternocleidomastoid, and the omohyoid muscles are dissected laterally.

The sternum is now exposed subperiosteally. Osteotomy of the sternum is performed with an oscillating saw taking care not to injure underlying vascular structures. A Gigli saw may also be used passing it underneath the sternum after reflecting away the parietal pleura off the undersurface. Complete median sternotomy is performed (5). Coating the bone edges with bone wax will decrease blood loss. The peritoneal cavity is located close to the tip of the xiphoid process. A complete sternotomy incision will need to avoid breeching this area.

A modified approach, which allows similar access to the cervicothoracic junction, involves partial median sternotomy (6). The sternum is divided through the manubrium to the second intercostal space. It is then divided to the left below the second rib or through the synostosis between the manubrium and body of the sternum.

The proximal and distal areas of dissection are now connected with division of the sternohyoid and thyrohyoid muscles. They are divided through their tendinous insertion on the underside of the manubrium for later repair. The sternocleidomastoid muscle may be left attached. The manubrium along with the clavicle and first and second ribs may now be retracted up and a chest or rib retractor inserted. Deep dissection is now undertaken.

Variations to this approach include an incision placed lateral to the midline overlying the sternoclavicular joint or clavicle on the left side. (7). In these approaches, the dissection varies in that the plane proceeds laterally to the sternohyoid and sternothyroid muscles but medial to the omohyoid and sternocleidomastoid muscles. The caudal dissection requires disarticulation of the sternoclavicular joint or osteotomy of the clavicle (7). These approaches can be associated with postoperative sternoclavicular joint instability and clavicular nonunion, respectively. Another disadvantage to approaches through the sternoclavicular joint or clavicle is that the first and second ribs remain attached to the sternum. The first and second ribs traverse the caudal area of dissection and may limit access to the thoracic spine beyond the T2 vertebra. If either of these approaches is used, the clavicle is retracted laterally to the field of dissection through the sternoclavicular joint or through the osteotomy site. The deep dissection is similar to that of the sternotomy approach described below.

2 Lateral Thoracotomy

For the lateral thoracotomy approach, the incision begins about one or two fingerbreadths medial to midscapula (Fig. 10). The incision follows along parallel to the

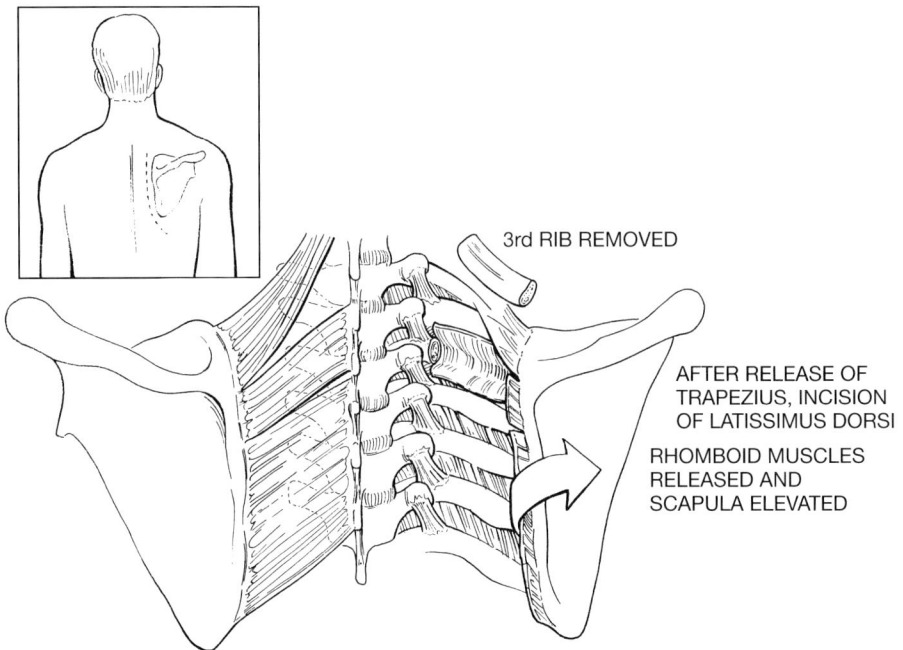

Figure 10 Lateral cervicothoracic exposure: superficial dissection with division of the latissimus and trapezius muscles, elevation of scapula, exposure and excision of third rib. Pleura in rib bed is incised and ribs are spread.

medial border and around the angle of the scapula, leaving a border for reattachment. The incision ends anteriorly at the level of the nipple line, stopping at the border of the pectoralis major. The incision proceeds through the skin and subcutaneous tissue encountering and cauterizing the lateral thoracic vein in the subcutaneous layer along the midaxillary line. Next encountered is the muscle layer. The long thoracic nerve and lateral thoracic artery are protected in the midaxillary line over the top of the serratus anterior and proceeding distally under the latissimus muscle. Small, medial cutaneous branches of the dorsal ramus of the thoracic spinal nerves may be encountered overlying the trapezius.

The dissection mobilizes the scapula for upward retraction by incising through the first muscle layer of the inferior trapezius. The underlying spinal accessory nerve is avoided as it descends out of the base of the skull innervating the trapezius along the undersurface. The incision is carried around anteriorly through part of the latissimus muscle. The next muscle layer consists of the rhomboid major along the medial border of the scapula. The inferior part of this muscle is incised along the scapular border. The rhomboid minor above may be left intact with sufficient scapular mobilization. The lower part of the serratus anterior around the angle of the scapula is also incised. The scapula can now be elevated superiorly out of the way.

Lateral thoracotomy to access the cervicothoracic junction requires excision and access through the bed of one of the upper three ribs. An approach through the bed of the first rib may be used for limited exposure to the upper thoracic spine. Generally the second or third rib is chosen. With increased kyphosis and depth of the wound overlying the thoracic spine, the third rib will permit greater access to the upper thoracic spine. This allows exposure of approximately C6 through T4 vertebrae.

The serratus anterior muscle attachment is subperiosteally elevated from the selected rib carefully protecting the overlying long thoracic nerve and, if needed, ligating the lateral thoracic artery. The periosteum of the selected rib is incised and elevated. The periosteum along the upper border of the rib is detached along with the intercostal muscle. The intercostal nerve, artery, and vein beneath the rib are protected during rib stripping. The intercostal muscles, external, internal, and innermost, are detached with subperiosteal stripping around posteriorly to the region of the paraspinal muscles. The rib section from costochondral junction to the border of the paraspinal muscles is cut and removed from its bed.

The periosteum and parietal pleura are now exposed in the bed of the excised rib. It is divided with attention to the underlying lung. Rib-spreading retraction can now be done. The left lung is deflated with a bifurcated endotracheal tube and packed away from the field of dissection with sponges. The deep dissection of the anterior spine below the parietal pleura can now be undertaken. A retropleural dissection has also been described. This involves blunt dissection of the parietal pleura away from the intercostal muscle layer and often requires resection of the rib more posteriorly to continue the plane of dissection posteriorly.

C Deep Dissection

1 Direct Anterior

Exposure of the anterior cervicothoracic spine involves deep dissection over lower cervical spine and upper thoracic spine. The lower cervical spine is exposed through the interval between the trachea and esophagus medially and the sternocleidomastoid muscle and carotid sheath laterally. This part of the dissection is essentially the approach of Robinson and Smith (8,9). The upper thoracic spine is exposed by careful dissection through the mediastinum and ligation of the left brachiocephalic vein. These two dissections will be joined to expose both the cervical and upper thoracic spine.

In the cervical dissection, the trachea is retracted toward the midline with the underlying esophagus. Blunt hand-held retractors are used while the plane is developed. The esophagus is confirmed by palpation of the esophageal tube within its muscular walls. The inferior thyroid artery and vein are ligated. The middle thyroid vein and accompanying artery may also need to be ligated as the midline structures are mobilized. The left recurrent laryngeal nerve is avoided and protected. It lies in the interval between the esophagus and trachea after ascending from underneath the arch of the aorta.

The caudal aspect of the dissection overlying the upper thoracic spine is developed. Blunt dissection of the mediastinum reveals the left brachiocephalic vein underneath the left side of the thymus. The left brachiocephalic vein lies anatomically at approximately the T1–T2 vertebral levels. This was noted in approximately 80% of the cases in one anatomical study (10). The arch of the aorta lies at approximately the T2–T3 vertebral levels as noted in 90% of cases studied (10). Retraction of the left brachiocephalic vein may be done safely to about the level of T2. Beyond this area, it may be necessary to ligate the left brachiocephalic vein to avoid excessive pressure with rupture of the vein (7). This will permit exposure to T3–T4 vertebral level. Also ligate and divide thymic branches as needed. Ligation of the left brachiocephalic vein may cause some postoperative swelling or venous congestion in the left arm. However, this has been noted to cause little morbidity (6).

The thoracic duct is protected within the deep field of dissection. It ascends along the anterior spine and enters the venous system on the left side between the subclavian and internal jugular veins in the region of C7 to T2 vertebra. Thoracic duct injury may cause a chylothorax postoperatively. The vertebral artery is another important structure located within the field of deep dissection. It lies lateral to the lower cervical spine. The vertebral artery most commonly enters the transverse foramen at the C6 vertebra. The vertebral artery lies anterior to the transverse process of the C7 vertebra.

With exposure to this level, the prevertebral fascia can be identified. The anterior vertebral bodies and endplate ridges can be identified with palpation. A localizing radiograph may be performed to confirm vertebral levels. The prevertebral fascia is incised longitudinally and elevated. The longus colli muscle is identified on either side of the spine inserting into each vertebra caudally to the T3 vertebral level. The longus colli muscle is elevated subperiosteally. Self-retaining retractors may be inserted under the edges of the longus colli muscle in the proximal part of the incision. Distally the arch of the aorta is protected and carefully retracted, as needed. The cervical sympathetic trunk and ganglia lies atop of the longus colli muscle lateral to spine. The stellate ganglion is located at the level of the T1 vertebra. Injury to the sympathetic nerves may result in left facial anhydrosis, ptosis, and meiosis of Horner's syndrome.

An extended exposure cephalad up to the level of C3 vertebra and caudal to about the level of T4 vertebra can be accomplished with this approach. Once adequate exposure of the necessary spinal segments has been obtained for the cervical and thoracic spine, the appropriate spinal procedure can be undertaken with protection of surrounding vital structures. Note that anatomical variation also exists as to the exact location of these structures.

2 Lateral Thoracotomy

Deep dissection of the lateral thoracotomy approach proceeds by reflecting away the parietal pleura. The left sympathetic trunk is also found parallel to the spine. The stellate ganglion lies in the vicinity of the first rib. Injury to the sympathetic trunk or ganglia is avoided as this may produce a left-sided Horner's syndrome.

Segmental arteries and veins along the thoracic vertebra are ligated and divided to mobilize the great vessels. The first and second intercostal arteries originate off the highest intercostal artery, which is a branch of the costocervical trunk from the left subclavian artery. Likewise, the left brachiocephalic vein gives off a branch to the highest intercostal vein from which arises the first and second intercostal veins. Additional vascular structures include the accessory hemiazygos vein, which runs along longitudinally to the left side of the spine. The thoracic duct ascends anterior to the spine crossing over to the left to empty into the venous system at the junction of the left subclavian and internal jugular vein. Injury to the thoracic duct can result in chylothorax. Control of the segmental vessels above and below the spinal segment allows the vasculature to be mobilized to the right off the spine. The midline structures including trachea and esophagus are retracted toward the opposite side. The arch of the aorta lies at about T2–T3. The vertebral artery enters the transverse foramen at C6 in most cases.

In contrast to an anterior thoracotomy approach, this exposure allows greater access to the thoracic spine and less exposure of the lumber spine. The accessed vertebrae generally span C6 through T4. An extended approach caudal to T4 can be undertaken with an additional rib dissection. Reaching cephalad to C6 is much more difficult.

D Wound Closure

1 Direct Anterior

After completion of the appropriate spinal procedure, the wound is inspected for adequate hemostasis. Bone graft and internal fixation is positioned to avoid pressure on vascular or neurological structures. Hemostatic agents are avoided in the area of the spinal canal to prevent swelling, pressure, and potential neurological compromise. A drain is inserted in the prevertebral space to prevent postoperative hematoma formation. The drain exits through the dissected interval over the top of the sterno-cleidomastoid muscle. It is placed through the skin lateral to the incision avoiding the area of the external jugular vein. Airway obstruction or neurological compromise is avoided with evacuation of postoperative fluid accumulation.

Self-retaining retractors are removed. The trachea and esophagus medially and sternocleidomastoid muscle and carotid sheath laterally are allowed to fall back into position closing the dissected interval. The great vessels are inspected for hemostasis. The sternotomy or partial sternotomy, depending on the approach, is closed. Sternal wires are used to secure the bone edges together. If access was gained through disarticulation of the sternoclavicular joint or osteotomy of the clavicle, then these routes need to be repaired. The sternoclavicular joint should be repaired with a heavy nonabsorbable suture. Pin fixation is contraindicated in this area because of its proximity to the great vessels and the potential of pin migration. Clavicular osteotomy is best repaired with plate fixation. Chest-tube drainage may be needed in the case of significant dissection involving the pleural cavity.

The sternothyroid and sternohyoid muscles are repaired to their tendinous insertion on the underside of the manubrium. Next the platysma muscle is sutured back together. The subcutaneous layer and skin are closed in routine fashion. Postoperative chest radiographs are used to check for potential pneumothorax. Postoperative care with incentive spirometry, cough, and deep breathing are prescribed. Drains are maintained and removed when drain decreased to acceptable levels.

2 Lateral Thoracotomy

The lateral thoracotomy incision is closed after spinal stability and desired fixation are achieved. The periosteal layer usually does not remain for closure. The pleural layer is closed if limited dissection preserves an adequate layer for reapproximation. Adequate hemostasis is necessary. This precludes any hemostatic agents or other space-occupying substance in the vicinity of the spinal cord. Absorbable substances may swell or expand and create compression on adjacent neurological structures.

A chest tube is necessary to adequately drain fluid accumulation. The chest tube prevents effusion and pneumothoraces during pleural healing. The chest tube is sutured to the skin with an added purse string suture for site closure when the tube is discontinued. The lung is reinflated with forced inspiration after packing removal.

The adjacent ribs are held together with a rib approximator. Pleura and intercostal muscles are closed in a watertight repair. Circumferential absorbable sutures around the upper rib and lower rib may be used to reinforce the repair. The neurovascular bundle below the rib is avoided. The scapula is brought down and the serratus anterior and rhomboid muscles are repaired. The latissimus and trapezius muscles are repaired next. Subcutaneous tissue and skin are closed.

Chest-tube suction is required for a few days. When drainage decreases to less than 100 cc per 24 h, the tubes are removed. The purse-string sutures serve to close the chest-tube site. An occlusive dressing is placed. Incentive spirometry and standard respiratory care aid in recovery from thoracotomy.

REFERENCES

1. Winter RB, Lonstein JE, Denis F, Leonard AS, Garamella JJ. Paraplegia resulting from vessel ligation. Spine 1996; 21:1232.
2. Vraney RT, Phillips FM, Wetzel T, Brustein M. Peridiscal vascular anatomy of the lower lumbar spine. Spine 1999; 24:2183–2187.
3. Capellades J, Pellise F, Rovira A, Grive E, Pedraza S, Villanueva C. Magnetic resonance anatomic study of iliocava junction and left iliac vein positions related to L5–S1 disc. Spine 2000; 25:1695–1700.
4. Faciszewski T, Winter RB, Lonstein JE, Denis F, Johnson L. The surgical and medical perioperative complications of anterior spinal fusion surgery in the thoracic and lumbar spine in adults. Spine 1995; 20:1592–1599.
5. Sundaresan N, Shah J, Feghali JG. A transsternal approach to the upper thoracic vertebrae. Am J Surg 1984; 148:473–477.
6. Darling GE, McBroom R, Perrin R. Modified anterior approach to the cervicothoracic junction. Spine 1995; 20:1519–1521.
7. Calderone RR. Spine anatomy and surgical approaches. In: Capen DA, Haye W, eds. Management of Spine Trauma. Philadelphia: Mosby, 1998:6–32.
8. Robinson RA, Smith GW. Anterolateral cervical disc removal and interbody fusion for cervical disc syndrome. Bull Johns Hopkins Hosp 1955; 96:223–228.
9. Robinson RA, Southwick WO. Surgical approaches to the cervical spine. Am Acad Orthoped Surg Instruct Course Lect 1960; 17:299–330.
10. Xu R, Grabow R, Ebraheim NA, Durham SJ, Yeasting RA. Anatomic considerations of a modified anterior approach to the cervicothoracic junction. Am J Orthoped 2000; 29: 37–40.

40

Anterior Thoracotomy and Corpectomy for Treatment of an Unstable Burst Fracture

LOUIS G. QUARTARARO, JUSTIN P. KUBECK, and ALEXANDER R. VACCARO

Thomas Jefferson University Hospital and the Rothman Institute, Philadelphia, Pennsylvania, U.S.A.

JOHN J. CARBONE

Johns Hopkins Bayview Hospital, Baltimore, Maryland, U.S.A.

ARJUN SAXENA

Jefferson Medical College, Philadelphia, Pennsylvania, U.S.A.

Anterior transthoracic decompression and fusion may be used for the treatment of thoracic and thoracolumbar spine fractures (T2 to L1), either as a single operative procedure or in conjunction with a posterior stabilization procedure. It is often utilized in the acute setting of a two- or three-column thoracic spinal fracture in a patient with an incomplete spinal cord injury and documented canal occlusion on spinal imaging. It is less frequently utilized for the delayed treatment of certain injuries, including late post-traumatic deformities (1–12).

I ANTERIOR DECOMPRESSION AND FUSION

An anterior thoracic corpectomy and fusion with or without instrumentation is best suited for patients with significant neural compression in the setting of an incomplete neurological deficit, particularly if a minimal kyphotic deformity exists. The anterior approach allows optimal visualization of the anterior thecal sac at the completion of a corpectomy. With the use of anterior instrumentation, it is possible to rigidly maintain correction of deformity and potentially avoid the need for a posterior stabilization procedure.

II SURGICAL TECHNIQUE

The transthoracic approach for trauma was first described by Paul and colleagues (10,13); it detailed techniques, and long-term results of this treatment have been published by Bohlman and associates (4,14).

A Positioning

The patient may be intubated with a double-lumen tube, so that the left and right mainstem bronchi may be ventilated separately. This allows for later collapse of one lung to provide adequate exposure of the spine. Often, however, a single lumen tube is adequate, with the lung easily retracted or packed off with lap sponges. The patient is usually placed in the right lateral decubitus position. The left chest is often chosen as the side of operation, assuming there are no contraindications or exposure-related considerations.

The thoracic and abdominal aorta sit, in general, anterior and to the left of midline along the thoracic spine. Following mobilization of the aorta, the left-sided approach is more convenient, because of the rigidity and strength of the thoracic aorta for retractors versus the vena cava on the right side.

Special care should be taken to place a pad just distal to the patient's downside axilla in order to prevent a stretch palsy of the brachial plexus. Also, an arm support should be used to hold the upper arm in a neutral position: forward flexion of 90° at the shoulder, neutral abduction–adduction, and almost straight at the elbow. Both arms should be adequately protected and padded, especially in the regions of the radial nerve in the posterior upper arm and near the ulnar nerve at the elbow. Forward flexion of more than 90° at the shoulder should be avoided to minimize the risk of brachial plexus palsy. Tape can be securely placed across the patient, both at the level of the greater trochanter and across the shoulder, and affixed to the table. A beanbag placed under the patient is also useful to help maintain this position.

The patient's entire flank, anterior chest, and posterior torso should be prepared from just inferior to the level of the axilla to inferior to the lateral iliac crest. Care should be taken to prepare the skin to the midline anteriorly and beyond the midline posteriorly. This minimizes the chance of disorientation during the operation and also makes it possible to perform an anterior transthoracic decompression and fusion and a posterior instrumentation and fusion simultaneously, if necessary.

B Exposure

The first step in a transthoracic approach is selecting the appropriate level. A standard AP and lateral thoracic spine film, demonstrating all ribs, is absolutely necessary when counting ribs for appropriate incision level. The surgeon needs to know whether the 12th rib is a palpable full-length rib or a short, nonpalpable rib with the first palpable rib being the 11th rib.

1 Upper Thoracic Spine Exposure

From T6 through T10, the incision should be made directly over the rib with the same number as the fractured vertebra (Fig. 1), or one level proximal. It is technically

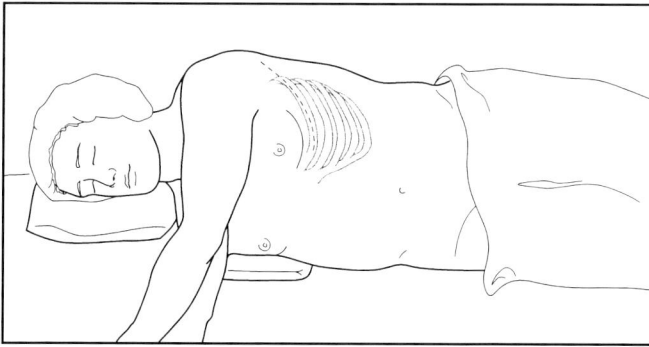

Figure 1   The patient is placed in a straight decubitus position with the shoulders extended forward 90 degrees, neutral in terms of abduction and adduction, with the elbows straight. A pad is placed under the downside axilla to protect the brachial plexus. The dotted line represents the starting incision over the rib that is at the same level or one level proximal to the fractured vertebrae.

easier to work distally than proximally. Removal of a rib one level higher works well, especially if the corpectomy involves more than one level. For fractures above T6, the skin incision should extend over the T6 rib anteriorly and laterally. Posteriorly, it should extend to the inferior tip of the scapula and then curve gently more cephalad, halfway between the medial border of the scapula and the midline spinous processes.

The incision should be made through the skin and subcutaneous tissues down to the deep fascia. From T6 through T10, the deep fascia and underlying muscles are incised in line with the skin incision down to the rib, which is stripped subperiosteally on both its outer and inner surfaces. The surgeon should be cautious concerning use of the electrocautery near the neurovascular bundle. A rib cutter is used to cut the rib at the costovertebral angle posteriorly and at the costochondral junction anteriorly. The remaining inner periosteum is then incised over the length of the rib bed. For T2–T5, it is important to note that the long thoracic nerve courses in the midaxillary line from the region of the axilla to its innervation of the serratus anterior muscle. Rather than cut this nerve and lose the innervation to the more caudal portion of the muscle, it is preferable to detach the serratus anterior muscle from the anterior chest wall and reflect it cephalad. This can be done to provide exposure up to the T3 rib, with additional exposure achieved by mobilization of the scapula. Division of the dorsal scapular muscles, rhomboids, and trapezius allows the scapula to be elevated and displaced laterally from the midline. This offers a simple method of gaining a more extensive thoracotomy through the bed of the third rib.

After the chest has been opened, the surgeon should place his or her hand in the chest in the midlateral line and count the cephalic and caudal ribs, because this is much more accurate than counting the ribs outside the chest wall. The surgeon should make certain that the rib removed is the rib that was planned for removal. The surgeon should also verify that the total number of ribs corresponds to that seen on a good-quality AP radiograph of the thoracic spine.

A self-retaining thoracotomy retractor is then inserted over moistened sponges in such a way that the neurovascular bundle of the cephalic rib and the neurovascular bundle from the removed rib are not compressed by the retractor. The chest retractor is opened slowly to minimize the chance of fracture of adjacent ribs. The lung is retracted with lap sponges and self-retaining retractors.

2 T10–L2 Exposure

When approaching the T10–T11 or T12 levels, the T10 rib should be dissected out. This is the last rib that is completely in the thoracic cavity. The T11 rib frequently has diaphragmatic insertions and requires more extensive takedown of the diaphragm, if this rib is resected.

The incision should be centered on the rib to be resected. Depending on the extensive nature of the surgery, the incision may need to be between 7 to 15 cm long. Using an electrocautery, the latissmus dorsi is split in a separate layer from the serratus. Finally the intercostal muscles are stripped off their insertion on the rib to be resected. The periosteum is then stripped off the rib with a Cobb elevator with care not to injure the underlying pleura.

For transthoracic retroperitoneal approaches, the retroperitoneal fat usually starts immediately at the tip of the 10th rib and can be swept anteriorly and inferiorly. The diaphragm is then incised along the thoracic wall, leaving a centimeter and a half of cuff tissue for later repair, especially the crus of the diaphram. Dissection is then taken back to the midbody of the L1 vertebral body, where it usually inserts. Significant caution should be exercised while elevating the diaphragmatic fibers from the L1 vertebral body, since they overlie the segmental vessels at the midportion of the body.

C Corpectomy

After the rib resection, the lung is generally packed superiorly with either lung retractors or moistened Lap sponges. The spine can be seen and palpated within the chest cavity. It is covered by the relatively thin and translucent parietal pleura. The rib base of the previously resected rib is traced down to its costovertebral junction. Remember that the rib inserts at the cephalic quarter of its own vertebra. This allows determination of the correct thoracic body to be removed. At this point, a spinal needle should be placed in a disk and a radiograph obtained to definitively identify levels.

The parietal pleural is then split at the midbody portion of the vertebral bodies and dissected free. The segmental vessels at the midbody of each thoracic body are then apparent. These segmentals can be tied off with 0-silk sutures and vascular clips. The vessels should be cut over the anterior third of the vertebral bodies so as not to interfere with collateral flow to the spinal cord, which enters the segmental vessels near the neuroforamen. Once the vessels are isolated and sectioned, the abdominal and thoracic aorta may be dissected off the spine by gentle bone dissection at the level of the disk spaces because of its avascular plane. Protective malleable retractors are placed between the spine and the aorta.

The disks above and below the vertebra to be resected can be removed with a scalpel, rongeurs, pituitaries, and currettes (Fig. 2). The vertebral body may then be removed with the use of a rongeur as well as gouges, osteotomes, and power burs

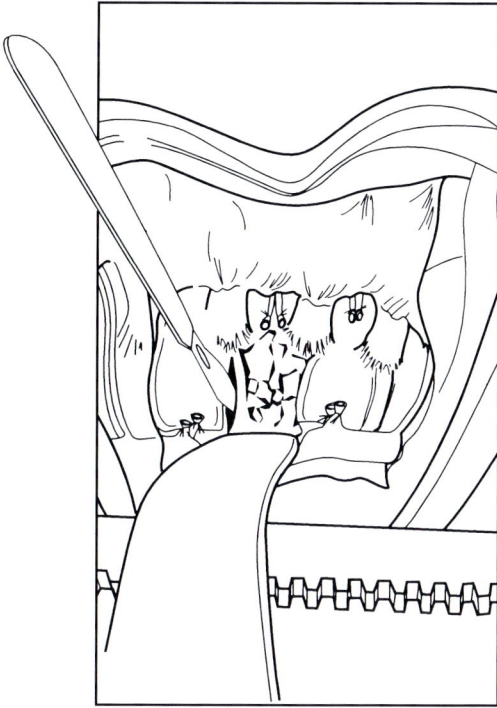

Figure 2   A scapel and rongeur are used to remove the disks above and below the level of the vertebral fracture.

(Fig. 3). Loupe magnification and a headlamp should be used for this procedure. In the case of an acute fracture with many loose pieces of bone, a large curette can be used to remove the bulk of the vertebral body. As the posterior margin of the vertebral body is approached, the red cancellous bone begins to be replaced by the white cortical bone, representing posterior cortex of the vertebral body. A high-speed bur may then be used to perforate the posterior cortex at the point of minimal neural compression (Fig. 4). Another technique to gain access to the spinal canal is to use a small Kerrison rongeur to enter through the adjacent disk space. Alternatively, one can begin by removing the pedicle and following the nerve root to the spinal cord. Once point of entry into the spinal canal has been made, the remainder of the posterior cortex of the vertebral body can be removed with appropriately shaped rongeurs and curettes (Figs. 5 and 6). This is often facilitated by the use of fine-angled curettes to allow the surgeon to push or pull the posterior cortex away from the spinal canal. This decompression should be performed from pedicle to pedicle to ensure that there is no residual spinal cord compression (Fig. 7). If the bone has been removed and the posterior longitudinal ligament does not bulge anteriorly, the ligament should be removed, while, at the same time, looking for other disk or bone fragments that may be causing continued compression of the dura. At the end of the decompression, the ligament or dura, or both, should be bulging anteriorly.

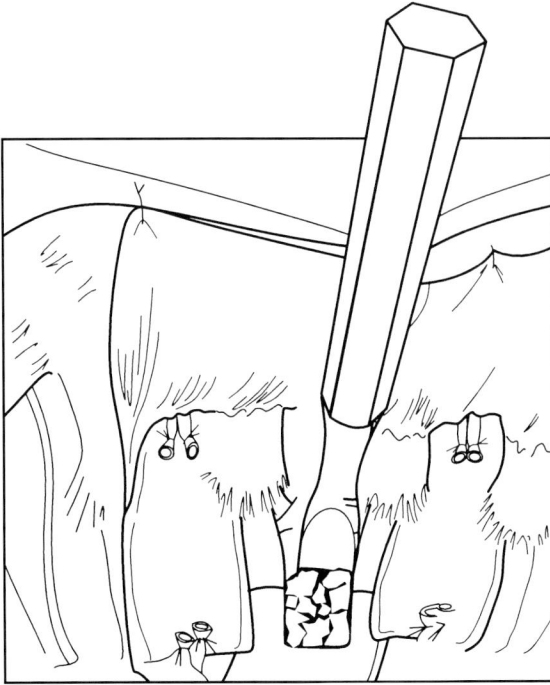

Figure 3 A chisel is utilized to excise the vertebral body back to its posterior cortex. During vertebral body resection, the chisel, osteotome, or gouge is held at a level perpendicular to the floor. Use of these instruments is limited to cancellous bone and should not be used once the cortex is encountered.

D Reconstruction

Choice of bone graft and technique vary from surgeon to surgeon. A trough may be cut into the vertebral bodies through the endplates above and below the area of decompression, or the endplates may be left largely intact, with just small burr holes drilled into them for the ingress of blood flow. Appropriate bone graft is then obtained for insertion across this level of decompression. The patient's tricortical iliac crest may be harvested. Another option, particularly if an injury is associated with minimal instability and the patient's rib is of adequate strength, is to impact three tiers of rib graft into this trough while an assistant pushes on the patient's gibbus to minimize the deformity. Alternatively, fresh frozen corticocancellous allograft (iliac crest or distal femur), or femoral or humeral shaft, can be used with good fusion success anteriorly. At the end of the decompression and bone grafting, there should be an adequate space between the neural elements and the bone graft, and there should be a posterior ridge on the vertebra both cephalad and caudad to the decompression to prevent migration of the bone graft toward the neural elements.

E Instrumentation Biomechanics

Gurr and colleagues (15) showed in an animal corpectomy model that the strength of the spine is markedly reduced after corpectomy in axial loading, flexion, and

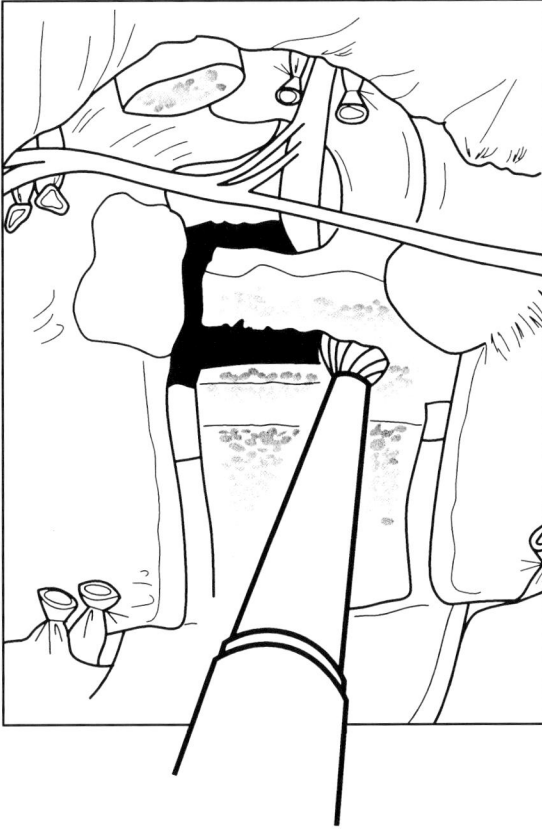

Figure 4 A high-speed burr can be used to perforate the posterior vertebral body cortex. A diamond-tipped burr can be utilized to minimize the chances of dural or neural injury.

rotation. The addition of an iliac crest graft increased stiffness, but still allowed three times the displacement with axial compression and torsional stiffness, and was less than one-third that of an intact spine. In trauma patients with significant osteoligamentous disruption, the addition of an anterior corpectomy confers additional instability. Therefore, an uninstrumented anterior transthoracic decompression and fusion should be reserved for those patients with significant neural compression and minimal instability only truly seen in a nontraumatic or degenerative disorder. As the degree of instability increases, it often becomes necessary to supplement the anterior decompression and fusion with either anterior or posterior instrumentation or a combination of both (10,16,17). Almost all patients should have postoperative immobilization in a TLSO, except, perhaps, those stabilized with rigid posterior segmental fixation devices.

F   Anterior Fixation

Anterior instrumentation following an anterior corpectomy and fusion has been available since the mid-1960s. Some of these instrumentation systems were devised pri-

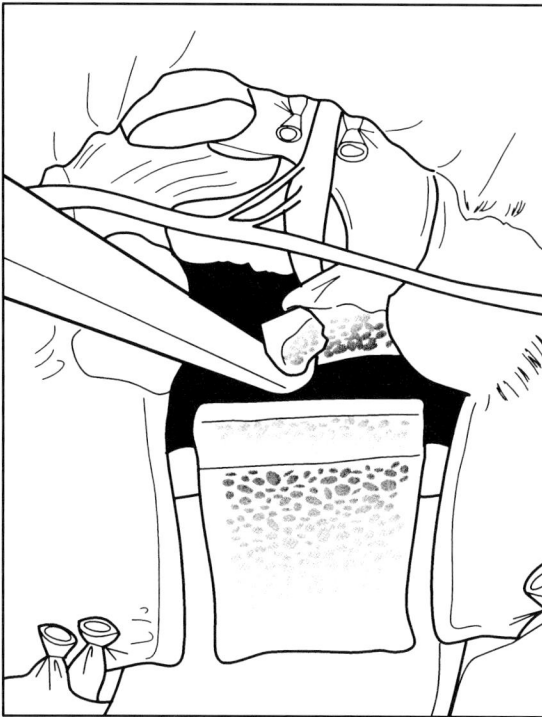

Figure 5   After entry into the spinal canal, the remainder of the posterior cortex of the fractured vertebral body is removed with appropriately shaped rongeurs.

marily for the treatment of spine deformity, while others, particularly the plating devices, were developed primarily for the treatment of spine trauma (10,18).

In the early 1990s, more sophisticated anterior plate systems were developed. These have significantly improved the quality of anterior fixation in the thoracic and thoracolumbar spine. Anterior plate fixation, however, is problematic at the L4, L5, and S1 levels because of the close proximity of the anterior abdominal vessels. Most of the current systems are based on the principle of two screws per vertebral level, with one screw placed posteriorly, parallel to the posterior cortical wall of the vertebral body, and the second angled obliquely from anterior to posterior in the body. This triangular arrangement improves pull-out strength. Most systems allow compression or distraction, which may improve incorporation of the graft anteriorly as well as the stability of the construct (10). Reported results have been good, with Kaneda reporting excellent results in 100% of patients in one study examining the use of the Kaneda device after anterior decompression in patients with neurological deficits (19). Gardner and associates (18) reported use of the CASP system for a variety of diagnoses, including acute burst fractures, with a fusion rate of 100%. Other authors, however, have noted high complication rates with anterior fixation (30%), as well as significant loss of initial deformity correction over time (50%) (15). Yuan and coworkers (20), reporting on their results with the use of the Syracuse I-Plate, cautioned that osteoporosis and significant posterior column disruption are both relative contraindications to anterior fixation.

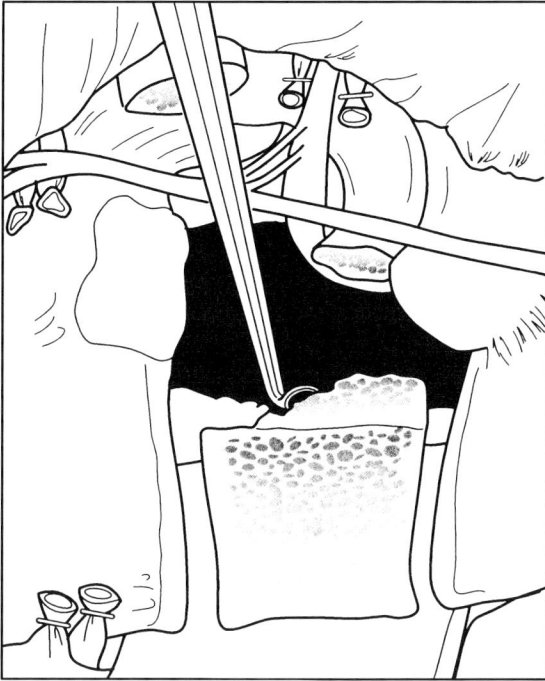

Figure 6   Same as Fig. 5, but with curettes.

After the corpectomy is completed, the appropriate-sized plate, or rod-screw construct, is selected. Two screws are placed at the level above and below the corpectomy. The posterior of the two screws is drilled parallel to the posterior cortex of the vertebral body. Care must be taken to understand precisely the orientation of the patient on the operating table and the resulting direction of drill placement. Placement of a Pennfield retractor over the posterior cortex through the neuroforamen aids in determination of the most posterior extent of the vertebral body. A bicortical hole is often drilled depending on the instrumentation system. The drill path is measured with a depth gauge to determine the proper screw length or bolt. The screws are then applied tightly into position and may then be used to apply distraction to the interspace, allowing restoration of body height at the injured level. Placement of the graft then ensues. The distraction can then be released and the proper-sized plate or rod selected so that it does not impinge on the open disk spaces above and below the stabilized levels. The plate or rod is placed over the bolts and the nuts are provisionally placed on the bolts. A slight compressive force is applied across the three levels, and the nuts are tightened down to maintain position. Finally, the anterior two screws are drilled and placed through the plate to complete the construct, or connected to a rod and the two rods cross-linked.

G   Closure

All malleable retractors are removed, and hemostasis is obtained before wound closure. The parietal pleura is reapproximated over the spinal instrumentation or bone

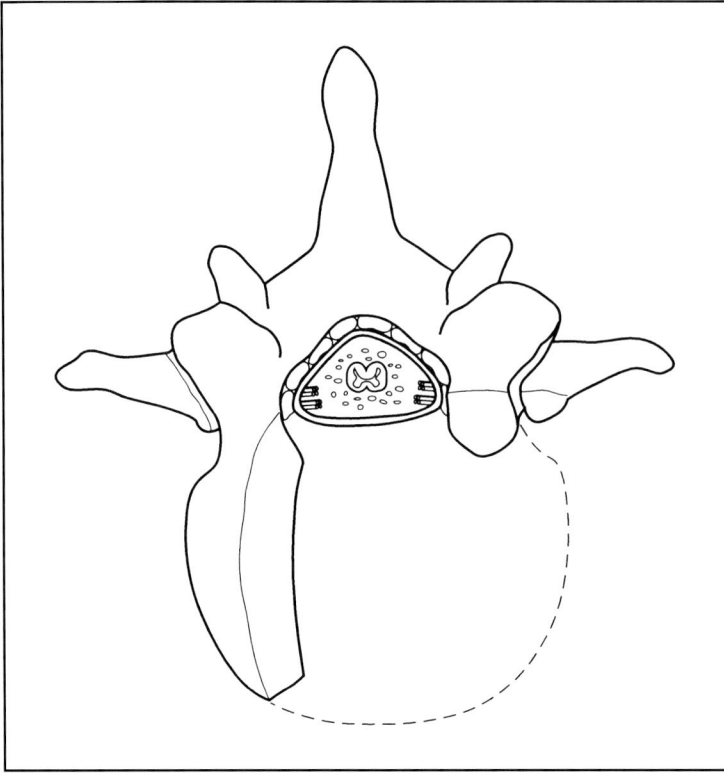

Figure 7 The bone resection at the end of decompression should extend from the pedicle on one side to the pedicle on the opposite side. At the end of neural decompression, the dura should bulge anteriorly in a uniform fashion from the endplate of the vertebra above to the endplate of the vertebra below and from pedicle to pedicle. If the dura does not bulge out concentrically, the surgeon should check for residual neural compression.

graft, if possible. If the diaphragm was taken down, it is important to reapproximate the crus and close the diaphragm. Multiple figure of eight #1 Vicryl sutures are placed at the site of the previous crus, and then a running #1 Vicryl suture is used to close the diaphragmatic separation. The free-hanging diaphragm is plicated with shorter suture bites on the thoracic wall, with longer suture bites on the diaphragmatic muscle itself.

Chest tube drainage is necessary for reinflation of the lung. Closure of the thoracic wall is accomplished in a layered fashion. The thoracotomy is closed with sutures placed above the cephalic rib and below the caudal rib, taking care to avoid the neurovascular bundle immediately beneath the caudal rib. A rib approximator is used to close the chest wall defect, and the pericostal sutures are tied. All of the muscles are sutured back to their original positions, including the serratus anterior if it was detached from the chest wall.

REFERENCES

1. Argenson C, Lovitt J, Camba PM et al. Osteosynthesis of thoracolumbar spine fractures with CD instrumentation. Proceedings of the Fifth International Congress on CD Instrumentation, Paris, June 1988, pp. 75–82.
2. Balasubramanian K, Ranu HS, King AI. Vertebral response to laminectomy. J Biomech 1978; 21:813–823.
3. Bohlman HH. Current concepts review: Treatment of fractures and dislocations of the thoracic and lumbar spine. J Bone Joint Surg 1985; 76A:165–169.
4. Bohlman HH, Freehafer A, Dejak J. The results of treatment of acute injuries of the upper thoracic spine with paralysis. J Bone Joint Surg 1984; 67A:360–369.
5. Cain JE, DeJong JT, Dinenberg AS et al. Pathomechanical analysis of thoracolumbar burst fracture reduction: A calf spine model. Spine 1993; 18:1647–1654.
6. Cammisa FP, Eismont FJ, Green AB. Dural laceration occurring with burst fractures and associated laminar fractures. J Bone Joint Surg 1989; 71A:1044–1052.
7. Cantor JB, Lebwohl NH, Garvey T et al. Nonoperative management of stable thoracolumbar burst fractures with early ambulation and bracing. Spine 1993; 18:971–976.
8. Fredrickson BE, Edwards WT, Rauschning W et al. Vertebral burst fractures: An experimental, morphologic, and radiographic study. Spine 1992; 17:1012–1021.
9. Harrington RM, Budorick T, Hoyt J et al. Biomechanics of indirect reduction of bone retropulsed into the spinal canal in vertebral fracture. Spine 1993; 18:692–699.
10. Browner BD, Jupiter JB, Levine AM, Trafton PG, eds. Skeletal Trauma: Fractures, Dislocations, Ligamentous Injuries, 2nd ed. Philadelphia: WB Saunders Co, 1988.
11. Willen J, Anderson J, Toomoka K et al. The natural history of burst fractures at the thoracolumbar junction. J Spinal Disord 1990; 3:39–46.
12. Zu Z, Mao-hua C, Tian-hua D. Unstable fractures of thoracolumbar spine treated with pedicle screw plating. Chin Med J (Engl) 1994; 107:281–285.
13. Paul RL, Michael RH, Dunn JE et al. Anterior transthoracic surgical decompression of acute spinal cord injuries. J Neurosurg 1975; 43:299.
14. Bohlman HH, Eismont FJ. Surgical techniques on anterior decompressions and fusion for spinal cord injuries. Clin Orthop 1981; 154:57.
15. Gurr KR, McAfee PC, Shih CM. Biomechanical analysis of anterior and posterior instrumentation systems after corpectomy: A calf spine model. J Bone Joint Surg 1988; 70A:1182–1191.
16. Been HD. Anterior decompression and stabilization of thoracolumbar burst fractures by the use of the Slot-Zielke device. Spine 1991; 16:70–77.
17. Been HD. Anterior decompression and stabilization of thoracolumbar burst fractures using the Slot-Zielke device. Acta Orthop Belg 1991; 57:144–161.
18. Gardner VO, Thalgott JS, White JI et al. The contoured anterior spinal plate system (CASP). Spine 1994; 19:550–555.
19. Kaneda K, Asano S, Hashimoto T et al. The treatment of osteoporotic-posttraumatic vertebral collapse using the Kaneda device and a bioactive ceramic vertebral prosthesis. Spine 1992; 17:S295–S303.
20. Yuan HA, Mann KA, Found EM et al. Early clinical experience with the Syracuse I-Plate: An anterior spinal fixation device. Spine 1998; 13:278–285.

41

Anterior Thoracolumbar Plating and Rodding Techniques

RAJIV TALIWAL and BERNARD A. RAWLINS

Hospital for Special Surgery, Weill Medical College of Cornell University, New York, New York, U.S.A.

I SURGICAL INDICATIONS

An anterior decompression of the thoracolumbar spine in the setting of trauma is indicated for an incomplete neurological deficit with canal compromise or the inability to achieve an indirect posterior reduction. Indications for surgery include the presence of a neurological deficit, anterior canal compromise, local kyphosis >30 degrees, significant loss of anterior vertebral height, or late pain due to malunion or nonunion. The advantage to this approach is a direct and more predictable decompression. The disadvantage of an anterior approach is its morbidity, particularly diminished pulmonary function in a trauma patient with associated thoracic injuries and limited reserves (1).

The ideal anterior fixation device should provide adequate mechanical stabilization while maintaining a low profile. This approach is most effective with intact posterior elements. Associated posterior column injuries are better treated with anterior and posterior fusion. For unstable three-column injuries in the neurologically intact patient, internal stabilization can decrease hospitalization and rehabilitation time, improve alignment, and decrease complications over nonoperative treatment (1).

II BIOMECHANICS

Using a dog corpectomy model, Zdeblick et al. compared anterior arthrodesis with and without instrumentation. The rate of fusion was significantly higher (86% vs. 29%) in the instrumented group. Biomechanically, the spines instrumented with the

Kaneda device were significantly stiffer (0.9 Nm/° vs. 0.65 Nm/°) in torsion than the uninstrumented group, with no significant difference in axial compression or flexural loading stiffness (2).

Gurr et al. compared anterior and posterior constructs in a calf corpectomy model, testing rotation, torque, axial displacement, and axial load across the spinal segment. In torsion and axial compression, the anterior Kaneda construct was as stiff as the posterior Cotrel-Dubousset (CD) or Steffee plate construct, and all three were as stiff as the intact spine. However, the Kaneda device only extended one level caudad and one level cephalad to the corpectomy, whereas the posterior CD and Steffee constructs required transpedicular fixation two levels caudad and two levels cephalad to achieve comparable stiffness (3).

Zdeblick et al. performed a biomechanical comparison of the Kaneda device, Texas Scottish Rite Hospital (TSRH) construct, Contoured Anterior Spinal Plate (CASP), and the Kostuik-Harrington device. They found the Kaneda and TSRH constructs effective in restoring spinal stability compared to the intact spine in axial compression (111.8 Nm, 130.2 Nm, 114.5 Nm); flexural strain (0.57%, 0.56%, 2.61%), and torsional stiffness (0.25, 0.19, 0.26). Both devices allowed distraction across the fracture site and then compression across the bone graft. The CASP system did not perform as well as the intact spine in axial load (89.8 Nm vs. 114.5 Nm). The Kostuik-Harrington construct was less stable in torsion (0.15 vs. 0.26) compared to the intact spine (4).

An et al. compared the biomechanical stability of two anterior rod and two anterior plate fixation systems with and without an interbody graft. With an interbody graft, all four devices (University Anterior Plate, Kaneda device, Z-Plate, and TSRH system) restored stability in flexion, extension, lateral bending, and torsion. Only the Kaneda device was stiffer in torsion than the intact spine. Without a structural graft, the University plate decreased motion in flexion, extension, and lateral bending, the TSRH system decreased flexion and lateral bending, and the Z-Plate decreased lateral bending only better than the intact specimen. Only the Kaneda device gave increased torsional stability with a graft, and was better overall in the absence of an interbody graft. In general, instrumentation restored stability in all directions with an interbody graft, with the Kaneda device having the best overall results, especially in torsion. Previous studies had shown the superiority of rod systems such as the Kaneda and TSRH systems. However, these implants are bulky and may theoretically increase the risk of injury to adjacent neurovascular structures. This study showed that plate systems such as University and Z-Plate performed similarly, although not as well, as previously tested rod systems (Kaneda and TSRH), and could be viable options for thoracolumbar instability (5).

Dick et al. evaluated four devices (Synthes Anterior Thoracolumbar Locking Plate (ATLP), Z-Plate, Kaneda device, and TSRH construct) without load-sharing bone graft to compare the fatigue strength and stiffness under the worst-case scenario. The fatigue life of the ATLP (80,000 cycles) was greater than the Z-Plate (26,500), and both were significantly greater than either the TSRH (6900) or Kaneda constructs (4400). The TSRH and Kaneda systems failed at the 3/16″ rod. Kaneda rods are threaded, further reducing strength to failure. The newer generation Kaneda device utilizes unthreaded rods with improved mechanics. The ATLP was stiffest in axial compression, lateral flexion, and torsion. The Kaneda device and Z-Plate were less stiff, and the TSRH system was least stiff in flexion and extension (6).

III TECHNIQUE

Adequate exposure is necessary to ensure proper placement of any instrumentation system. It is important to visualize the proximal and distal vertebral body fully, taking care not to disrupt the junctional disk. Exposure should be proximal enough so that the wound edge does not misguide the alignment of the surgeon's instruments and cause a screw to be inserted obliquely. Exposure should be posterior enough to identify the base of the pedicle and adequately evaluate the anterior–posterior extent of the vertebral body and the location of the spinal canal. Using blunt dissection, the spine can be exposed circumferentially. The decompression is performed, as discussed previously. The disks above and below the fracture are excised, taking care not to damage the intact endplates.

All current anterior thoracolumbar fixation systems utilize anterolateral vertebral body screws for fixation points. Snyder et al. evaluated the strength and rigidity of different methods of anterior spinal screw fixation. Using 6.5-mm fully threaded cancellous screws, they compared unicortical screws, bicortical screws, bicortical screws with a washer, and bicortical screws with a staple. Each of the four screw constructs failed by cutting through the vertebral body in the coronal plane and partially pulling out. The bicortical screw with staple was the strongest and most rigid form of fixation. The staple may contribute to stability by providing a rigid buttress for the screw, increasing surface area of contact with the vertebral body, and resisting tilt or vertical displacement via the staple prongs (7).

Most current devices require a staple as part of the fixation construct to direct the screw. This staple invariably increases surface area of contact with the vertebral body and protects the screw against bending moments (7). Staple size is selected to maximize coverage of the body so that all staple edges are well within the margins of the bone. Placement of the staple on the vertebral body should ensure that the direction of the posterior screw is not angled in the direction of the spinal canal. An awl is used to initiate a starting hole through the staple by penetrating the near cortex. The authors' preferred technique is to tap to a length within the vertebral body that would not penetrate the opposite deep cortex. The tapped hole is then palpated with a ball-tipped probe to confirm no violation of the opposite cortex. The hole is then tapped an additional 5 mm and checked again with a ball-tipped probe to identify if the opposite cortex has been penetrated. If this is the case, a screw of the last chosen tap length is used, otherwise the previous step is repeated. This will usually provide a safe technique for bicortical purchase without direct visualization. We prefer bicortical fixation for its ability to maximize fixation.

There are alternate methods to assessing screw length. One can expose the vertebral body circumferentially and manually palpate the opposite cortex. A C-shaped guide can be placed around the anterior vertebral body to the opposite side to ''catch'' the tap as it comes through the opposite cortex. Others advocate using the diameter of the vertebral body at the endplate after the corpectomy or diskectomy as a guide to screw length. The vertebral body is shaped such that its diameter is larger closer to the endplate and smaller in its midportion. Therefore, using the disk space as a guide can markedly overestimate the vertebral body diameter, particularly in a degenerative spine.

IV   ROD SYSTEMS

A   Kaneda Anterior Spinal System

This is a stainless steel double-rod system. Using the previous technique, the screws are placed in a converging configuration in each vertebral body. The posterior screw is angled about 10 to 15 degrees anterior (away from the spinal canal) and parallel to the endplate. The anterior screw is placed almost directly transversely across the body and parallel to the endplate. The triangular convergence increases pull-out strength and adds stability to the construct. The staples are aligned in a trapezoidal pattern with the anterior screws farther apart. This puts the anterior screws closer to the proximal and distal endplates, respectively, to allow the relatively stronger end-plate bone to support the anterior column of the construct. Closed screws are inserted proximally and distally. Using a distractor, the kyphotic deformity is corrected. Bone grafting is preformed as previously discussed. It is important to note that anterior devices should be load sharing, and offer significantly greater stability when the appropriate-sized graft is utilized (8). The posterior threaded rod is inserted with two inner locking nuts placed between the two vertebral screws. Outer nuts are applied and tightened, and the inner nuts lock into the eyelet. Two transverse couplers are added for stability by creating a box configuration (Fig. 1). The Kaneda device is biomechanically stable in flexion, extension, lateral bending, and torsion (5). This is partly because the cross-link gives it a stable rectangular configuration. The system allows a reduction of the fracture and then provides graft compression. Although it is higher profile than plate systems, there have been no reports to date of neurovascular injuries secondary to the Kaneda device (9).

B   TSRH

This is a stainless steel single- or double-rod system. Application of the double-rod device is similar to the Kaneda system. After decompression, the posterior screw is placed beginning near the posterior margin of the vertebral body and aiming 20 degrees away from the canal. The anterior screw is placed in the diagonally opposite corner of the vertebral body perpendicular to the floor. This ensures a triangular configuration between the two screws in the same vertebral body and increases pull-out strength. The anterior screws are placed further apart in a trapezoidal pattern. Distraction can be applied via a provisional rod placed between the anterior screws. The TSRH eyebolts are attached and the double-rod construct is assembled. Care should be taken to ensure that the rod seats into the eyebolt fully to maximize connection to the screw. Cross-link plates can then be applied to increase rigidity of the system. The TSRH rod system is capable of fracture reduction and then subsequent graft compression after insertion of the screws. Variable length can be achieved because of the rod construct. As with all rod constructs, it has a higher profile than plate systems, particularly if the double-rod construct with cross-link is applied.

C   AO Anterior Titanium Rod

This rod system is somewhat different in that the montage is preassembled prior to insertion. The construct is placed on the lateral surface of the vertebral body and provisionally held with fixation pins. This plate guides the direction of the screw

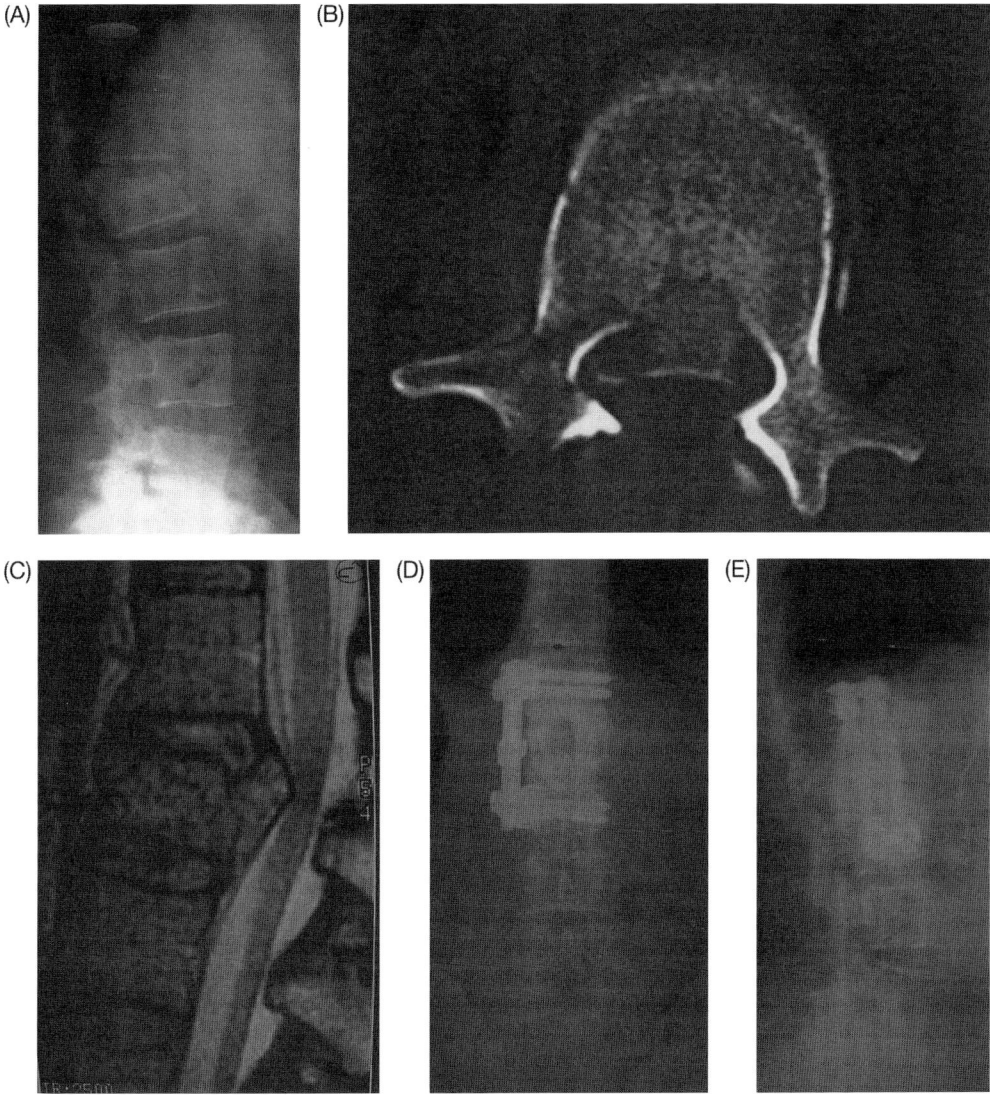

Figure 1 A 45-year-old female involved in a motor vehicle accident sustained an L2 burst fracture without neurological deficit. Patient had an anterior decompression and fusion from L1 to L3 using Kaneda instrumentation. (A) Lateral radiograph demonstrates L2 burst fracture with loss of anterior height. (B) CT scan shows retropulsed fragment with 50% canal compromise. (C) MRI illustrates canal encroachment by retropulsed fragment. (D) Anteroposterior radiograph at 2 years follow-up demonstrates Kaneda instrumentation in place. (E) Lateral radiograph illustrates restoration of sagittal alignment.

and, once applied, all screws are fixed in their trajectory. It is critical that the plate is initially applied to take into account the eventual direction of the vertebral body screws. The drill guide is seated into the screw hole and must be directed according to the angle of the plate to ensure proper fit of the screw. This system precludes fracture realignment before placement of the rods. Once applied, though, the graft can be compressed via the locking nuts on the rods. This is a titanium system with the added advantage of being MRI compatible.

V PLATE SYSTEMS

A Contoured Anterior Spinal Plate

After adequate decompression, the distance between endplates can be opened by (1) flexing the OR table, (2) placing manual pressure on the posterior apex of the kyphosis, or (3) using a distractor device. Bone graft is then sized and inserted as previously discussed. The CASP requires realignment of the spine prior to application. An appropriately-sized plate is contoured to the vertebral body. A minimum of three 6.5-mm fully threaded cancellous screws is placed in the two end vertebral bodies. Screws are directed transversely across the vertebral body, parallel to one another. The heads are not locked into the plate, and the plate does not predetermine the angle. This construct is unable to provide compression across the graft. It serves to buttress the graft, and is less effective than the intact spine in axial compression (89.8 Nm vs. 114.5 Nm) and torsion (0.19 vs. 0.26) (4). The advantage of using the CASP is the low profile and lateral position on the vertebra. The authors recommend bicortical fixation to maximize fixation, particularly in osteopenic bone.

B Z Plate

This is a titanium, MRI-compatible construct. It consists of slots at the superior end and fixed holes at the inferior end of the plate. There is a radius of curvature to match the curve of the vertebral body. The system is top loading for ease of application. Fixation to the vertebral body is with bolts (rigid interface with plate) and screws (semirigid interface with plate). The more prominent bolts are placed posteriorly as in other systems, taking care to aim away from the spinal canal. Once placed, the bolts can be used to provide distraction. The plate is then applied and the bolts partially tightened. The slots then allow for compression across the graft. Anterior screws are then placed convergent to the posterior bolts in each vertebral body and the construct is tightened and locked into place by crimping the nuts on the bolts. As a plate, it offers the benefits of low profile and lower theoretical risk to the surrounding neurovascular structures. This system can be used to distract the fracture and then compress across the graft before final fixation. Biomechanically, it has comparable stiffness to rod systems (5).

C Anterior Thoracolumbar Locking Plate

This titanium, MRI-compatible plate construct is very similar in nature to the Ventrofix titanium rod system. The plate guides the angle of the vertebral body screws. Once the initial screws are inserted, the remaining screws must be placed in a predetermined position directed by the plate. One must obtain reduction of the fracture with placement of the bone graft before the plate is applied in situ. The first two screws (4.0 mm) are placed into the two oval-shaped compression holes in the plate. As these screws are sequentially tightened, the plate is able to compress across the bone graft. Once in the compressed position, four static vertebral body screws (7.5 mm) are inserted, making sure the posterior screws are aimed away from the spinal canal. The compression screws can then be removed. This leaves the construct locked in a compressed position. The vertebral body screws lock into the plate, thereby increasing the rigidity of the construct. This is a very rigid plate with biomechanical properties exceeding those of rod systems (6). It has a relatively low profile compared to rod systems, but is bulky in comparison to other plates.

The fundamentals of anterior thoracolumbar instrumentation are common to all systems. Screws provide fixation to the vertebral body, preferably in a bicortical manner. The number of fixation points, number of cortices (unicortical vs. bicortical), and screw angle are potential options. There are two major systems, rods and plates. Each system has its advantages and disadvantages. Some systems require reduction of the fracture and bone grafting first, then application of the instrumentation in situ. Other systems allow for placement of the vertebral body screws, distraction across the fracture site, placement of the intervening bone graft, and then compression across the bone graft. Though fracture realignment can be performed through some instrumentation systems, we prefer to use endplate distractors and manual pressure over the kyphotic apex to aid in reduction and minimize the chance of screw cut out. Plate systems tend to compress via a mechanism applied through the vertebral body screws. Rod systems allow for screw placement first and then compression via a mechanism involving the screw–rod connector.

The profile of anterior instrumentation is important to consider. Given the nature of the local neurovascular structures, it is important to use an implant with a low profile while maintaining adequate biomechanical stability. Historically, bulky implants have led to catastrophic complications secondary to aortic erosions (1). Plates offer the advantage of having a lower profile compared to rods. Biomechanical studies have confirmed the viability of low-profile plates when compared to rod systems in stress testing (5).

When determining the length of the construct, rods offer a unique advantage over plates. Plates are available in a finite number of sizes, and the surgeon may need to adjust his construct based on the size of the plate in relation to the ultimate position of the vertebral body screws in relation to the endplates. Rods have no such limitation, and the vertebral body screw may be placed independent of the position of the final construct. In a rod system, the screws are placed first, then the rod is cut to match the construct. The surgeon should be careful to avoid excessive preloading of the construct, which might place the spine in kyphosis.

It is important to note that most biomechanical studies on instrumentation are performed using an in vitro model. This may or may not translate into clinical success. Instrumentation is only a means to obtaining a solid bony arthrodesis. It is important for the surgeon to understand the design characteristics of a particular instrumentation system when choosing which system will best meet the needs of the patient.

REFERENCES

1. McCullen G, Vaccaro A, Garfin S. Thoracic and lumbar trauma: Rationale for selecting the appropriate fusion technique. Orthop Clin N Am 1998; 29(4):813–828.

2. Zdeblick T, Shirado O, McAfee P, DeGroot H, Warden K. Anterior spinal fixation after lumbar corpectomy: A study in dogs. J Bone Joint Surg 1991; 73A:527–534.
3. Gurr K, McAfee P, Shih C. Biomechanical analysis of anterior and posterior instrumentation systems after corpectomy. J Bone Joint Surg 1988; 70A:1182–1191.
4. Zdeblick T, Warden K, Zou M, McAfee P, Abitbol J. Anterior spinal fixators: A biomechanical in vitro study. Spine 1993; 18(4):513–517.
5. An H, Lim T, You J, Hong J, Eck J, McGrady L. Biomechanical evaluation of anterior thoracolumbar spinal instrumentation. Spine 1995; 20(18):1979–1983.
6. Dick J, Brodke D, Zdeblick T, Bartel B, Kunz D, Rapoff A. Anterior instrumentation of the thoracolumbar spine: A biomechanical comparison. Spine 1997; 22(7):744–750.
7. Snyder B, Zaltz I, Hall J, Emans J. Predicting the integrity of vertebral bone screw fixation in anterior spinal instrumentation. Spine 1995; 20(14):1568–1574.
8. Kaneda K, Taneichi H, Abumi K, Hashimoto T, Satoh S, Fujiya M. Anterior decompression and stabilization with the Kaneda device for thoracolumbar burst fractures associated with neurologic deficits. J Bone Joint Surg 1997; 79A:69–83.
9. Ghanayem A, Zdeblick T. Anterior instrumentation in the management of thoracolumbar burst fractures. Clin Orthop Rel Res 1997; 335:89–100.

42

Thoracolumbar Anterior Strut Fusion Techniques Following Corpectomy for Trauma

CHRISTOPHER J. DeWALD

Rush Medical College, Rush Presbyterian St. Luke's Medical Center and Cook County Hospital, Chicago, Illinois, U.S.A.

JAMES BICOS

Rush Medical College, Rush Presbyterian St. Luke's Medical Center, Chicago, Illinois, U.S.A.

I INTRODUCTION

The ideal treatment methods for thoracolumbar spinal instability have been debated for many years. A conservative approach adapted by Stanger, Nicoll, and Guttmann was well accepted by the majority of physicians in the middle of the twentieth century (1–3). A more aggressive surgical approach (i.e., fusion, described in 1911) was found to be effective in the management of spinal tuberculosis (4,5). Modern contemporary surgical techniques have led to the explosion of sophisticated posterior segmental internal fixation and anterior column replacement devices, which have found utilization in the treatment of a variety of spinal disorders unresponsive to conservative treatment.

Holdsworth pioneered the concept of stable and unstable spinal injuries, and treated unstable spinal injuries using plates bolted to the spinous processes (6). The technique and benefits of anterior spinal surgery for thoracolumbar trauma is predicated on the need to address anterior column instability and potential neural compression from the anterior approach. Anterior interbody devices designed to distract or maintain interbody spatial relationships function by restoring sagittal alignment and stability while maintaining foraminal height and spinal canal patency (7–16).

589

Currently, with the widespread availability of allograft bone tissue and new synthetic materials, the surgeon has a variety of choices and techniques for thoracolumbar interbody fusion procedures.

Following an anterior decompression for a thoracolumbar fracture, an anterior interbody device is now selected to reconstruct the anterior spinal column. The surgeon must decide the type of graft or device to place in the interbody space and whether or not adjunctive anterior or anterior and posterior instrumentation is also necessary. Most pure axial compression injuries without associated posterior column disruption can be stabilized using an anterior strut device and anterior instrumentation alone (14,17). Anterior spinal injuries that also include posterior column injury such as flexion distraction–type fractures may require the addition of posterior instrumentation (Fig. 1A–D).

II   CHOICE OF ANTERIOR SPINAL COLUMN INTERBODY DEVICE

The type of anterior column interbody device to reconstruct the anterior spinal column includes any structure that has adequate load-bearing or load-sharing capacity for the requirements of the thoracolumbar spine. Load-bearing strut devices support the anterior spine. They may span from endplate to endplate and can be made of autogenous bone (i.e., iliac crest, fibula, or rib), allogeneic bone (i.e., iliac crest, femur, humerus, or fibula), or a synthetic or metallic material (i.e., titanium, ceramic, or carbon fiber cages). Load-sharing strut grafts are typically utilized as an inlay support within a trough and can also be autogenous bone (i.e., iliac crest, fibula, or rib), allogeneic bone (i.e., fibula or iliac crest), or a synthetic or metallic material. Load-bearing struts can often be stabilized using anterior instrumentation alone, whereas load-sharing struts often require adjunctive posterior instrumentation to maintain proper construct stability (14,17,18–20).

III   LOAD-BEARING STRUTS

The choice of load-bearing strut is mostly surgeon dependent; however, each device has its own merits and strengths. Autogenous iliac crest is the gold standard strut graft for an anterior column deficit. Autogenous strut grafts have shown excellent arthrodesis rates and should be considered for nearly all anterior spinal column defects (14,18,21,22). However, autogenous iliac crest struts are limited by the length

——>

Figure 1   L3 vertebrae of a 46-year-old man with an incomplete neurological injury sustained from a fall. This CT axial cut across the pedicles reveals significant canal compromise and a lamina fracture that has entrapped the dura. (A) A lower CT cut reveals significant posterior column injury with grossly widened facet joints at the L3/4 level. (B) This case was initially approached posteriorly to stabilize the three-column injury and explore the spinal canal. A dural tear was found within the lamina fracture at L3 and repaired. The spinal canal was decompressed through a left transpedicular approach. (C) A staged anterior support strut was inserted because of the severe comminution and vertebral height loss. An anterior single Kaneda rod was used for additional stabilization of the cage.

(A)

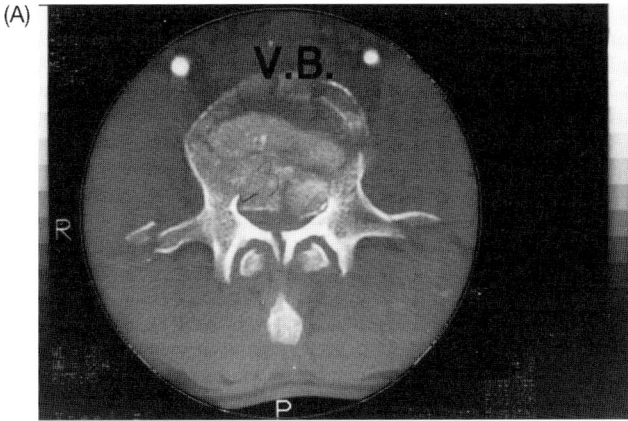

(B)

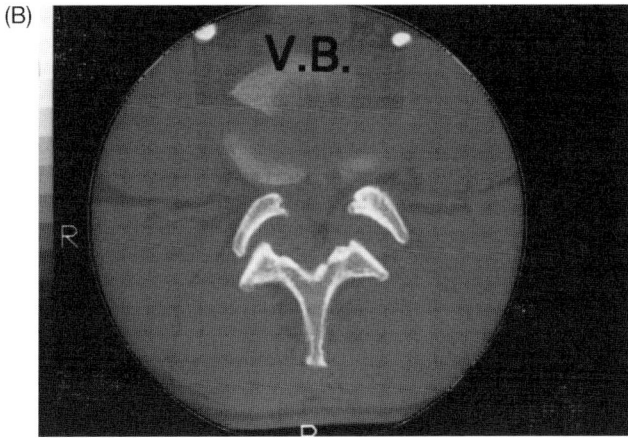

(C)

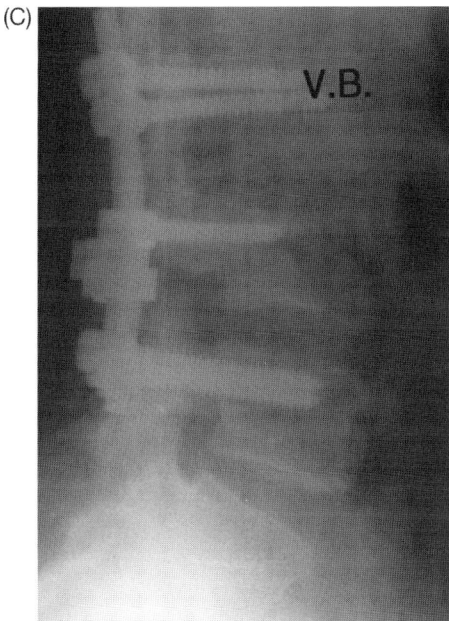

(D)

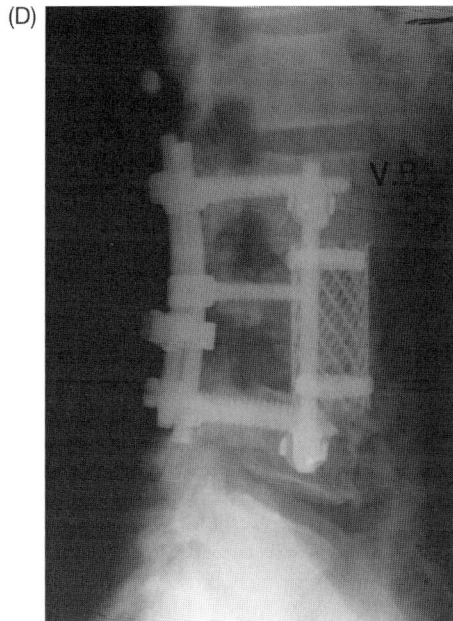

of the strut required and therefore the morbidity associated with its harvesting. Currently, the benefits and success of newer alternative strut devices, such as titanium mesh cages, have resulted in the decreased need for using iliac tricortical grafts for many anterior column reconstructive procedures.

Allograft bone has been used as a substitute for autogenous bone in many reconstructive procedures because of its abundance or lack of graft harvest morbidity. Allografts have been shown to have greater success in the anterior spine where the graft is under compression. Arthrodesis using allografts has shown great success as an interbody strut graft for degenerative spinal conditions. Femoral rings packed with autogenous cancellous bone have become a common choice for anterior interbody fusions. The use of fresh frozen allograft bone as long segment strut grafts has performed satisfactorily in spinal tumor and fracture reconstructive surgery with arthrodesis rates reported as high as autogenous strut grafts (23,24). The use of an allograft strut not only provides a good support for the anterior spine but also allows ample space for placement of autogenous bone around the allograft. One of the drawbacks to the use of fresh frozen allograft bone is its availability. Fortunately, bone banks are growing in number and size with the growing popularity of anterior spinal surgery. The obvious concern with allograft bone is the risk of viral transmission (25). Fortunately, the risk of viral transmission of fresh frozen allograft bone has been estimated at one in a million.

Allograft strut grafts, especially of iliac crest origin, are useful in osteopenic bone where the patient's own bone is of poor quality and metallic cages would cut deeply into the adjacent vertebral endplates.

Femoral shaft allografts have demonstrated excellent supportive strength and peripheral incorporation in clinical practice. The medullary canal of the femur can be packed with morselized bone graft or with autologous strut grafts to provide a good source of autogenous bone graft to the construct (Fig. 2A–C). Allograft bone in and of itself is also a potential source of healing bone that may incorporate into the host bone. The main advantage of femoral shaft allografts as an anterior strut is the length of graft that can be utilized. Femoral shafts can easily span over two corpectomy sites whereas an iliac crest allograft is usually adequate for a single-level corpectomy. The greatest disadvantage of femoral shaft allografts is the strong cortical bone of the femur. The diameter of the femoral shaft usually fits within the vertebral body circumference and does not always rest on the harder bone of the outer ring of the bony endplate as an iliac strut will do. Often an edge of the femoral shaft will cut into the endplate of the adjacent vertebral body. As with titanium mesh cages, it is important that the patient's adjacent endplates are sufficiently hard and intact to support the interbody graft. Because of this, femoral shaft allografts are often used in the same clinical situations as metallic mesh cages.

Prosthetic interbody devices were developed to provide the advantage of structural support without the need to harvest a large autogenous bone graft as well as to avoid the use of cadaveric allograft bone. As with the various allograft struts, each prosthetic device has particular clinical scenarios where it is most efficacious. Bioactive ceramic or carbon fiber spacers have a broader surface area and a modulus of elasticity closer to bone that lend themselves to less subsidence. Ceramic blocks are specifically utilized in osteoportic or metastatic patients for this purpose. They have been used commonly in Japan with satisfactory results (26,27). The blocks are rectangular and are placed into the corpectomy site within the midbody portion of the

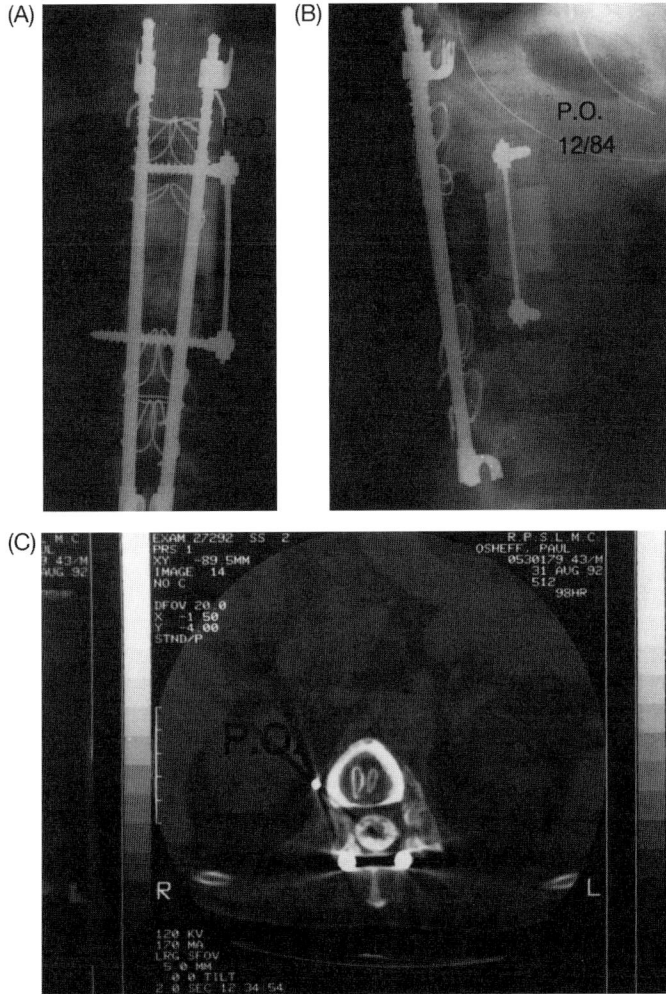

Figure 2 (A,B) AP and lateral plain radiographs of a corpectomy and reconstruction of a plasmacytoma at T12. A femoral shaft allograft is used as a load-bearing graft. Notches have been developed into the allograft to lock into the host vertebrae in a tongue-and-groove fashion. In addition, autogenous rib struts have been passed through the canal of the femoral shaft and inlayed into a trough within the host bone of the contiguous endplate (see AP view). (C) An axial CT scan revealing the femoral shaft allograft with the autogenous rib struts within its medullary canal.

vertebral body in a similar fashion as an iliac crest strut graft, resting across the edges of the endplates. Bioactive ceramic blocks allow for bony ingrowth into the periphery of the block. The main disadvantage of ceramic blocks is that they cannot be altered or trimmed, although different sizes are available.

Despite the drawbacks of metallic mesh cages (i.e., subsidence in osteopenic vertebral endplates), specific devices such as the Harms' cage have become a popular choice for anterior column reconstruction of large anterior spinal defects. It is a strong and extremely versatile anterior strut support for anterior spinal column defects, particularly for trauma patients and also in metastatic disease where a circumferential approach is contemplated (24,28). It is especially useful in younger patients where a strong spinal stabilization construct is needed. Its greatest advantage is its versatility in sizes with multiple diameters and its ability to provide interdigitation of the edges of the cage within strong bony endplates of the adjacent vertebral bodies (Fig. 3A–D). The cage can be trimmed and shaped quite easily in large or smaller millimeter increments by cutting the prongs of the cage down. The subsidence of the mesh prongs into the vertebral endplates provides additional torsional stability to the spinal construct (29). Unfortunately, the countersinking of the "pickets" or prongs of the mesh cage into the vertebral endplates is a real concern in osteoporotic patients. Usually, such subsidence is of little clinical significance with only a mild loss of sagittal contour. On occasion, however, significant subsidence may lead to the loss of spinal stability and stable fixation of the spinal implant. Endplate covers are available for the different cage diameters and do provide some resistance to continued subsidence.

Titanium mesh cages are hollow and allow packing with autogenous bone graft from the fractured vertebral body or sacrificed rib from the surgical approach without the added surgical morbidity of an additional bone graft incision. These sources of autogenous bone graft are packed into and around the hollow mesh cage while the cage provides the structural support for the anterior spinal column. Adherence to proper decortication and arthrodesis techniques along with moderate use of local autogenous rib and fractured vertebral body in traumatic injuries can provide almost similar arthrodesis success to that of an autologous strut graft reconstruction.

A Technique of Placing a Load-Bearing Strut Interbody Graft or Device

If using adjunctive instrumentation, Kaneda recommends placing vertebral body screws above and below prior to the removal of the fractured vertebral body to prevent additional cancellous bleeding expected from the corpectomy site (14). Others remove the intervertebral disks prior to placement of an anterior fixation device to get a better orientation of the spatial relationship of the vertebral bodies. This allows easier placement of the screws parallel to the endplates. In using the Kaneda system as an example, two screws are placed in each vertebral body using a vertebral

Figure 3   (A) MRI of a 55-year-old man who sustained a L1 burst fracture from a fall while intoxicated. Significant neural compression was evident. (B) CT scan revealing neural compression and comminution of the vertebral body. (C) AP radiograph showing bicortical screw fixation of the contiguous vertebral bodies. On this first standing radiograph after surgery, the mild indentation of the Harms cage into the endplates can be seen. The diameter of the cage is wide enough to span from the opposite pedicle to the near pedicle. It is particularly important in osteopenic bone to choose a larger diameter cage to sit more on the periphery of the vertebral body. (D) Lateral radiograph revealing morselized bone placed anterior to the cage after the cage has been packed with autogenous bone. This amount of bone placed anterior to the cage has caused the retained anterior longitudinal ligament to bow anteriorly.

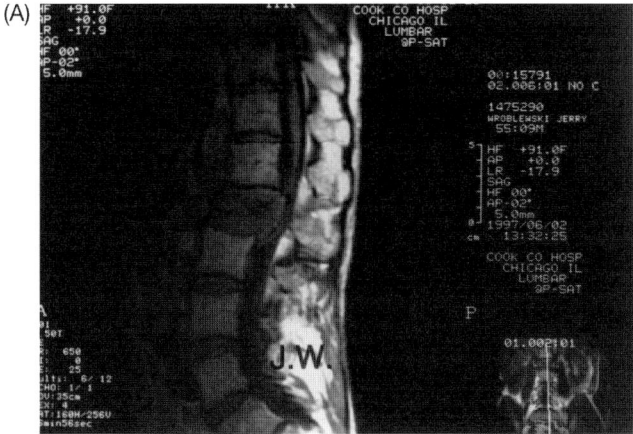

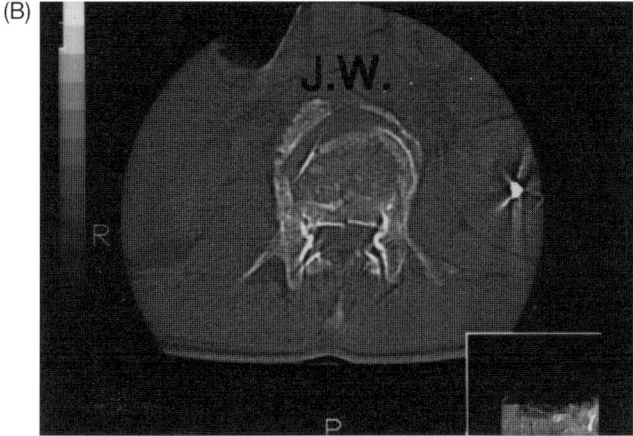

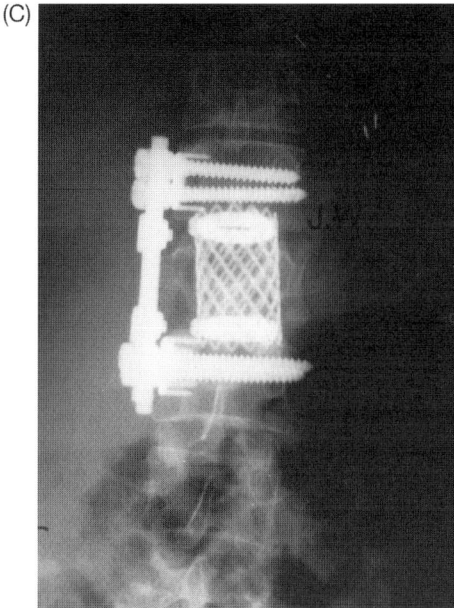

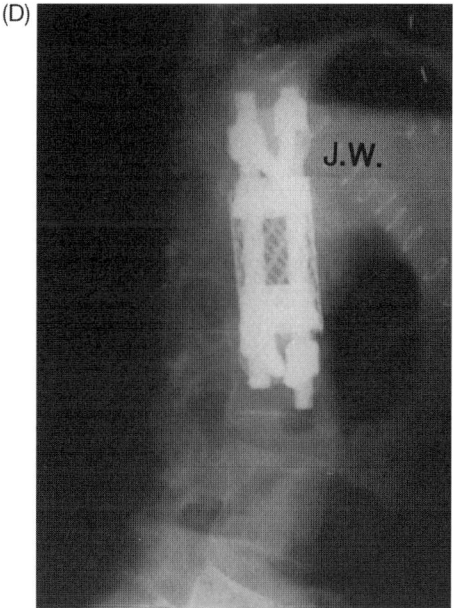

body staple to assist in the proper spacing of the screws (Fig. 4). The screws should be placed in a bicortical manner, although some instrumentation systems, such as the anterior thoracolumbar locking plate of Synthese, advocates a unicortical screw purchase with their device. Bicortical fixation is recommended in the majority of the systems in cancellous vertebral body bone for stable fixation and adequate compression strength to minimize screw loosening during distraction or compression maneuvers.

The technique of safe bicortical screw placement relies on the surgeon's finger to feel the tap or screw exiting the contralateral cortex of the vertebral body. In using this technique, the surgeon can triangulate the screws for proper angular insertion, while keeping the screws parallel to the exposed vertebral body endplates. In addition, the surgeon is ensured that the screw angle does not encroach the spinal canal.

An awl is used to penetrate the vertebral cortex. Next, with gentle blunt dissection, the surgeon's finger is placed around the vertebral body to the opposite side. One can usually feel the rib articulation or the transverse process on the contralateral vertebral body side. This maneuver is quite easy to perform in the lower thoracic spine down to the L1 vertebral body level, but as the diaphragmatic crus is reached, it becomes more difficult. The vertebral body is tapped to the opposite cortex until the tap is felt with the surgeon's finger. The tap is calibrated to show the appropriate screw length. Alternatively, a depth gauge can be used. The screw should be long enough for one or two screw threads to penetrate the contralateral cortex (Fig. 5). A distraction device may now be used through the screw heads to obtain distraction and reduction via ligamentotaxis (Fig. 6).

The remaining retropulsed bone of the fractured vertebral level is removed back to the posterior longitudinal ligament. Usually it is not necessary to remove the posterior longitudinal ligament unless there is either MRI or visual evidence of bony

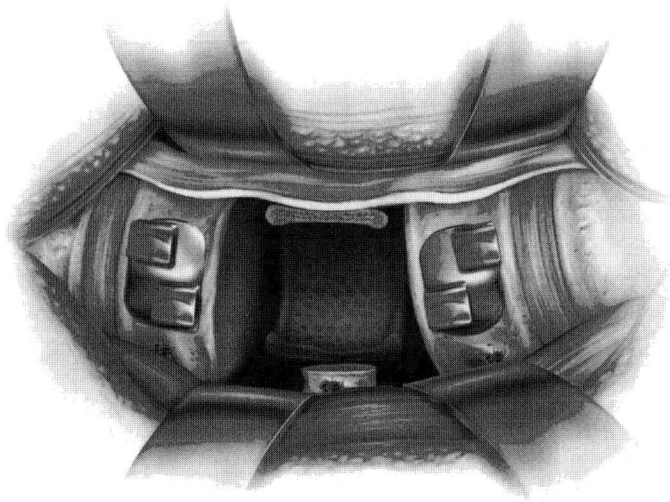

Figure 4   In this drawing, vertebral body screws have been placed at one level above and one level below the fractured vertebrae, and subsequent corpectomy has been performed. Proper spacing of the screws in the lateral aspect of the vertebral bodies is assured by use of a vertebral body staple.

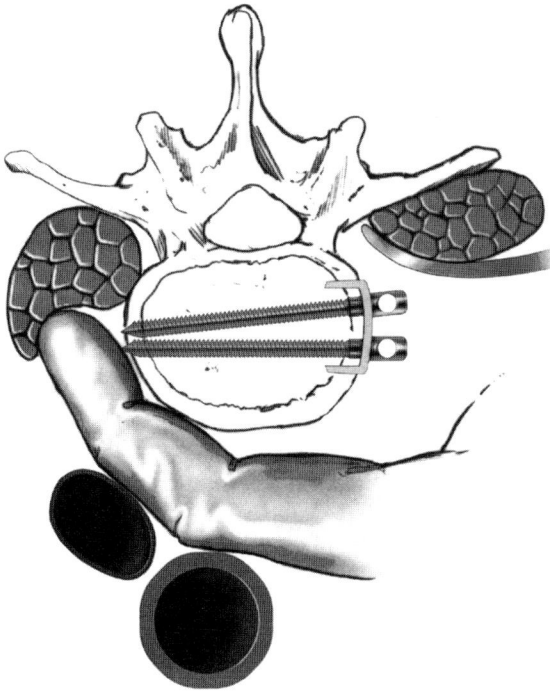

Figure 5 As depicted in the drawing, vertebral body screw length is safely determined by tapping the body until the tap is felt by a bluntly placed finger on the opposite cortex. The descending aorta and inferior vena cava are protected by this finger during screw placement. The screws have been placed through a vertebral body staple.

rupture through the ligament. Removing the posterior longitudinal ligament will expose the epidural veins, which can bleed quite profusely. If the ligament needs to be removed, a thrombin-soaked gel foam can be placed against the exposed dura to help control the bleeding. An epinephrine-soaked sponge can also be placed within the corpectomy site and held with slight pressure against the remaining cancellous vertebral bone in order to control cancellous bleeding. This should be done for 5 min to obtain hemostasis and provide better visualization of the surgical field. Great care should be taken to avoid excessive pressure on the thecal sac.

Following adequate spinal canal decompression and hemostasis, the interbody strut graft is now placed. The length of the distracted corpectomy site is measured from endplate to endplate. Distraction is performed until the anterior longitudinal ligament and the adjacent annulus is taut. Therefore, the anterior longitudinal ligament and the anterior annulus of the adjacent disks should not be destroyed to prevent overdistraction of the fracture site.

B   Endplate Preparation

The endplates are next prepared for placement of the chosen interbody strut device. The cartilaginous endplate is completely removed down to the hard bony endplate until bleeding occurs. Great care should be taken not to destroy or remove the bony

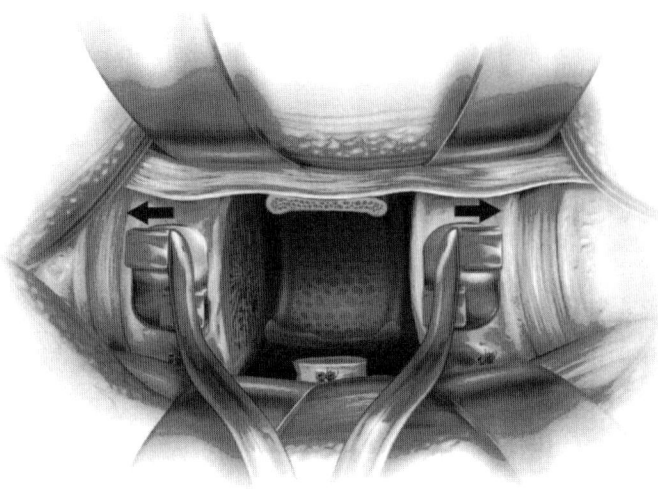

Figure 6 In preparation for strut graft placement, the corpectomy site is distracted with a device fitting on the previously placed vertebral body screw heads as shown in the drawing.

endplate. The majority of the bony endplate must be left intact in order to provide a firm platform for docking of the interbody corpectomy strut. Some authors have suggested removing the bony endplate to expose bleeding cancellous bone for better healing (30). Although this method may work in theory, the cancellous bone may not be strong enough to support the strut graft and the compressive forces seen in the anterior thoracolumbar spine. An additional anatomical consideration in placing the graft is the concavity of the vertebral body endplate. This requires that the lateral lip of the vertebral body at the entrance site of the graft be removed using a lexel rongeur or osteotome to provide a flat grafting surface.

The strut graft can now be placed within the corpectomy site. The graft is countersunk 2 to 3 mm deep to the ipsilateral vertebral body edge and should span the diameter of the vertebral body. At the time of insertion of the interbody graft, the surgeon can place his hand on the patient's back to provide a lordotic force against the posterior aspect of the spine, easing the insertion of the strut (Fig. 7). After proper seating of the graft, the distraction device is removed. The strut graft should be checked for stability and should not be able to be moved within the corpectomy site.

The remaining rib graft or vertebral body bone which was removed during the surgical exposure or decompression can now be used as bone graft around the strut device. This supplemental graft can be placed anterior to the strut graft, between it and the remaining anterior vertebral body wall (Fig. 8A,B). The anterior impacted morselized graft also helps to further stabilize the strut graft itself. Alternatively, the rib can be cut the same length as the corpectomy site and can either be placed anterior or lateral to the iliac strut graft or metallic cage. In addition, if enough room exists, one or two rib segments, in addition to the strut device, can be impacted within the endplates, providing additional strut support. Although the Kaneda device has a

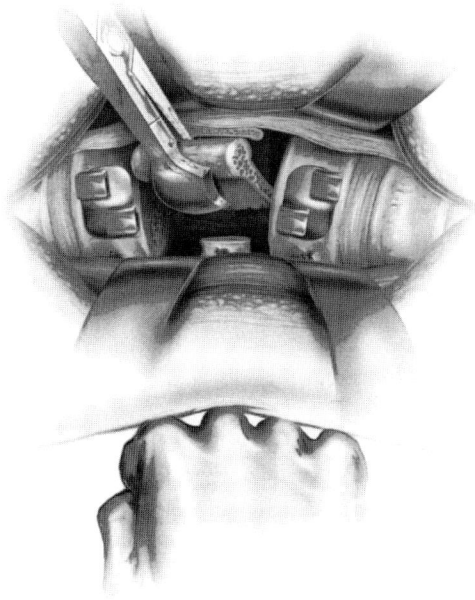

Figure 7 The interbody strut graft is placed into the corpectomy site under distraction, as shown in the drawing. A fist pushing on the patient's back under the surgical level can apply a lordotic force, thereby increasing the distraction and aiding in graft placement.

higher lateral profile as compared to plate constructs, it allows for an abundant amount of bone graft to be placed beneath the rods (Fig. 9A,B).

The anterior plate or rod is fitted to the vertebral screws and compression is applied while the screws are tightened. Usually, the anterior interbody device is slightly larger than the measured anterior defect (approximately 1–2 mm), anticipating some mild compression across the strut device. If the strut is undersized and compression is applied, kyphosis will occur across the fracture site. A few millimeters of compression should provide adequate stability across the strut. The final tightening of the plate or rod is now performed (Fig. 10A–C).

IV LOAD-SHARING STRUT GRAFTS

A load-sharing graft is placed through the endplates of the bordering vertebral bodies. It has the ability to be stable in terms of preventing graft dislodgement in the absence of anterior instrumentation. Load-sharing strut devices usually require the addition of adjunctive posterior instrumentation for adequate stability. Occasionally, both posterior and anterior instrumentation are required to provide adequate construct strength. This grafting technique had been the standard anterior spinal column reconstruction method prior to the advent of anterior internal fixation. This is also a viable reconstructive alternative when the spinal pathology only requires an arthrodesis and not a corpectomy or decompression.

(A)

(B)

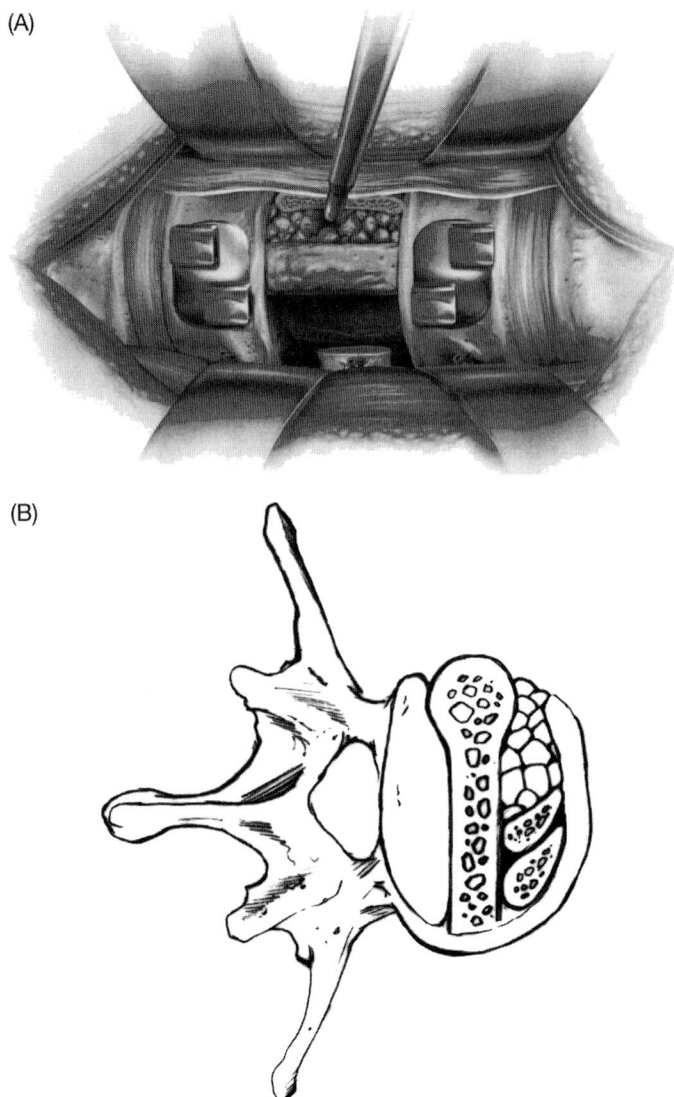

Figure 8   (A,B) Morselized bone graft is placed anterior to the strut graft between it and any remaining anterior vertebral wall. This both stabilized the strut graft initially and allows for further osteoconduction and osteoinduction.

Load-sharing strut grafts do not rest on the vertebral endplates, but are keyed into a trough or peg hole in the adjacent vertebral bodies. Any thin strut may be utilized as a load-sharing graft by inlaying the strut into the trough. The vascular bed of the cancellous bone of the adjacent vertebral bodies provides an excellent osteogenic environment for bony healing (30,31). Autogenous iliac crest or fibula are the most commonly used load-sharing grafts (Fig. 11) (30–32). Autogenous rib grafts are also used as an inlay load-sharing strut, but are better-suited because of

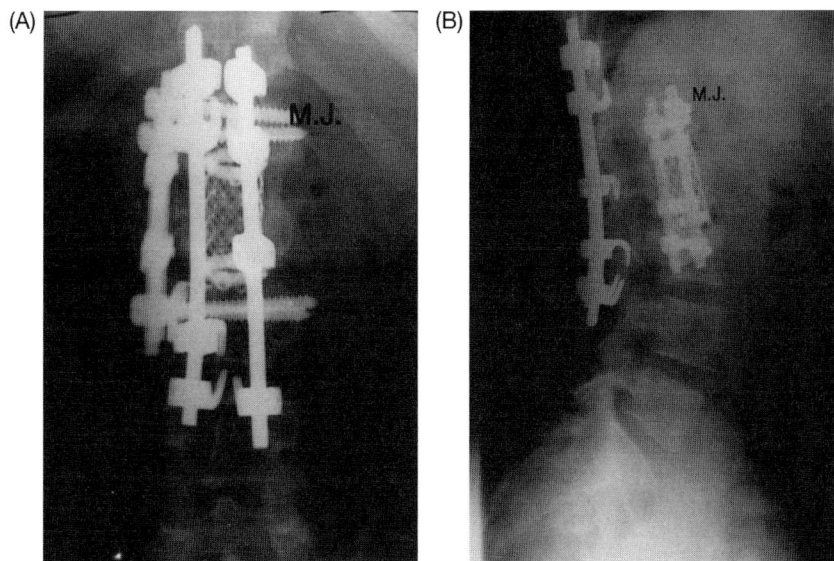

Figure 9 (A) AP radiograph of a burst fracture treated by anterior decompression and stabilization followed by a staged posterior instrumentation and fusion. Note the rib graft utilized anteriorly adjacent to both sides of the Harms cage. (B) Postoperative lateral radiograph shows the appropriate cage size and remaining anterior vertebral body. A posterior claw configuration is utilized for further stabilization, staggering the hooks to decrease the amount of canal intrusion near the injury.

their size and shape as a true interbody strut across a single disk space. Allograft iliac crest or fibula can also be used as inlay strut grafts and have been shown to incorporate well into host bone (Fig. 12) (24).

The inlay graft functions by maintaining the height of a corpectomy site but often does not provide enough anterior column stability without adjunctive instrumentation. This is due to the lack of support of the adjacent vertebrae endplate. In these cases, it is often advisable that posterior instrumentation be applied either prior to or following the anterior column reconstruction procedure.

A Technique of Load-Sharing Strut Placement

The technique of developing a trough and inserting an inlay graft is the same, regardless of the type of load-sharing device chosen. The anterior portion of the vertebrae should be left intact along with the anterior longitudinal ligament during the corpectomy procedure. After the corpectomy and decompression have been performed and the endplates of the adjacent vertebral bodies have been prepared as described above, a trough is made by cutting a small slot of bone out of the lateral aspect of the adjacent vertebral bodies (Fig. 13). The trough is made 1 cm in width or the approximate width of the chosen inlay strut graft to be used and typically placed midbody, but can be moved anteriorly or posteriorly depending on the clinical situation. The depth of the trough is dependent on the type of strut utilized, but is

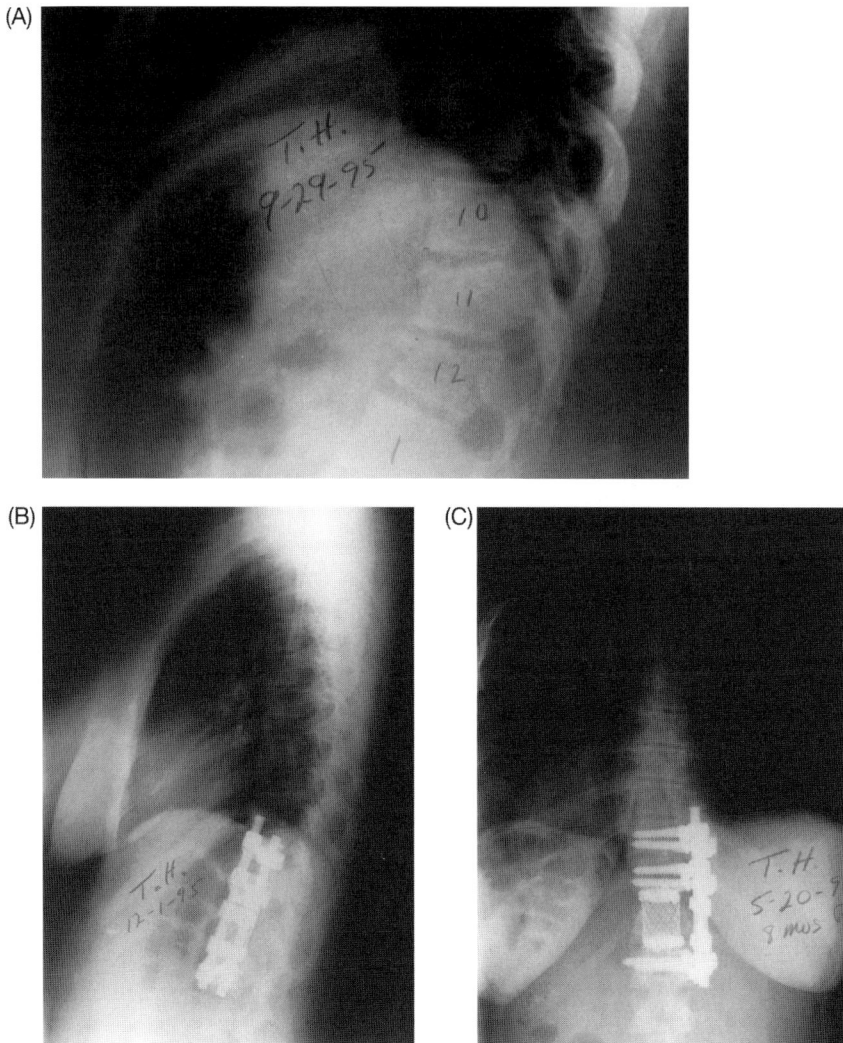

Figure 10 (A) A lateral radiograph of a 15-year-old girl with an incomplete neuro-logical injury sustained from a fall. A burst fracture T12 and a superior endplate compression fracture at T11 are noted. Anterior decompression was decided upon. (B,C) Postoperative AP and lateral radiographs revealing restored vertebral height and sag-ittal contour. The Kaneda instrumentation was used in a segmental fashion to include the compression fracture at T11 after diskectomy of the T10/11 disk and insertion of autogenous rib graft.

typically two-thirds the lateral width of the vertebral body. The length of the trough made into the vertebral bodies is also determined by the spinal pathology. The trough is altered to the length of strut needed and the desired degree of spinal alignment correction, if necessary. The trough is kept within the proximal half of the vertebral body if adjunctive anterior instrumentation is to be used also. Often the inlay strut

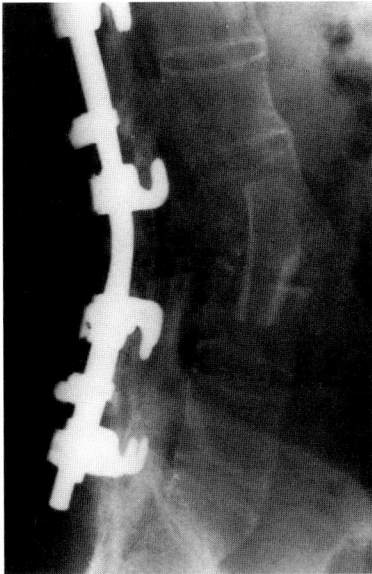

Figure 11 A patient with ankylosing spondylitis following a posterior osteotomy and inlay grafting using a large autogenous iliac crest bone graft.

will come to contact the vertebral screws of the anterior instrumentation preventing further migration of the inlayed strut graft.

The entire strut trough is measured while the kyphotic deformity is held in a corrected position. A ventrally directed force on the posterior aspect of the spine will correct the kyphotic deformity. A vertebral body or laminar spreader can be used to hold the spinal correction, but the spreader must be placed on the solid endplates of the remaining vertebral bodies. Care must be taken not to fracture the endplates while using the spreader, especially if the bone is osteoporotic or concern exists about the integrity of the endplate. The trough is measured using a ruler or calipers and the inlay strut graft is cut 3 to 5 mm longer than what was measured in the corrected position. The graft is then typically trimmed to approximately 2 mm longer than measured. It is best to use a mini oscillating saw to trim the strut graft in small increments so as not to fracture the strut. As the spine is distracted by a ventrally directed force from the posterior aspect of the spine, the superior end of the strut is keyed into the trough. The opposite end of the strut is impacted at its bottom end to countersink the superior graft end into the superior vertebral bone until the inferior graft end slides past the edge of its own vertebral trough. The superior graft end can now be impacted into the depth of the trough made. The strut graft usually holds the corpectomy site in the corrected position. The lordosing force can now be relaxed while a second strut is configured to the same length as the first. The second strut is placed on top of the first in the same manner. Additional struts are utilized if enough room exists. If an iliac crest graft is chosen, it is usually used as single inlay graft.

It is preferable to keep the anterior longitudinal ligament intact to prevent overdistraction and to provide a pocket for additional bone graft to be placed. Mor-

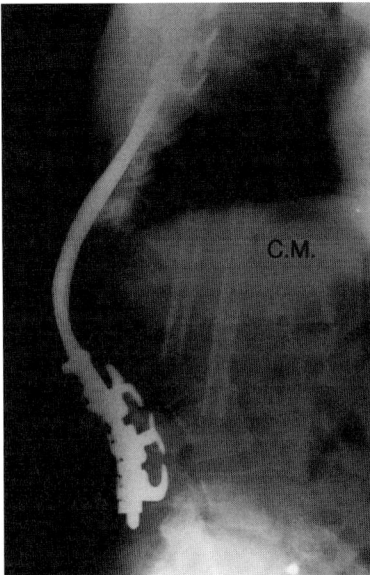

Figure 12 A lateral radiograph of a 36-year-old woman with spinal tuberculosis and subsequent sever kyphosis. Two long fibular allograft struts are inserted in an inlay fashion into troughs developed in the vertebral bodies inline with the vertical sagittal axis. In severe kyphosis the struts will span across a few vertebrae as demonstrated.

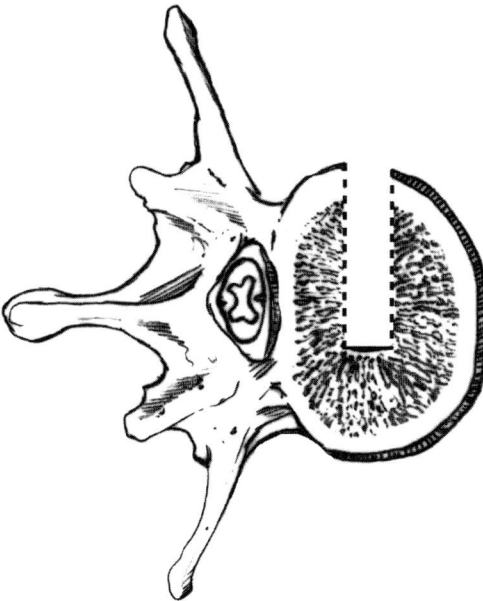

Figure 13 As shown in the drawing, troughs are made in the vertebral bodies above and below the corpectomy site to accommodate the future strut graft. The trough is typically made to extend two-thirds the lateral width of the vertebral body.

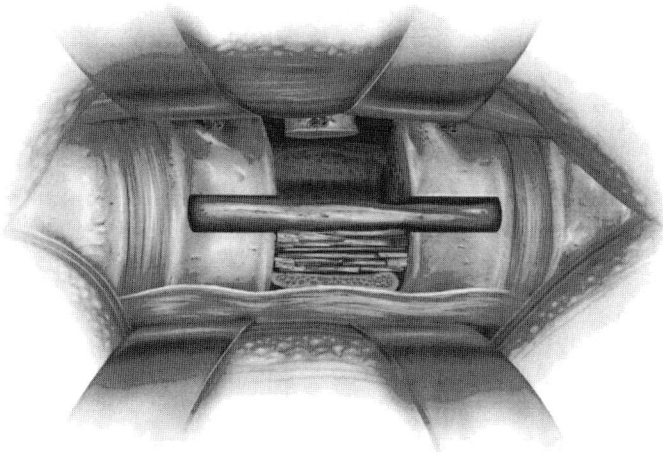

Figure 14 In this drawing, the load-sharing strut graft is placed into the troughs in the superior and inferior vertebral bodies spanning the corpectomy site. Morselized bone graft is placed anterior to the strut graft and beneath any remaining anterior vertebral body wall.

selized bone graft is packed anterior to the inlayed strut up against the remaining anterior vertebral body and anterior longitudinal ligament (Fig. 14). The remaining anterior vertebral body acts as a vascularized bone bed providing an osteoinductive source to the arthrodesis construct. The packed morselized bone helps to secure the inlayed graft. The inlayed load-sharing strut is now quite secure within the anterior and posterior walls of the host's vertebral bodies, which prevents it from kicking out anteriorly or posteriorly into the spinal canal. Since the inlayed strut is sitting on cancellous vertebral bone, it is expected that a small amount of subsidence will occur. It is imperative, therefore, that the troughs are long enough within the adjacent vertebral bodies to prevent excess subsidence and not too long as to violate the far endplate of the vertebral body

It is usually necessary to augment this grafting technique with posterior instrumentation. Cutting a trough in the vertebral body can occasionally result in a fracture of the vertebral wall or endplate. Thus, the strength of the posterior spinal instrumentation is critical. If pedicular posterior instrumentation is used, care should be taken not to displace the anterior struts with a transversing screw. A hook system placed in a claw configuration can also be used.

Finally, an attractive alternative is a combination of both techniques described above: combining the keyed fit of an inlayed strut and its increased osteogenic potential with the endplate support of a load-bearing strut. Using this type of construct, the troughs can be made smaller and the load-bearing strut can be fashioned in a tongue-and-groove fashion to also fit within the trough.

REFERENCES

1. Guttmann L. Surgical aspects of the treatment of traumatic paraplegia. J Bone Joint Surg 1949; 31B:339–403.

2. Nicoll EA. Fractures of the dorso-lumbar spine. J Bone Joint Surg 1949; 31B:376–394.

3. Stranger JK. Fracture-dislocation of thoracolumbar spine. With special reference to reduction by open and closed operations. J Bone Joint Surg 1947; 29:107–118.

4. Albee FH. Transplantation of a portion of the tibia into the spine for Pott's disease: A preliminary report. J Am Med Assoc 1911; 57:885–886.

5. Hibbs RA. An operation for progressive spinal deformities: A preliminary report of three cases form the service of the orthopaedic hospital. NYork Med J 1911; 93:1013–1016.

6. Holdsworth FW. Fractures, dislocations and fracture-dislocations of the spine. J Bone Joint Surg 1970; 52:1534–1551.

7. Bagby GW. Arthrodesis by the distraction-compression method using a stainless steel implant. Orthopedics 1988; 11:931–944.

8. Cloward RB. Lesions of the intervertebral disks and their treatment by fusion methods: The painful disk. Clin Orthop 1963; 27:51–77.

9. Cloward RB. The treatment of ruptured lumbar intervertebral disks by vertebral body fusion. J Neurosurg 1953; 10:154.

10. Crock HV. Anterior lumbar interbody fusion. Clin Orthop 1982; 165:157–163.

11. Harmon PH. Anterior excision and vertebral body fusion operation for intervertebral disk syndromes of the lower lumbar spine: Three to five year results in 244 cases. Clin Orthopaed 1963; 26:107–127.

12. Hodgson AR, Stock FE, Fang HSY, Ong GB. Anterior spine fusion: The operative approach and pathologic findings in 412 patients with Pott's disease of the spine. Br J Surg 1960; 48:172–178.

13. Hoover NW. Methods of lumbar fusion. J Bone Joint Surg 1968; 50A:194–209.

14. Kaneda K, Abumi K, Fujiya M. Burst fractures with neurologic deficits of the thoracolumbar spine. Results of anterior decompression and stabilization with anterior instrumentation. Spine 1984; 9(8):788–795.

15. Stauffer RN, Coventry MB. Anterior interbody lumbar spine fusion. J Bone Joint Surg 1972; 54A:756–768.

16. Wiltberger BR. Intervertebral body fusion by the use of posterior bone dowel. Clin Orthop 1964; 35:69–79.

17. Kaneda K, Taneichi H, Abumi K, Hashimoto T, Satoh S, Fujiya M. Anterior decompression and stabilization with the Kaneda device for thoracolumbar burst fractures associated with neurologic deficits. J Bone Joint Surg 1997; 79(A):69–83.

18. Bradford DS, McBride GG. Surgical management of thoracolumbar spine fractures with incomplete neurologic deficits. Clin Orthop 1987; 218:201–216.

19. Dunn, HK. Anterior stabilization of thoracolumbar injuries. Clin Orthopaed Related Res 1984; 189:116–124.

20. Haas N, Blauth M, Tscherne H. Anterior plating in thoracolumbar spine injuries. Indications, techniques and results. Spine 1991; 16(3 Suppl):s100–111.

21. McAfee PC, Bohlman HH, Yuan HA. Anterior decompression of traumatic thoracolumbar fractures with incomplete neurological deficit using a retroperitoneal approach. J Bone Joint Surg 1985; 67(A):89–104.

22. Bridwell KH, Lenke LG McEnery KW, Baldus C, Blanke K. Anterior structural allografts in thoracic and lumbar spine. Spine 1995; 20:1410–1418.

23. DeWald CJ, Mardjetko SM, Hammerberg KW, DeWald RL. Anterior spinal column reconstruction using the MOSS titanium mesh cage. Presented at NASS annual meeting, Minneapolis, 1994.

24. Singh K, DeWald CJ, Hammerberg KW, DeWald RL. Long segment structural allografts in the management of large anterior spinal column defects. Clin Orthop (in press).

25. Kaneda K, Asano S, Hashimoto T, Satoh S, Fujiya M. The treatment of osteoporotic-posttraumatic vertebral collapse using the Kaneda device and a bioactive ceramic vertebral prosthesis. Spine 1992; 17(8):295–303.

26. Kaneda K. Reconstruction with a ceramic vertebral prosthesis and Kaneda device following subtotal or total vertebrectomy in metastatic thoracic and lumbar spine. In: Bridewell KH, DeWald RL, eds. The Textbook of Spinal Surgery. Philadelphia: JB Lippincott, 1997.

27. Merk H, Koch H, Liebau C, Baltzer A, Dragendorf L, Grasshoff H. (Implantation of a Harms titanium mesh cylinder for vertebral body replacement in spinal metastases) (German). Z Orthop Ihre Grenzgebiete 2000; 138(2):169–173.

28. Lee SW, Lim TH, You JW, An HS. Biomechanical effect of the anterior grafting devices on the rotational stability of spinal constructs. J Spinal Disord 2000; 13(2):150–155.

29. Hollowell JP, Vollmer DG, Wilson CR, Pintar, FA, Yoganandan N. Biochemical analysis of thoracolumbar interbody constructs. How important is the endplate? Spine 1996; 21(9):1032–1036.

30. Bradford DS, Ganjavian S, Antonious D, Winter RB, Lonstein JE, Moe JH. Anterior strut grafting for the treatment of kyphosis. Review of experience with forty-eight patients. J Bone Joint Surg 1982; 64A:680–90.

31. Bradford DS, Winter RB, Lonestein JE, Moe JH: Techniques of anterior spine surgery for the management of kyphosis. Clinical Orthop 1977; 128:129–139.

32. Cotler HB, Cotler JM, Stoloff A, et al. The use of autografts for vertebral body replacement of the thoracic and lumbar spine. Spine 1985; 10(8):748–756.

43

Management of Spine Fractures in Special Conditions: Ankylosing Spondylitis

MICHAEL J. BOLESTA

University of Texas Southwestern Medical Center, Dallas, Texas, U.S.A.

GLENN R. RECHTINE

University of Florida, Gainesville, Florida, U.S.A.

I PATHOPHYSIOLOGY OF ANKYLOSING SPONDYLITIS

Ankylosing spondylitis is an inflammatory enthesopathy that has a predilection for males. It does not follow simple Mendelian genetics, but the predisposition to the disorder is inherited. Many, but not all, patients with ankylosing spondylitis are HLA-B27 positive. Conversely all individuals who are HLA-B27 positive do not develop this disorder, indicating variable penetration and the role of yet unknown environmental factors that modulate the expression of the genetic substrate.

It typically begins with axial pain and stiffness, which is worse in the morning. All radiographs are initially normal. The first site of radiographic abnormality is usually the sacroiliac joint. The joint surfaces become irregular and then later will fuse, a harbinger of the spine's fate.

The disease follows a variable course. In the early phases, individuals will find relief with anti-inflammatory medication and positioning. Knowledgeable primary care providers and rheumatologists will wisely counsel patients to avoid pillows beneath the head and lower extremities to prevent loss of cervical and lumbar lordosis. Although this flexed posture is more comfortable for patients in the early and middle phases of the disease, fusion in this position is biomechanically disastrous. It places the center of gravity anterior to the sacrum and predisposes the patient to a progressive chin-on-chest deformity and a stooped posture.

In the late phase, the inflammation subsides. In milder forms of the disorder, spinal mobility is preserved. Spinal fusion occurs in the final stage of fully expressed ankylosing spondylitis. The properly managed patient will be erect with the head centered over the pelvis. If lumbar and cervical lordosis have been maintained along with normal kyphosis, the risk of developing secondary deformity is low. Those who fuse in a poor position may not suffer an acute fracture but the ankylosed spine is paradoxically weak from associated osteoporosis (1–3). Although it is radiographically fused, stress fractures occur and result in gradual remodeling and progressive cervical or thoracic kyphosis. Studies of individuals in the early phase of the disease demonstrate reduced bone mineral density as compared to age-matched controls (2,3). This osteoporosis likely results from a hyperemia of the inflammatory enthesopathy. The inflammation involves the ligamentous attachments to the spinal column with relative sparing of the appendicular skeleton. Coxarthrosis sufficient to warrant a total hip arthroplasty is an exception to this general rule. The measured osteoporosis occurs both in the lumbar spine and the femoral neck (2,3), but involves the thoracic and cervical spine as well.

Studies of patients with advanced disease and widespread ankylosis also have osteoporosis. When measured by DEXA, bone mineral density in the femoral neck is decreased but is increased or normal in the lumbar spine (2). This is factitious as the flowing osteophytes of the typical bamboo spine falsely elevate the measured density. The spine is osteoporotic and stiff, which prevents unique challenges when fractures occur. Not all patients' progress to total ankylosis, but even severely involved individuals usually retain motion at the occipitocervical and atlantoaxial articulations. Since all motion occurs at these levels, some individuals will develop instability of the occipitocervical or atlantoaxial joints.

II FRACTURES IN ANKYLOSING SPONDYLITIS

Fractures in the patient with ankylosing are unique in many ways. They can occur at any level of the spine but, like adults without ankylosing spondylitis, there is a high incidence in the lower cervical, cervicothoracic, and thoracolumbar junctions (4–8). Unlike the normal spine where externally applied moments may be dissipated through normal adjacent segments, the ankylosed spine resembles a diaphyseal injury in a long bone. The long lever arms involved generate large forces. Even physiological loading may result in late displacement.

Another factor unique to these individuals is the presence of osteoporosis, which is advanced relative to age-matched controls (1–3). Osteoporotic bone does heal but makes internal fixation more challenging.

As in their normal counterparts, fracture may occur in the setting of high-energy trauma (8). In this setting, displacement and neurological injury are more common. As in normal counterparts, the clinician must be alert to the presence of other fractures at noncontiguous levels (5,9).

Because of the many factors discussed already, fracture can occur with low-energy, even trivial, trauma (4,7,8,10,11). Displacement is less likely in the acute phase, although displacement can occur because of the long lever arms. The osteopenia and occurrence of many injuries at the cervical thoracic junction make the diagnosis difficult. Since these individuals often have chronic pain, they may not seek attention or health care providers may dismiss the new complaints (10). Hence, the diagnosis may be delayed (9,10,12).

Third, stress fractures can occur in these osteoporotic individuals (8). When the spine ankyloses in an unfavorable position, these insufficiency fractures will often heal but recur, leading to a gradual, but progressive kyphosis. They do not invariably heal, however, and the nonunion can be characterized by sufficient osteolysis as to simulate a malignant process (13). These insufficiency fractures are mentioned for completeness but are outside the purview of this text.

One unique component of spinal fracture in this group of patients is a much higher incidence of clinically significant epidural hematomata (14–16). This likely represents a combination of multiple factors. The osteoporosis itself leads to more bleeding, probably from the reduced bone volume and relative increase in hemopoietic and vascular tissue. Another factor is the long lever arms leading to increased motion and clot instability. In the setting of low-energy trauma, the surrounding soft-tissue envelope is not disrupted. The blood cannot dissipate into the surrounding tissues and enter the spinal canal instead. This may lead to spinal cord compression. In the absence of coagulopathy, significant epidural hematoma producing a neurological deficit is unusual in a spine without ankylosis.

Less well recognized but highlighted in a recent report is disk herniation contributing to neurological dysfunction (14). The onset of ankylosing spondylitis occurs in young adulthood, often before significant disk degeneration and narrowing can occur. Hence, the trauma can occur through and about relatively preserved disks, which can then herniate with cord compression. This may be concomitant with a large epidural hematoma (14).

Fractures in osteoporotic bone are notoriously difficult to diagnose, particularly if there is minimal displacement or in a region of the spine difficult to image, such as the cervicothoracic junction. Larger individuals are also more challenging. In the trauma setting, it is more difficult to image the lower cervical spine in a supine patient. CT scan is used in many trauma centers to image the spine when plain radiographs are inadequate but can miss fractures in the transverse plane, particularly minimally displaced ones.

Surgical reconstructions may be helpful when there is a neurological deficit. Intrathecal contrast will also provide useful information in this setting.

Bone scan should be considered if plain radiographs and CT are equivocal. The clinician should be aware of false negatives, however.

MRI may be the modality of choice for diagnosis of occult fractures in ankylosing spondylitis (17). Marrow edema will be noted early after injury. The preferred sequences are the inversion recovery fat suppression or the diffusion weighted image. Furthermore, MRI will easily diagnose epidural hematoma as well as status of the spinal cord.

Spinal cord injury is the most severe complication in this group of patients. In one series, one-third presented with a significant neurological deficit (8). Another third developed spinal cord injury in delayed fashion. This reflects the long lever arm, the potential for late displacement, as well as the development of large epidural hematoma.

Clinically, these individuals have chronic spinal pain. Given the fragility and potential of the ankylosed spine for late neurological catastrophe, all patients with advanced ankylosing spondylitis who present with any history of trauma and complaints of new or worsened spinal pain must be presumed to have a fracture until proven otherwise (Fig. 1) (9,10,12). Multiple radiographic modalities should be employed and the patient's spine immobilized throughout the evaluation. Individuals with preexisting deformity pose an unusual challenge in immobilization. The standard teaching is to immobilize them in their premorbid alignment. No attempts should be made to realign the kyphotic cervicothoracic spine lest the clinician produce a fracture dislocation or epidural hematoma with significant, often irreversible, quadriplegia. Family members and friends may be able to provide photographs of the patient, which will aid immobilization in the proper position. In the cervical spine, halo traction may be used with the minimal amount of weight necessary to support the head. Disimpaction of the fracture and overdistraction will produce dangerous instability. The entire spinal column must be assessed, looking for noncontiguous injuries.

III MANAGEMENT OF SPINAL FRACTURE IN ANKYLOSING SPONDYLITIS

This is one of the more controversial areas. Advanced ankylosing spondylitis is a rare condition and reported series are small. Proponents of both nonoperative and operative management can be found.

A Nonoperative

Cervical and cervicothoracic injuries, which are nondisplaced and neurologically intact, may be managed with kinetic bed therapy (Roto-Rest bed) initially. Once evaluation is complete and discomfort has subsided, the patient may be converted to a halo ring and vest (8,14). This is most applicable in individuals who have mild to no premorbid deformity.

Cervical injuries in the deformed patient may be managed in halo traction as mentioned above. Care must be taken to avoid disimpaction or distraction of the fracture, as that may destabilize the spine and may increase epidural bleeding (14). The vector of the halo traction should place the head in the premorbid condition. Nursing care is quite challenging. Pulmonary toilet must be aggressive given the restrictive lung disease from ankylosis of the rib cage. Several weeks of immobilization are necessary before converting to a halo cast. Off-the-shelf vests will not fit these individuals. No attempt is made to correct the cervicothoracic kyphosis. Some authors suggest that correction may be performed gradually (14).

Thoracic injuries are good candidates for kinetic bed therapy lasting 4 to 6 weeks, followed by orthotic management until clinical and radiographic healing is complete (18,19). This may not be possible if the patient has significant cervical or thoracic kyphosis. Standard bedrest with meticulous nursing care may be an option, but surgery with internal fixation may be preferable in this subgroup of patients.

Another indication for nonsurgical management is the patient with severe medical comorbidities. Patients with ankylosing spondylitis, complete spinal cord injury presenting late may also be candidates for nonsurgical treatment, particularly if they have developed other complications, such as pneumonia and pressure ulceration in the region of the potential stabilization.

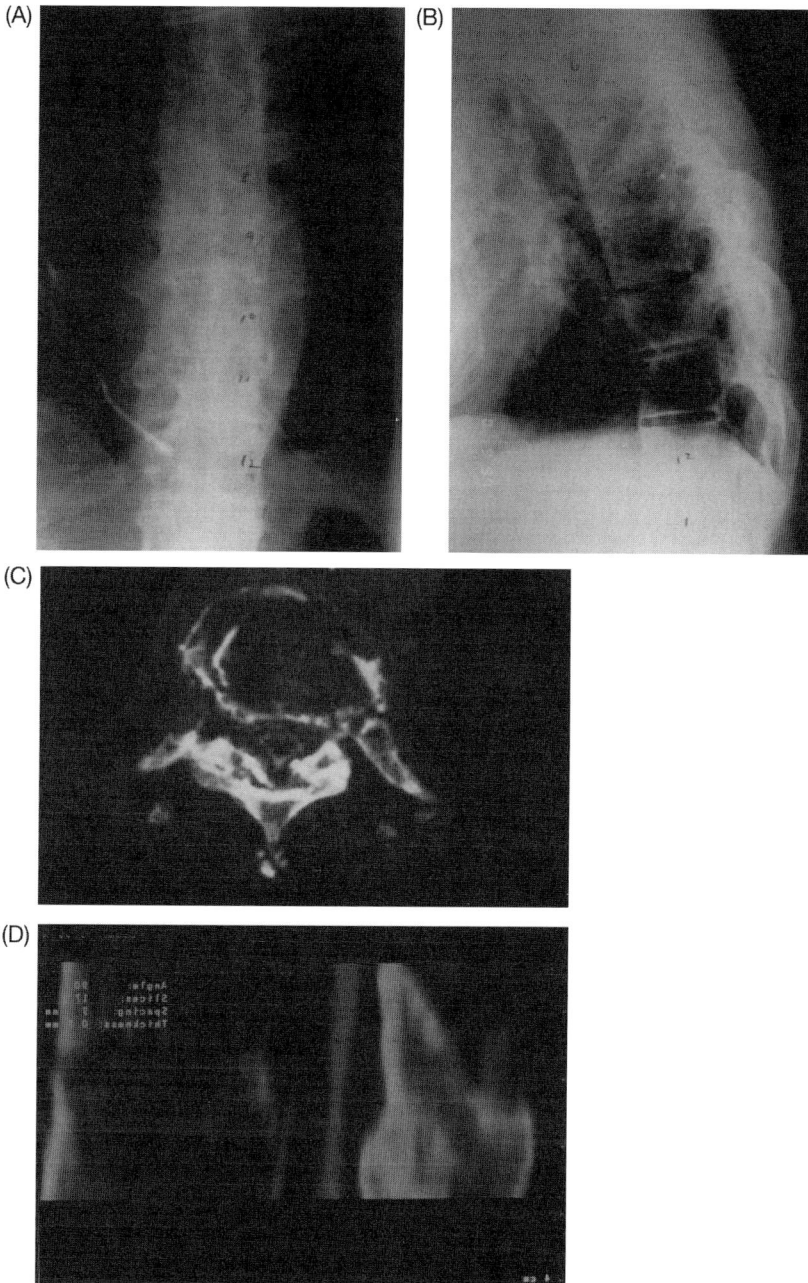

Figure 1   (A) An anteroposterior view of a 79-year-old man with long-standing ankylosing spondylitis who fell while cutting down a tree several weeks prior to presentation. He complained of back pain and was ambulatory. He fractured through the T9–10 disk space. Note the paravertebral hematoma. His pacemaker precluded a MRI. (B) On the lateral radiograph, the fracture is minimally displaced. (C) CT through the fracture demonstrating narrowing of the thecal sac. (D) Minimal displacement of the fracture with suggestion of an epidural hematoma constricting the thecal sac. The treating physicians placed patient in a TLSO.

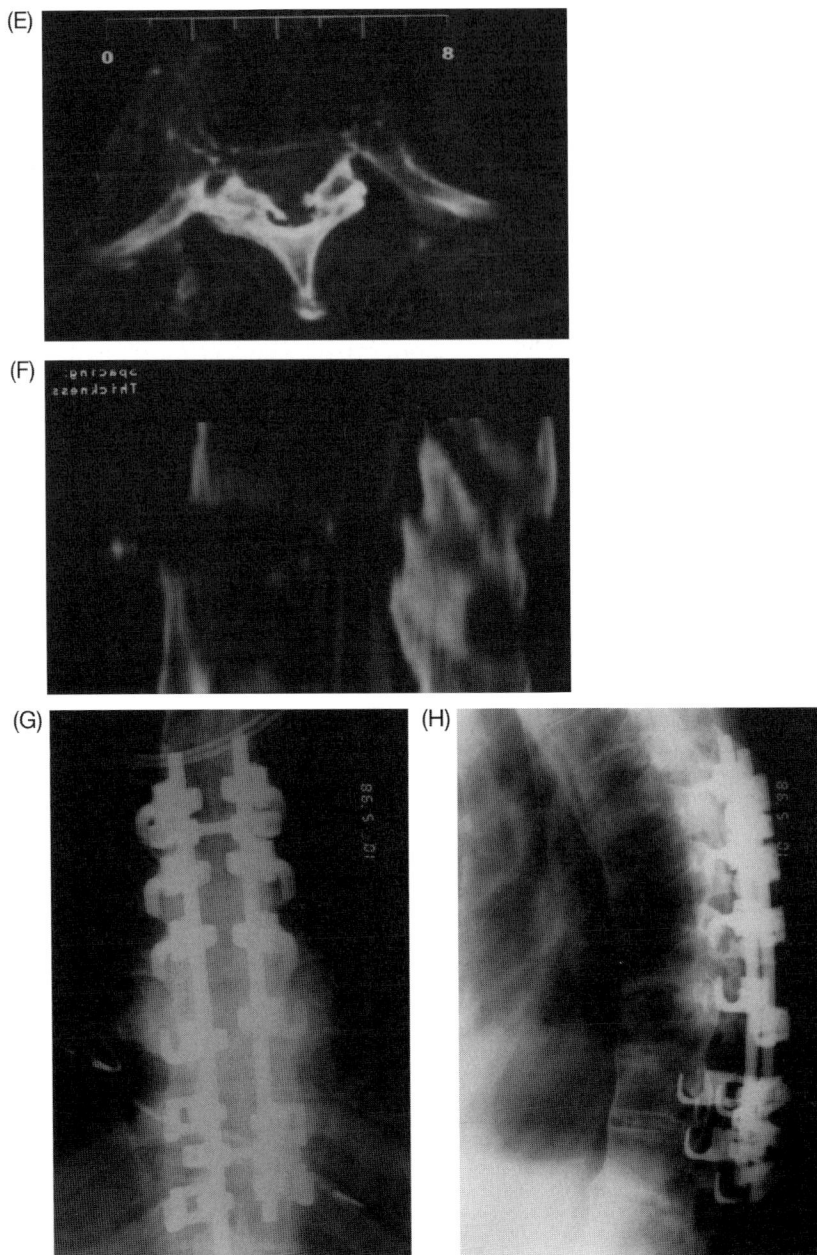

Figure 1 (E) Five days later, patient was noted to be paraparetic and unable to walk. CT with intrathecal contrast shows no dye at the level of the fracture. (F) Sagittal reformatting reveals posterior translation and distraction through the fracture with cord compression. Patient was transferred for operative management, where he underwent posterior decompression and stabilization. Organizing hematoma was found to contribute to the neural compression. (G) An anteroposterior view 1 year postoperatively. (H) The lateral radiograph shows fracture reduction and healing. The patient regained near normal strength in his lower extremities, but ambulation was limited because of persistent dorsal column dysfunction.

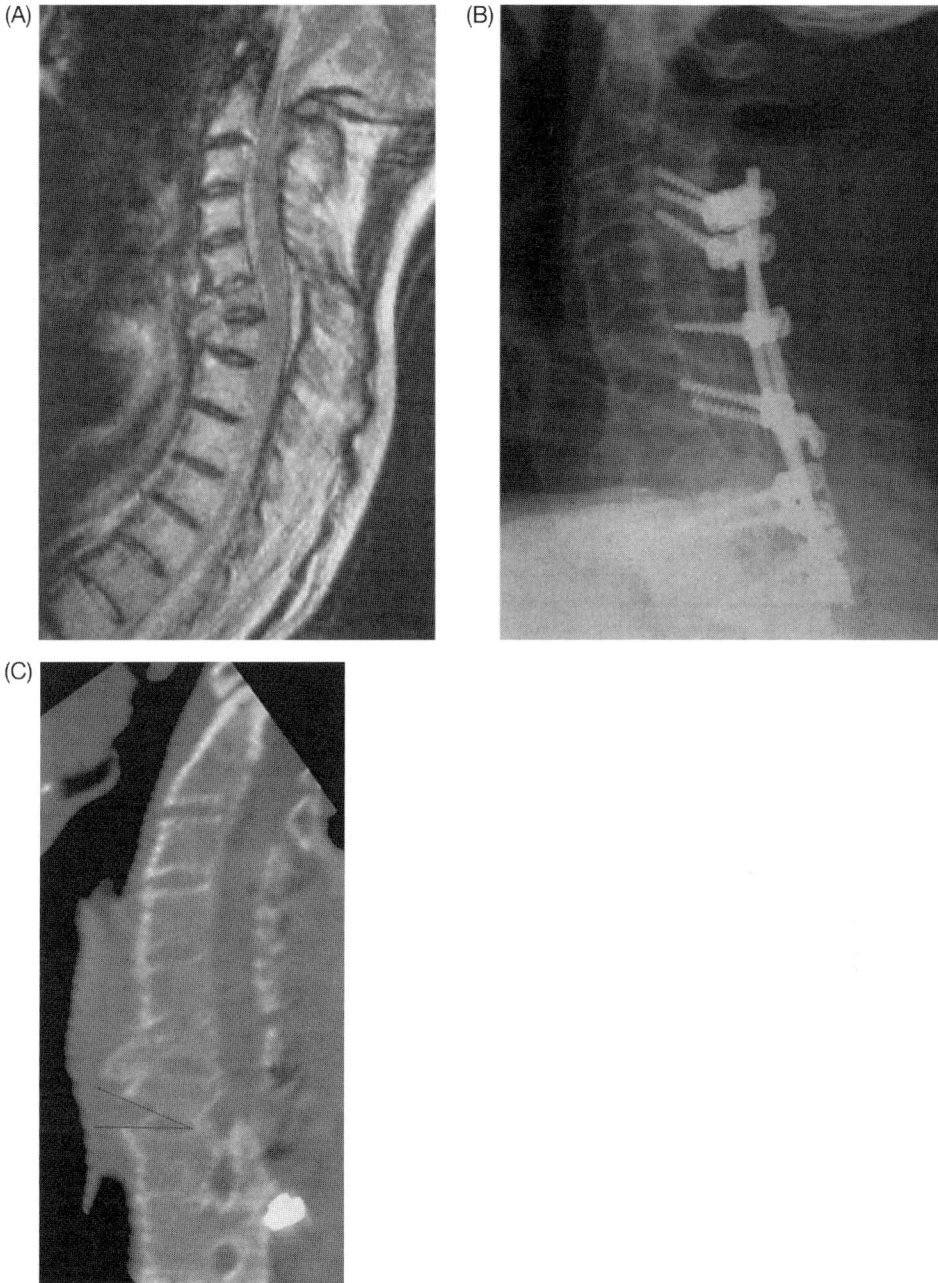

Figure 2   (A) Sagittal MRI of a 42-year-old male with ankylosing spondylitis who had been in a fight 6 months prior to the study. He complained of neck pain and increasing deformity. Bone scan was normal. He was followed for 2 months and strongly urged to cease all tobacco use. The MRI was ordered when he developed hyperreflexia and LE instability. There are fractures of C6 and C7, and kyphosis. (B) Postoperative lateral radiograph following an osteotomy at C7–T1. The kyphosis has been corrected. (C) Postoperative sagittal reconstruction demonstrating 30-degree correction.

Nonoperative management in the paralyzed patient with ankylosing spondylitis may have significantly shorter length of stay and, therefore, a significantly lower cost of care (20).

B   Operative Management

Indications for surgery include widely displaced fractures, unstable fracture, those associated with a progressive neurological deficit, those with a large epidural hematoma, incomplete spinal cord injury, and patients with significant deformity (5,8,14,21). Severely deformed patients may not be amenable to bedrest or orthotic management; they are not simple to position for surgery either. Depending on the level of the fracture, some surgeons would consider concomitant correction of deformity, although this is controversial.

Injuries may be approached anteriorly or posteriorly, although most reports are with posterior fixation. The advantage of the posterior approach is the ability to expose a large segment of the spine and obtain fixation at multiple segments. Since the ligamentum flavum is also ossified and the facet joints ankylosed, traditional hook sites in the thoracic spine are not available. Multiple transverse process hooks are an option. Transpedicular instrumentation and spinous process wires are also possibilities. In the cervical spine, lateral mass fixation is a good option (Fig. 2).

The anterior approach may be useful for some displaced fractures, some cervical injuries, and perhaps for decompression (8). The attendant osteoporosis severely limits the quality of fixation. Anterior instrumentation alone is probably insufficient in the cervical, thoracic, and lumbar spine. If an anterior approach is used, it is usually supplemented with a posterior approach. Again, however, the amount of published data is very limited. These statements are based on the known quality of the bone, the limitation of modern anterior devices and clinical biomechanics.

Regardless of the instrumentation, most clinicians would favor additional support in the form of an orthosis or cast for at least 6 to 12 weeks and probably longer. The standard complications seen with operative management are present in this group of patients. A more difficult problem is that of osteoporosis. Loss of fixation is a significant threat best addressed by multiple points of fixation intraoperatively and protecting the patient postoperatively with the orthoses until there is definite radiographic evidence of healing and clinical reduction if not absence of pain. In summary, this is a very challenging group of patients both in diagnosis and management. It is a rare condition and may benefit from referral to a spinal trauma center (8).

REFERENCES

1. Cooper C, Carbone L, Michet CJ, Atkinson EJ, O'Fallon WM, Melton LJ, 3rd. Fracture risk in patients with ankylosing spondylitis: a population based study. J Rheumatol 1994; 21:1877–1882.
2. Donnelly S, Doyle DV, Denton A, Rolfe I, McCloskey EV, Spector TD. Bone mineral density and vertebral compression fracture rates in ankylosing spondylitis. Ann Rheum Dis 1994; 53:117–121.
3. Mitra D, Elvins DM, Speden DJ, Collins AJ. The prevalence of vertebral fractures in mild ankylosing spondylitis and their relationship to bone mineral density. Rheumatology (Oxford) 2000; 39:85–89.

4. Bernd L, Blasius K, Lukoschek M. Spinal fractures in ankylosing spondylitis. Z Orthop Ihre Grenzgeb 1992; 130:59–63.
5. Fox MW, Onofrio BM, Kilgore JE. Neurological complications of ankylosing spondylitis. J Neurosurg 1993; 78:871–878.
6. Kiwerski J, Bobryk A, Wozniak E. Spinal fracture in the course of spondylarthritis ankylopoietica (Bechterew disease). Chir Narzadow Ruchu Ortop Pol 1990; 55:23–30.
7. Kovacs Z, Siko I, Vajda O. Fracture of the lower thoracic spine in ankylosing spondylitis. Magy Traumatol Orthop Helyreallito Seb 1992; 35:305–309.
8. Olerud C, Frost A, Bring J. Spinal fractures in patients with ankylosing spondylitis. Eur Spine J 1996; 5:51–55.
9. Finkelstein JA, Chapman JR, Mirza S. Occult vertebral fractures in ankylosing spondylitis. Spinal Cord 1999; 37:444–447.
10. Hunter T, Forster B, Dvorak M. Ankylosed spines are prone to fracture. Can Fam Physician 1995; 41:1213–1216.
11. Karasick D, Schweitzer ME, Abidi NA, Cotler JM. Fractures of the vertebrae with spinal cord injuries in patients with ankylosing spondylitis: imaging findings. Am J Roentgenol 1995; 165:1205–1208.
12. Milicic A, Jovanovic A, Milankov M, Savic D, Stankovic M. Fractures of the spine in patients with ankylosing spondylitis. Med Pregl 1995; 48:429–431.
13. Albertsen AM, Jurik AG. Posttraumatic spinal osteolysis in ankylosing spondylitis as part of pseudoarthrosis. A case report. Acta Radiol 1996; 37:98–100.
14. Rowed DW. Management of cervical spinal cord injury in ankylosing spondylitis: the intervertebral disc as a cause of cord compression. J Neurosurg 1992; 77:241–246.
15. Van de Straete S, Demaerel P, Stockx L, Nuttin B. Spinal epidural hematoma and ankylosing spondylitis. J Belge Radiol 1997; 80:109–110.
16. Wozniak E, Bronarski J. Injuries of the cervical spine and spinal cord in patients with ankylosing spondylitis—diagnosis using magnetic resonance imaging. Chir Narzadow Ruchu Ortop Pol 1995; 60:353–358.
17. Iplikcioglu AC, Bayar MA, Kokes F, Gokcek C, Doganay OS. Magnetic resonance imaging in cervical trauma associated with ankylosing spondylitis: report of two cases. J Trauma 1994; 36:412–413.
18. Hartman MB, Chrin AM, Rechtine GR. Non-operative treatment of thoracolumbar fractures. Paraplegia 1995; 33:73–76.
19. Rechtine GR, II, Cahill D, Chrin AM. Treatment of thoracolumbar trauma: comparison of complications of operative versus nonoperative treatment. J Spinal Disord 1999; 12:406–409.
20. Apple DF, Jr, Anson C. Spinal cord injury occurring in patients with ankylosing spondylitis: a multicenter study. Orthopedics 1995; 18:1005–1011.
21. Hertlein H, Schams S, Lob G. Extension-distraction injury of the lumbar spine in Bechterew's disease. Unfallchirurgie 1991; 17:259–263.

44

Spinal Injuries in the Setting of Diffuse Idiopathic Skeletal Hyperostosis

LOUIS G. QUARTARARO and ALEXANDER R. VACCARO

Thomas Jefferson University Hospital and the Rothman Institute, Philadelphia, Pennsylvania, U.S.A.

JOHN J. CARBONE

Johns Hopkins Bayview Hospital, Baltimore, Maryland, U.S.A.

I   INTRODUCTION

Diffuse idiopathic skeletal hyperostosis (DISH), as its name implies, is a condition characterized by a generalized (diffuse) abundant ossification of ligaments (skeletal hyperostosis) of unknown etiology (idiopathic). The spine is the most commonly affected area of the body. The longitudinal ligaments of the spine, in particular the anterior longitudinal ligament (ALL), are most often affected. Exuberant ossification and bony spurring is also seen at ligament and tendon insertions throughout the body. In particular, DISH patients demonstrate calcifications at ligamentous insertions involving the iliac crests in 66% of patients, and the ischial tuberosities, lesser trochanters, and greater trochanters in 53%, 42%, and 36%, respectively.

II   PREVALENCE

Other than a slight decrease in the range of motion of the spine, DISH is often asymptomatic, and thus most affected patients are unaware of it. The incidence of DISH in the general population has been studied in autopsy and radiographic studies (1,2). The prevalence of DISH in males over 50 years is 25%, and in females over 50 is 15%. In the over-70 population, males display a prevalence of 35% and females

26%. DISH is less commonly seen in African-American and Native-American populations (2).

III RADIOGRAPHY

The classic radiographic description of diffuse idiopathic skeletal hyperostosis describes flowing calcification or ossification of the anterolateral margin of at least four contiguous vertebral bodies (Fig. 1). In addition, there must be preservation of disk height in the involved areas and absence of sclerosis or fusion of the sacroiliac joints (3). This is important in distinguishing DISH from ankylosing spondylitis, a condition appearing similar on x-ray, but having fused SI joints.

Interestingly, the calcifications are seen anterolaterally, on the right side only. It is believed that the pulsating of the aorta precludes formation of calcifications on the left side. This is supported by the observation that patients with situs-inversus have left-sided calcifications.

Thoracic vertebrae are involved in 100% of DISH patients, with the lumbar segments involved 68 to 90% of the time and the cervical segments 65 to 78% of the time.

IV PATHOPHYSIOLOGY

DISH, in its earliest stages, involves ossification of the ALL adjacent to the mid-portion of the vertebral bodies. As the calcification becomes more extensive, it forms anteriorly directed, irregularly shaped, strong, thick bony bridges of the disk space, anchored firmly to the proximal and distal thirds of each vertebral body. The middle third of the body is thus the weak link, and is understandably the most vulnerable to traumatic forces. Therefore, most fractures occur through the vertebral bodies. Fractures have been reported at the ends of solidly fused segments, and, less commonly, through the disk space (4).

In contrast, ankylosing spondylitis patients demonstrate ossification at the periphery of the vertebral body, extending toward the annulus fibrosis, forming bridging syndesmophytes. Chondroid metaplasia and disk calcification result in weakening of the disk space. It is thus the area most prone to fracture in these patients, distinguishing it from DISH.

The distinction between DISH and ankylosing spondylitis is important for several reasons. Ankylosing spondylitis patients sustain more fractures than DISH patients. However, DISH patients have an increased incidence of spinal cord damage because of the presence of juxtaposed, rigidly fused spinal segments. These segments produce longer lever arms, and are highly unstable. Minimal trauma has been shown to produce fractures in these patients. This population must be carefully evaluated using advanced imaging modalities such as CT and/or MRI after seemingly minor accidents, for spinal fracture (3,5–7).

V MECHANISM OF INJURY

Hyperextension fractures of the thoracolumbar spine, although rare in a normal individual, are the main fracture mechanism in the DISH patient. The long lever arms

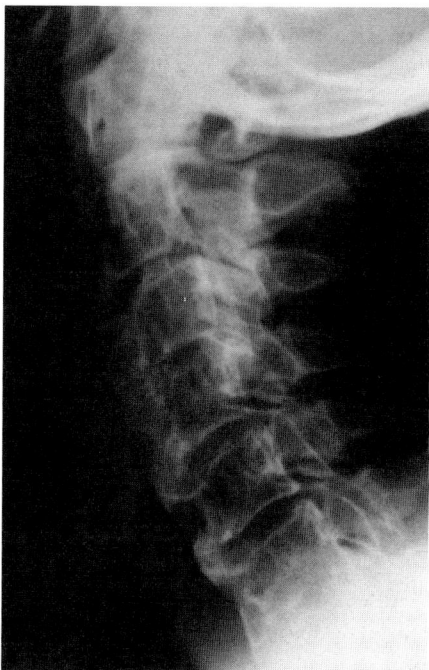

Figure 1 A lateral plain radiograph of the cervical spine revealing evidence of diffuse idiopathic skeletal hyperostosis. Note the flowing ossification involving the anterior longitudinal ligament with bridging osteophytes over the disk space with preservation of disk space height.

of the fused segments place high stresses on the anterior column, making it susceptible to failure under minimal forces (3,6–8).

VI   DIAGNOSIS

It is often difficult to demonstrate a spinal fracture in patients with DISH because of the excessive bone formation or associated osteoporosis. CT and/or MRI are therefore frequently useful in these patients with back pain, even after minor trauma. MRI is often a more sensitive modality for detecting vertebral body edema or disk disruption, as a CT scan with its gantry aligned in the plane of a fracture may miss nondisplaced transverse fractures.

VII   TREATMENT

There is relatively little written in the literature on the treatment of fractures in DISH patients. Any fracture suspected in such patients should be immediately immobilized and reduced, if necessary, especially when associated with neurological compromise (6,7,9). Displaced fractures, late diagnosis, nonunion, or osteolysis of the spine are further indications for stabilization (4).

Posterior segmental instrumentation is usually the mainstay of treatment in the common hyperextension-type fracture pattern seen in this patient population (Fig.

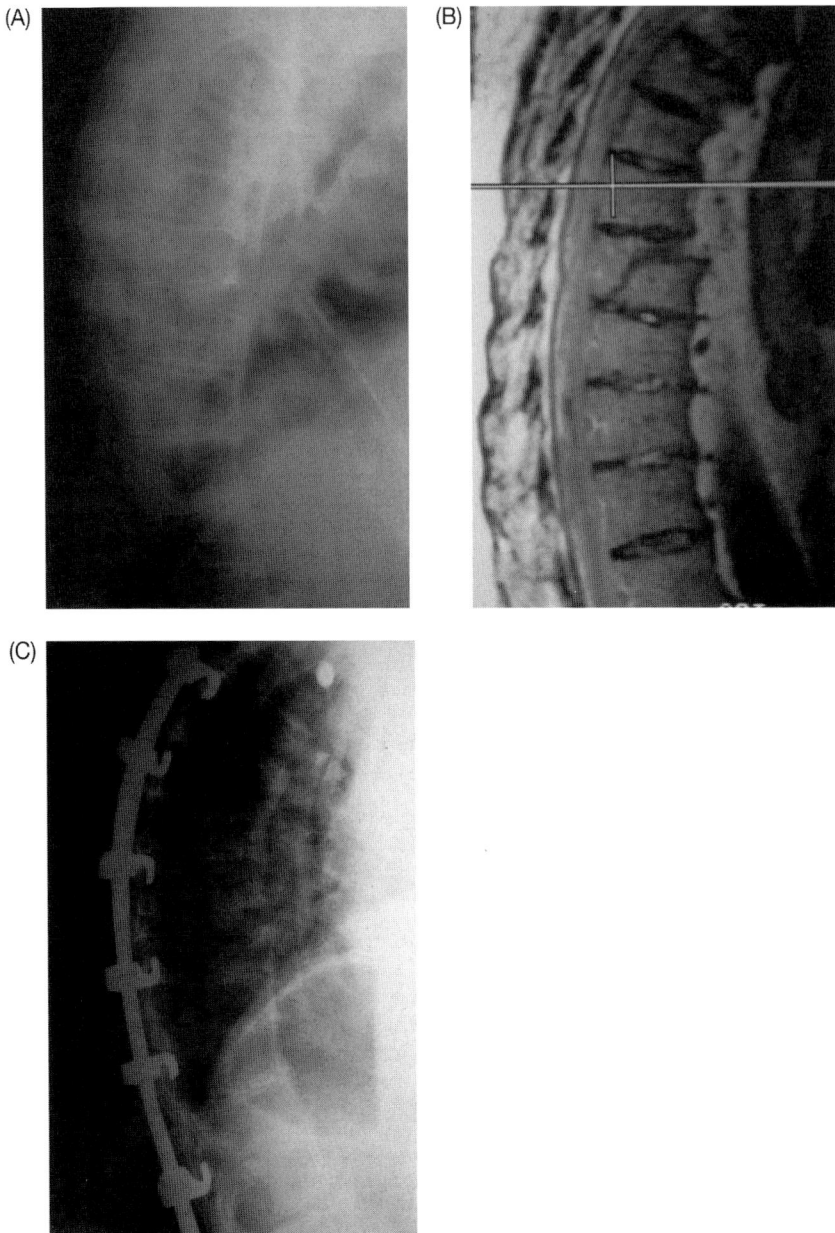

Figure 2 (A) Lateral plain radiograph of the thoracic spine demonstrating a distraction extension injury of the T7–T8 vertebral levels with fracture extension into the T8 body in a patient with diffuse idiopathic skeletal hyperostosis. (B) A sagittal plane MRI demonstrates clearly the fracture line traversing anteriorly through the T7–T8 disk space and coursing posteriorly into the T8 body. (C) The patient underwent closed postural reduction of his spinal fracture by prone positioning over lami-rolls, followed by a multisegmental posterior fixation involving rods and hooks to prevent any displacement at the fracture site.

2A–C). Great care must be taken in patient positioning so that further fracture displacement does not occur, resulting in neurological embarrasment. Any distraction of the spine should be avoided, due to the lack of competency of the anterior column (anterior longitudinal ligament). Even minimal distraction from anterior graft placement may lead to spinal cord tension, and possible neurocompromise. In situ fixation of the realigned spine is the technical strategy that should be sought.

Bracing alone is often ineffective in patients with displaced fractures because of the instability caused by the long lever arms of the adjacent spinal columns. Several studies have cited late spinal malalignment and neurological compromise with brace or cast treatment. In a study by Hendrix, two-thirds of patients in which the initial diagnosis and stabilization was delayed developed paraplegia (3). Burkus reviewed four patients with thoracolumbar spine fractures in the setting of DISH; three patients treated with a posterior spinal stabilization procedure went on to an uncomplicated fusion, while one patient treated in a brace incurred severe neurological deterioration and poor spinal algnment (9). However, some authors do recommend nonoperative treatment involving bedrest and brace treatment for stable, minimally displaced injuries (7).

VIII CONCLUSION

DISH is an ossifying spinal disorder common in the population. Relevant literature on the treatment of spine fractures in this group is minimal. Surgical intervention is the treatment of choice in displaced or unstable injuries. Patients presenting with back pain and DISH after minor trauma must be carefully worked up for an occult fracture, even in the presence of "negative" x-rays.

REFERENCES

1. Boachie-Adjei O, Bullough PG. Incidence of ankylosing hyperostosis of the spine (Forestier's disease) at autopsy. Spine 1987; 12(8):739–743.
2. Weinfeld RM, Olson PN, Maki DD, Griffiths HJ. The prevalence of diffuse idiopathic skeletal hyperostosis in two large American midwestern metropolitan hospital populations. Skeletal Radiol 1997; 26(4):222–225.
3. Hendrix RW, Melany M, Miller F, Rogers LF. Fracture of the spine in patients with ankylosis due to diffuse skeletal hyperostosis: Clinical and imaging findings. Am J Roentgenol 1994; 162(4):899–904.
4. Mikles MR, Vaccaro AR, Rau CM, Cotler JM, Balderston RA. The treatment of thoracolumbar spinal fractures in patients with diffuse idiopathic skeletal hyperostosis: A review. Jefferson Orthop J 1995; 24:41–44.
5. Colterjohn NR, Bednar DA. Identifiable risk factors for secondary neurologic deterioration in the cervical spine injured patient. Spine 1995; 20(21):2293–2297.
6. Meyer PR. Diffuse idiopathic skeletal hyperostosis in the cervical spine. Clin Orthop 1999; 359:49–57.
7. Paley D, Schwartz M, Cooper P, Harris WR, Levine AM. Fractures of the spine in diffuse idiopathic skeletal hyperostosis. Clin Orthop 1991; 267:22–32.
8. Israel Z, Moosheiff R, Gross E, Muggia-Sullam M, Floman Y. Hyperextension fracture-dislocation of the thoracic spine with paraplegia in a patient with diffuse idiopathic skeletal hyperostosis. J Spinal Disord 1994; 7(5):455–457.
9. Burkus JK, Denis F. Hyperextension injuries of the thoracic spine in diffuse idiopathic skeletal hyperostosis. A report of four cases. J Bone Joint Surg Am 1994; 76(2):237–243.

45

Klippel-Feil Syndrome

WILLIAM MITCHELL

Jefferson Medical College, Philadelphia, Pennsylvania, U.S.A.

GREGORY J. PRZYBYLSKI

Northwestern University, Chicago, Illinois, U.S.A.

Klippel-Feil syndrome (KFS) classically describes the patient with fused cervical vertebrae and the clinical triad of a short neck, low posterior hairline, and decreased range of motion of the neck. Although this constellation of attributes was originally recognized in 1912 (31,32), identification of the syndrome in additional patients facilitated development of a classification scheme based upon the extent of spinal fusion segments. Since only half of patients with KFS will have the classic triad, congenital fusion of two or more vertebrae has become synonymous with KFS. For example, patients with type I KFS have an extensive cervical and upper thoracic segmentation failure. In contrast, patients with type II KFS have only an isolated one- or two-segment fusion. Finally, patients with type III KFS have associated thoracic or lumbar fusion.

I EPIDEMIOLOGY

The actual incidence of KFS remains elusive, since many patients are asymptomatic. The prevalence of the disease is estimated to range from 0.02–0.7%, based upon a symptomatic population study (18), a cadaveric analysis (8), and a radiographic review (8). There is a slight female predilection of 1.5:1 and a variable age at presentation (18). Younger patients are typically diagnosed with KFS during evaluation of a spinal deformity from a large segmentation abnormality, a neurological deficit from a craniocervical abnormality, or incidentally during evaluation of an associated anomaly. In contrast, older patients present with neurological deficits or organ system dysfunction. However, the vertebral segmentation abnormalities often lead to identification of the syndrome. Rostral fusions often present earlier with pain (11), whereas caudal fusions manifest later in life from adjacent hypermobility or degenerative changes (20,34). Diminished cervical range of motion is common, occurring in 50 to 76% of patients with KFS. Typically, lateral bending and rotation are the most restricted motions (26,37,66). However, compensation from a hypermobile adjacent segment may account for the normal range of flexion and extension that may be observed. Although only 20% of patients will develop neurological symptoms before 5 years of age, nearly two-thirds will be symptomatic before age 30 (20).

In addition to vertebral abnormalities, 60% of patients will also have one or more associated anomalies in other organ systems (4). The most common anomalies involve the musculoskeletal, craniofacial, nervous, genitourinary, and cardiovascular systems (2,21,35,47). Segmentation occurs between the third and eighth week of fetal life, concurrent with developmental changes in these organ systems. Musculoskeletal anomalies include torticollis, scoliosis, kyphosis, Sprengel's deformity (failure of scapular descent), and rib anomalies. Congenital scoliosis can be seen in 60% of patients with KFS (18,20,26,63,66). Conversely, patients with congenital scoliosis and kyphosis have a 25% increased risk of segmentation defects of the cervical spine (25,49,68). Consequently, cervical spine radiographs should be obtained in patients with congenital scoliosis, as 20% will have KFS (69). Moreover, the compensatory curve has a high propensity to progress (24,26). Sprengel's deformity is seen in 20 to 50% of patients (18,20,26,37,66). Rib anomalies occur in one-third (20,37,66), with 15% involving cervical ribs (18,20,59). Craniofacial and neurological anomalies include hearing loss, deafness, and synkinesis. Moreover, 15 to 36% of patients with KFS have hearing dysfunction (26,37,66), which is usually sensorineural deafness. However, one-third may have conductive abnormalities from abnormal ossicles (29,38,47,58), and 15 to 20% of patients will have synkinesis (24,66). Significant renal abnormalities, typically unilateral renal agenesis, have been seen in 25 to 35% of patients with KFS (26,37,41,54,66). Finally, 14 to 29% of patients have cardiovascular abnormalities, many of which can be identified as a murmur on auscultation (26,66). Cardiovascular anomalies include ventricular or atrial septal defect, valvular abnormalities, and a persistent patent ductus arteriosus.

II PATHOGENESIS

Several theories about the pathogenesis of KFS have been proposed including vascular disruption, global fetal insult, primary neural tube abnormality, genetics, and facet segmentation failure. Although a subclavian artery disruption (7) could cause abnormal segmentation at 6 to 7 weeks of gestation, with sporadic incidence and variable findings including hearing abnormalities, this does not explain other abnormalities unrelated to subclavian disruption. A global fetal insult similar to VATER (5) may occur, given that KFS is nonrandom in nature and no single insult can account for its effects. Further support comes from a study in which one-third of rabbits subjected to hypoxia at 9 to 11 days of gestation developed vertebral anomalies (10). Overdistention of the neural tube in the precartilaginous sclerotome stage may foster congenital fusion (49). Gunderson et al. suggest a genetic predisposition since patients with specific subtypes of KFS had a higher frequency of the disease observed in other family members (22). In fact, Clark et al. proposed a gene locus on chromosome 8q that segregates C2–C3 and vocal cord impairment (9). Furthermore, Gray et al. found that 10% of patients reported had a family history of the disease (20). Several syndromes have been associated with KFS. For example, Treadwell et al. described a 50% frequency of congenital cervical spine fusion in 38 patients sustaining fetal alcohol syndrome (65). In addition, Avon et al. identified congenital fusions in 10% of patients with Goldenhar syndrome (1).

III DIAGNOSIS

Radiographic studies have shown that a single level of fused vertebrae is most common (14,18,66), and the majority of congenital fusions involve fewer than three levels (20). A variety of anterior, lateral, and posterior patterns of fusion have been observed in half of the patients, whereas an isolated anterior fusion is seen in 20% (3,6,20,22,24,28,31,33,40,46). The morphology of the abnormal vertebrae includes a wide and flat body (13) with a hypoplastic or absent intervertebral disk space (11,26,66). Although patients with KFS may have a normal canal size, congenital stenosis (12,15,16,47,49,53,56) and more frequent spondylosis and hypermobility at an adjacent segment (23,25,49,53,56) have been described. While spinal stenosis may be observed at the level of segmentation abnormality (43,53), it occurs more frequently at adjacent levels from degenerative changes (33). However, others found stenosis below (56), but not at, the fusion level (49,53). For example, Pizzutillo (51) reported a higher frequency of spinal stenosis adjacent to a segmentation defect when compared with controls. Traumatic odontoid fractures in patients with KFS have been associated with atlanto-occipital or upper cervical fusion. It has been suggested that the limitation of flexion and extension increases the strain on atlantoaxial ligaments, increasing the risk of odontoid fracture (36).

Asymptomatic patients with KFS during infancy usually develop acute neck pain after a traumatic event during adolescence (45). Additional symptoms include chronic persistent pain, radiculopathy, myelopathy, and sometimes sudden death from minor trauma (12,17,20,39,42,43,44,53,55,60,62,67). Pain may be related to adjacent level hypermobility and spondylotic degeneration of abnormal articulations (40, 42,50). For example, stenosis has been noted at adjacent segments (12,15,16,23, 25,34,43,48,49,51,53,56). In addition, spondylotic and diskogenic changes may occur at junctional segments adjacent to fused (Fig. 1) vertebrae from hypermobility (36,52). Accelerated degenerative disk disease, instability, and stenosis increase the risk of traumatic spinal cord injury (36). Karasick et al. found 9 of 14 consecutive patients with KFS who sustained trauma developed a neurological injury. Although the defective segmentation patterns were not described, the propensity of neurological sequelae from trauma were identified (30). The predisposition to spinal cord injury may result from the altered biomechanics of the long lever arm of the fused segments with the hypermobile adjacent intervertebral joints (21). However, there does not appear to be an increased risk of spinal fracture, other than the odontoid process in patients with upper cervical segmentation abnormalities. Neurological deficit, instability, and pain refractory to conservative therapy may be indications for decompression and fusion.

IV CLASSIFICATION

There have been several proposed methods to identify patients that may be at risk of neurological injury. For example, Nagib et al. attempted to identify asymptomatic

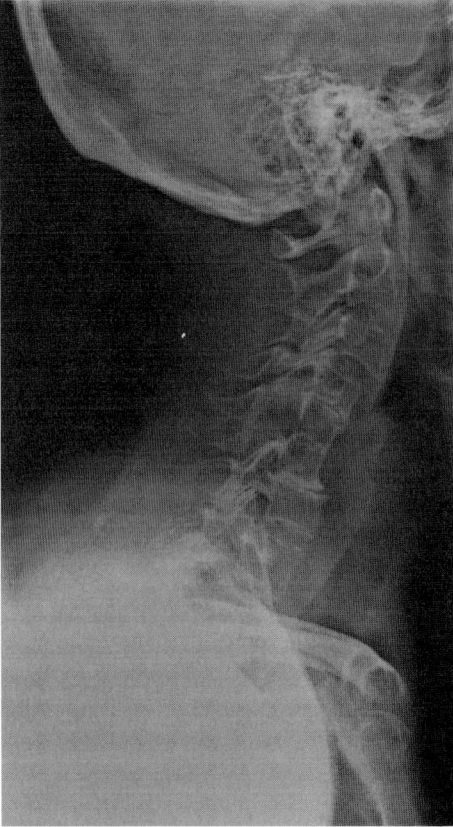

Figure 1   Lateral cervical radiograph of a 71-year-old woman with progressive cervical myelopathy. Imaging reveals C5–C6 block vertebrae with severe spondylosis at the adjacent intervertebral joints. No subluxation was seen on dynamic radiographs.

patients at risk of becoming symptomatic and described three patterns that predispose patients with KFS to developing neurological deficits (43,44). After observing 21 patients over 20 years, only 9 developed neurological sequelae. A classification based upon the segmentation abnormalities was proposed (Table 1). While patients with type I abnormalities are at risk for subluxation, patients with type II disease are at risk for foramen magnum encroachment. Stenosis and hypermobility may predispose the patient to developing quadriplegia after minor trauma (53). In fact, others have

Table 1   Classification Scheme Based on
Segmentation Abnormalities

Type I	Two fusions separated by an intervening disk.
Type II	Craniocervical anomalies with congenital fusion below C2.
Type III	Fusion at one or more levels with stenosis.

Source: Refs. 44, 45.

reported patients with two fused vertebrae separated by a functional intervening disk (Fig. 2) developing quadriplegia (12,40,42). In contrast, craniovertebral anomalies and congenital cervical fusion are the most common cause of upper cord injury in these patients (27,39,40,42,57,60). For example, MacRae et al. reported 16 of 25 patients with occipitalization of the atlas had long tract signs. Moreover, 11 also had C2–C3 congenital fusion (38). Finally, spinal cord injury in patients with stenosis and congenital fusion has also been reported (17,23,53). In a series of patients with transient quadriplegia, Torg et al. reported 4 of 32 had KFS with stenosis (64).

Another classification system was suggested by Pizzutillo et al. after reviewing 111 patients with KFS (50). The authors concluded that neurological sequelae may occur in patients with a hypermobile cervical spine or iniencephaly (incomplete posterior cervical spine closure). A classification scheme based on spinal mobility was proposed (Table 2). Five of 111 patients developed neurological deficits. Four of five had instability of the upper cervical spine. However, 12 patients with degenerative changes or instability of the lower cervical spine had pain without a neuro-

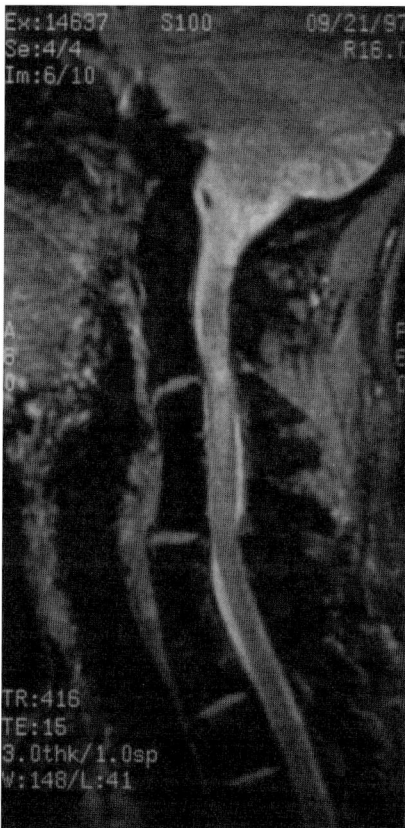

Figure 2   Sagittal magnetic resonance image of a 23-year-old man who sustained a blow to the head, resulting in quadriparesis. Imaging reveals C34 stenosis with blocked vertebrae above and below the intervening C34 intervertebral disk. Abnormal signal in the spinal cord is seen at the level of stenosis. No fracture was identified.

Table 2 Classification Scheme Based on Spinal Mobility

Type I	Normal range of motion in flexion and extension without hypermobility
Type II	Excessive range of motion of the upper cervical segment or presence of basilar invagination or iniencephaly
Type III	Hypermobility or degenerative changes of the lower cervical spine
Type IV	Combination of Types II and III

Source: Ref. 52.

logical deficit. A treatment algorithm based upon this classification system was proposed. Patients with type I spinal mobility (1/3) should be observed. In contrast, those with type II spinal mobility (1/3) are at increased risk and should be examined annually. Moreover, these patients should also avoid high-impact loading activities and contact sports. Finally, patients with type III spinal mobility are at risk for progressive degenerative disease and should only be treated symptomatically.

Yet there are patients with KFS who have suffered neurological sequelae ranging from radiculopathy to quadriplegia to death from minor trauma, but do not fit into these high-risk groups (12,14,34,62). Graaff evaluated 145 patients with cervical myelopathy (19). Patients with craniocervical anomalies with congenital fusion below C2 were excluded. Eight of 145 had an isolated C2–C3 fusion and one had a C2–C3 fusion and a C5–C6 fusion. All nine had quadriparesis and upper extremity dysfunction.

In conclusion, all patients with KFS should be carefully observed. Radiographic imaging of the entire spinal axis is important in order to identify the various spinal abnormalities that may occur. For example, craniocervical anomalies including occipitalization of the atlas, basilar impression, os terminale, os odontoidium, hypoplastic dens may be found (39,43,44,61,66). In addition, thoracic, lumbar, and sacral abnormalities have been reported (26,55). Magnetic resonance imaging may be helpful in detecting hindbrain abnormalities as well as stenosis (56). If dynamic lateral cervical radiographs are performed, stability may be evaluated. Pizzutillo (50) and Nagib (43) have proposed classifications to identify patients with KFS at high risk of injury. Both schema use hypermobility or the risk of instability as a major factor. However, there is no standard treatment paradigm recommended for asymptomatic patients with KFS. These patients must be followed clinically and radiographically for signs of instability. However, if specific fusion patterns (two fused segments with an intervening disk or a fusion and an occipitocervical abnormality) are observed, perhaps earlier treatment addressing potential instability should be considered.

REFERENCES

1. Avon SW, Shively JL. Orthopaedic manifestations of Goldenhar syndrome. J Pediatr Orthop 1988;8:682–686.
2. Baga N, Chusid EL, Miller A. Pulmonary disability in the Klippel-Feil syndrome. Clin Orthop 1969;67:105–110.
3. Baird PA, Robinson GC, Buckler WSJ. Klippel-Feil syndrome. Am J Dis Child 1967; 113:546–551.

4. Beals RK, Robbins JR, Rolfe B. Anomalies associated with vertebral malformations. Spine 1993;18:1329–1332.
5. Beals RK, Rolfe B. Current concepts review. VATER association. J Bone Joint Surg Am 1989;71:948–950.
6. Bernini F, Elefante R, Smaltino F, Tedeschi G. Angiographic study on the vertebral artery in cases of deformities of the occipitocervical joint. Am J Roentgenol 1969;107: 526–529.
7. Bouwes Bavnick JN, Weaver DD. Subclavian artery supply disruption sequence: hypothesis of a vascular etiology for Poland, Klippel-Feil, and Mobius anomalies. Am J Med Genet 1986;23:903–918.
8. Brown MW, Templeton AW, Hodges FJ. The incidence of acquired and congenital fusion in the cervical spine. Am J Roentgenol 1964;92:1255–1259.
9. Clark RA, Singh S, McKenzie H, et al. Familial Klippel-Feil syndrome and paracentric inversion inv(8)(q22.2q23.3). Am J Hum Genet 1995;57:1364–1370.
10. Degnehardt KH, Klodetzxy L. Malformaciones de la columna vertebrale y del esbozo de la corda dorsalis. Actua Pediatr Barcelona 1956;7:1.
11. Dolan KD. Developmental abnormalities of the cervical spine below the axis. Radiol Clin North Am 1977;15:167–175.
12. Elster AD. Quadriplegia after minor trauma in the Klippel-Feil syndrome. A case report and review of the literature. J Bone Joint Surg Am 1984;66:1473–1474.
13. Erskine CA. An analysis of the Klippel-Feil syndrome. Arch Pathol 1946;41:269–281.
14. Epstein JA, Carras R, Epstein BS, Levine LS. Myelopathy in cervical spondylosis with vertebral subluxation and hyperlordosis. J Neurosurg 1970;32:421–426.
15. Epstein JA, Carras R, Hyman RA. Cervical myelopathy caused by the developmental stenosis of the spinal canal. J Neurosurg 1979;15:489–496.
16. Epstein NE, Epstein JA, Benjamin V, et al. Traumatic myelopathy in patients with cervical spinal stenosis without fracture dislocation. Methods of diagnosis, management, and prognosis. Spine 1980;5:489–496.
17. Epstein NE, Epstein JA, Zilkha A. Traumatic myelopathy in a seventeen-year-old child with cervical spine stenosis (without fracture or dislocation) and a C2-3 Klippel-Feil fusion. Spine 1984;9:344–346.
18. Gjorup PA, Gjorup L. Klippel-Feil's syndrome. Dan Med Bull 1964;11:50–53.
19. Graaff R. Congenital block vertebrae C2-3 in patients with cervical myelopathy. Acta Neurochir 1982;61:111–126.
20. Gray SW, Romaine CB, Skandalakis JE. Congenital fusion of the cervical vertebrae. Surg Gynecol Obstet 1964;118:373–385.
21. Guilles JT, Miller A, Bowen JR, et al. The natural history of Klippel-Feil syndrome: clinical, roentgenographic, and magnetic resonance imaging findings at adulthood. J Pediatr Orthop 1995;15:617–625.
22. Gunderson CH, Greenspan RH, Glaser GH, Lubs HA. The Klippel-Feil syndrome: genetic and clinical reevaluation of cervical fusion. Medicine 1967;46:491–512.
23. Hall, JE, Simmons ED, Danylchuk K, et al. Instability of the cervical spine and neurologic involvement in Klippel-Feil syndrome. A case report. J Bone Joint Surg Am 1990;72:460–462.
24. Hensinger RN: Congenital anomalies of the cervical spine. Clin Orthop Rel Res 1991; 264:16–38.
25. Hensinger RN, Fielding JW. The cervical spine. In: Morrissy RT, ed. Pediatric Orthopedics, 3rd ed. Philadelphia: JB Lippincott, 1990:703–737.
26. Hensinger R, Lang JE, MacEwen GD. Klippel-Feil syndrome: a constellation of associated anomalies. J Bone Joint Surg Am 1974;56:1246–1253.
27. Herring JA, Bunnel WP. Instructional case. Klippel-Feil syndrome with neck pain. J Pediatr Orthop 1989;9:343–346.

28. Illingworth RS. Attacks of unconsciousness in association with fused cervical vertebrae. Arch Dis Child 1956;31:8–11.
29. Jarvis JF, Sellars SL. Klippel-Feil deformity associated with congenital conductive deafness. J Laryngol Otol 1974;88:285–289.
30. Karasick D, Schweitzer ME, Vaccaro AR. The traumatized cervical spine in Klippel-Feil syndrome: imaging features. Am J Radiol 1998;170:85–88.
31. Klippel M, Feil, A. Un cas d'absence des vertebres cervicales avec cage thoracique remontant jusqu'a la base du crane. Nouv Icon Salpetriere 1912;25:223–250.
32. Klippel M, Feil A. The classic. A case of absence of cervical vertebrae with the thoracic cage rising to the base of the cranium (cervical thoracic cage). Clin Orthop Rel Res 1975;109:3–8.
33. Koop SE, Winter RB, Lonstein JE. The surgical treatment of instability of the upper part of the cervical spine in children and adolescents. J Bone Joint Surg Am 1984;66:403–411.
34. Lee CK, Weiss AB: Isolated congenital cervical block vertebrae below the axis with neurological symptoms. Spine 1981;6:118–124.
35. MacEwan D. The Klippel-Feil syndrome. J Boint Joint Surg Br 1975;57:261–267.
36. MacMillan M, Stauffer ES. Traumatic instability in the previously fused cervical spine. J Spinal Disord 1991;4:449–454.
37. McElfresh E, Winter R. Klippel-Feil syndrome. Minn Med 1973;56:353–357.
38. McLay K, Maran AGD. Deafness and the Klippel-Feil syndrome. J Laryngol Otol 1969;83:175–184.
39. McRae DL, Barnum AS. Occipitalization of the atlas. Am J Roentgenol 1953;70:23–46.
40. Michie I, Clark M. Neurological syndromes associated with cervical and craniocervical anomalies. Arch Neurol 1968;18:241–247.
41. Moore WB, Matthews TJ, Rabinowitz R. Genitourinary anomalies associated with Klippel-Feil syndrome. J Bone Joint Surg Am 1975;57:355–357.
42. Mosberg WH Jr. The Klippel-Feil syndrome. Etiology and treatment of neurologic signs. J Nerv Ment Dis 1953;117:479–491.
43. Nagib MG, Maxwell RE, Chou SN. Identification and management of high-risk patients with Klippel-Feil syndrome. J Neurosurg 1984;61:523–530.
44. Nagib MG, Maxwell RE, Chou SN. Klippel-Feil syndrome in children: clinical features and management. Child's Nerv Syst 1985;1:255–263.
45. Ogden JA. Skeletal injury in the child, 2nd ed. Philadelphia: WB Saunders, 1990.
46. Ogden JA, Conlogue G, Phillips S, et al. Sprengel's deformity: radiology of the pathological deformation. Skeletal Radiol 1979;4:204–211.
47. Palant DI, Carter BL. Klippel-Feil syndrome and deafness. Am J Dis Child 1972;123:218–221.
48. Payne EE, Spillane JD. The cervical spine: an anatomicopathological study of 70 specimens (using a special technique) with particular reference to the problem of cervical spondylosis. Brain 1957;80:571–596.
49. Pizzutillo PD. Klippel-Feil syndrome. In: Cervical Spine Research Society Editorial Committee, ed. The Cervical Spine, 2nd ed. Philadelphia: JB Lippincott, 1989:258–271.
50. Pizzutillo PD, Mandell GA, Schoedler S. Spinal stenosis and the Klippel-Feil syndrome. Proceedings of the 58th Meeting of the American Academy of Orthopaedic Surgeons, 1991.
51. Pizzutillo PD, Woods MW, Nicholson L. Risk factors in Klippel-Feil syndrome. Orthop Trans 1987;11:473–482.
52. Pizzutillo PD, Woods M, Nicholson L, MacEwen G. Risk factors in Klippel-Feil syndrome. Spine 1994;19:2110–2116.

53. Prusick VR, Samberg LC, Wesolowski DP. Klippel-Feil syndrome associated with spinal stenosis. A case report. J Bone Joint Surg Am 1985;67:161–164.
54. Ramsey J, Bliznak J. Klippel-Feil syndrome with renal agenesis and other anomalies. Am J Roentgenol 1971;113:460–463.
55. Rish BL. Klippel-Feil syndrome: case report. Va Med 1982;109:520–521.
56. Ritterbusch JF, McGinty LD, Spar J, et al. Magnetic resonance imaging for stenosis and subluxation in Klippel-Feil syndrome. Spine 1991;16:S539–S541.
57. Rouvreau MD, Glorion C, Langlais J, et al. Assessment and neurologic involvement of patients with cervical spine congenital synostosis as in Klippel-Feil syndrome: study of 19 cases. J Pediatr Orthop 1998;7:179–185.
58. Sakai M, Shinkawa A, Miyake H, et al. Klippel-Feil syndrome with conductive deafness and histological findings of removed stapes. Ann Otol Rhinol Laryngol 1993;92:202–206.
59. Sherk HH, Uppal GS. Congenital bony anomalies of the cervical spine. In: Frymoyer JW, ed. The Adult Spine: Principles and Practice. New York: Raven Press, 1991:1015–1037.
60. Shoul MI, Ritvo M. Clinical and roentgenological manifestations of the Klippel-Feil syndrome (congenital fusion of the cervical vertebrae, brevicollis). Am J Roentgenol 1952;68:369–385
61. Southwell RB, Reynolds AF, Badger VM, Sherman FC. Klippel-Feil syndrome with cervical cord compression resulting from cervical subluxation in association with an omo-vertebral bone. Spine 1980;5:480–482.
62. Strakx TE, Baran E. Traumatic quadriplegia associtaed with Klippel-Feil syndrome: discussion and case reports. Arch Phys Med Rehab 1975; 56:363–365.
63. Thomsen MN, Schneider U, Weber M, et al. Scoliosis and congenital anomalies associated with Klippel-Feil syndrome types I–III. Spine 1997;22:396–401.
64. Torg JS, Pavlov H, Genuario SE, et al. Neurapraxia of the cervical spinal cord with transient quadriplegia. J Bone Joint Surg Am 1986;68:1354–1370.
65. Tredwell SJ, Smith DF, Macleod PJ, Wood BJ. Cervical spine anomalies in fetal alcohol syndrome. Spine 1982;7:331–334.
66. Van Kerckhoven MF, Fabry G. The Klippel-Feil syndrome: a constellation of deformities. Acta Orthop Belg 1989;55:107–118.
67. Whitehouse GH, Harrison RJ. Klippel-Feil syndrome. Proc R Soc Med 1970;63:287–288.
68. Winter RB, Erickson DL, Lonstein JE, et al. Segmental spinal dysgenesis: a report of 20 cases. Proceedings of the 58th Meeting of the American Academy of Orthopaedic Surgeons, 1991.
69. Winter RB, Moe JH, Lonstein JE. The incidence of Klippel-Feil syndrome in patients with congenital scoliosis and kyphosis. Spine 1984;9:363–366.

46

Osteoporotic Fractures of the Spine

JOHN P. KOSTUIK

Johns Hopkins University Medical Center, Baltimore, Maryland, U.S.A.

I INTRODUCTION

Osteoporosis is a major public health concern in the industrialized world. It is estimated that 25 million women in the United States have osteopenia or osteoporosis. The lifetime risk of death is equal to that of breast cancer as a result of fractures.

Osteoporosis should be considered as a preventative disorder and not a disease. The course of bone loss and fracture can be altered through various therapies.

The impact of osteoporosis is significant to families and patients as a result of pain, deformity, dependency, depression, fear of falling and premature death.

Considerable demographic trends in aging Americans are occurring. Baby boomers are not aging gracefully. The elderly, over 65, and the very old, over 80, are the fastest growing proportions of our population. It is estimated that by the year 2020, more than 30% of the U.S. population will be over the age of 65. The median age of the U.S. population will increase from the mid-twenties in 1970 to approximately 40 by the year 2025.

Osteoporosis is a disease of aging. At age 50, at least 10% of people have osteoporosis; and by age 65, the rate rises to between 20 and 25%; and by age 75, to 40%. Greater than 50% of patients with osteoporosis will sustain some form of fracture, of which vertebral compression fractures are the most common. As a prevalence of common diseases of aging, osteoporosis ranked third, behind heart disease and arthritis, but ahead of such things as depression, diabetes, cancer, Alzheimer's disease, and Parkinson's disease.

In 1984, it was estimated that 0.6 million people were at risk of spinal fractures from osteoporosis at the cost of approximately 6 billion dollars. In 1997, the cost had risen to an estimated 13 billion dollars, and by the year 2050, the cost of care for osteoporotic spinal fracture is estimated to be as high as 240 billion dollars.

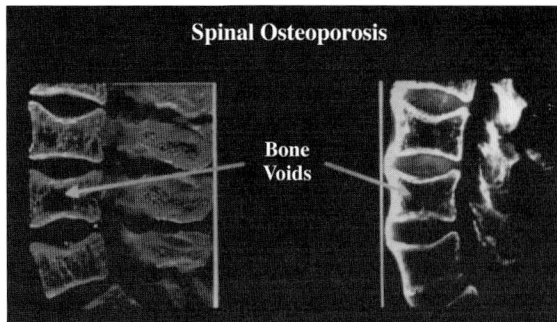

Figure 1 Pathological and radiological evidence of osteoporosis.

Osteopenia is a radiological descriptive term meaning "reduced radio density" and indicates, at least 30% reduction in total bone mass. Major implications are decreased vertebral body strength. Osteoporosis is a syndrome characterized by decreased amounts of normal bone leading to increased susceptibility to fracture. Peak bone mass is reached somewhere shortly before the age 30, and thereafter decreases both in males and females. Because of bone voids, the osteoporotic spine may develop kyphosis, vertebral wedging, concave fractures, and scalloped endplates. The cortical shell is responsible for 10% of vertebral body compressive strength (Figs. 1 and 2).

Osteoporosis is of two types: primary osteoporosis (type 1), which is a post-menopausal osteoporosis that occurs starting 3 to 8 years following menopause as result of estrogen deficiency. Primary osteoporosis (type II), is senile osteoporosis, seen in men and women over the age 70; it is related to aging and perhaps to long-term calcium deficiency (Fig. 3) Currently, it is estimated that there are between 30 to 35 million people at risk of osteoporosis, of which 700,000 will sustain vertebral fractures, more than 200,000 will require narcotics, and 150,000 will require hospitalization.

A number of myths and legends versus reality exist about osteoporosis and spinal fractures. The reality is that most of these fractures are painful. Greater than

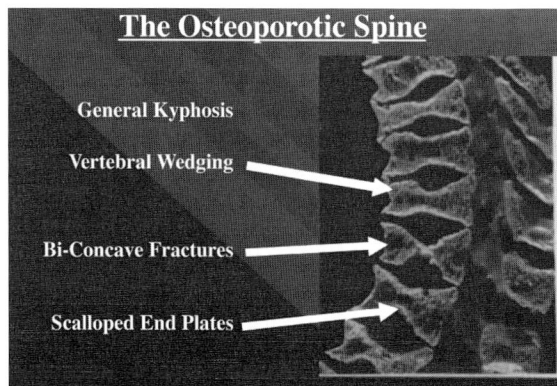

Figure 2 Pathological picture of fractures in the osteoporotic spine.

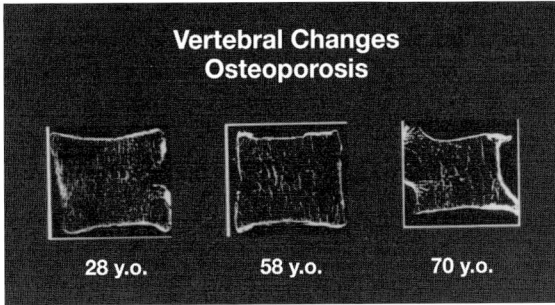

Figure 3   Progressive osteoporosis.

200,000 people per year with osteoporotic fractures require narcotics, and it is known that 150,000 require hospital admission. Sixty percent of people do get better within 3 months. Bed rest as a treatment is bad since 10% of bone mass loss may occur within 2 weeks.

The natural history is not clearly understood. In a recent study of osteoporotic fractures in 9000 women older than 65 years of age, with follow-up greater than 8 years, there were 1915 with fractures at baseline. The study was adjusted for age,

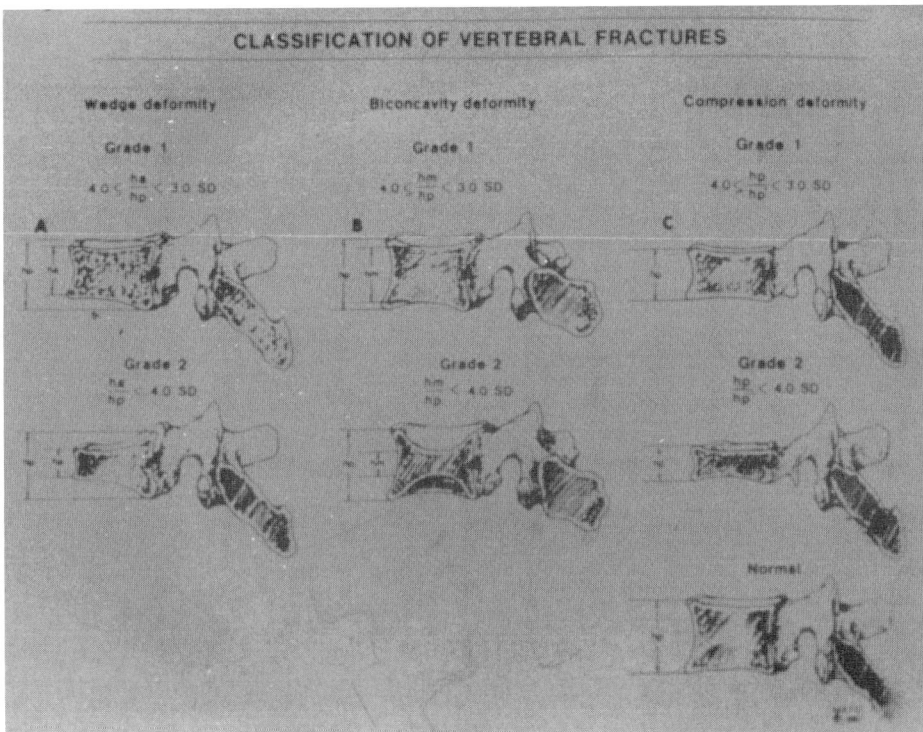

Figure 4   Classification of vertebral fractures showing types—wedges, biconcave, and compression.

comorbidities, and smoking. It is noted that if you had one fracture, the average increase in kyphosis was 12 degrees, there was a decrease in vital capacity of approximately 9%, and an increased risk of further fractures of >500%. Any fracture resulted in a 23% increase in mortality, a severe fracture in 37% increase in mortality, and increased risk of pulmonary death of at least 300%. The myths to be dispelled are that these fractures do not disable people or hurt much; people should rest until they heal, and there are no long-term problems.

An anterior/posterior x-ray and lateral x-ray of the thoracic and lumbar spine may be all that is necessary to diagnose osteopenia, and it may help to establish baseline bone density. Plain x-rays may also help with the classification of fracture types (Fig. 4). MRI, of course, is most helpful and may show a decrease in marrow fat signal; it can assess canal compromise and show evidence of osteonecrosis. In order to assess whether fracture is a new or old, a bone scan may be of value.

II PREVENTION AND MEDICAL TREATMENT

The current treatment consists of a careful assessment of the patient including neurological examination, deformity, osteoporotic risks, radiographs, and consideration of other studies such as a CT scan, MRI, and bone scanning as indicated.

The current treatment options of symptomatic spinal osteoporotic fractures include prevention, medical management, including analgesics, bracing, and surgical intervention particularly for chronic pain and neurological problems. The problem with the many current treatments is that prevention does not reverse severe cases. With symptomatic control, deformity remains, often with chronic pain. Surgical intervention is invasive and often subject to fixation failure. The main means of prevention is exercise. Building bone mass when young with adequate calcium and Vitamin D intake and weight-bearing exercises can lead to prevention provided postmenopausal care is used, including estrogen and calcium replacement. It is recognized that if a female engages in a weight-bearing exercise for 20 min, four times a week, 10 years prior to menopause, she will not develop primary osteoporosis. These exercises can include spinal exercises, walking, isometric and abdominal exercises,

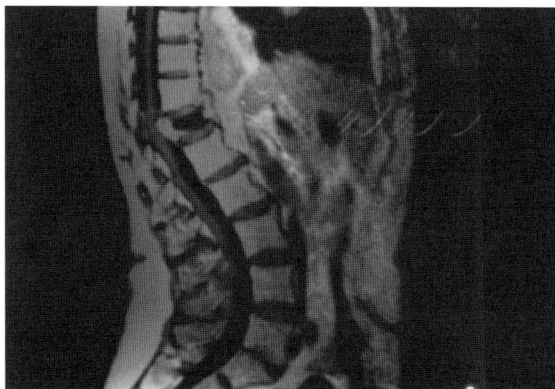

Figure 5 Compression, burst fracture, T12, in a 72-year-old female with severe osteoporosis and neurological signs and symptoms.

water exercises, being on one's feet 4 to 6 h a day, light free weights, and proprioceptive skills.

Other preventive measures, postmenopausal, include hormone replacement with estrogens. There is no doubt that estrogen therapy unequivocally reduces fractures, and if there are no contraindications, all women at risk should be considered for estrogen therapy. Estrogen therapy prevents rapid postmenopausal bone loss but does not increase bone density. This is recommended as a primary treatment and may be combined with progesterone. Controversy continues to exist as to its contraindications with the history of cancer. Estrogen use in postmenopausal osteoporotic women

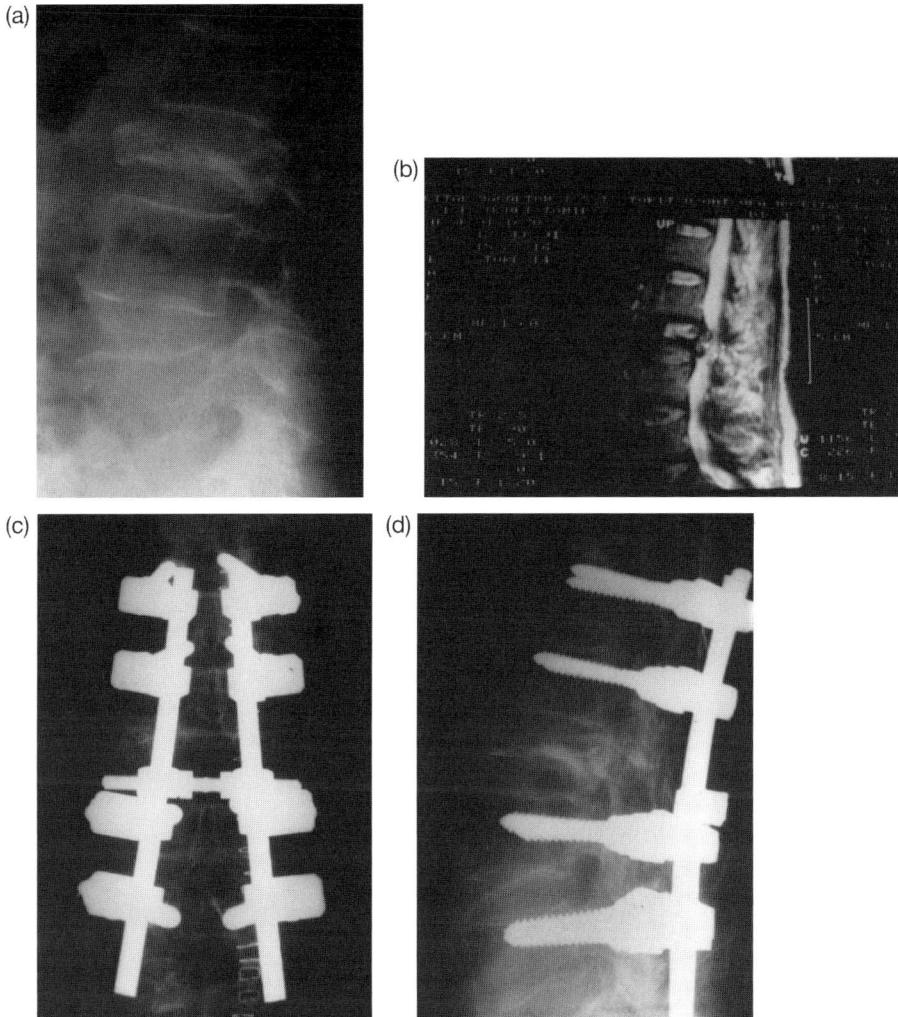

Figure 6 (a) Severe osteoporotic compression with pain, instability and neurological sequelae; (b) MRI of same case demonstrating cauda equina compression; (c) postoperative anterior-posterior radiograph; (d) postoperative lateral radiograph; decompression via posterior decancelization; nonradiopaque cement was used for pedicle screw retention.

with at least one vertebral fracture has been shown to decrease subsequent fracture risk by 125%.

Intranasal calcitonin is indicated in the elderly patient group with low bone mass who cannot or refuse to take estrogens. This may result in an increased bone density, particularly in the spine, with a plateau effect at about 18 months. Calcitonin is also available in the injectable form, and it requires subcutaneous injections every 2 weeks. It has been shown to increase bone mass. In addition, intranasal calcitonin may have an analgesic effect.

Antiosteoclastic drugs such as Alendronate or biphosphonate therapy are available. The effect on fracture incidence reduction is not yet clear with the use of

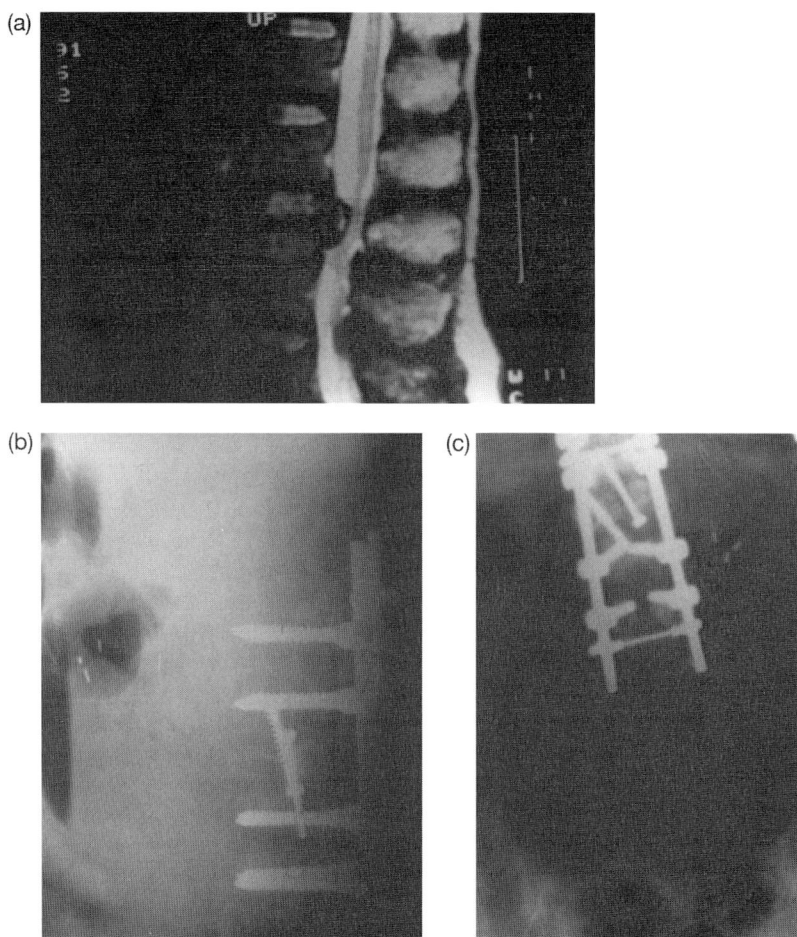

Figure 7 (a) Preoperative MRI demonstrating severe compressive burst fracture with cord compression; (b) lateral postoperative radiograph; decancelization of the body was performed using a posterior approach; reinforced PMMA was used to replace body anteriorly; pedicle screws were reinforced with PMMA; a posterior approach was used as the patient was too ill for an anterior approach; (c) anterior-posterior radiograph of the same patient.

biphosphonates, and it does have few side effects. Oral alendronate (Fosamax) has been shown to decrease fracture risk about 35% as well as having analgesic effect in fresh fractures. It does, however, have a high rate of gastrointestinal effects and must be taken very specifically; it is contraindicated if there is reflux.

Intravenous Pamidronate does increase bone mass as well and it requires infusions every 2 to 3 months.

Selective estrogen receptor modulators are the newest drug class in prevention.

Calcium supplements should be between 1200 to 1500 mg per day. Radiographs should be used for follow-up and for progression.

A study evaluating the efficacy of calcium and vitamin D in 1255 postmenopausal women with osteoporosis was undertaken. At inception, 265 had no prevalent fractures, 926 had one to five prevalent fractures, and 64 had greater than five prevalent fractures. All patients received 1000 mg of calcium and 400 IU of vitamin D and were followed annually for 5 years. At follow-up, a significant reduction of fractures occurred in patients receiving 200 IU of calcitonin.

IV FRACTURE TYPE

The majority are due to axial compression failure (Fig. 4). They may be wedged with anterior column collapse; they may retain their relative square to trapezoidal

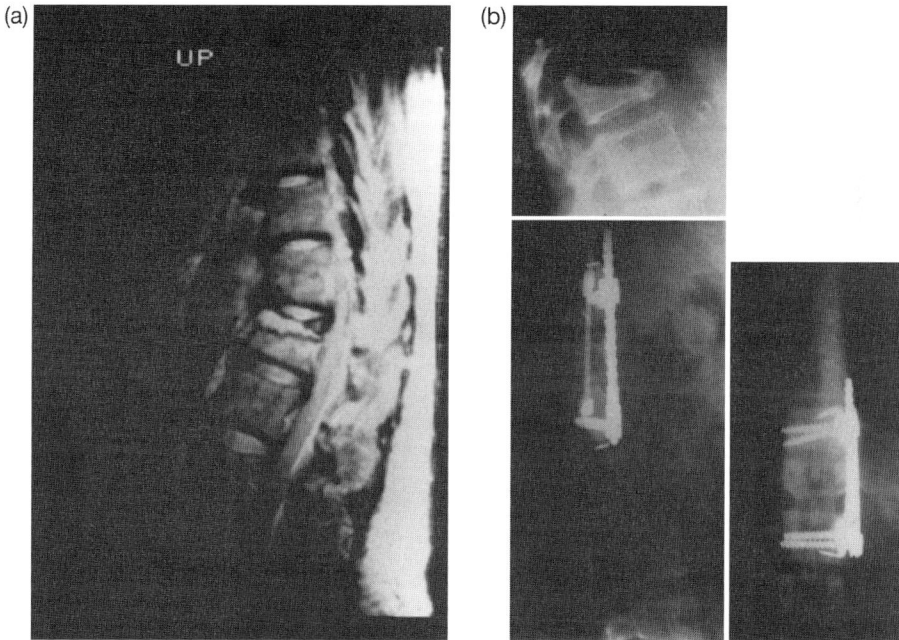

Figure 8   (a) Compression fracture with neurological sequelae at the thoracolumbar junction; (b) an anterior approach was performed; a corpectomy was done and replaced with an autologous iliac crest strut graft (an allograft could have been used as well).

(a)

(b)

(c)

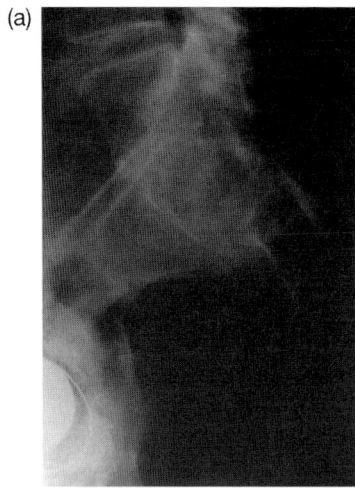

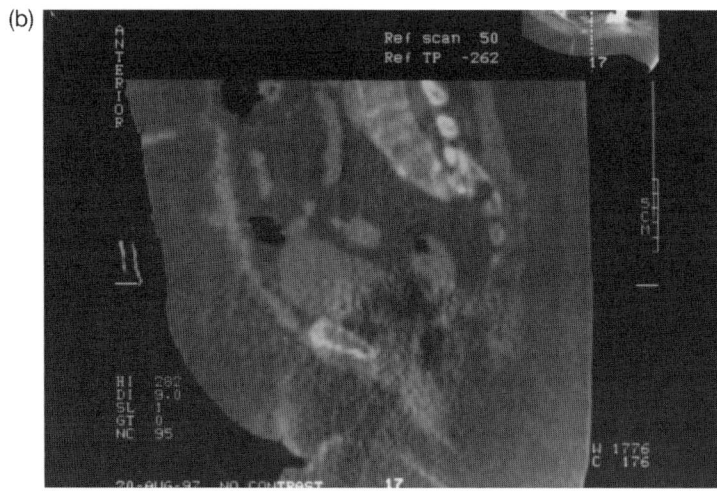

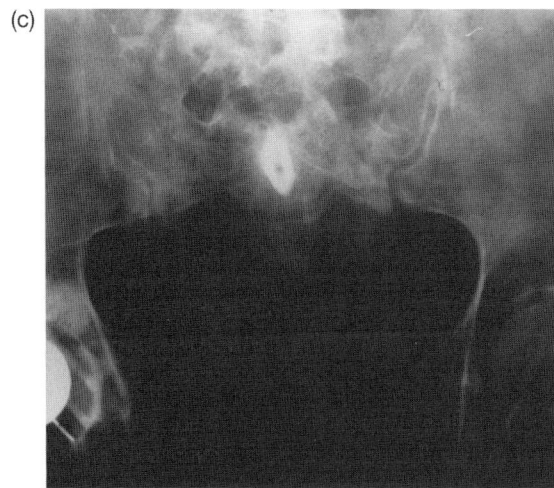

Figure 9 (a) Osteoporotic fracture of the sacrum with nonunion; (b) CT scan demonstrates the fracture; (c) a fibular allograft was used anteriorly to fix the fracture that healed uneventfully.

shape with associated biconcave endplate failure; or they may be crushed with anterior and middle column failure, the so-called "burst fractures" (Fig. 5). The implications for the latter are the potential for instability and neurological compromise.

The upper thoracic spine is most commonly affected, of which 50% are asymptomatic. The pain is more prevalent with fractures in the lumbar spine. Progressive collapse may ensue secondary to avascular necrosis. Patients with thoracic fractures may experience radicular pain and this always precedes any motor deficit secondary to cord compression. A neurological deficit or radicular symptoms may develop weeks or months following the initial fracture. Delayed collapse may be insidious and progressive. There is no doubt that the posterior cortex of the vertebral body is more involved than it was previously felt, resulting in the so-called "burst fracture" (Fig. 5). As a result, all osteoporotic fractures should be followed for a minimum of 1 year. It is important to rule out osteomalacia, particularly in the elderly living in inner cities or in places where access to regular sunlight may be difficult.

IV BRACING

Bracing is often poorly tolerated in the elderly, women in particular, as many of them are thin and do not tolerate the skin irritation of appropriate bracing. Corset-type bracing may be valuable in the lumbar spine, but more rigid bracing is necessary in the thoracolumbar area. Because of rib support and inadequacy of bracing, upper thoracic fractures generally are not helped by bracing.

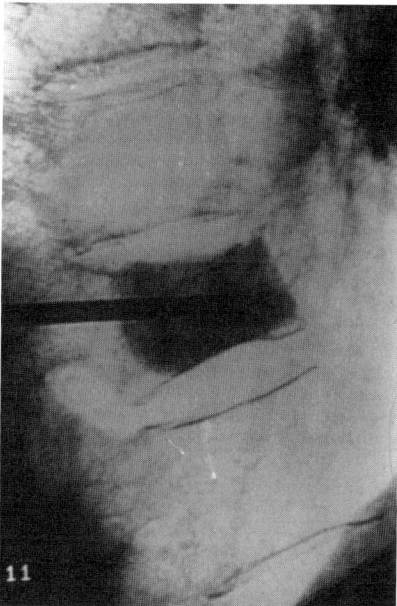

Figure 10   Vertebroplasty done via pedicle-lateral view.

V ANALGESICS

Analgesics remain the mainstay of symptomatic control. Strong narcotics or long-standing narcotics should be avoided in the elderly as these often result in confusion. In addition, preventive measures, noted previously, should be administered.

VI NUTRITION

Nutrition should be assessed to rule out osteomalacia and to assess adequate nutrition for prevention. This is particularly important preoperatively. Serum albumin, total lymphocyte count, calorie count, and serum transferrin should all be assessed.

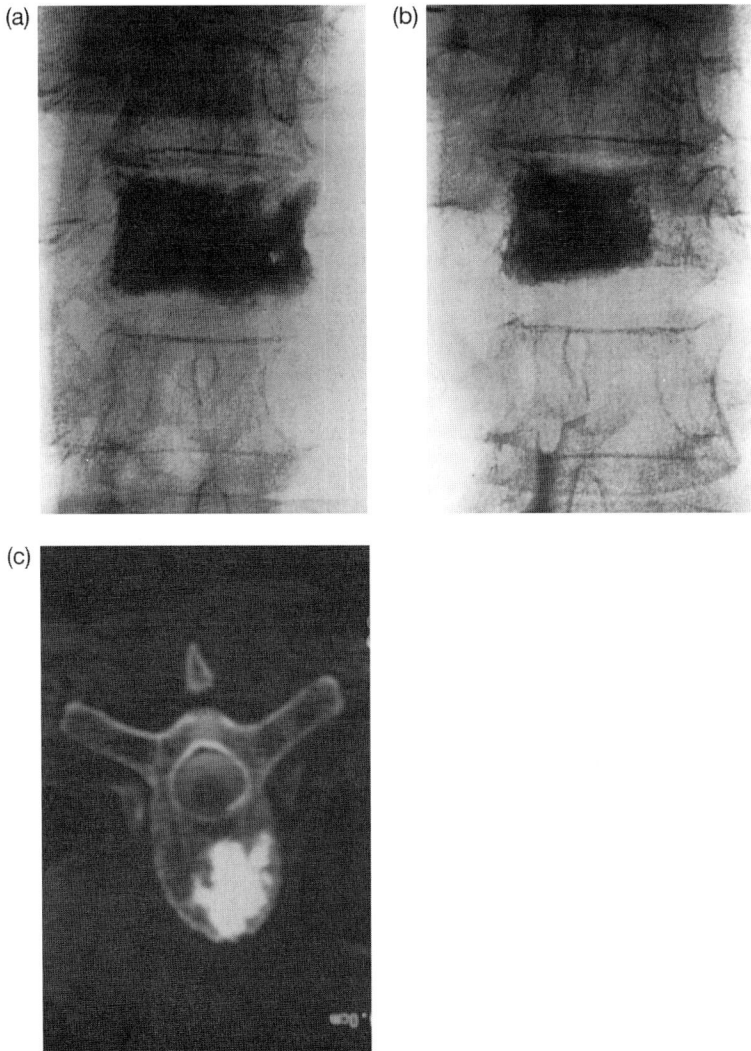

Figure 11   (a) Anterior-posterior view of vertebroplast performed via pedicles—bilateral; (b) anterior-posterior view of unilateral pedicle infection; (c) axial CT postvertebroplasty.

VII SURGICAL INDICATIONS

Indications for surgery include progressive deformity with intractable pain and burst fractures with neurological deficit which are rare; progressive deformity with spinal stenosis; and instability associated with symptoms of spinal stenosis.

Although surgery is not commonly indicated, at the present time the indications and numbers are rapidly increasing because of the changing aging demographics of our population, as pointed out earlier in this chapter.

Critical surgical concepts include the fact that there is greatly decreased mechanical strength of bone in an osteoporotic individual. The pedicle is the strongest point for fixation. Anterior cortex fixation is important in the sacrum, and far cortex fixation is important for anterior screw fixation in vertebral bodies proximal to the sacrum. In anterior approaches, the sacral promontory is a better point of fixation than the ala. Methyl methacrylate supplementation of vertebral body may be important as well, and it will be discussed later.

Surgery should be individualized to the patient and his or her comorbidities. Ideally, for burst fractures with neurological problems, the anterior approach is preferred, but may be contraindicated in severe respiratory depression. Other approaches may include posterior approaches, posterolateral decompression, an egg shell pro-

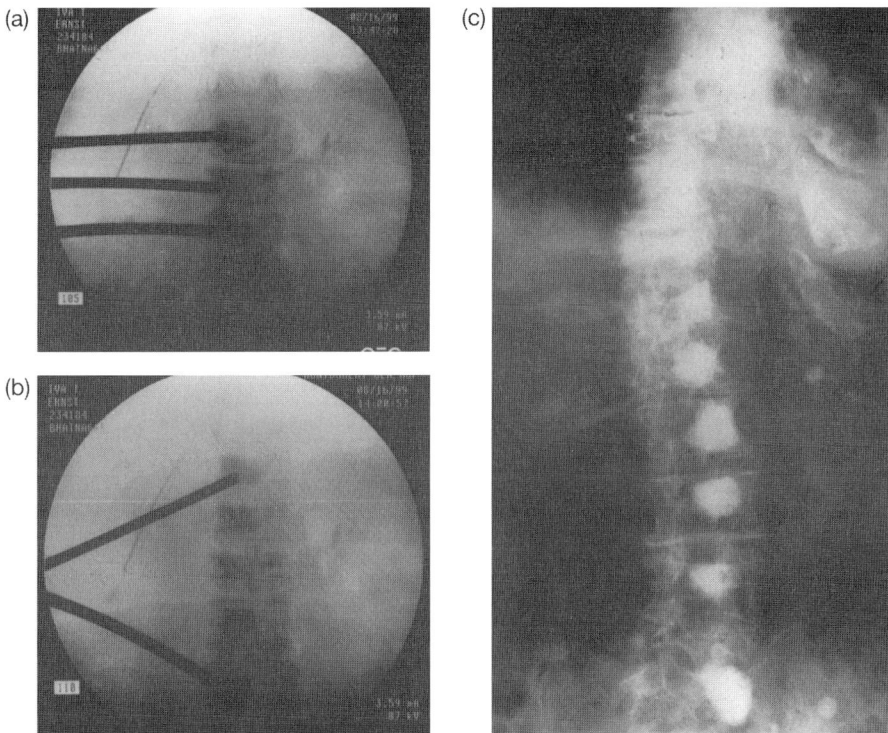

Figure 12   (a) Multiple level posterolateral approach to vertebroplasty, a quicker and safer approach than vertebroplasty via the pedicle; (b) five-level vertebroplasty via posteriolateral approach; we generally advocate no more than three levels at a time; (c) seven-level posterolateral vertebroplasty done in two stages.

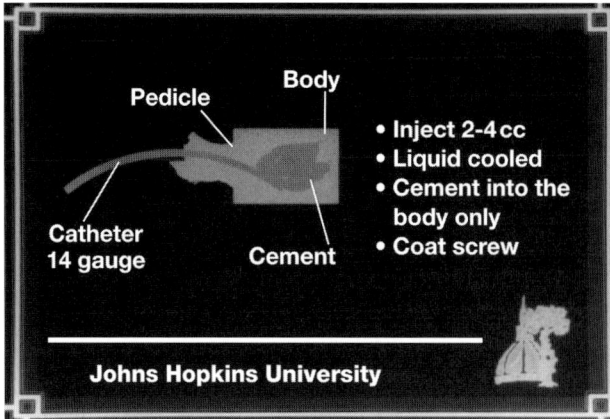

Figure 13 Diagram of acute fracture; pedicle injection of PMMA; note all cement is in the body; none should be placed in the pedicle; this is the method for pedicle screw reenforcement.

cedure (decancelization), or a combination of approaches (Figs. 6a–d; 7a–c; 8a,b.

Technical considerations in spinal fixation must be considered. Osteoporosis does affect fixation. There is an increased risk of laminar fracture and pullout when hooks are used. Pullout is less with screws. A maximal diameter of pedicle screw should used because of the thin pedicle cortex that exists in the osteoporotic spine.

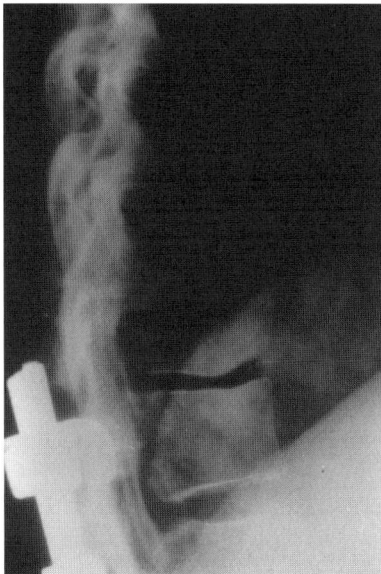

Figure 14 Osteoporotic stress fracture above instrumentation, which stopped at the thoracolumbar junction, unfortunately resulting in kyphus.

Continued low back and pelvic pain should include ruling out the possibility of occult sacral fractures (Fig. 9a–c) and pelvic fractures.

VIII   VERTEBRAL BODY AUGMENTATION

Intravertebral injections were initially done for sclerosis of vascular lesions preoperatively in the early 1980s and were found to be therapeutic for tumor pain. In 1984, polymethyl methacrylate was injected into the vertebral bodies for the treatment of aggressive angioma, resulting in pain relief and stability. The use of poly-

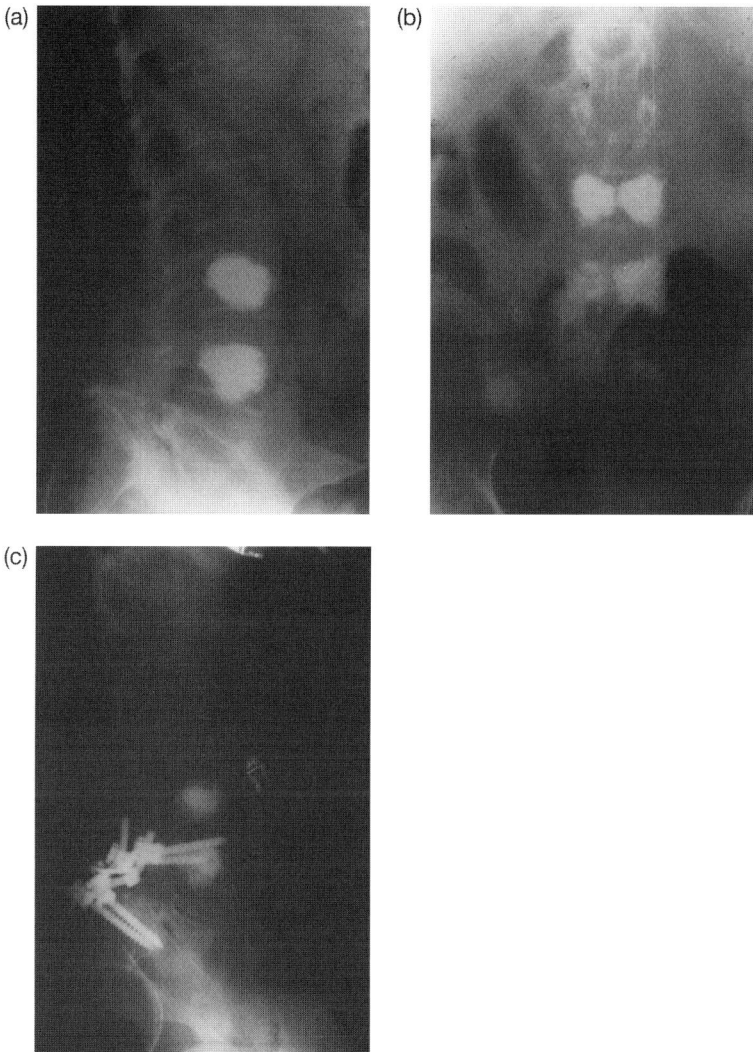

Figure 15   (a) AP and (b) lateral post-preoperative vertebroplasty in a 32-year-old male with spondylolisthesis. (c) Postoperative stabilization, most cephalad vertebroplasty was to prevent fracture at a level of increased stress; most caudal level was to hold proximal screws.

methyl methacrylate for vertebral compression fractures was reported in France in 1991, with about 75 to 80% satisfactory results for relief of pain. A series in 1996 was reported in 22 patients. Injections were not without risk, with 2 of 22 patients developing neurological problems. At this time, it was recognized that the posterior cortex must be intact prior to vertebral body injection. In a more recent study of 37 French patients, 36 had good lasting pain relief with no neurological problems. There was evidence on CT scanning of some extraosseous polymethyl methacrylate in 20%. There have been no long-term reports on the effect of polymethyl methacrylate injections for osteoporotic compression injuries. Anecdotally, this has been used for vertebral screw fixation anteriorly for more than 25 years by the author with no evidence of any untoward problems reported. In a review of the first 20 patients with compression fracture at Johns Hopkins treated transpedicularly in 1997 and 1998, 25 of 27 treated levels had good pain relief with no neurological problems. Two patients did develop fractures at other levels at a later time. More recently, 300 more patients have been treated (Figs. 10, 11a–c).

Studies in our laboratory in 1991, looked at stiffness related to osteoporotic controls using 3, 6, and 9 cc of polymethyl methacrylate augmentation of the vertebral body. Vertebral stiffness increased 40, 45, and 60%, respectively. Energy to fracture increased 2.5 times with 3 cc augmentation, and 3 times for 6 cc augmentation. Compressive strength improved between 33 to 100%. Further studies of energy to fracture using a unilateral pedicle injection with 3 cc indicated improvement of 40% and, with 6 cc, 150% improvement. A bilateral injection with 5 cc was

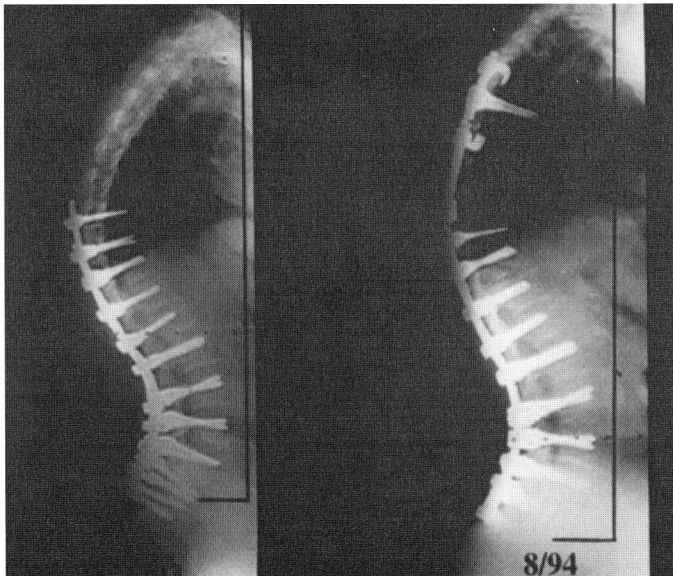

Figure 16 Female, age 62, with osteoporosis and deformity; fusion was initially stopped at thoracic apical kyphosis; a fracture occurred at the level proximal to the uppermost screw; this is wrong—extension and correction to the proximal thoracic spine was necessary and should have been performed initially.

equivalent or slightly greater than a unilateral 6 cc injection. Further experimental studies were done on pedicle screw augmentation. These were randomized by pedicle to a control group with no PMMA injection and a direct injection of 1 cc of polymethyl methacrylate into the vertebral body via the pedicle. Screw diameters of 5, 6, and 7 mm were assessed.

Augmentation of 1 cc increased the pullout strength by 100%, 2 cc by 400%, and 3 cc by 1000%.

The traditional augmentation of the vertebral body has been via the pedicle. More recently, Bhatnagar has advocated a posterolateral approach that is safer, more rapid, and equally effective (Fig. 12a–c).

Intraoperatively polymethyl methacrylate can be introduced into the vertebral body via a 14-gauge catheter injecting 2 to 4 cc of polymethyl methacrylate (Figs. 13–18). A variety of polymethyl methacrylates can be used, including the standard materials used for joint replacement, which, if left in the refrigerator an hour prior to injection, renders them more liquid and slower to set. Cranioplasty has been advocated as used primarily by neuroradiologists. Injection must be very slow since this is quite liquid and subject to flow outside of its intended point. Cement should not be injected directly into the pedicle, as studies have shown a variety of incidences of pedicle hole perforation as high as 20% during screw hole preparation.

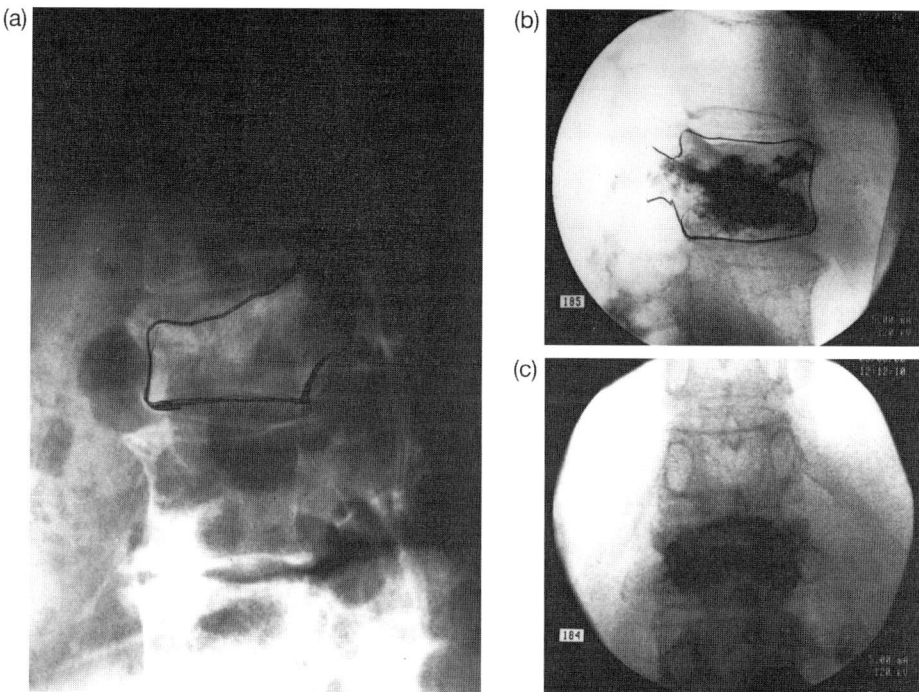

Figure 17 (a) Compression fracture, L1, in a 62-year-old female with severe osteoporosis; (b) postoperative kyphoplasty; vertebral body height restored; PMMA injected; (c) anterior-posterior of the same.

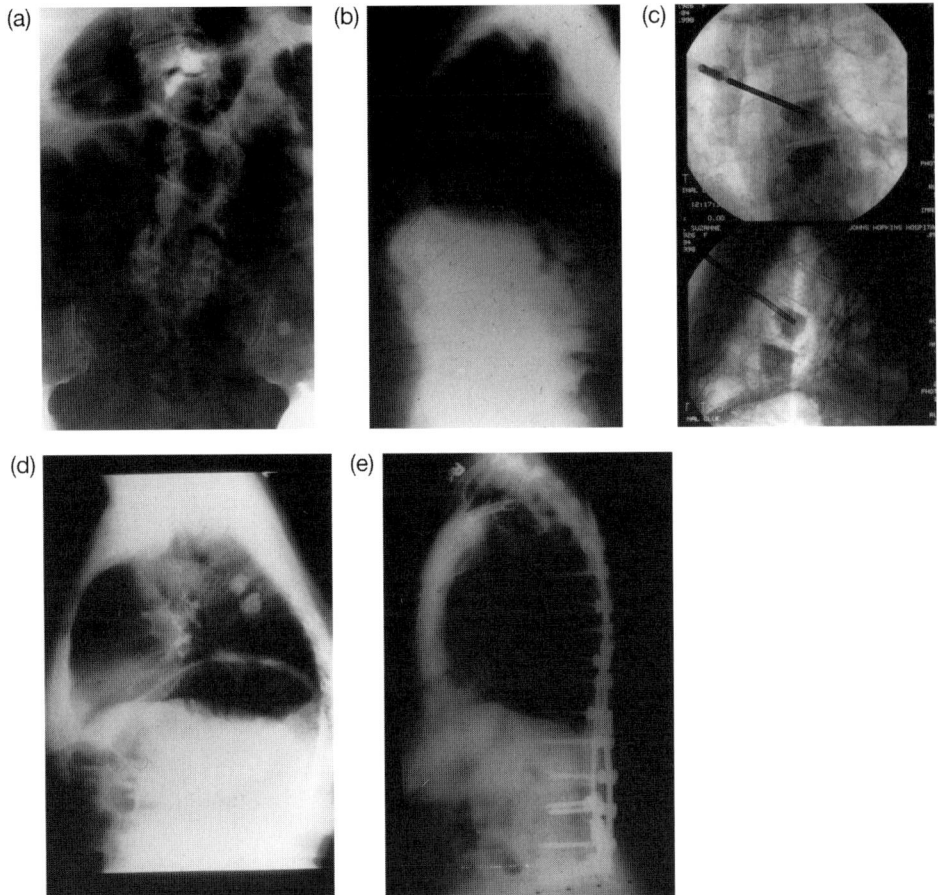

Figure 18 (a) Female aged 73; six previous operations; severe osteoporosis with scoliosis; (b) kyphosis and pseudoarthrotosis; (c) vertebroplasty performed preoperatively in the upper thoracic spine to and in screw retention (see Fig. 18e) and prevention of proximal vertebral body collapse; (d) lateral x-ray of same showing vertebroplasty; (e) postoperative lateral indicating excellent correction of kyphosis; patient is more then 2 years postoperative with excellent pain relief and no loss of correction.

IX AUGMENTATION FOR VERTEBRAL BODY OSTEOPOROTIC FRACTURES

The ideal vertebral body for augmentation is one that has collapsed less than 50%. Avascular collapse or significant collapse beyond this is not amenable to augmentation therapy. The main problem is the natural history since at least 60% of fractures are asymptomatic within a few months of their onset. It is also important to follow these fractures closely following their presentation to make sure that further collapse is not happening in the first few months.

X OTHER INDICATIONS FOR VERTEBRAL BODY AUGMENTATION

In addition to the treatment of osteoporotic vertebral body fractures, as indicated, other uses include augmentation of vertebral bodies for pedicle screw fixation and prevention of the toping-off syndrome (Figs. 14, 15a–c, 16).

XI KYPHOPLASTY

Although augmentation of vertebral body may help alleviate pain, deformity is not corrected. Recently, a technique using balloon expansion of the compressed vertebral body via a pedicle approach has been advocated for reduction of the deformity and restoration of vertebral body height followed by augmentation of the void created by the balloon with polymethyl methacrylate (Fig. 17a–c).

Indications remain unclear, and currently it is advocated for compression fractures with 50% loss of height or less, within the first 4 to 6 weeks of fracture. In some cases, particularly steroid-induced, the time has been extended up to 6 months from the time of fracture.

Although the initial results seem promising, the real question remains as to what is the natural history of such a fracture. It is recognized that the vast majority of the osteoporotic compression fractures will be pain-free without major sequela, which brings to question the timing of such intervention. Currently, clinical trials on balloon expansion of compression fractures with the above indications are underway, and, hopefully, answers will be provided.

SUGGESTED READING

1. Al-Assair I, Perez-Iligueras A, Forensa J, Munoz A, Cuesta F. Percutaneous vertebroplasty: a special syringe for cement injection. Bone 1999;25(suppl):11S–15S.
2. Arden N, Cooper C. Present and future of osteoporosis: epidemiology. In: *Osteoporosis: Diagnosis and Management*. St. Louis: Mosby, 1988:1–16.
3. Bai B, Jarwazi I, Kummer F, Spivak J. The use of an injectable, biodegradable calcium phosphate bone substitute for the prophylactic augmentation of osteoporotic vertebrae and the management of vertebral compression fractures. Spine 1999;24:1521–1526.
4. Barr J, Br M, Lemley T, McCann R. Percutaneous vertebroplasty for pain relief and spinal stabilization. Spine 2000;25:923–928.
5. Beckenbaugh R, Tressler H, Johnson E. Results of hemiarthroplasty of the hip using a cemented femoral prosthesis: a review of 109 cases with an average follow up of 36 months. Mayo Clin Proc 1977;52:349–353.
6. Belkoff S, Fenton F, Mathis J. Biomechanical comparison of two bone cements for use in vertebroplasty. 45th Annual Meeting, Orthopaedic Research Society, Feb.1–4, 1999, Anaheim, California.
7. Belkoff S, Maroney M, Fenton D, Mathis J. An in vitro biomechanical evaluation of bone cements used in percutaneous vertebroplasty. Bone 1999;25(suppl):23S–26S.
8. Belkoff S, Mathis J, Drbe E, Fenton D. Biomechanical evaluation of a new bone cement for use in vertebroplasty. Spine 2000;25:1061–1064.
9. Bhatnagar M, Mathur S, Mess C. Case report: fatal pulmonary embolism caused by acrylic cement: an unseen complication in vertebroplasty (to be submitted).
10. Chiras J, Depriester C, Weill A, Sola-Martinez M, Deramond H. Percutaneous vertebroplasties; technique and indications. J Neuroradiol 1977;24:45–59.
11. Convery F, Gunn D, Hughes J et al. The relative safety of PMMA. J Bone Joint Surg 1975;57A:57–64.

12. Coper C, Atkinson F, Jacobsen S, O'Fallon W, Melton L. Population study of survival following osteoporotic fractures. Am J Epidemiol 1993;137:1001–1005.
13. Cortet B, Cotten A, Boutry N, et al. Percutaneous vertebroplasty in patients with osteolytic metastases or multiple myeloma. Rev Rhum 1997:177–183.
14. Cotton A, Dwarte F, Cortet B, et al. Percutaneous vertebroplasty for osteolytic metastases and myeloma: effect of the percentage of lesion filling and the leakage of methyl methacrylate at clinical follow up. Radiology 1996;200:525–530.
15. Cunin G, Boissonet H, Petite H, Blanchat C, Guillemin G. Experimental vertebroplasty using osteoconductive granular material. Spine 2000;25:1070–1076.
16. Cyteval C, Sarrabere M, Roux J, et al. Acute osteoporotic vertebral collapse: open study on percutaneous injection of acrylic surgical cement in 20 patients. Am J Roentgenol 1999;173:1685–1690.
17. DePriester C, Deramond H, Toussaint P, Jhaveri H, Galibert P. Percutaneous vertebroplasty: indications, technique and complications. Semin Musculoskelet Radiol 1997;1: 285–296.
18. Deramond H, Wright N, Belkol TS. Temperature elevation caused by bone cement polymerization during vertebroplasty. Bone 1999;25(suppl):17S–21S.
19. Duncan J. Intraoperative collapses or death related to the use of acrylic cement in hip surgery. Anesthesia 1989;44:149–153.
20. Dunnagan S, Know M, Deaton S. Osteoporotic compression fracture with persistent pain: treatment with percutaneous vertebroplasty. The Journal 1999;96:258–259.
21. Einhorn T. Verbebroplasty: an opportunity to do something really good for patients. Spine 2000;25:1051–1052.
22. Enneking F. Cardiac arrest during total knee replacement using a long-stem prosthesis. JCA 1995;7:253–263.
23. Ferris B, Kinsella M. Fatal complications of the surgical treatment of distal fractures of the femur. Injury. Br J Accident Surg 1984:16:207–208.
24. Feydy A, Congard C, Miaux Y, et al. Acrylic vertebroplasty in symptomatic cervical hemangiomas: Report of 2 cases. Neuroradiology 1996:38:389–391.
25. Gangi A, Kastler, Dietermann J. Percutaneous vertebroplasty guided by a combination of CT and fluoroscopy. AJNR 1994:15:83–86.
26. Garfin S, Mennelstein I, Mirkovic S, Sandhu H, Vaccaro A. Challenges of spine fixation in the adult. NASS Annual Meeting, Oct. 31, 1998.
27. Grados F, Hardy N, Cayrolle G et al. Treatment of vertebral compression fractures by vertebroplasty (abstract). Rev Rhum (Engl. Ed) 1997;64:38.
28. Ide C, Gangi A, Rimmelin A, et al. Vertebral hemangiomas with spinal cord compression: the place of preoperative percutaneous vertebroplasty with methyl methacrylate. Neuroradiology 1966:38:585–589.
29. Jasper I, Deramond H, Mathis J, Belkoff S. The effect of monomer-to-power ratio on the material properties of cranioplastic. Bone 1999;25(suppl):27S–29S.
30. Jensen M, Evans A, Mathis J, Kallmes D, Cloft H, Dion J. Percutaneous polymethylmethacrylate vertebroplasty in the treatment of osteoporotic vertebral body compression fractures: technical aspects. AJNR 1997;18:1987–1904.
31. Kostuik J. The Adult Spine: Principles and Practice. Philadelphia: Lippincott, 1998:661–677.
32. Martin J, Sugiu J, Ruiz D. Vertebroplasty: clincal experience and follow up results. Bone 1999;25(suppl):11S–15S.
33. McLaughlin R, Difazio C, Hakala M, et al. Blood clearance and acute pulmonary toxicity of methylmethacrylate in dogs after simulated arthroplasty and intravenous injection. J Bone Joint Surg 1973;55A:1621–1628.
34. Orsini E, Richard R, Mullen J. Fatal fat embolism during cemented total knee arthroplasty: A case report. CJS 1986;29:385–386.

35. Padovani B, Kasriel O, Brunner P, Peretti-Viton P. Pulmonary embolism caused by acrylic cement: a rare complications of percutaneous vertebroplasty. ANJR 1999;20: 375–377.
36. Philips H, Cole P, Letton A. Cardiovascular effects of implanted acrylic bone cement. Br Med J 1971;3:460–461.
37. Taurel P, Cyteval C, Sarrabere M, et al. Acute osteoporotic vertebral collapse: open study of percutaneous injection of acrylic surgical cement in 20 patients. Am J Roentgenol 1999;173:1685–1690.
38. Tohmeh A, Mathis J, Fenton D, Levin A, Belkoff S. Biomechanical efficacy of unipedicular versus bipedicular vertebroplasty for the management of osteoporotic compression fractures. Spine 1999;24:1772–1766.
39. Wasnich U. Vertebral fracture epidemiology. Bone 1996;18:1795–1835.
40. Weill A, Chibras J, Simon J, Rose M, Sola-Martinez T, Eukaoua F. Spinal metastases: indications for and results of percutaneous injection of acrylic surgical cement. Radiology 1996;199:241–247.
41. Wijn de J, Slooff T, Driessens F. Characterization of bone cements. Acta Orthop Scand 1975;46:38–51.
42. Wilson D, Myers E, Mathis J, et al. Effect of augmentation on the mechanics of vertebral wedge fractures. Spine 2000;25:158–165.
43. Wolff A, Dixon A. Fractures in osteoporosis. Osteoporosis: A Clinical Guide, 2nd ed. St. Louis: Mosby, 1998:153–176.

47

Gunshot Wounds to the Spine

ROBERT F. HEARY

UMDNJ–New Jersey Medical School, Newark, New Jersey, U.S.A.

CHRISTOPHER M. BONO

University of California at San Diego, San Diego, California, U.S.A.

I INTRODUCTION

With the rise of violence throughout the world, the incidence of gunshot wound injuries continues to increase (1). Among the most troublesome are gunshot wounds to the spine, which account for 13 to 17% of all spinal cord injuries (SCIs) each year (2,3). Most common in the thoracic region, they are perhaps most devastating in the cervical spine where the potential for severe neurological impairment is greatest (2,4). Spinal gunshot wounds occur most frequently in young males between the ages of 15 and 34 years (3,5,6). Spinal cord injuries resulting from gunshot wounds are more likely to result in complete sensorimotor paralysis compared with SCIs from blunt trauma (1). Of victims of gunshot wounds resulting in SCI, approximately half result in paraplegia and half in tetraplegia (7). Like spinal cord injuries in general, incomplete injuries from gunshot wounds have much better prognoses (8).

II CLINICAL SIGNIFICANCE OF BALLISTICS AND BULLET DESIGN

According to the formula $KE = 1/2\ mv^2$ (where KE = kinetic energy, m = mass, and v = velocity), the energy of the bullet is influenced by both the mass and the speed of the bullet. As the equation dictates, increases in velocity have exponential effects on the energy of the injury. Thus, by convention, muzzle velocities between 1000 to 2000 ft/s are considered low energy, while speeds greater than 2000 to 3000 ft/s are considered high energy (9,10). Low-velocity, low-energy firearms include pistols and handguns. High-velocity, high-energy weapons include military assault rifles

655

such as the AK-47 and M-16. In contrast, shotguns are low-velocity weapons that incur high-energy wounds because of the combined mass of the numerous fired pellets (11). In addition, shotgun wounds are further complicated by the presence of large pieces of "wadding" that accompany the metallic fragments (11).

In general, civilian gunshot wounds are considered low energy. However, the reader is cautioned in this assumption. An increasing frequency of high-energy injuries is being reported in the nonmilitary population (12). Greater availability of military-type firearms, especially among the criminal element, is a contributing factor. In 1995, high-velocity weapons accounted for 16% of all homicides in New York City (13). Close-range gunshots lose less energy during transit and therefore transfer more energy to the victim. Differentiation between high and low-energy injuries is crucial, as the treatments are distinct.

Bullet energy is not the sole determinant of the extent of injury. Fragmentation of the missile can increase the zone of tissue destruction. Hollow-point bullets "explode" on impact, leading to multiple fragments that deviate from the linear path of the intact member. The phenomenon of yaw refers to the tumbling of a bullet along its longitudinal axis. Longer bullets have a tendency for greater yaw, which can further increase the circumference of destruction. In its midpath, one can imagine the bullet turned 90 degrees to its long axis so that it is, in effect, being pulled through the tissues sideways. Bullets can be nonjacketed, partially jacketed, or fully jacketed. Fully jacketed bullets exhibit little deformation with firing and are intended for long-range attacks. They are highly precise and incur clean exit and entrance wounds. Partially jacketed or nonjacketed missiles expand on impact and, like hollow-point bullets, exponentially extend the circumference of tissue damage. Such designs are intended for close-range targets.

Varying materials have been used to produce bullets. Most bullets are composed of a lead core, which may be combined with a number of different metals, to achieve a desired hardness. Similarly, the jacketing material can be copper, brass, or nickel. These substances can have both systemic and local toxicities on tissues. More commonly seen in synovial joints of the extremities, lead poisoning has been reported with bullets lodged in the intervertebral disk (14). Though cerebrospinal fluid would intuitively be an effective solvent, systemic lead elution with bullets in the intramedullary substance of the spinal cord can occur. In cases of retained lead bullets, lead levels can be measured periodically. Notwithstanding other clinical factors, significant increases in lead levels and characteristic hematopoietic changes can be an indication for bullet removal. In actual clinical practice, bullets very rarely need to be removed because of lead toxicity.

In vivo experiments in monkeys have demonstrated the local necrotic effect of copper on brain tissue (15). Extrapolating to human spinal cords, it is believed that copper bullets would have a similar effect. Some authors recommend removal of copper-containing bullets from the spinal canal (5,16). The clinical challenge is determining the material of the bullet, which, in many instances, is not known.

III EVALUATION

A Acute Examination

Initial focus of the gunshot victim must address all life-threatening injuries. Maintenance of airway, breathing, and circulation (ABCs) is paramount. Consideration may be particular to the region of injury. Gunshots to the neck are frequently complicated by tracheal injuries that can necessitate emergent intubation or tracheostomy (17). Action should not be delayed for radiological evaluation of the cervical spine, as the overwhelming majority of fractures are inherently stable (18–20). Standard intubation techniques are preferred, as fiberoptic intubations are time consuming and, ultimately, rarely necessary. Carotid and vertebral artery perforations are suspected with pulsatile neck bleeding. Immediate vascular consultation to restore cerebral blood flow is beneficial, as temporary stents placed in the emergency situation can enable definitive repair at a later time. Pharyngeal and esophageal wounds must also be detected and evaluated as they are often associated with infections. In particular, large hypopharyngeal lacerations are associated with a higher rate of infection. Endoscopic techniques have been used effectively and expediently for surveillance in the acute setting (17). Open surgical exploration is mandatory to repair any documented esophageal injuries.

The thoracic spine is the most commonly affected region with gunshot wounds (4). The lungs, heart, and great vessels are at risk with such injuries. Careful chest auscultation can detect asymmetric breath sounds indicating hemothorax or pneumothorax. Cardiac monitoring, including distal pulses, can suggest heart perforation, aortic disruption, or tamponade. Until stabilization of ventilation and hemodynamics is completed, the evaluation of a thoracic spine injury is secondary. Similarly, the examination of the abdomen is focused on suspected vascular or viscus injuries. In particular, colonic perforations that occur prior to the missile passing through the back are associated with a high rate of spinal infection (3,21–24). Though numerous organs exist in the pelvic area, sacral gunshots are most often complicated by hemorrhage (25).

Following a posterior gunshot to the sacral region, sterile packing of the posterior bullet hole using methyl cellulose and bone wax have been reported effective in facilitating tamponade (25). Likewise, emergent angiographic embolization can diminish or halt uncontrollable bleeding. Unfortunately, this embolization may result in possible devascularization of neural structures (25).

B   Evaluation of the Spinal Injury

After patient stabilization by the trauma team, focus is turned toward the spinal injury. Witnesses, emergency medical technicians, or law enforcement officers can offer useful information about the direction of the injury, the type of weapon or bullet, and the proximity of the shot. Often, the patient can account for the number of shots fired. The need for immediate cervical stabilization with a collar is usually not necessary.

The patient must be stripped of all clothing. Entrance and exit wounds should be examined thoroughly. Often, only an entrance hole can be found as the bullet is lodged in tissue. The entrance hole may be differentiated from the exit wound. As a bullet pierces the skin from the outside, the margins of the wound are cleaner and more defined. Upon exit, the bullet can take a more random path (i.e., yaw, fragmentation) and has more of a "blown out" appearance. In the abdomen, it is critical to determine the path traveled by the bullet. Though deep probing is not recommended, superficial inspection for imbedded pieces of clothing or foreign materials is useful. After sterile wound care and dressing, radiopaque markers (e.g., electrocardiogram leads) are placed over all wounds. This facilitates roentgenographic deduction of the gunshot path.

The physical exam should continue as for all other spinal trauma. All spinous processes must be palpated for tenderness and crepitus. An in-depth neurological exam including motor, sensory, reflexes, and anal sphincter tone is mandatory and must be documented precisely. In the intubated or unconscious patient, neurological testing is limited. However, if paralytic agents have not been administered, then deep tendon and bulbocavernosus reflexes can still be elicited.

C   Imaging

Two orthogonal plain radiographic views of the spine can help detect gunshot fractures and locate bullet fragments. Using the radiopaque bullet markers, the bullet path can be traced. Damage must be suspected to structures along the missile path. Bullet location may be in the soft tissues, the intervertebral disk, the vertebra, or within the spinal canal. Parameters such as vertebral body height, interpedicular distance, and adjacent segment kyphosis can be measured, although gunshots rarely cause unstable spine fractures (5). In the awake, neurologically intact patient in whom spinal stability is in question, dynamic flexion extension views may be obtained.

The necessity of imaging the cervical spine after gunshot wounds to the head and face has been questioned in a number of recent articles. In a series of 53 consecutive patients sustaining gunshots to the cranium, none had cervical spine fractures (26). Similarly, Kennedy et al. (18) found wounds limited to the calvaria had no concomitant cervical spine trauma in 105 cases. However, with gunshots extending outside the calvaria, 10% sustained a cervical spine fracture. Kihtir and associates (20) studied the association of cervical injuries with gunshot wounds to the face. Dividing the face into three zones, spinal fractures were noted in 10% and 20% of midface (maxillary) and orbital (frontal) injuries, respectively, while none were noted after gunshots to the lower face (mandibular region). From these data, it would appear that gunshots to the maxilla and orbits carry the highest risk for concomitant cervical spinal trauma and that radiographic imaging should be pursued more aggressively after such incidents.

After the level of the bullet and/or fracture has been determined by plain films, computerized tomography (CT) should be obtained. Currently, this is the modality of choice for spinal gunshot trauma (27). CT images allow better localization of the bullet within the vertebral segment and can more clearly demonstrate foreign bodies in the spinal canal. Thin slices (1 to 3 mm) are used to evaluate the integrity of the bony elements. Of note, images are often obscured by artifact when metallic bullet fragments are present (28,29). This can limit the amount of detail appreciable.

The use of magnetic resonance imaging (MRI) to evaluate gunshots of the spine is controversial. Bullet migration from the pull of the strong magnet is a relevant issue and can possibly lead to further neurological or soft-tissue damage. This issue remains theoretical, as numerous reports of MRI after gunshot wounds to the spine have not supported this concern (28–30). The advantages of MRI over CT include markedly less artifact, better soft-tissue imaging, and coronal, sagittal, and axial visualization of the neural elements (29). Although these advantages are attractive, the use of MRI should be on an individual and patient-specific basis. For example, bullets lodged in a vertebral body may have less propensity to migrate than intracanal fragments. However, these contentions remain unproven in a controlled scientific study. In the authors' experience, the most frequent complaint with MRI is that the patient may feel a sensation of heat from the bullet, which may cause the study to be aborted. This is particularly common with jacketed bullets.

IV INITIAL TREATMENT

The initial treatment of the gunshot wound victim is an integral part of the trauma evaluation. As discussed above, maintenance of ABCs is the primary goal. Management can be facilitated with the use of a structured algorithm. Bishop et al. (4) examined the results of a comprehensive treatment scheme for both blunt and penetrating chest and abdominal trauma. The authors noted substantially higher mortality for cases in which treatment deviated from the algorithm. Interestingly, 60% of the deviations that lead to death occurred in gunshot wound victims, while 81% of deaths that occurred without deviations were after gunshot wounds. Although the benefits of such programmed decision trees are obvious, it would appear that its impact on the outcome after gunshot wounds is minimal. Among the most common causes of death were exsanguination and hypoxemia from massive hemothorax.

A Antibiosis

Tetanus prophylaxis must be considered in all instances of spinal gunshot wounds. If there is any question regarding the patient's most recent immunization, the gunshot wound victim should receive tetanus prophylaxis in the emergency department at the time of the initial evaluation.

Although some authors advocate bullet wound cultures (16), there is currently no support of this practice in the literature. Extrapolating from evidence of long bone open wounds, the utility of wound culture is minimal (31). Broad-spectrum antibiosis should be initiated as soon as possible. Previous theories that bullets become heat sterilized upon firing have been discounted (32). In addition, bullet entry can exhibit a vacuum effect in which outside air and contents may be pulled into the wound. Recommendations for the duration of antibiosis vary. For gunshot wounds not complicated by viscus perforations, it is generally recommended to maintain 48 to 72 h of prophylaxis. This must be considered in regard to clinical evidence of infection both in spinal and extraspinal regions.

Viscus perforations carry a higher risk of infection (21–24,33). Rates of infection are highest with colonic wounds that occur prior to the bullet entering the spine (22). It is thought that the stomach and small bowel are sterile, although case reports of spinal infection have been documented (33). After colonic perforation, the lowest infection rates have been documented with antibiotics continued for 7 to 14 days after injury (21,23). Bullet removal and surgical debridement have been associated with higher rates of infection (34). Barring other indications, such as neurological deterioration or lead toxicity, bullet extraction is not advocated to decrease the infection risk (3).

The role of antibiotic prophylaxis after esophageal and upper airway perforation is less clear. Pooled secretions in the hypopharynx are thought to increase the propensity for infection with gunshot wounds to this area (17). The decision to explore these wounds is usually based on the size of the lesion, as small rents can effectively be treated nonoperatively. To the authors' knowledge, there are no controlled studies of the duration of antibiotic prophylaxis after upper airway injuries associated with gunshot wounds. Notwithstanding evidence of frank infection or meningitis, it is prudent to extend prophylaxis for 48 to 72 h.

V   SPECIFIC INJURIES

A   Gunshot Wound—Cerebrospinal Fluid Leak

In the initial treatment of gunshot wound patients, the bullet entry site should be treated with debridement of any devitalized skin and superficial soft tissues. If a cerebrospinal fluid (CSF) leak appears to be present, then a lumbar subarachnoid drain should be placed. In cases where a persistent CSF leak or fistulae is present through the bullet entry or exit sites at the level of the skin, consideration of open surgery must be entertained (21,22,35,36). Due to the risk of meningitis resulting from a persistent CSF leak, the treatment would involve a laminectomy with repair of the dural violation either primarily or with use of a dural graft (35,37). In these relatively rare instances, placement of a temporary lumbar subarachnoid drain following the laminectomy may be beneficial to supplement the dural repair.

B   Gunshot Injury—No Neurological Deficit

In addition to the principles of antibiosis described above, the treatment of gunshot wounds to the spine with a neurologically intact patient is similar to those from blunt trauma. Especially in the neurologically intact patient, spinal stability must be assessed.

Static radiographs and imaging are helpful. Using the three-column theory of Denis (38), disruption of two or more columns may indicate spinal instability. In contrast to blunt trauma, however, two- or even three-column disruption is less likely to result in instability. In Denis' original work, the proposed mechanisms of injury implied an abrupt acceleration/deceleration of the body/spine in space. With gunshot wounds, the body/spine can be considered stationary and the bullet is the directional force. In the best-case scenario, a through-and-through bullet wound will only damage those structures that lie directly in its effective path. Low-energy gunshots have a narrower circumference of damage than high-energy wounds. These factors influence the amount of spinal instability after gunshots to the spine. These concepts can be likened to the magician who pulls a tablecloth from a table set with glasses and plates. The bullet acts as the tablecloth. If pulled very quickly, the glasses and plates (i.e., spinal elements) stay in place. If he pushes the table abruptly (i.e., motor vehicle accident), the contents will surely fall and break.

In the awake, cooperative, neurologically intact patient, dynamic lateral radiographs can be obtained. Careful flexion and extension of the spine can demonstrate pathological mobility of adjacent spinal segments. In the cervical spine, commonly used criteria for radiographic instability are greater than 11 degrees of angulatory change or more than 3.5 mm of translation between flexion and extension views (39). In the L5–S1 segment, more than 5 mm of translation or 15 degrees of angulation is considered unstable (39). In cases of instability, the affected segments can be stabilized with a variety of instrumentation and fusion constructs, which is beyond the scope of this chapter.

Interestingly, the majority of cases of unstable spines after gunshot wounds have been associated with overly aggressive decompression (8). Fortunately, there are few indications for decompression in a neurologically intact patient. Frequently cited indications are for the treatment of lead intoxication from the bullet or contact of a copper-jacketed missile with the neural elements (5,14,16,35,40). Routine removal of the bullet is not warranted for transcolonic injury and is associated with a high rate of complications.

C   Gunshot Injury—Neurological Deficit

A spinal cord injury from a gunshot wound is a devastating injury to the patient, family, and society. In a study by Roye, et al. in 1988, the average hospital costs for survivors of cervical level injury were greater than 50,000 dollars (2). High-level complete injuries may leave patients ventilator dependent, requiring highly specialized units for prolonged care. Gunshot wounds more frequently result in complete (ASIA class A) injuries, which may be paraplegia or tetraplegia depending on the level. Incomplete injury can present in a variety of manners, including Brown-Sequard, central cord, anterior cord, or, in rare cases, cruciate hemiplegic syndrome (41).

1   Steroids

The use of corticosteroids in spinal cord–injured patients after gunshot wounds has recently been examined (42,43). Levy and associates (43) retrospectively studied 252 cases of both complete and incomplete gunshot spinal cord injuries. Administration of methylprednisolone according to NASCIS-2 protocol did not significantly affect neurological prognosis. Similarly, Heary et al. (42) demonstrated that administration of either methylprednisolone or dexamethasone regimens did not significantly improve the neurological recovery of patients with either complete or incomplete injuries compared to those receiving no steroids. Interestingly, the incidence of pancreatitis was statistically greater in patients who received methylprednisolone, while gastrointestinal complications were highest in those who received dexamethasone. Though these data were not randomized, prospective analyses, they offer compelling evidence that emergent corticosteroid infusion does not have a role in the treatment of spinal cord injury after gunshot wounds.

2   Decompression

The first rule of medicine is "do no harm." This philosophy should be kept in mind in the management of a patient with a neurological deficit after a gunshot wound to the spine. A natural tendency for surgeons is to feel compelled to remove bullets and decompress the spinal canal. However, the clinical benefit of these actions is inconsistent and is not without complications.

In both complete and incomplete spinal cord injuries, the role of decompression has been studied. Stauffer et al. (8) reviewed 185 cases of gunshot paralysis, half of which were treated with laminectomy and half with observation only. The authors documented no appreciable return of neurological function after both surgery and nonoperative management for complete lesions. With incomplete injuries, 71% of decompressed spines and 77% of nonsurgically treated spines demonstrated neural improvement. Incomplete lesions to the lumbar spine and thoracolumbar junction had better neurological recovery than more cranial levels, regardless of whether surgery was performed. Although an antibiotic regimen was not documented, four wound infections and six spinal fistulae were reported in the operative group as well as six cases of late spinal instability. There were no cases of infection, cerebrospinal fluid fistula, or spinal instability in the nonsurgically treated patients. Both groups had a high incidence of causalgia (19% and 15% for operative and nonoperative groups). In support of a nonoperative approach, Robertson and Simpson (36) reported no neurological improvements with lumbar laminectomy versus nonsurgical treatment in 30 patients with gunshot wounds to the cauda equina region. A high rate of postoperative complications was reported. In no case did the authors report an intracanal bullet.

In a more recent prospective study, Waters and Atkins (44) demonstrated statistically significant motor improvement after surgical decompression from the T12 to L4 levels compared with nonoperatively treated spines. Importantly, only patients with bullets lodged within the spinal canal were included. At more rostral sites in the thoracic and cervical regions, surgical removal of the bullet and decompression of the neural elements had no significant effect (Fig. 1). No case of infection was reported in either group.

The timing of surgery is an important consideration. Cybulski et al. (45) documented substantially higher rates of infection and arachnoiditis if decompressive

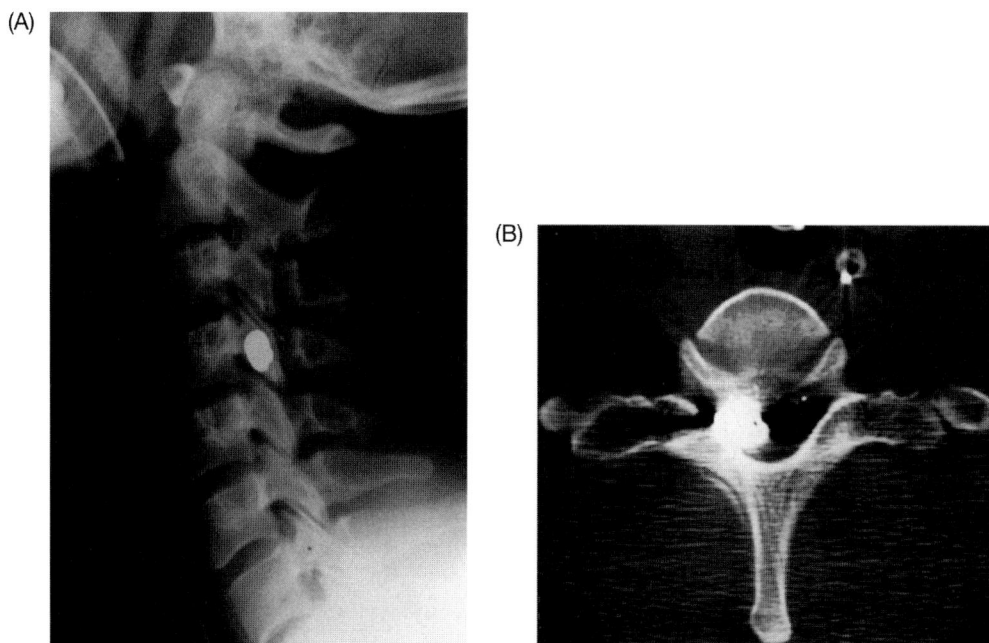

Figure 1 (A) Lateral cervical radiograph of a patient who sustained a gunshot wound to the neck with the bullet entering from the posterolateral side. The patient had a complete neurological deficit at the C4 level. There were no associated pharyngeal, tracheal, or vascular injuries. (B) An axial CT image demonstrates an intracanal bullet. The patient was treated nonsurgically with little neurological recovery.

laminectomy of the lumbar spine was performed more than 2 weeks from injury. If warranted, and if the patient can medically tolerate a surgical procedure, the bullet should be removed within 5 to 10 days of the initial injury. Regardless of the level of injury, most authors agree that a documented progression of a neurological deficit, although quite rare, is an indication for bullet removal.

D Gunshot Wounds with Herniated Disks

A herniated disk after a gunshot wound to the spine is a rare, but significant, cause for neurological compromise (46). By lodging in the intervertebral space, it is postulated that the pressure in the nucleus pulposus is increased. With a defect in the posterior or posterolateral annulus, the disk material can be expelled into the canal or foramen to compress the spinal cord or nerve root. Treatment recommendations are similar to those for other acute disk herniations. Significant, acute neurological deficits can be ameliorated with disk excision. Herniations associated with the cauda equina syndrome are a surgical emergency. Bullet removal is neither necessary nor indicated unless it can be easily removed without further jeopardizing surrounding neural or bony supporting structures.

E High-Energy Gunshot Wounds

The authors strongly emphasize that the above recommendations are relevant to low-energy gunshots. High-energy rifle and shotgun wounds are associated with significantly more soft tissue devitalization and a larger zone of injury (11, 47). From experience with United States combat troops in Panama, Parsons et al. (47) advocated aggressive surgical debridement after such injuries. Likewise, Splavski (12) and others reported low complication rates (14%) in spinal injuries treated with wide debridement and decompressive laminectomy during the Croation War in the early 1990s. Although not controlled, comparative studies, the authors highlighted that the decompression does not likely affect neurological recovery. With the increasing prevalence of gang and terrorist acts worldwide, the use of high-energy weapons has necessitated adaptation of military surgical tactics to the civilian population who are subjected to these types of injuries (12).

VI LATE SEQUELAE AND COMPLICATIONS

Lead intoxication is a rare complication of spinal gunshot wounds (14,40,48). Elution from bullets bathed in spinal cerebrospinal fluid is rare. Synovial fluid is a more effective solvent (40,49). Bullets in close proximity to facet joints or the intervertebral disk may be more likely to cause lead intoxication. The diagnosis is often missed and requires a high level of suspicion. Peripheral blood lead levels can detect increases and bone marrow biopsy can confirm hematopoietic alterations. Treatment with chelating agents, such as dimercaprol and calcium disodium edetate, is initiated immediately followed by carefully planned bullet removal.

Besides neurological deficit, pain is probably the most common long-term complication of gunshot wounds with spinal cord injury. In particular, conus medullaris and cauda equina level lesions are associated with a high rate of pain (50). The incidence of pain is not reduced with bullet removal (44). Pain is mediated by spontaneous discharges from deafferentated dorsal horn neurons and can be conservatively managed with oral neuroleptic medication such as amitriptyline (Elavil) or gabapentin (Neurontin). These medications have been demonstrated to be successful in the treatment of neuropathic pain syndromes. In unresponsive cases, a vascularized omental pedicle graft can be surgically transplanted to the affected cord level (51). Pain may be relieved by increasing the neurovascularity of the region as well as by altering the neurotransmitter milieu. As a last resort, the DREZ (dorsal root entry zone) procedure surgically removes the nociceptive dorsal rootlets. Spaic et al. (50) have documented excellent results with this maneuver in six patients with pain recalcitrant to omental transplant after thoracolumbar gunshot wounds.

Other long-term sequelae can occur. Bullet migration can cause neurological deficits months to years after the initial injury (52,53). Kuijlen and associates (52) documented neurogenic claudication 11 years after a gunshot wound to the abdomen. The bullet migrated from the paraspinal muscles at the L3 level into the spinal canal where it effectively disintegrated into multiple fragments causing a diffuse inflammatory reaction. The patient responded favorably to a decompressive laminectomy. Conway et al. (53) reported a case of cauda equina syndrome after a bullet previously lodged in the intervertebral disk migrated into the spinal canal 9 years after injury. Again, decompressive laminectomy was effective. Numerous other reports of bullet migration have been documented within the spinal canal, within the dura, and in a caudal-to-cranial direction (54–56). Bullet migration is not always associated with neurological deficit and, as such, bullet removal must be assessed on an individual basis.

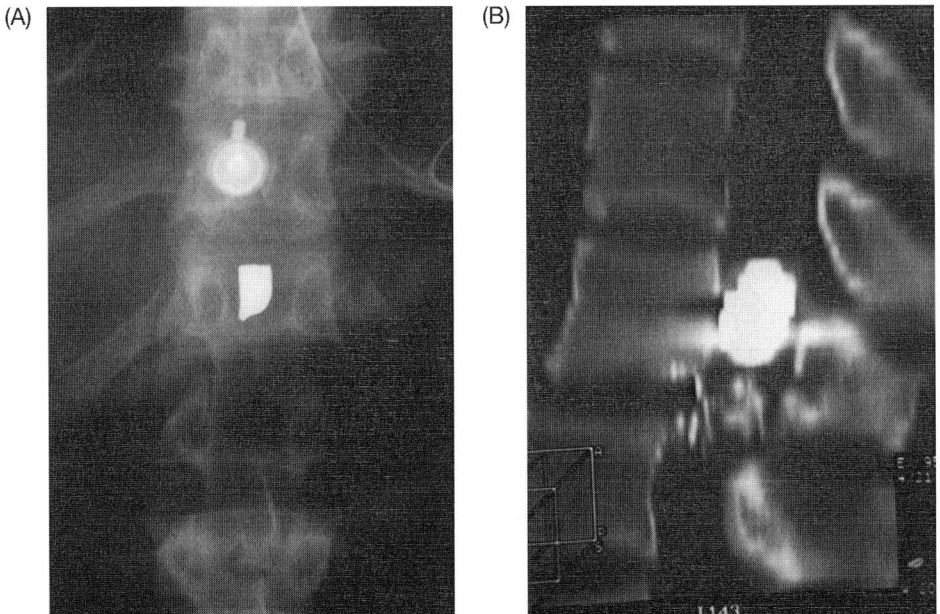

Figure 2 (A) The anteroposterior radiograph of the lumbar spine demonstrates a midline bullet at the T12 level after a gunshot wound to the back in a patient with a stable, incomplete, neurological deficit. (B) Sagittal CT reformations clearly show the bullet lying in the spinal canal. The patient was taken to the operating room for posterior decompression. The bullet was easily removed.

VII SUMMARY

Civilian gunshot wounds are usually the result of low-velocity weapons. Tetanus prophylaxis is routinely indicated, as are antibiotics for any injuries with dural violations. Steroids are of no proven benefit in the management of gunshot wound injuries and should not be administered.

(A)

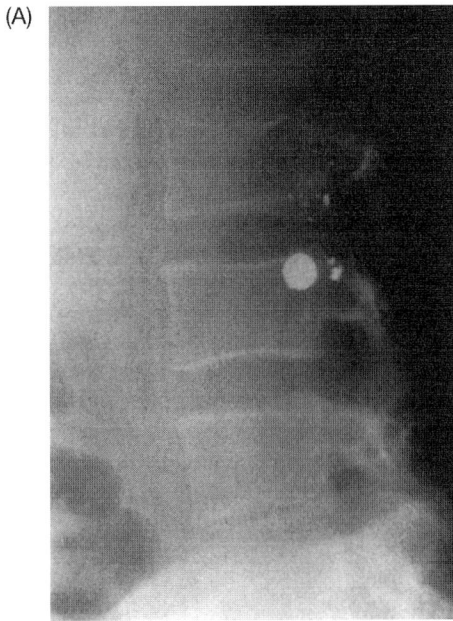

(B)

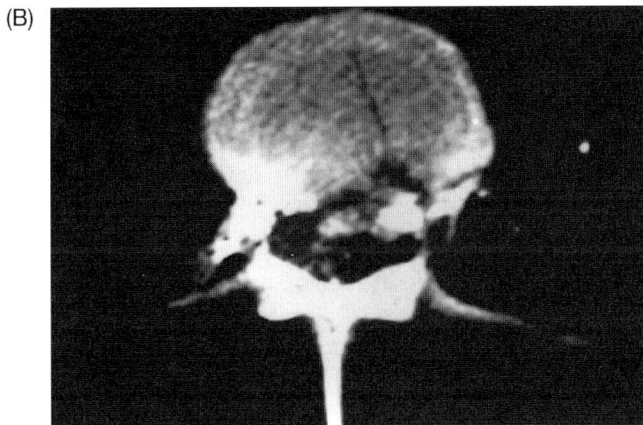

Figure 3 (A) After a gunshot wound to the left flank, the patient presented with complete neurological deficit at the L3 level. The lateral radiograph displays a bullet at the level of the posterior vertebral body of L3. (B) Axial CT images were helpful in detecting retropulsed bony fragments, which were compressing and displacing the cauda equina to the contralateral side. The patient's spinal canal was adequately decompressed without removal of the anterior bony fragments. Surgical stabilization or fusion was not required after laminectomy.

Spine surgery has very little role in the treatment of civilian gunshot wounds. The neurological status is very rarely affected favorably by decompressive spinal surgery. Likewise, spinal instability resulting from a civilian gunshot wound is extremely rare. As such, open surgical intervention for patients with spinal cord injuries resulting from civilian gunshot wounds is reserved for patients with progressive neurological deterioration, persistent CSF fistulae, or, in some cases, incomplete spinal cord injuries with active neural compression from either a bullet, an intervertebral disk, or a hematoma within the spinal canal (Fig. 2).

Patients with cauda equina injuries from civilian gunshot wounds have been shown to have better overall results than patients with spinal cord injuries and, as a result, spine surgery in these instances may impact favorably on the long-term neurological outcome (Fig. 3). Despite the overall dismal results with respect to neurological improvement following civilian gunshot wounds, the decision to pursue an open surgical intervention needs to be made on a case-by-case basis.

REFERENCES

1. Farmer JC, Vaccaro AR, Balderston RA, Albert TJ, Cotler J. The changing nature of admission to a spinal cord injury center: violence on the rise. J Spinal Disord 1998; 11: 400–403.
2. Roye WP, Dunn EL, Moody JA. Cervical spinal cord injury—a public catastrophe. J Trauma 1988; 28:1260–1264.
3. Lin SS, Vaccaro AR, Reich SM, Devine M, Cotler JM. Low-velocity gunshot wounds to the spine with an associated transperitoneal injury. J Spinal Disord 1995; 8:136–144.
4. Bishop M, Shoemaker WC, Avakian S, James E, Jackson G. Evaluation of a comprehensive algorithm for blunt and penetrating thoracic and abdominal trauma. Am Surg 1991; 57:737–746.
5. Yoshida GM, Garland D, Waters RL. Gunshot wounds to the spine. Orthop Clin North Am 1995; 26:109–116.
6. Isiklar ZU, Lindsey RW. Gunshot wounds to the spine. Injury 1998; 29:SA7–12.
7. Young JA, Burns PE, Bowen AM. Spinal Cord Injury Statistics: Experience of the Regional Spinal Cord Injury Systems. Phoenix: Good Samaritan Medical Center 1982: 1–152.
8. Stauffer ES, Wood RW, Kelly EG. Gunshot wounds of the spine: the effects of laminectomy. J Bone Joint Surg 1979; 61A:389–392.
9. Fackler ML. Wound ballistics and soft-tissue wound treatment. Techniques Orthop 1995; 10:163–170.
10. Janzon B, Seeman T. Muscle devitalization in high-energy missile wounds and its dependence on energy transfer. J Trauma 1985; 25:138–144.
11. Simpson RK, Venger BH, Fischer DK, Narayan RK, Mattox KL. Shotgun injuries of the spine: neurosurgical management of five cases. Br J Neurosurg 1988; 2:321–326.
12. Turgut M, Ozcan OE, Gucay O, Saglam S. Civilian penetrating spinal firearm injuries of the spine. Results of surgical treatment with special attention to factors determining prognosis. Arch Orthop Trauma Surg 1994; 113:290–293.
13. Zawitz MW. Guns used in crime. Washington, DC: US Department of Justice: Bureau of Justice Statistics Selected Findings 1995; NCJ-148201.
14. Grogan DP, Bucholz RW. Acute lead intoxication from a bullet in an intervertebral disc space. J Bone Joint Surg 1981; 63A:1180–1182.
15. Cushid JG, Kopeloff LM. Epileptogenic effects of metal powder implants in the motor cortex in monkeys. Int J Neuropsychiatr 1968; 3:24–28.

16. Eismont FJ. Gunshot wounds of the spine. In: Levine A, Lampert R, Garfin S, Eismont F, eds. Spine Trauma. Philadelphia: WB Saunders, 1998:525–543.
17. Fetterman BL, Shindo ML, Stanley RB, Armstrong WB, Rice DH. Management of traumatic hypopharyngeal injuries. Laryngoscope 1995; 105:8–13.
18. Kennedy FR, Gonzalez P, Beitler A, Sterling-Scott R, Fleming AW. Incidence of cervical spine injury in patients with gunshot wounds to the head. South Med J 1994; 87:621–623.
19. Kupcha PC, An HS, Cotler JM. Gunshot wounds to the cervical spine. Spine 1990; 15: 1058–1063.
20. Kihtir T, Ivatury RR, Simon RJ, Nassoura Z, Leban S. Early management of civilian gunshot wounds to the face. J Trauma 1993; 35:569–575.
21. Roffi RP, Waters RL, Adkins RH. Gunshot wounds to the spine associated with a perforated viscus. Spine 1989; 14:808–811.
22. Romanick PC, Smith TK, Kopaniky DR, Oldfield D. Infection about the spine associated with low-velocity missile injury to the abdomen. J Bone Joint Surg 1985; 67:1195–1201.
23. Kumar A, Wood GS, Whittle AP. Low-velocity gunshot injuries of the spine with abdominal viscus trauma. J Orthop Trauma 1998; 12:514–517.
24. Kihtir T, Ivatury RR, Simon R, Stahl WM. Management of transperitoneal gunshot wounds of the spine. J Trauma 1991; 31:1579–1583.
25. Naude GP, Bongard FS. Gunshot injuries of the sacrum. J Trauma 1996; 40:656–659.
26. Chong CL, Ware DV, Harris JH. Is cervical spine imaging indicated in gunshot wounds to the cranium? J Trauma 1998; 44:501–502.
27. Kaiser MC, Capesius P. Gunshot wounds to the spine as evaluated by CT-scanning. Two illustrative case reports. Comput Radiol 1985; 9:121–124.
28. Bashir EF, Cybulski GR, Chaudhri K, Choudhury AR. Magnetic resonance imaging and computed tomography in the evaluation of penetrating gunshot injury. Spine 1993; 18: 772–773.
29. Ebraheim NA, Savolain ER, Jackson WT, Andreshak TG, Rayport M. Magnetic resonance imaging in the evaluation of a gunshot wound to the cervical spine. J Orthop Trauma 1989; 3:19–22.
30. Finitsis SN, Falcone S, Green BA. MR of the spine in the presence of metallic bullet fragments: is the benefit worth the risk? Am J Neuroradiol 1999; 20:354–356.
31. Gustilo RG. Current concepts in the management of open fractures. Inst Course Lect 1987; 36:359–366.
32. Wolf AW, Benson DR, Shoji H, Hoeprich P, Gilmore A. Autosterilization in low-velocity bullets. J Trauma 1978; 18:63.
33. Hales DD, Duffy K, Dawson EG, Delamarter R. Lumbar osteomyelitis and epidural and paraspinous abscesses. Case report of an unusual source of contamination from a gunshot wound to the abdomen. Spine 1991; 16:380–383.
34. Heary RF, Vaccaro AR, Mesa JJ, Balderston RA. Thoracolumbar infection in penetrating injuries to the spine. Orthop Clin North Am 1996; 27:69–81.
35. Wigle RL. Treatment of asymptomatic gunshot injuries to the spine. Am Surg 1989; 55: 591–595.
36. Robertson DP, Simpson RK. Penetrating injuries restricted to the cauda equina: a retrospective review. Neurosurgery 1992; 31:265–269.
37. Gentleman D, Harrington M. Penetrating injury of the spinal cord. Injury 1984; 16: 7–8.
38. Denis F. The three columns of the spine and its significance in the classification of acute thoracolumbar spine injuries. Spine 1983; 8:817–831.
39. White AA, Panjabi MM. Clinical biomechanics of the spine. Philadephia: Lippincott-Raven, 1990.

40. Linden MA, Manton WI, Stewart RM, Thal ER, Feit H. Lead poisoning from retained bullets. Pathogenesis, diagnosis, and management. Ann Surg 1982; 195:305–313.
41. Ciappetta P, Salvati M, Raco A, Artico M. Cruciate hemiplegia: a clinical syndrome, a neuroanatomical controversy. Report of two cases and review of the literature. Surg Neurol 1990; 34:43–47.
42. Heary RF, Vaccaro AR, Mesa JJ, Northrup BE, Albert TJ, Balderston RA, Cotler JM. Steroids and gunshot wounds to the spine. Neurosurgery 1997; 41:576–583.
43. Levy ML, Gans W, Wijesinghe HS, SooHoo WE, Adkins RH, Stillerman CB. Use of methylprednisolone as an adjunct in the mangagement of patients with penetrating spinal cord injury: outcome analysis. Neurosurgery 1996; 39:1141–1148.
44. Waters RL, Adkins RH. The effects of removal of bullet fragment retained in the spinal canal. A collaborative study by the National Spinal Cord Injury Model Systems. Spine 1991; 16:934–939.
45. Cybulski GR, Stone JL, Kant R. Outcome of laminectomy for civilian gunshot injuries of the terminal spinal cord and cauda equina:. Neurosurgery 1989; 24:392–397.
46. Robertson DP, Simpson RK, Narayan RK. Lumbar disc herniation from a gunshot wound to the spine. A report of two cases. Spine 1991; 16:994–995.
47. Parsons TW, Lauderman WC, Ethier DB, Gormley W, Cain JE, Elias Z, Coe J. Spine injuries in combat troops—Panama, 1989. Mil Med 1993; 158:501–502.
48. Cagin CR, Diloy-Puray M, Westerman MP. Bullets, lead poisoning, and thyrotoxicosis. Ann Intern Med 1978; 89:509–511.
49. Machle W. Lead absorption from bullets lodged in tissues. J Am Med Assoc 1940; 115:1536–1541.
50. Spaic M, Petkovic S, Tadic R, Minic L. DREZ surgery on conus medullaris (after failed implantation of vascular omental graft) for treating chronic pain due to spine (gunshot) injuries. Acta Neurochir 1999; 141:1309–1312.
51. Clifton GL, Donovan WH, Dimitrijevic MM, Allen SJ, Ku A, Potts J, Moody FG, Boake C, Sherwood AM, Edwards JV. Omental transposition in chronic spinal cord injury. Spinal Cord 1996.
52. Kuijlen JM, Herpers MJ, Beuls EA. Neurogenic claudication, a delayed complication of a retained bullet. Spine 1997; 22:910–914.
53. Conway JE, Crofford TW, Terry AF, Protzman RR. Cauda equina syndrome occurring nine years after a gunshot injury to the spine. A case report. J Bone Joint Surg 1993; 75:760–763.
54. Gupta S, Senger RL. Wandering intraspinal bullet. Br J Neurosurg 1999; 13:606–607.
55. Jeffery JA, Borgstein R. Case report of a retained bullet in the lumbar spinal canal with preservation of cauda equina function. Injury 1998; 29:724–726.
56. Oktem IS, Selcuklu A, Kurtsoy A, Kavuncu IA, Pasaoglu A. Migration of bullet in the spinal canal: a case report. Migration of bullet in the spinal canal: a case report 1995; 44:548–550.

48

Management of Spinal Fractures in Polytrauma Patients

ROBERT F. McLAIN

The Cleveland Clinic Foundation, Cleveland, Ohio, U.S.A.

I INTRODUCTION

Most spine fracture patients can be treated in a timely fashion, at the surgeon's discretion, with a reliably satisfactory outcome. This chapter discusses treatment of the most severely injured segment (10%) of spine trauma patients—those patients whose lives depend on rapid resuscitation, mobilization, and prevention of pulmonary and thromboembolic complications. These patients can deteriorate very rapidly after admission, and may not be suitable for delayed surgery for weeks thereafter, if ever. While urgent surgery is not necessary or efficacious in every severe spinal fracture, there are no compelling reasons to withhold surgery on these patients when other conditions press for urgent treatment.

A major impediment to rapid stabilization is the pervasive prejudice that polytraumatized patients are too ill to undergo spinal surgery. The fear that these patients are "too sick" for spine surgery is unfounded, and they are likely only to get sicker with delayed treatment and prolonged recumbency.

Trauma remains the leading cause of death in individuals 1 to 45 years of age. The most common causes of death in patients with otherwise survivable injuries include hemorrhage, pulmonary insufficiency, adult respiratory distress syndrome (ARDS), and pneumonia, sepsis, and thromboembolic disease (10). Although the trauma literature clearly shows that urgent stabilization of long-bone injuries has reduced both morbidity and mortality among polytrauma patients, many physicians still feel that urgent spinal surgery is dangerous in severely injured patients (8–10, 30,45). An unstable spinal fracture exposes the patient to the same hazards as a segmental femur or pelvic fracture—pain, systemic shock, enforced recumbency and

669

pulmonary impairment, inability to mobilize the patient—and delayed treatment of a spinal fracture can result in the same complications dealt with in extremity polytrauma.

There is now good evidence that the incremental risk of acute spinal surgery is not great, while the risk imposed by delay and prolonged recumbency is significant. Current segmental instrumentation systems—far more rigid than nonsegmental systems in use just a decade or so ago—allow surgeons to take advantage of early surgery to aggressively mobilize injured patients. The purpose of this chapter is not to endorse urgent surgery as the *best* treatment for spinal fractures. However, urgent surgical treatment (within 24 h of injury) does not endanger polytrauma patients, and it does allow surgeons to apply the principles of trauma care proven to reduce morbidity and mortality in extremity skeletal trauma.

II INCIDENCE AND DEMOGRAPHICS

Approximately 80% of the thoracic and thoracolumbar fractures treated in an acute care environment can be managed nonoperatively. Indications for surgical treatment remain (1) an unstable thoracic or thoracolumbar spine fracture, as determined by neurological injury; sagittal angulation of 25 degrees or more relative to adjacent levels; axial compression of 50% of vertebral height or more; multiple contiguous fractures; and/or three-column spinal injury resulting in acute instability (16) or (2) potentially unstable fractures in a patient with *multiple associated injuries.*

Polytrauma can be defined as significant injury (requiring hospitalization and active management) to two or more major organ systems, of which, in this case, the spine is one. Injury Severity Scores (ISS) calculated using the Revised Abbreviated Injury Scale (13) provide an objective way of ranking and comparing the magnitude of injury in patients with multisystem trauma. In this system, a score from $0-5$ is assigned to each organ system, with 0 being no injury, and 5 being the most severe injury. The three highest scores are squared and then summed to provide a final injury severity score. Unsurvivable injuries are automatically given a score of 75.

The highest ISS score any isolated injury can generate is 25. Therefore, a score of 27 would indicate that a patient had at least one major associated injury in addition to their spinal fracture. For example, the maximum score for an *isolated* spine fracture, with complete spinal cord injury, would be 5, which would give an ISS of 25 ($5^2 + 0 + 0 = 25$). An ISS threshold of 27 excludes those patients with isolated spinal column injuries or spinal injuries associated with only a minor secondary injury (ileus or minor laceration) ($5^2 + 1^2 + 0 = 26$). Any patient with a score of 27 or greater would, by definition, have sustained significant injuries to at least two major organ systems.

The combination of severe, multisystem injury and thoracolumbar fracture is seen in less than 4% of acute spine fracture patients presenting to the trauma center (37). Even among operative cases, polytrauma is atypical and seen in fewer than 15% of cases. Polytrauma spine patients are predominantly male, predominantly young, and demographically typical of blunt and penetrating trauma populations throughout the United States. Their spinal injuries, however, are uniformly more serious, as a group, than those seen in any *unselected* series of spine fractures, (4,6,17,23,39,43,48). In a series of consecutive spine fractures treated with segmental instrumentation, 74% of patients were injured in automobile or motorcycle accidents, either as drivers, passengers, or pedestrians (37). This is an increased percentage of motor vehicle (high-speed, high-energy injuries) compared to the 43–68% reported in other large series (18,32,37,39,43,52). Of these patients, 41% suffered an additional vertebral fracture at the time of injury, compared to 7–10% in other series (52). The large number of associated injuries and the high ISS further attest to the severity of the trauma in this patient group.

Patients with stable fractures, thoracic compression, or stable burst fractures, and some lumbar burst fractures can be treated nonoperatively or with nonsegmental systems. Harrington rods, with or without Drummond wires, can be used for single-level thoracic fractures in otherwise stable patients (12,22). Pedicle screw systems such as the AO Fixateur Interne (Synthes, Paoli, PA) have been used in single-level thoracolumbar burst fractures (21); and plate and screw systems can be used in one- and two-level lumbar burst fractures (20,50).

III ASSESSMENT

Whether acting as a member of a team of trauma specialists or alone in the emergency department, an orderly, stepwise approach to assessment and management will limit the likelihood of missing a significant injury. In evaluating the polytrauma patient, regardless of neurological status, the surgeon must rapidly: (1) assess vital functions—airway, bleeding, circulation; (2) manage initial shock or life-threatening injuries while protecting the spine; (3) stabilize the spinal column and protect the neural elements; and (4) initiate a diagnostic workup for suspected spinal injury.

IV INITIAL ASSESSMENT AND ABCs

In any trauma situation, the highest priority is to save the patient's life. In some circumstances, the threat to life is obvious, from hemorrhage, visceral trauma, etc., and in others it is not.

Unstable thoracic and thoracolumbar fractures are usually high-energy injuries. Anywhere from 40–80% of these injuries result from motor vehicle accidents, either as drivers or passengers of automobiles, as riders of motorcycles, or as pedestrians struck by motor vehicles (18,33,34,37,39,43,52). Other causes of spine fractures include falls from height, penetrating trauma, and massive crush injuries, as when a worker is caught beneath a collapsing wall. In such high-energy injuries, polytrauma is common. In our experience, patients with unstable thoracolumbar fractures average two major associated injuries in addition to their spinal fracture, with some patients presenting with as many as six associated injuries (37).

Common injuries associated with thoracolumbar and thoracic fracture reflect the nature of the traumatic event. **Intrathoracic injuries** include pneumo- and hemothorax caused by rib fractures or bronchial disruption, myocardial contusion, and great vessel injury from blunt trauma and rapid deceleration, hemopericardium, and cardiac tamponade, and diaphragmatic rupture and acute hiatal hernia due to rapidly increased intra-abdominal pressure. These injuries are often associated with thoracic fractures and fracture dislocations. Tension pneumothorax and cardiac tamponade can be rapidly fatal, but auscultation assessing bilateral breath sounds and heart sounds will identify either problem. Both conditions impair cardiac output and the patient will be shocky and cyanotic. In tension pneumothorax, the breath sounds will be absent or diminished on the side of the pneumothorax, and the esophagus and mediastinum may deviate to the opposite side. In cardiac tamponade, the neck veins will be distended. A plain chest x-ray will confirm the hemo/pneumothorax, diaphragmatic rupture, and may show widening of the mediastinum associated with a great vessel injury. If multiple rib fractures are seen, particularly with first rib and clavicle fractures, consider getting an angiogram to study the aortic arch. Rapid placement of a chest tube will relieve the pneumo- or hemothorax, and oxygenation and cardiac output will immediately improve. Pericardiocentesis will eliminate the cardiac tamponade, and rapidly improve circulatory function.

Intra-abdominal injuries are also common in thoracolumbar injuries, and are particularly common in flexion distraction or "seatbelt" fractures (1,28). Solid viscera may be ruptured when compressed between the body wall and a solid object striking the abdomen, or they may be torn from their attachments when the body is suddenly and rapidly decelerates. A rigid abdomen, a drop in hematocrit, and abdominal pain and tenderness are clear indications for emergent evaluation. In a stable patient with no evidence of shock, abdominal CT can rule out an abdominal injury. Particular attention should be paid to patients with seatbelt injuries; the association of lapbelt abrasions with the classic flexion distraction fracture should alert the physician to a high likelihood of intra-abdominal injury. Because the fracture is caused as the body is flexed forward over the lapbelt, visceral injuries ranging from splenic rupture to mesenteric avulsions can be found in between 40 and 60% of patients (24,47). It is prudent to get a general surgical assessment of the patient whenever a flexion distraction injury is suspected.

Thoracic and thoracolumbar fractures are very commonly associated with other **skeletal injuries**. In motor vehicle accidents and falls from height, fractures of the femurs, tibias, and feet are common. Up to 40% of patients will have another, noncontiguous spinal fracture. Upper extremity fractures are less common. Major pelvic fractures are rare and usually seen only after massive trauma or crush injury. Hemorrhage associated with multiple long-bone fractures can lead to shock (10).

Injuries to the head and neck should be carefully assessed in the emergency room, and the cervical spine should be protected throughout the initial evaluation and emergency procedures. Unconscious patients and those with an altered level of consciousness cannot be relied upon for an accurate history or report of symptoms, and should be protected as though their neck was unstable (Fig. 1) (36,41). Head injuries may be evaluated by MRI or CT prior to anesthesia if surgery is needed, or may be observed if otherwise stable.

Shock occurs for a variety of reasons. In any situation, rapid vascular access and fluid resuscitation are the crucial initial treatment for spinal trauma patients. **Hemorrhagic, hypovolemic shock** is eminently life-threatening, and must be recognized and corrected quickly. Young patients present with tachycardia and peripheral vasoconstriction as primary symptoms; hypotension may not occur until blood loss is severe and vascular collapse occurs. Older patients do not compensate as well, and tachycardia and hypotension occur early on. Place a foley catheter to monitor urine output, and rapidly assess common sites of bleeding—open wounds, intra-abdominal and intrathoracic hemorrhage, and long-bone and pelvic fractures. **Neurogenic shock** may be seen in spinal cord–injured patients. Neurogenic shock results from loss of normal vasomotor tone. Patients with neurogenic shock manifest hypotension and tachycardia just as seen in patients with hemorrhagic shock, but have

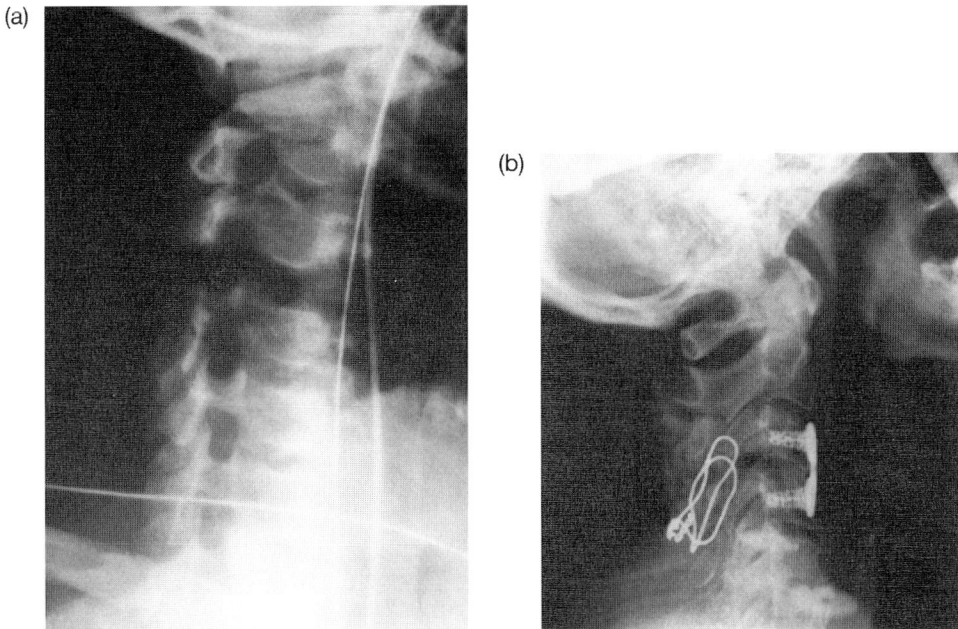

Figure 1 Cervical dissociation after high-speed collision. Patient admitted with closed head injury, thoracic and abdominal injuries, combative and intoxicated. (a) Initial lateral views failed to show the injury, but this oblique view, taken following laparotomy, splenectomy, and hemicolectomy demonstrates the complete disruption of anterior, posterior, and lateral restraints. (b) Although the cervical injury was not diagnosed until after extensive surgical intervention, strict spinal cord precautions were maintained throughout all transfers and procedures. The patient suffered no neurological injury and underwent successful stabilization using anterior and posterior fixation.

warm, well perfused skin and peripheral tissues. Vasopressors may be needed to manage the patient with neurogenic shock. **Cardiogenic shock** may result from any condition that reduces cardiac output, such as cardiac tamponade, tension pneumothorax, or myocardial injury or infarction.

V PROTECTING THE PATIENT

From the time of the initial assessment to the conclusion of the diagnostic workup and initiation of treatment, the spinal column and spinal cord must be protected. This is particularly important in the polytrauma patient who may be unconscious, may require emergency anesthesia and surgical care, and must be moved repeatedly in order to manage other life-threatening injuries (36). Plain radiographs of the cervical spine are mandatory before intubating the patient. If injury is seen or suspected, a fiberoptic nasotrachial intubation is the safest.

Until the spine is cleared, the patient should be maintained on a full-length backboard with the neck immobilized in a hard cervical collar. Transfer of the patient is safest on a spine board or slide board, but should always be carried out with sufficient personnel to make the transfer smoothly and without struggling. When log-rolling the patient, the team must coordinate efforts to see that the shoulders and pelvis move together as a unit. If the patient is hemodynamically stable and does not require emergency procedures, he or she may be transferred to a firm mattress and maintained at strict spinal precautions until the workup is completed. Precautions include strict supine positioning, log-rolling side to side every 2 h for skin care, and periodic reexamination of neurological status. A Roto-rest bed may simplify skin care and positioning if bed rest is required for more than a day or two (40). Head-injured and combative patients may need to be sedated and intubated to avoid self-inflicted spinal cord injury (Fig. 2).

VI INITIAL SPINAL EVALUATION

Check the chest wall, pelvis, and hips for stability, and examine the abdomen for seat-belt abrasions. A global assessment of motor/sensory function should be rapidly focused to specifically assess any areas of deficit. If the patient cannot cooperate, carefully observe and note spontaneous movements and withdrawal responses. Perform a rectal exam to assess rectal tone, voluntary rectal control, and the bulbocavernosus reflex. Log-roll the patient so that the spine can be palpated for step-offs, tenderness, or kyphosis, and examine the skin for abrasions and lacerations. If an incomplete deficit exists, assess the area of pain radiographically before moving the patient.

A **formal physical examination** and history may not be possible until the patient has been stabilized hemodynamically and has recovered from initial resuscitation. When the patient is alert and cooperative, a formal motor/sensory/reflex examination should be repeated, if necessary, and a detailed history of the accident obtained.

The history should focus on mechanism of injury, presence or absence of neurological symptoms, and previous spinal trauma, surgery, or symptoms. Knowledge of the injury mechanism can help identify associated injuries and provide clues to the level of instability to be expected. A lapbelted patient in a head-on collision is likely to suffer a flexion distraction injury, for instance, and must be assessed for cardiac contusion and visceral injuries. A patient ejected from a car or motorcycle frequently presents with a more complex fracture pattern caused by a combination of torsional and axial forces experienced when they impacted the ground.

If the patient can recall the event it is important to elicit any history of transient paresthesias or paralysis from the time of injury. If the patient cannot give the details of the event, carefully review field notes to see whether the patient had abnormal findings at the accident site. These notes are often gross evaluations only, however, and a patient with a severe cauda equina injury can still ''move all four.''

The physical examination for the spinal injured patient focuses on a careful, complete neurological assessment. Having examined the musculoskeletal system in the emergency department, the physician now takes the time to carefully reexamine the extremities for tenderness and pain, and examines the back again to determine the level of discomfort, the presence of step-offs or gaps between the spinous processes, and to assess the quality of the integument over the area of injury.

Document a complete motor and sensory examination. Test each motor group of the lumbar and sacral plexuses independently and compare to the contralateral group. When extremity injuries are present, the examiner must make an educated

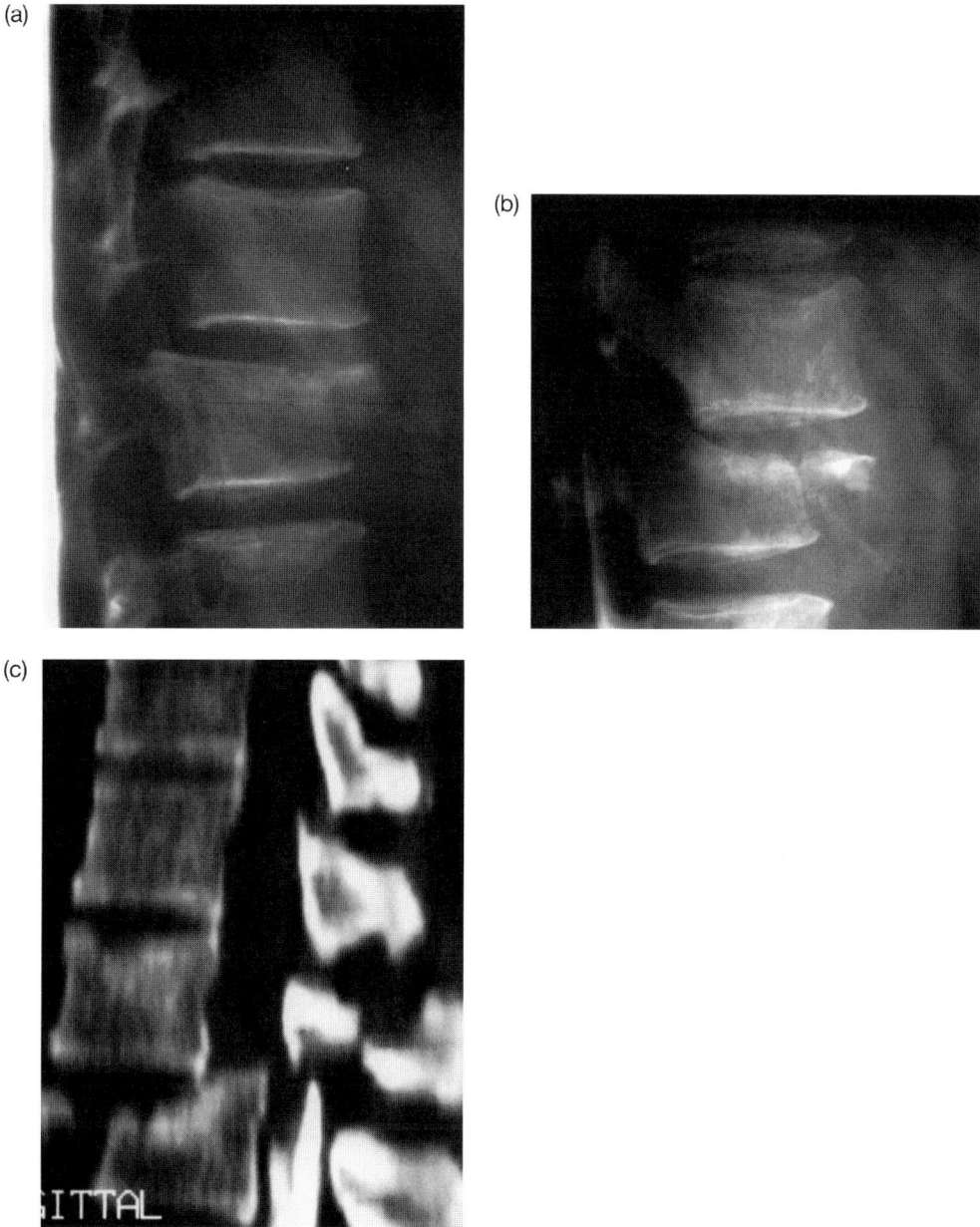

Figure 2 (a) Lateral view of an L1–L2 fracture sustained when the patient fell from a roof. Patient also sustained a head injury and pulmonary contusion, but had no neurological injury. (b) Following admission, patient was placed on spinal precautions. Intoxicated and combative, the patient became paraplegic after he got out of bed and scuffled with police. (c) Preoperative myelogram demonstrates complete dye cutoff at level of fracture dislocation. Patient experienced little neurological recovery after re-duction, decompression, and fusion.

assessment as to whether the patient is clinically weak or limited in effort by pain. The examiner must also determine whether the pattern of weakness is consistent with a cord lesion, a root lesion, or a peripheral nerve injury.

Begin the sensory examination at the upper extremities and proceed down the chest wall seeking a level of anesthesia root by root down to the sacrum. Patients with thoracic cord injuries will have an anesthetic level at or just below their fracture. If the anesthetic level and the recognized fracture do not correlate, obtain an MRI to determine the real cause of the cord impairment. Each dermatome in the lower extremities should be tested for light touch and pin-prick sensation.

Check reflexes at both the knees and ankles. *Hyperactive reflexes* suggest disinhibition due to a spinal cord injury. *Absent reflexes in an isolated distribution* suggest an incomplete cord lesion or root injury. *Complete absence of reflexes* suggests either spinal cord shock or a complete cauda equina injury. Spinal cord shock occurs at the time of injury, and may persist for 72 h. During spinal cord shock, the neurological examination remains unreliable—an incomplete injury may be masked by the overriding effects of shock. Once shock resolves and caudal reflexes return, the examination provides clear prognostic value: incomplete injuries have potential for improvement, complete injuries have almost none. The bulbocavernosus reflex is the most reliable level for testing reflex return as it tests the most caudal segment of the spinal cord.

Plain radiographs should include AP and lateral views of the thoracic spine and/or the lumbosacral spine depending on the symptomatic level (53). On occasion, standard thoracic films will cut off T12–L1, and lumbosacral films will start at L1, giving an inadequate view of the most frequently injured level. If fracture of the thoracolumbar junction is suspected, AP and lateral radiographs should be repeated, centered at the T12 level. In stable fractures—compression fractures, mild burst fractures, and mild flexion distraction injuries—plain radiographs will be sufficient to allow definitive treatment and no further diagnostic studies will be needed. In unstable spine fractures, however, additional imaging studies are often indicated.

Unstable fractures—severe burst fractures, fracture dislocations, significant flexion distraction injuries, and any fracture with a neurological deficit—require further study to assess the extent of bony disruption, spinal cord impingement, canal compromise, and/or cord injury. CT provides the most definitive information on bony characteristics such as fracture pattern and comminution (21). The transverse cuts of the CT scan can completely miss flexion distraction injuries, however. MRI is superior for soft tissue details such as cord injury, cord compression, disk herniation, and ligamentous disruption. MRI has the added benefit of scanning the entire thoracolumbar spine and picking up noncontiguous fractures, cord injury, or epidural hematoma at levels other than the primary fracture. Longitudinal MRI cuts show the soft-tissue disruption and bony separation of flexion distraction injuries well.

VII SURGICAL TREATMENT

A Timing of Surgery

Patients should be treated according to the standards of polytrauma management (10) insuring adequate fluid resuscitation, early and aggressive intervention for visceral injuries, and a concerted effort to stabilize skeletal injuries and mobilize each patient as soon as possible. All polytrauma patients should be treated within the first 48 h of admission. Many patients may undergo spinal stabilization in combination with other emergent operative procedures, at the time of admission. Patients with incomplete or progressive neurological injuries are treated as soon as medically stable. Initiate steroid therapy in the emergency room for all patients with neurological deficit, in accordance with the Second National Acute Spinal Cord Injury Study (11).

Accepted indications for urgent spinal surgery include:

1. Progressive neurological deficit.
2. Unreduced spinal dislocation with neurological deficit.
3. Severe deformity or kyphosis compromising the overlying skin or ability to position the patient.
4. Extensive polytrauma predisposing to pulmonary/metabolic derangements if patient is not mobilized.
5. Associated injuries that dictate emergent surgical treatment.
6. Chest trauma and pulmonary contusions that predictably result in pulmonary deterioration (29).

The principal indication for early surgical intervention in polytrauma patients is to permit early mobilization and eliminate the hazards presented by bed rest and recumbency (Table 1). Delayed spinal stabilization (more than 72 h after injury) is not consistent with the basic tenets of modern trauma management. If the patient is adequately resuscitated, hemodynamically stable and likely to deteriorate over the first 48 h of hospitalization, surgery will be safer earlier than later, and these patients are stabilized urgently. This is particularly true if the patient is already in the operating room.

Since segmental spinal instrumentation systems offer superior versatility and reliability of fixation compared to the nonsegmental rod-hook systems prevalent just a decade or so ago, surgeons can mobilize patients rapidly, obtaining an upright posture, improved cardiopulmonary function, and a reduced risk of pneumonia, venous thrombosis, or urosepsis. Properly stabilized, all patients should be upright in bed or a cardiac chair immediately following spinal instrumentation (37). The nursing

Table 1 Injury and Perioperative Characteristics of Urgent and Early Treatment Groups

	Urgent group	Early group	
Mean age (years)	27.5 (16–46)	30.0 (18–58)	NS
Mean ISS	42 (27–75)	36 (27–50)	NS
% with neurological injuries	71%	54%	NS
Mean time to OR	9.7 h	35.0 h	P < .00001
Mean op time (post)	5.18 h	5.60 h	NS
Mean op time (comb)	12.0 h	13.25 h	NS
Mean EBL (post)	1432 cc	1600 cc	NS
Mean EBL (comb ant/post)	6812 cc	4000 cc	NS
Mean EBL (total)	2966 cc	1877 cc	NS
Perioperative deaths	1/14	1/13	NS
ARDS	0/14	1/13	NS

staff and associated services must be dedicated to the goal of mobilizing the patient as soon as surgery is complete.

Several studies have shown that aggressive early treatment of long-bone fractures reduces morbidity and mortality in polytrauma patients (7,30,42). Stabilizing femoral fractures within 24 h of injury significantly reduces pulmonary dysfunction, ARDS, pulmonary emboli, and pneumonia, as well as ventilator days and length of hospitalization (8). By comparison, 10 days of recumbent traction essentially doubled the duration of pulmonary failure relative to patients with immediate femoral rodding (45). While surgeons agree on the value of immediately stabilizing long-bone and pelvic fractures in polytrauma patients, urgent spinal stabilization has not been universally endorsed.

Urgent spinal stabilization does appear to reduce morbidity in severely injured patients, compared either to previous surgical series or to common experience based on ISS. In a review of polytrauma patients undergoing urgent (<24 h) versus early (>24 but <48 h) spinal stabilization, the benefits of urgent treatment were demonstrated relative to both early treatment and historical experience with delayed treatment (37). Although the mean ISS for the urgent treatment group was higher than for the early group (42 vs. 36), there was no difference in the operative time, rate of complications, morbidity, or mortality. Urgently treated patients averaged 1.1 Frankel grades of improvement compared to 0.57 for patients treated early. All three patients with full neurological recovery were in the urgent treatment group. Estimated blood loss was significantly higher in the urgently treated group (mean 2966 cc's vs. 1877 cc's), reflecting, in part, that four of six combined anterior/posterior procedures were done in the urgent group. There were no pneumonias and only one case of adult respiratory distress syndrome. Despite the high injury scores in both early and urgent groups (10 with ISS > 40), there were only two deaths, one of which was due to unsurvivable injuries. Complication rates for both urgent and early treatment groups were lower than in previous surgical series (17,23,39,44,48).

1   Mortality

The LD50 (level at which 50% mortality would be expected) for patients in this age group is an ISS = 40. The mean ISS for polytrauma/spine fracture patients overall was 39 (range 27–75) (37). Ten patients in our study had an ISS > 40; they had more associated injuries, more life-threatening injuries, and a higher incidence of neurological injury. Among the nine patients with an ISS > 40 and *survivable* injuries, mortality was only 11%. Our 20% overall mortality in this specific subgroup was significantly better than expected (2,3,15,51).

2   Blood Loss

Stauffer has shown that surgical blood loss is reduced by two-thirds if surgery can be delayed 48 h after injury (49). Benefits of urgent stabilization must be balanced against this increased blood loss. In our series, blood loss for urgent *posterior* procedures was comparable to that reported for patients undergoing delayed treatment (19,37). Patients undergoing urgent *anterior* decompression often experienced brisk hemorrhage, however, primarily from torn epidural vessels and fresh fracture.

3   Neurological Recovery

Unexpectedly, neurological improvement was better in the urgent treatment group than in the early treatment group; all three patients with complete neurological recovery, and both of those with more than two grades of recovery were treated within the first 24 h of their injury. The numbers involved are too small to suggest a statistically significant difference, and the recovery in these patients cannot be used to argue that urgent treatment might provide improved recovery in complete spinal cord injuries. In fact, because it is frequently impossible to distinguish complete from incomplete lesions in urgently treated patients, any urgently treated group is likely to contain some apparently "complete" injuries, which would improve spontaneously. This will bias any comparison to patients treated at a later time when spinal shock has resolved. Nonetheless, concerns that urgent intervention might *compromise* neurological recovery are clearly not substantiated.

In our series, neurological recovery was more directly related to early intervention and fracture reduction than to the method of decompression. There was no clear relationship between anterior decompression and neurological recovery. Canal compromise can be improved through indirect reduction (46), and remodeling improves canal diameter over time, regardless of treatment (38). An incomplete neurological deficit in the face of persistent compression remains an indication for direct surgical decompression (6,14,26,32).

VIII SPECIFIC TREATMENT CONSIDERATIONS

A Triage and Priorities

The primary and overriding goal of polytrauma care is to save the patient's life, in other words, to prevent death due to immediate threats such as hemorrhage, shock, and hypoxia, as well as subsequent and delayed threats such as thromboembolism, sepsis, and pneumonia. Properly prioritized, initial treatment will effectively stop bleeding, restore ventilation, reverse shock, and stabilize the musculoskeletal system sufficiently to allow aggressive mobilization, providing an upright chest and normalizing hemodynamics. If the patient remains supine at the end of the day, the primary goal has not been met.

With this in mind, procedures must be prioritized to provide the greatest incremental benefit for the time allowed. Life-threatening injuries must be addressed immediately, at the same time that hypovolemia, hypoxia, and shock are being medically corrected. Open fractures, dislocations, and vascular injuries are also addressed as emergencies, although final reconstruction may be put off to a later, staged procedure. Next, long-bone and spinal fractures must be stabilized to allow transfers and mobilization. Finally, definitive care of intra-articular fractures, fractures of the hands, arms, and feet, and ligamentous injuries are treated on an elective basis.

B Intra-Abdominal and Intrathoracic Injuries

Visceral injuries within the thoracic or abdominal cavities can result in lethal hemorrhage. Exploration and repair or control of these injuries take precedence over all other aspects of care. Coordinate care with the general surgical team, however, since the spine service may be able to complete a formal decompression and reconstruction of the fracture through the laparotomy or thoracotomy used to treat the visceral trauma.

C Open Fractures and Dislocations

Treat open fractures and unreduced dislocations as true emergencies. Splint fractures of the upper extremity, hands, and feet, and transport for irrigation and debridement as soon as hemodynamically stable. Perform a closed reduction of any unreduced dislocation in the emergency department, and splint in the reduced position. Unless the patient has a progressive spinal cord or cauda equina deficit, irrigate, debride, and stabilize open fractures before formally addressing the spine fracture.

D Concomitant Femur Fractures

A healthy patient may lose as much as four units of blood into an unstabilized femur fracture. With bilateral femur fractures, a patient can literally exsanguinate into their thighs. Place a tibial traction pin in the emergency department and maintain traction throughout any preliminary radiographic or clinical evaluations, or emergent surgical procedures. Stabilize the fracture as soon as possible: if the patient requires emergent surgery for other injuries, plan to fix the fracture during that anesthetic. Otherwise, fix the fracture as a semiemergent procedure, within the first 24 h after the injury, and address the spine fracture according to neurological status and the stability and level of the injury.

If the patient has a progressive neurological deficit, maintain femoral traction from the end of the operative table, and carry out the necessary spinal decompression and instrumentation first. Once the spine is stabilized, perform a standard femoral rodding to control the fracture and allow immediate mobilization. Patients with highly unstable cervical fractures should also be considered for spinal fixation as the first procedure. If the patient has no neurological injury, or a complete but stable deficit, consider fixing the femur fracture initially. With the patient supine on the back board or O.R. table, perform a retrograde intramedullary rodding through the knee. This procedure can be carried out without turning the patient or transferring him to a fracture table. If the proper personnel are available, proceed with definitive spinal stabilization after that. If the spine team cannot be assembled at that time of night, it is prudent to return the patient to the floor or intensive care unit for up to 24 h, until the proper personnel are available.

E Other Extremity Injuries

Humerus fractures can generally be splinted and treated definitively at the surgeon's discretion. If vascular access is an issue in a patient with bilateral upper extremity injuries, urgent stabilization with an intramedullary device or external fixator will free up the arm for intravenous or arterial access. Upper extremity fractures and dislocations should be given serious attention—if the patient is rendered paraplegic or paraparetic by their spinal injury, this upper extremity will have to function as a *weight-bearing, high-demand limb* for the rest of his life.

Vascular injuries should be given priority over spinal stabilization except in the rare case of a progressive neurological injury. Even then, consideration should be given to placing a shunt or performing a vascular repair to save the dysvascular extremity before proceeding with a prolonged spinal operation. In a Level 1 trauma center, it may be possible to have two surgical teams simultaneously address both problems.

F   Pelvic Fractures

Unstable pelvic and spine fractures are rarely seen in the same patient. When they do occur concomitantly, the patient has usually been exposed to massive trauma (Fig. 3), and stabilization of the two injuries is a life-saving proposition. Placement of an

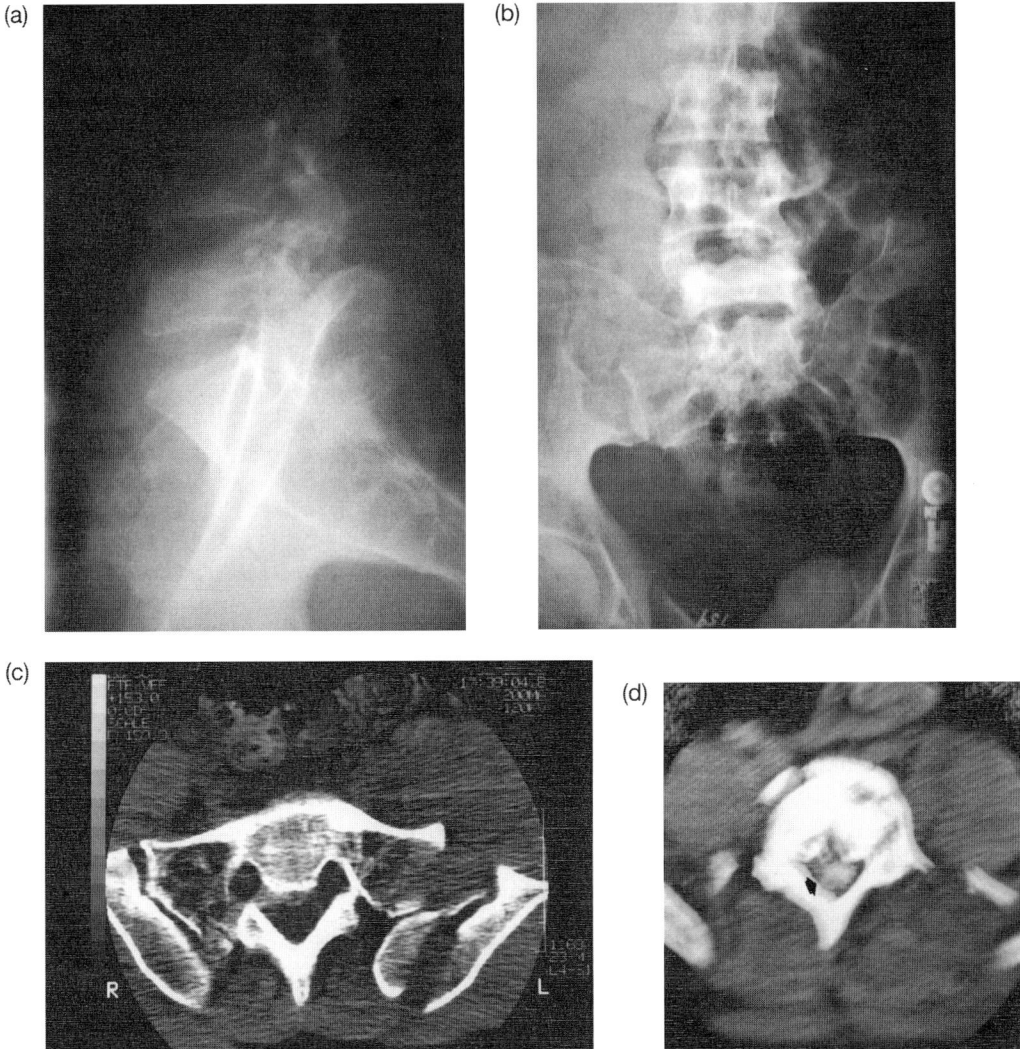

Figure 3   Severe spinopelvic trauma: 19-year-old construction worker trapped under a collapsing wall, and found in a hyperflexed position with his head and shoulders pinned between his feet. (a) Lateral radiograph shows L5 burst fracture with deceptively little axial collapse. (b) Anterior view shows vertebral collapse as well as the widely disrupted sacroiliac joint on the left, and the sacral ala fracture on the right. (c,d) Computed tomography confirmed the extent of the pelvic and sacroiliac disruption, and demonstrated large vertebral fragments retropulsed across the full diameter of the canal.

(e)   (f)

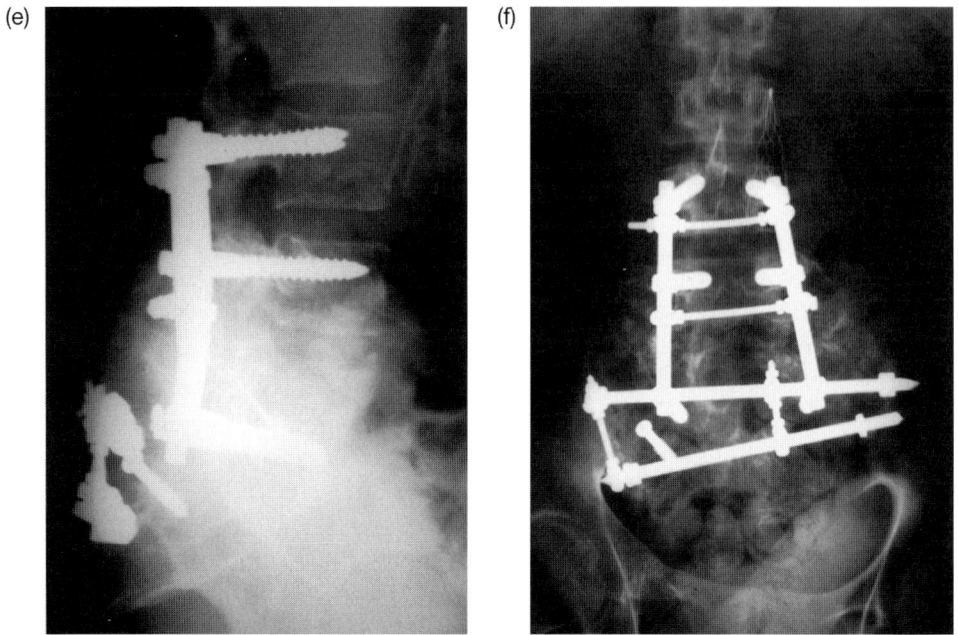

Figure 3   (e,f) A progressive neurological deficit necessitated an emergent anterior decompression. Patient underwent staged anterior and posterior spinal procedures, and a sacropelvic reconstruction with transsacral bars. Excellent neurological recovery was obtained, with the patient requiring only an ankle-foot orthosis for independent ambulation.

anterior pelvic fixator will interfere with prone positioning for any spinal procedure, but newer percutaneous pelvic clamps may provide provisional stability until the spine can be stabilized. However, it is better if both the pelvic instability and the spinal condition can be definitively stabilized at the same operation. Pubic ramus disruption or diastasis may be stabilized through a small Pfannensteil incision, or by extending the laparotomy incision distally if laparotomy is needed. Percutaneous sacroiliac screw fixation can be carried out under fluoroscopic control, restoring the integrity of the pelvic ring. An anterior thoracolumbar or lumbar decompression and reconstructing can then be performed without repositioning the patient.

IX   INSTRUMENTATION

The instrumentation placed at the time of initial stabilization must be sufficient to allow aggressive mobilization of the patient without the benefit of a brace or body cast. Preliminary fixation or partial instrumentation of the fracture should be avoided, as there is no guarantee that the patient will be able to return to the O.R. for completion of the instrumentation in a timely fashion. Successful construct patterns for fracture stabilization have been refined, and segmental spinal instrumentation has been used for a variety of thoracic and thoracolumbar spinal fractures (27,34,35, 48). McBride reported good results in thoracic and thoracolumbar fractures treated with longer hook and rod constructs (33) and short-segment pedicle instrumentation (SSPI) constructs have been recommended for treatment of lumbar fractures (25,35).

If the fracture is severely comminuted, the anterior spinal column may need to be reconstructed with an anterior graft before the patient can be fully mobilized. The risk of sagittal collapse following instrumentation is related to the level and severity of the fracture, the approach taken, and the construct chosen. Sagittal collapse following fracture reduction is common, particularly around the thoracolumbar junction, with authors reporting progression of relative kyphosis of between 12 and 19 degrees (5,27,31). Although Dimar reported sagittal collapse after combined anterior and posterior reconstruction (19), anterior reconstruction generally eliminates sagittal collapse and should be carried out at the initial procedure, if possible. If that is not possible at the time of stabilization, augmenting posterior fixation with additional hooks is recommended (54).

X CAVEATS

Polytrauma patients should be treated in a level 1 trauma center. The need to treat complex spinal injuries at any time of the day or night is just one more reason that multiply injured patients need to be consistently triaged to those centers where acute care is immediately and reliably available. Unless the surgical team can complete the treatment plan, including rigid spinal instrumentation that will allow the patient to sit up and participate in pulmonary and rehabilitation therapy, aggressive surgical intervention will expose the patient to the risks of surgery without providing the benefits of the proper procedure. Urgent laminectomy, for instance, may or may not provide some benefit in terms of neurological injury. If stabilization is not provided at the time of decompression, however, the patient will be left at an increased risk of pulmonary and thromboembolic complications, and may even suffer greater neurological injury due to spinal instability or collapse.

Similarly, if the nursing staff and intensive care/general surgical staff are not comfortable mobilizing a patient after surgical treatment, the benefits of that surgery will not be fully realized. Education of your associates is important to your success with this aggressive surgical approach.

XI SUMMARY

The spine surgeon treating polytrauma patients must work in tandem with experienced general surgical and orthopedic trauma services to manage multisystem injuries. Urgent stabilization of the spine will increase blood loss during surgery. The inability to use hypotensive anesthesia in a polytraumatized patient, development of coagulopathy or diathesis following serial surgical procedures, the need to expose and debride the fresh fracture site, and traumatic and surgical disruption of epidural and segmental vessels all contribute to intraoperative hemorrhage. Despite this, patients treated urgently fare better than those treated in a standard time frame, and often do as well as patients with isolated spinal injuries.

REFERENCES

1. Anderson PA, Montesano PX, Rechtine G. Flexion distraction and Chance thoracolumbar spine fractures. J Orthop Trauma 1989; 3:160–170.

2. Baker SP, O'Neill B, Haddlon W. The injury severity score: A method for describing patients with multiple injuries and evaluating emergency care. J Trauma 1974; 14:187–196.
3. Baker SP, O'Neill B. The injury severity score: An update. J Trauma 1976; 16:882–885.
4. Benson DR, Burkus JK, Montesano PX, Sutherland TB, McLain RF. Unstable thoracolumbar and lumbar burst fractures treated with the AO fixateur interne. J Spinal Disord 1992; 5(3):335–343.
5. Benzel EC. Short-segment compression instrumentation for selected thoracic and lumbar spine fractures: the short-rod/two-claw technique. J Neurosurg 1993; 79(3):335–340.
6. Bohlman HH, Freehafer A, Dejak J. The results of treatment of acute injuries of the upper thoracic spine with paralysis. J Bone Joint Surg 1985; A67(3):360–369.
7. Bohlman HH. Treatment of fractures and dislocations of the thoracic and lumbar spine. J Bone Joint Surg 1985; 67A(1):165–169.
8. Bone LB, Bucholz R. The management of fractures in the patient with multiple trauma. J Bone Joint Surg 1986; 68A(1):945–949.
9. Bone LB, Johnson KD, Weigelt J, Scheinbeng R. Early vs. delayed stabilization of fractures: A prospective, randomized study. J Bone Joint Surg 1989; 71A(1): 336–340.
10. Bone, LB. Management of Polytrauma. In: Chapman MW, ed. Operative Orthopaedics, 2nd ed. Philadelphia: J.B. Lippincott Co., 1993:299–304.
11. Bracken MB, Shepard MJ, Collins WF, et al. A randomized, controlled trial of methylprednisolone or naloxone in the treatment of acute spinal cord injury. Results of the Second National Acute Spinal Cord Injury Study. N Engl J Med 1990; 322:1405–1411.
12. Bryant CE, Sullivan JA. Management of thoracic and lumbar spine fractures with Harrington distraction rods supplemented with segmental wiring. Spine 1983; 8(5):532–537.
13. Civil ID, Schwab CW. The abbreviated injury scale, 1985 revision: A condensed chart for clinical use. J Trauma 1988; 28:87–90.
14. Clohisy JC, Akbarnia BA, Bucholz RD, Burkus JK, Backer RJ. Neurologic recovery associated with anterior decompression of spine fractures at the thoracolumbar junction (T12-L1). Spine 1992; 17(8 Suppl):S325–330.
15. Copes WS, Champion HR, Sacco WJ, Lawnick MM, Keast SL, Bain LW. The injury severity score revisited. J Trauma 1988; 28:69–77.
16. Denis F. The three column spine and its significance in the classification of acute thoracolumbar spinal injuries. Spine 1983; 8(8):817–831.
17. Dickman CA, Yahiro MA, Lu HT, Melkerson MN. Surgical treatment alternatives for fixation of unstable fractures of the thoracic and lumbar spine. A meta-analysis. Spine 1994; 19(20 Suppl):2266S–2273S.
18. Dickson JH, Harrington PR, Erwin WD. Results of reduction and stabilization of the severely fractured thoracic and lumbar spine. J Bone Joint Surg 1978; 60A(6):799–805.
19. Dimar JR 2nd, Wilde PH, Glassman SD, Puno RM, Johnson JR. Thoracolumbar burst fractures treated with combined anterior and posterior surgery. Am J Orthoped 1996; 25(2):159–165.
20. Ebelke DK, Asher MA, Neff JR, Kraker DP. Survivorship analysis of VSP spine instrumentation in the treatment of thoracolumbar and lumbar burst fractures. Spine 1991; 16(8 Suppl):S428–432.
21. Esses SI, Botsford DJ, Wright T, Bednar D, Bailey S. Operative treatment of spinal fractures with the AO internal fixator. Spine 1991; 16(3 Suppl):S146–150.
22. Flesch JR, Leider LL, Erickson DL, Chou SN, Bradford DS. Harrington instrumentation and spine fusion for unstable fractures and fracture-dislocations of the thoracic and lumbar spine. J Bone Joint Surg 1977; 59A(2):143–153.

23. Fletcher DJ, Taddonio RF, Byrne DW, Wexler LM, Cayten CG, Nealon SM, Carson W. Incidence of acute care complications in vertebral column fracture patients with and without spinal cord injury. Spine 1995; 20(10):1136–1146.
24. Gertzbein SD, Court-Brown CM. Rationale for the management of flexion-distraction injuries of the thoracolumbar spine based on a new classification. J Spinal Disord 1989; 2(3):176–183.
25. Gillet P, Meyer R, Fatemi F, Lemaire R. Short Segment Internal Fixation Using CD Instrumentation with Pedicular Screws: Biomechanical Testing. The 6th Proceeding of the International Congress on Cotrel-Dubousset Instrumentation. Montpellier: Sauramps Medical, 1989:19–24.
26. Golimbu C, Firooznia H, Rafii M, Engler G, Delman A. Computed tomography of thoracic and lumbar spine fractures that have been treated with Harrington instrumentation. Radiology 1984; 151(3):731–733.
27. Graziano GP. Cotrel-Dubousset hook and screw combination for spine fractures. J Spinal Disord 1993; 6(5):380–385.
28. Gumley G, Taylor TK, Ryan MD. Distraction fractures of the lumbar spine. J Bone Joint Surg [Br] 1982; 64(5):520–525.
29. Hanley EN, Simpkins A, Phillips ED. Fractures of the thoracic, thoracolumbar and lumbar spine: classification, basis of treatment, and timing of surgery. Sem Spine Surg 1990; 2:2–7.
30. Johnson KD, Cadambi A, Seibert GB. Incidence of adult respiratory distress syndrome in patients with multiple musculoskeletal injuries. Effect of early operative stabilization of fractures. J Trauma 1985; 25:375–384.
31. Kramer DL, Rodgers WB, Mansfield FL. Transpedicular instrumentation and short-segment fusion of thoracolumbar fractures: a prospective study using a single instrumentation system. J Orthopaed Trauma 1995; 9(6):499–506.
32. McAfee PC, Bohlman HH, Yuan HA. Anterior decompression of traumatic thoracolumbar fractures with incomplete neurological deficit using a retroperitoneal approach. J Bone Joint Surg 1985; 67A(1):89–104.
33. McBride GG. Cotrel-Dubousset rods in spinal fractures. Paraplegia 1989; 27(6):440–449.
34. McBride GG. Cotrel-Dubousset rods in surgical stabilization of spinal fractures. Spine 1993; 18(4):466–473.
35. McLain RF, Sparling E, Benson DR. Early failure of short-segment pedicle instrumentation for thoracolumbar fractures. A preliminary report. J Bone Joint Surg 1993; 75(2):162–167.
36. McLain RF, Benson DR. Missed cervical dissociation—Recognizing and avoiding potential disaster. J Emerg Med 1998; 16(2):179–183.
37. McLain RF, Benson DR. Urgent surgical stabilization of spinal fractures in polytrauma patients. Spine 1999; 24:1646–1654.
38. Mumford J, Weinstein JN, Spratt KF, Goel VK. Thoracolumbar burst fractures. The clinical efficacy and outcome of nonoperative management. Spine 1993; 15:955–970.
39. Place HM, Donaldson DH, Brown CW, Stringer EA. Stabilization of thoracic spine fractures resulting in complete paraplegia. A long-term retrospective analysis. Spine 1994; 19(15):1726–1730.
40. Rechtine GR, Cahill D, Chrin AM. Treatment of thoracolumbar trauma: comparison of complications of operative vs. nonoperative treatment. J Spinal Disord 1999; 12:406–409.
41. Reid DC, Henderson R, Saboe L, Miller JDR. Etiology and clinical course of missed spine fractures. J Trauma 1987; 27:980–986.
42. Rogers FB, Shackleford SR, Vane DW, Kaups KL, Harris F. Prompt fixation of isolated femur fractures in a rural trauma center: a study examining the timing of fixation and resource application. J Trauma 1994; 36:774–777.

43. Saboe LA, Reid DC, Davis LA, Warren SA, Grace MG. Spine trauma and associated injuries. J Trauma 1991; 31(1):43–48.
44. Schlegel J, Bayley J, Yuan H, Fredricksen B. Timing of surgical decompression and fixation in acute spinal fractures. J Orthoped Trauma 1996; 10:323–330.
45. Seibel R, LaDuca J, Hassett JM. Blunt multiple trauma (ISS 36), femur traction, and the pulmonary failure-septic state. Ann Surg 1985; 202:283–295.
46. Shuman WP, Rogers JV, Sickler ME, Hanson JA, Crutcher JP, King HA, Mack LA. Thoracolumbar burst fractures: CT dimensions of the spinal canal relative to postsurgical improvement. Am J Roentgenol 1985; 145(2):337–341.
47. Smith WS, Kaufer H. Patterns and mechanisms of lumbar injuries associated with lap seat belts. J Bone Joint Surg 1969; 51A:239–254.
48. Stambough JL. Cotrel-Dubousset instrumentation and thoracolumbar spine trauma: a review of 55 cases. J Spinal Disord 1994; 7(6):461–469.
49. Stauffer ES. Thoracolumbar fractures: Principles of treatment. Presented at Scoliosis Research Society. Baltimore, MD, September, 1988.
50. Steffee AD, Biscup RS, Sitkowski DJ. Segmental spine plates with pedicle screw fixation. A new internal fixation device for disorders of the lumbar and thoracolumbar spine. Clin Orthopaed Related Res 1986; 203:45–53.
51. Swiontkowski MF. The multiply injured patient with musculoskeletal injuries. In: Rockwood CA, Green DP, Bucholz RW, Heckman JW, eds. Fractures in Adults. New York: Lippincott-Raven, 1995:121–158.
52. Tasdemiroglu E, Tibbs PA. Long-term follow-up results of thoracolumbar fractures after posterior instrumentation. Spine 1995; 20(15):1704–1708.
53. Wenger DR, Carollo JJ. The mechanics of thoracolumbar fractures stabilized by segmental fixation. Clin Orthopaed Related Res 1984; 189:89–96.
54. Yerby S, Ehteshami J, McLain RF. Offset laminar hooks decrease bending moments on pedicle screws during in-situ contouring. Spine 1997; 22:376–381.

49

Management of Post-Traumatic Syringomyelia

ROBERT J. KOWALSKI and EDWARD C. BENZEL

The Cleveland Clinic Foundation, Cleveland, Ohio, U.S.A.

I INTRODUCTION

Interest in spinal cord injury dates back to the time of Galen. Galen experimented by making longitudinal and transverse cuts to the spinal cord of animals (1). Most modern advancements, however, can be credited to the pioneering work of Guttmann, including the opening of the first dedicated spinal unit in 1944 at Stoke Mandeville Hospital in England (2).

With the advances made in the treatment of spine trauma, we find ourselves with new challenges. Now that patients are surviving longer, they are developing longer term complications. This chapter examines the phenomenon of post-traumatic syringomyelia.

Spinal cord cavities are generally divided into those that are expansions of the central canal (i.e., hydromyelia) and those that are separate from the central canal (i.e., syringomyelia) (3,4). Some have proposed the term syringohydromyelia, which encompasses both entities. However, within the limits of current understanding, post-traumatic cavities seem to arise from the gray matter, hence, the preferred term, post-traumatic syringomyelia. Usage of this term includes cavities that may communicate with the central canal. Syringomyelia is further classified into communicating and noncommunicating types, referring to the presence, or lack thereof, of a direct communication with the fourth ventricle. Thus, post-traumatic syringomyelia is a noncommunicating form of syringomyelia that may result from penetrating or nonpenetrating trauma (3). The cystic cavity is typically found in the structurally weakest portion of the spinal cord—the gray matter, particularly the dorsal horns. The cavity is not lined with ependymal cells, but contains fluid that is indistinguishable from cerebrospinal fluid.

Although Estienne first described cavitation of the spinal cord in 1546, it was not until the 1800s that others associated clinical signs with the pathology and first used the term syrinx (Gr. syrinx = tunnel) (5). Barnett et al. was the first to publish an extensive monograph based on his experience with 591 paraplegic patients. He utilized the term ''post-traumatic cystic myelopathy'' (6).

II EPIDEMIOLOGY

The incidence of post-traumatic syringomyelia identification has increased with improved outcomes in the treatment of spinal cord injury and the advent of the MRI. As it is often a late phenomenon, reported incidences vary with the length of follow up in a given series. Most series fall in the range of 1 to 4.5%, with complete quadriplegics accounting for the majority of cases (7).

III PATHOPHYSIOLOGY

The observed post-traumatic spinal cord pathology exists on a spectrum from arachnoiditis, to microcystic degeneration, to syringomyelia. The highly variable time course and often protracted interval between injury and clinical presentation may indicate that several causative factors may be at work. Another difficult question is whether different factors are involved in formation as opposed to enlargement. Approximately 50% of injured spinal cords show small cavities on imaging studies (3,8), while only one-tenth of these patients develop symptomatic syringes (9). One commonly agreed upon initiating event is a hematoma of the spinal cord, known as hematomyelia. As the hematoma itself resolves, a cavity of necrotic debris is left behind, possibly capable of inciting further damage through the production of toxic substances. The adjacent spinal cord parenchyma undergoes myelomalacia. Ischemia with concomitant production of free radicals may contribute to the process as well.

Alterations in the CSF flow dynamics have a significant impact on syrinx progression, as well as on syrinx formation. CSF pathway blockage may be the result of mechanical obstruction from intradural as well as extradural sources. Arachnoiditis, through the production of adhesions, also directly alters the CSF flow. Additionally, adhesions may exert a ball valve effect, trapping CSF and allowing subsequent pulsations to force fluid into the cord parenchyma (3,10). CSF may also accumulate through dilated Virchow-Robin spaces, resulting from glial damage. Alternate theories include the coalescence of microcysts that form following the initial trauma. The syrinx is often located at the level of the injury, but there may also be intervening normal levels.

IV CLINICAL PRESENTATION

The clinical presentation of syringomyelia does not vary with etiology, only with axial and transverse extent. Onset is variable and may range from a few months to over 20 years (11). Pain is so pervasive a symptom of syringomyelia that its presence in the neck or upper extremities in a paralyzed patient often leads to a presumptive diagnosis. Increased intra-abdominal or intrathoracic pressure, such as that induced by straining, coughing, sneezing, or Valsalva maneuvers, may exacerbate symptoms. Additional sensations include hypalgesia, dysesthesia, and electric shocklike or burning pain (12). These phenomena may occur in a radicular distribution. In cases of progression, the symptoms migrate, leaving the previous area anesthetic.

Motor function loss is typically a late finding following anterior horn cells atrophy. When the cervical spinal cord is involved, arm muscles weaken and reflexes are diminished. In incomplete lesions, distal weakness and spasticity may progress, along with deterioration of bowel and bladder function. Sensory deficits are predominantly asymmetrical. Motor deficits are often more easily appreciated on physical examination, while pain and temperature deficits in the classic capelike distribution often leave patients with telltale scars. The aforementioned findings are more evident with cervical spine injuries.

V EVALUATION

Imaging studies usually show the cavity to be emanating from the trauma focus (fracture, etc.). It usually extends rostrally and/or caudally. When the cavity extends caudally in a complete lesion, hyperhidrosis may be the only symptom. Traditional myelography often fell short from a diagnostic perspective in cases of post-traumatic syringomyelia since it often lacked the requisite spinal cord enlargement necessary for diagnosis. Postmyelography CT increases the sensitivity, but still suffers some of the same shortcomings (13). MRI, with its ability to visualize the rostral and caudal extent of the pathology and even delineate septations, has become the gold standard (Fig. 1) (14). By permitting earlier diagnosis, MRI may help improve outcome as well. Cine MRI has added the ability to demonstrate CSF dynamics (Fig. 2). Ultrasound can be a useful intraoperative tool, but is limited to the extent of a previously performed laminectomy (15).

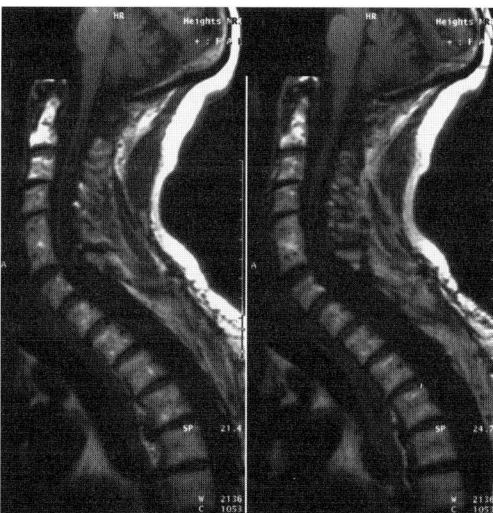

Figure 1   Sagittally T1-weighted MRI revealing a septated syrinx.

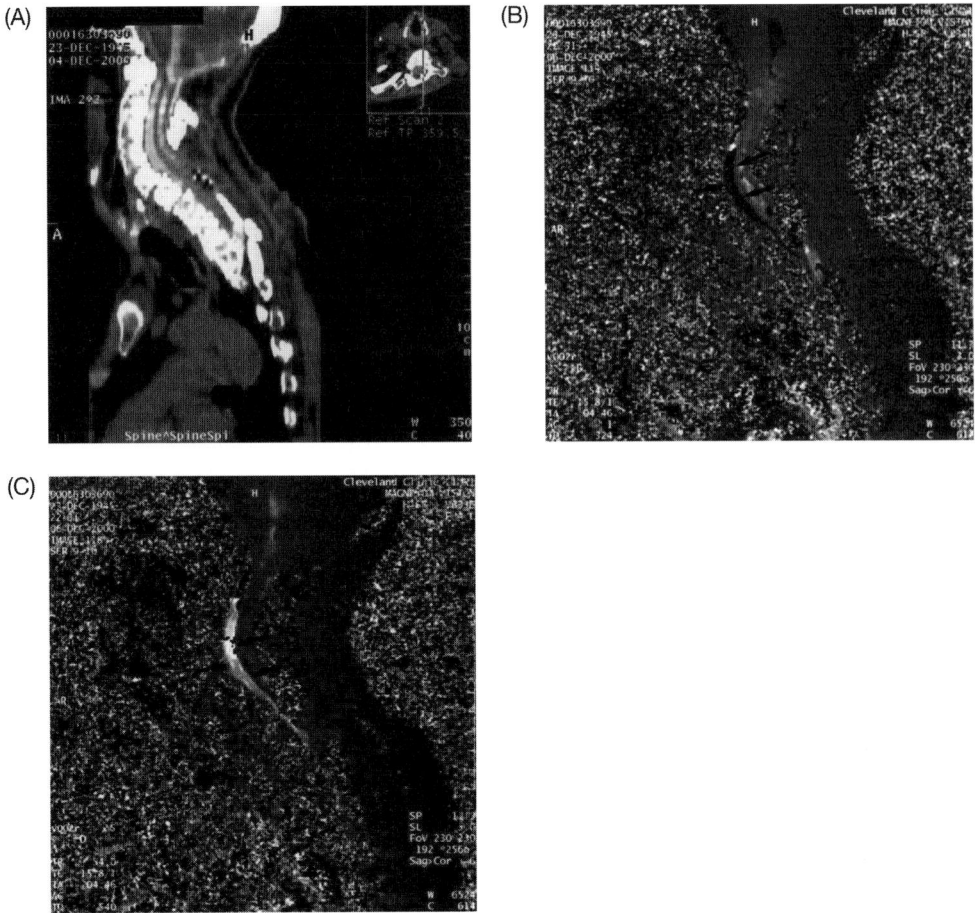

Figure 2 Imaging of a patient with a cervical syrinx and a concurrent history of trauma and a Chiari I malformation. (A) Sagittally reconstructed CT reveals mild cervical subluxation and evidence of a prior suboccipital decompression (note the shunt artifact, arrow). (B, C) Cine MRI reveals the actual site of obstruction is the previous Chiari decompression instead of at the site of trauma as hypothesized (bidirectional flow represented by the black-and-white signal).

VI MANAGEMENT

A History

The number of different approaches used throughout history, in and of itself, is a testimonial to the lack of consensus regarding the most appropriate treatment. Myelotomy, needle aspiration, decompressive laminectomy, tube syringostomies, and even omental transfers have all had their proponents at one time or another.

Barnett et al. examined the role of cordectomy and silastic tube syringostomy (16). Using a tube to divert the fluid into an area of normal subarachnoid space seemed logical and slowly gained acceptance. While initial results were encouraging, there were those who had reservations about its long-term efficacy. They believed that the cause of the problem—disruption of normal CSF pathways—ought to be the primary target.

Percutaneous cyst aspiration is plagued by reaccumulation. Aspiration, however, may be beneficial in patients who are not operative candidates and may provide useful diagnostic information if symptoms resolve (7). Simple myelotomy also has the same inherent reaccumulation potential.

B Surgical Technique

1 Reestablishment of CSF Pathways

Williams and Sgouros believed that shunting is rarely the entire solution (11). They espoused attacking the source of the problem, "deactivating" the cyst by lysing adhesions and remodeling any abnormal anatomy to reestablish CSF pathways (17). Specifically, this requires the creation of a large subarachnoid space with concurrent untethering of the cord through lysis of adhesions. The procedure begins with a wide laminectomy uncovering the extent of scarring, usually at least two levels above and below the site of injury. The dura mater is opened in the midline with care taken not to injure the distorted and possibly displaced spinal cord. The spinal cord in the vicinity of the cyst tends to be avascular and often takes on a bluish hue. Using the operating microscope and microsurgical dissection techniques, the dura mater is first dissected free. Next, the arachnoid layer is divided along with any adhesions and then dissected away from the pia. A neuroendoscope may be utilized as well. If the spinal cord is still under tension, the dentate ligaments may be incised. Meticulous hemostasis is paramount, as blood products could form the nidus for additional scarring. Finally, the dura is closed using one of two methods (Fig. 3). Utilizing a dural graft, the dura mater is closed. Some advocate "tenting" it with tacking sutures to the paraspinous muscles creating an enlarged subarachnoid space (18). The other option, advocated by Williams, involves the creation of a pseudomeningocele by leaving the dura open and suturing the edges to the paraspinous muscles (19). This is not a commonly utilized strategy. Both strategies theoretically restore a patent CSF pathway around the site of pathology.

2 Shunting Procedures

The procedure is begun by utilizing good standard laminectomy or laminotomy techniques. Often, one level of exposure is all that is required. Exposure should be wide enough to reveal both dorsal root entry zones, but with care taken to avoid destabilizing the spine. The first decision is, "where to make the myelotomy." While the midline and at the dorsal root entry zone are two standard approaches, often the local anatomy will reveal a thinned, avascular area with little risk of producing a new neurological deficit. The operating microscope and intraoperative ultrasound provide useful assistance. Entering the caudal-most extent of the cavity will allow utilization of the hydrostatic column of fluid while also minimizing the neurological level of any iatrogenic injury. Utilizing different locations for the durotomy and myelotomy will minimize potential tethering from dural scarring. The location of the distal end of the catheter is a matter for debate. Shunts in this setting are low flow and therefore subject to a higher incidence of obstruction and subsequent failure. This, combined with the risk of neurological injury on insertion, makes shunting procedures less than desirable.

(A)

(B)

(C)

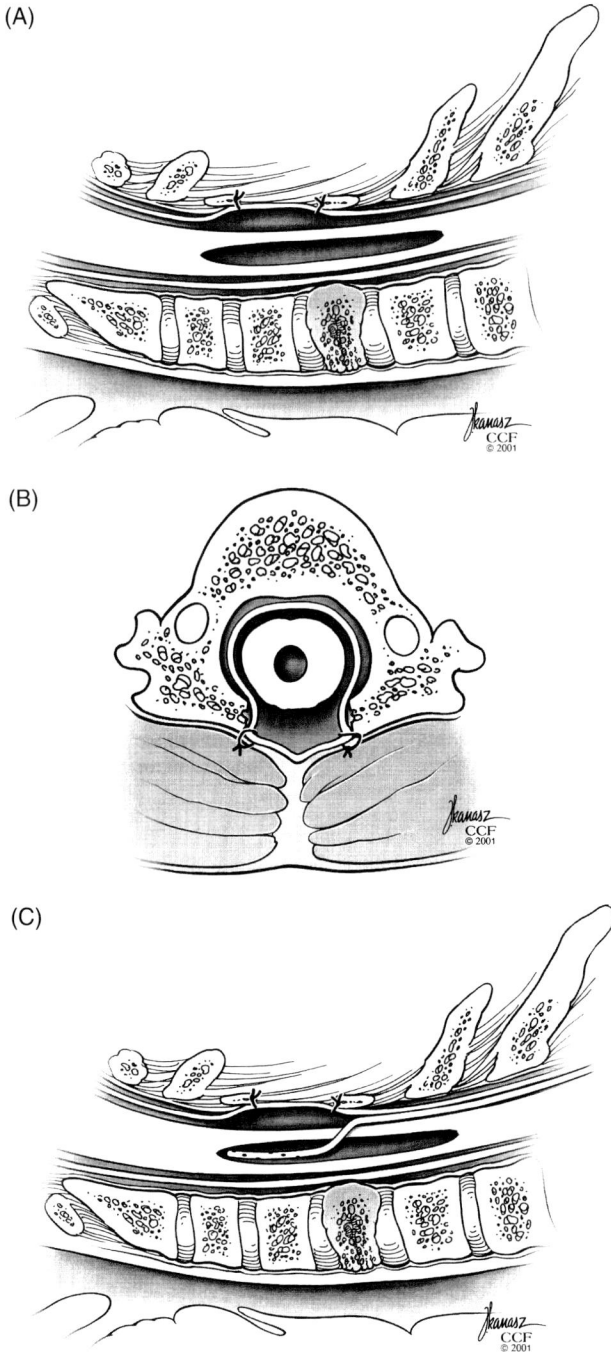

Figure 3   (A) Sagittal view of a post-traumatic syrinx. After detethering, the dura may be tacked to the paraspinal musculature creating a pseudomeningocele or closed with a duraplasty. (B) Axial view showing optional duraplasty. (C) Sagittal view of a post-traumatic syrinx after detethering with the addition of a syringosubarachnoid shunt.

Syringosubarachnoid. The distal end is threaded into the caudal surrounding subarachnoid space. Final placement should always take into account local conditions. Areas of frank arachnoiditis should be avoided. The tube should be secured to both the arachnoid and the dura mater, and the dura closed in a watertight fashion. One of the advantages of this approach is that it only requires one incision. A drawback is the high incidence of arachnoid adhesions in post-traumatic syringomyelia that may result in shunt obstruction (20). Also of concern is the fact that the syrinx and subarachnoid pressures have not been shown to differ significantly.

Syringoperitoneal. The principles are similar to the more familiar ventriculoperitoneal shunt except the quantity of fluid and pressure are much lower, requiring very low pressure systems. Utilizing the prone position for the intraspinal portion necessitates repositioning the patient or, alternately, using a lateral position. The distal end is brought through a new durotomy, tunneled through the subcutaneous tissue, and placed intraperitoneally, similar to a VP shunt. Several advantages are inherent with this approach. The intraspinal pressure fluctuations that result from coughing, sneezing, etc., are eliminated. Also, obstruction from arachnoid adhesions are avoided and, if a distal revision is required, no intraspinal portion is required.

Syringopleural. The pleural cavity also avoids complicating arachnoid adhesions and allows exposure from the prone position. The inherent physiology of the pleural cavity, whereby negative pressures are generated, will assist in keeping the cyst collapsed (21). Care must be taken to traverse the superior aspect of the rib in order to avoid damaging the neurovascular bundle. Several steps may be taken to minimize the incidence of pneumothorax, such as utilizing the smallest exposure of parietal pleural possible, using copious irrigation, and tying off the suture during a Valsalva maneuver (21,22). Pleural CSF effusions are occasionally problematic. Tube thoracostomy drainage of such accumulations, particularly utilizing negative pressures, should be avoided in the face of a functioning syringopleural shunt for fear of complications related to thecal sac overdrainage.

C Cordectomy

Patients who have a complete spinal cord injury are potential candidates for a complete cord transection (19). Exposure of the cord is achieved using the same principles as above. After identifying the level of maximum spinal cord injury, a caudal 1-to-2 cm section is removed, incorporating the distal end of the cavity. Additional untethering and/or shunting may be added as needed. Caution must be exercised at the cervical level, where the potential of iatrogenically increasing the level of injury may be catastrophic. Some patients may find the finality of cordectomy to be unpalatable in light of current and ongoing transplant research.

VII OUTCOME

Patients, even after successful obliteration of the cavity, may still experience neurological decline from an entity termed progressive post-traumatic noncystic myelopathy (PPNM). Edgar et al. postulated that this was the result of arachnoiditis induced by pooling blood dorsolaterally (9). Treatment involves the reestablishment of CSF pathways as described above.

Some retrospective studies have reported slightly better outcomes utilizing the syringoperitoneal shunt over other shunts, but a definitive prospective trial is lacking (23,24). Edgar et al. reported a 10 to 15% rate of early shunt malfunction in the hands of experienced surgeons, with rates as high as 50% with less experience. He also believed that most failures occur at the proximal end secondary to tissue debris and scar. Thus, any push for extraspinal diversion may be unwarranted (9).

Typical complications after intradural surgery, such as infection, wound dehiscence, and DVTs occur with comparable rates. Additional morbidities include worsening of the neurological deficit, shunt obstruction, low-pressure headaches, and an increased incidence of CSF leaks when tubes transverse the dura mater.

The overall efficacy of surgical treatments results in approximately 50% of patients experiencing some level of improvement and an additional 20 to 30% with a halt in the progression of their symptoms. A postoperative MRI establishes syrinx resolution (or lack thereof) and serves as a baseline for future follow-up. Unfortunately, radiographic cure does not always equate to clinical cure (25,26). There is a tendency for gliosis to progress even after cyst decompression. In general, motor, sensory, and even pain are more likely than not to improve, with spasticity enjoying a more modest level of improvement (27).

REFERENCES

1. Prindergast JS. The background of Galen's life and activities, and influences on his achievements. Proc R Soc Med 1930; 23:1131–1148.
2. Guttmann L. History of the National Spinal Injuries Centre, Stoke Mandeville Hospital, Aylesbury. Paraplegia 1967; 5:115–126.
3. Backe HA, Betz RR, Mezgarzadeh M, et al. Post-traumatic spinal cord cysts evaluated by magnetic resonance imaging. Paraplegia 1991; 29:607–612.
4. Morioka T, Kurita-Tashima S, Fujii K, et al. Somatosensory and spinal evoked potentials in patients with cervical syringomyelia. Neurosurgery 1992; 30:218–222.
5. Finlayson AI. Syringomyelia and related conditions. In: Joynt RJ, ed. Clinical Neurology, Vol 3. Philadelphia: J.B. Lippincott, 1989:1–17.
6. Barnett HJM, Botterell EH, Jousse AT. Progressive myelopathy as a sequel to traumatic paraplegia. Brain 1966; 98:159–174.
7. Levy R, Rosenblatt S, Russel E. Percutaneous drainage and serial magnetic resonance imaging in the diagnosis of symptomatic posttraumatic syringomyelia: case report and review of the literature. Neurosurgery 1991; 29:429–433.
8. Sett P, Crockard AH. The value of magnetic resonance imaging in follow up management of spinal injury. Paraplegia 1991; 29:396–410.
9. Edgar R, Quail P. Progressive post-traumatic cystic and non-cystic myelopathy. Br J Neurosurg 1994; 8:7–22.
10. Cho KH, Iwasaki Y, Imamura H, et al. Experimental model of posttraumatic syringomyelia: the role of adhesive arachnoiditis is syrinx formation. J Neurosurg 1994; 80:133–139.
11. Sgouros S, Williams B. Management and outcome of posttraumatic syringomyelia. J Neurosurg 1996; 85:197–205.
12. Shannon N, Symon L, Logue V, et al. Clinical features, investigation and treatment of posttraumatic syringomyelia. J Neurol Neurosurg Psychiatry 1981; 44:35–42.
13. Kan S, Fox AJ, Vinuela F. Delayed metrizamide CT enhancement of syringomyelia: postoperative observations. Am J Neuroradiol 1985; 6:613–616.

14. Sze G. MR imaging of the spinal cord: current status and future advances. Am J Roentgenol 1992; 159:149–159.
15. Robertson DP, Narayan RK. Intraoperative endomyelography during syrinx drainage: technical note. Neurosurgery 1992; 30:246–249.
16. Barnett HJM, Jousse AT. Nature, prognosis and management of post-traumatic syringomyelia. In: Barnett HJM, Forster JB, Hudgson P, eds. *Syringomyelia. Major Problems in Neurology*. Philadelphia: W.B. Saunders, 1973.
17. Teddy PJ, Lustgarten L. Post-traumatic syringomyelia. In: Kaye AH, McL Black P. *Operative Neurosurgery*, Vol 2. London: Harcourt Publishers imited, 2000:1981–1993.
18. Klekamp J, Batzdorf U, Samii M, Bothe HW. Treatment of syringomyelia associated with arachnoid scarring caused by arachnoiditis or trauma. J Neurosurg 1997; 86:233–240.
19. Williams B, Terry AF, Jones F, et al. Syringomyelia as a sequel to traumatic paraplegia. Paraplegia 1981; 19:67–80.
20. Van den Bergh R. Pathogenesis and treatment of delayed post-traumatic syringomyelia. Acta Neurochir 1991; 110:82–86.
21. Ram Z, Findler G, Tadmor R, et al. Syringopleural shunt for the treatment of syringomyelia. Technical note. Spine 1990; 15:231–233.
22. Pitts LH. Technique for syringopleural shunting for the treatment of syringomyelia. Spine 1990; 15:985.
23. Barbaro NM, Wilson CB, Gutin PH et al. Surgical treatment of syringomyelia. Favourable results with syringoperitoneal shunting. Neurosurgery 1984; 61:531–538.
24. Peerless SJ, Durward OJ. Management of syringomyelia. A pathophysiological approach. Clin Neurosurg 1982; 30:531–576.
25. Aschoff A, Kunze S. 100 years of syrinx-surgery—a review. Acta Neurochir 1993; 123:157–159.
26. Foo D, Bignami A, Rossier AB. A case of post-traumatic syringomyelia. Neuropathological findings after 1 year of cystic drainage. Paraplegia 1989; 27:63.
27. Umbach I, Heilporn A. Review article: post-spinal cord injury syringomyelia. Paraplegia 1991; 29:219–221.

50

Management of Post-Traumatic Deformity

ROBERT J. KOWALSKI and EDWARD C. BENZEL

The Cleveland Clinic Foundation, Cleveland, Ohio, U.S.A.

I INTRODUCTION

Deformation, both in its initiation and progression, requires the presence of at least one unstable motion segment. In addition, there must be a pathological stressor acting upon the spine. This may be absolute, resulting from the application of supraphysiological forces, or relative, whereby normally benign forces create pathological stresses when acting on an already deformed spine. The latter circumstance is summed up by the phase "deformity begets deformity."

The correction of spinal deformity requires the simultaneous consideration of several objectives: deformity correction, prevention of further deformity, restoration of balance in both of the sagittal and coronal planes, optimization of cosmesis, and restoration and preservation of neurological function (1). Failing to consider any of the above may prevent a successful outcome.

The knowledge of basic spine biomechanics is essential to achieving a good outcome. Identifying the instantaneous axis of rotation (IAR) and the neutral axis is fundamental in determining first, if surgical correction is indeed warranted, and then, assisting in construct design (2). The prevention of kyphotic deformation progression with a ventral approach requires the construct to be placed ventral to the neutral axis. Similarly, a dorsal approach requires dorsal placement. Increasing the distance from the neutral axis, thereby increasing the moment arm, results in a more effective construct. Conversely, in the case where there is minimal deformation and axial loading is the paramount concern, a graft should be placed in line with the neutral axis.

Spine deformities are often complex, being composed of more than one defor-

697

mation type and more than one component problem. A complex solution can be achieved through combining component strategies for each aspect. It is helpful when faced with a complex deformity to keep two simple guidelines in mind. First, try to understand the forces at play in creating the deformity. This is necessary because the correction is essential to counter or reverse those forces, thereby neutralizing the pathology. Second, remember that while complete correction is often the goal, it is not necessarily required to alleviate the patient's symptoms.

II REGION-SPECIFIC STRATEGIES

The human spine is composed of several regions that have unique biomechanical and geometrical properties and thus it is appropriate to consider strategies in a region-specific manner. Accordingly, the following regions are addressed here: the craniocervical junction and upper cervical spine, lower cervical spine, cervicothoracic junction, thoracic spine, thoracolumbar junction, lumbar spine, and the lumbosacral region.

A Craniocervical Junction and Upper Cervical Spine

The high degree of mobility and biomechanical complexity of this region leave it subject to deformities in the coronal, sagittal, and axial planes, with kyphosis, spondylolisthesis, and subsidence being the most common results. While many cases may be corrected with nonoperative strategies, deformity reduction, and occipitocervical fusion are occasionally required. Additional region-specific techniques include the resistance of an angular bending moment through transarticular C1–C2 screw fixation. This strategy prevents rotation. Occasionally, a transoral spinal canal decompression for the release of dislocated C1–C2 joints is required (3).

B Lower Cervical Spine

Deformity correction in the lower cervical spine presents some unique opportunities as well as challenges when compared to the thoracic and lumbar spine. The ease of both ventral and dorsal access is offset by the relatively poor fixation points available. Strategies for each of the fundamental planes are discussed.

1 Coronal Plane Deformities

Fortunately, scoliotic deformity of the cervical spine is relatively uncommon. The applicable strategies of concave distraction and convex compression, as well as the use of the derotation maneuver is thus rarely required. The introduction of rod-and-screw constructs to cervical spine surgery, however, has facilitated the utilization of these techniques when necessary.

2 Sagittal Plane Deformities

Sagittal plane deformities are relatively common and consist of kyphosis, subsidence, and spondylolisthesis.

Cervical Spine Kyphosis and Subsidence.   Kyphotic cervical spine deformities are often accompanied by vertebral body height loss (subsidence) such as that found in a wedge compression fracture. Further loading, even at nonpathological levels, may promote deformation progression secondary to the substantial bending moment resulting from the extended moment arm. Deformation progression may be further complicated by progressive myelopathy.

Ventral, dorsal, or a combined approaches can all be utilized in cervical spine kyphosis. A ventral approach provides the opportunity to address both neural compression and spine deformation. It has the added benefit that if deformity correction is not mandatory, a ventral decompression may be all that is necessary. A ventral decompression or diskectomy can be used to facilitate deformity correction by "relaxing" the spine.

Several dorsal techniques, originally developed for the thoracic and lumbar spine, may also be used for cervical kyphotic deformation reduction. One example is the crossed-rod technique (Fig. 1A). This can be enhanced by vertical interbody distraction (Fig. 1B). This can be applied via lateral mass screw fixation techniques. As mentioned previously, the effectiveness of a dorsal approach can often be maximized when it is combined with a ventral release procedure. Weakening or disrupting the dorsal tension band will tend to exaggerate sagittal plane deformations. Clinically, this is most commonly seen in the wake of a laminectomy and, to a lesser degree, laminoplasty (4).

Cervical Translation Deformation.   Cervical spine subluxation can be managed by both ventral and dorsal approaches. The fear of an inadvertent retropulsion of disk material into the spinal canal has resulted in many surgeons preferring at least to begin with a ventral procedure, if not to rely on it solely (5,6). A common approach begins with a diskectomy, followed by distraction of the disk interspace to disengage the locked facet joints, and fixation and fusion upon the achievement of normal

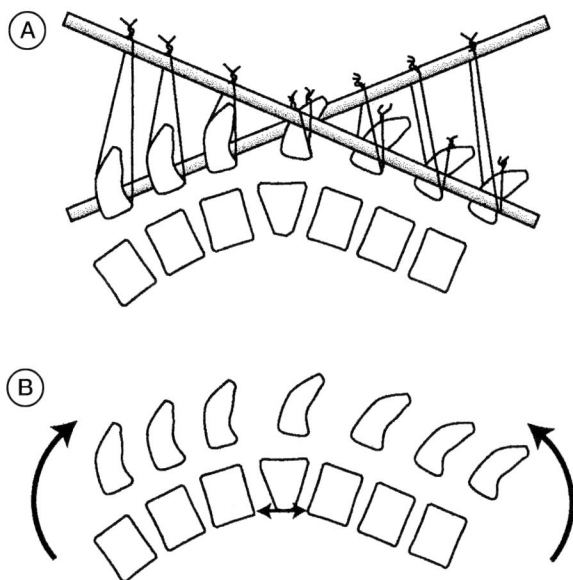

Figure 1   Correction of kyphosis with (A) the crossed-rod technique supplemented with (B) ventral interbody distraction (straight arrows) producing an applied bending moment (curved arrows).

alignment (Fig. 2). Several tools are available, including a specifically developed tool by Cloward, a disk interspace spreader, and even a simple curette. Caspar pins may be used as well. They provide the advantage of enabling the correction of a rotational deformity, as would be present with a unilateral locked facet.

Dorsal strategies must often begin with a partial resection of the facet joint. This iatrogenic destabilization of the facet joint, and accompanying traumatic destabilization, often obligates the incorporation of an additional motion segment into the fusion. Reduction of the deformity and internal fixation complete the procedure. Occasionally, deformity correction is unattainable from a dorsal approach alone. If neural decompression has been achieved, it may be acceptable to fuse and instrument in the nonreduced position.

In certain cases, a failed initial attempt at ventral reduction may require a combined ventral–dorsal–ventral approach (540°). This provides ventral decompression and both ventral and dorsal stabilization (Fig. 3).

C Cervicothoracic Junction

Beyond the more externally apparent transition from cervical lordosis to thoracic kyphosis, there is more profound structural change in this region. Smaller unprotected cervical vertebral bodies transition to the larger thoracic vertebral bodies that are protected by the rib cage. Biomechanical considerations are further complicated by geometrical, implant–bone interface integrity, and ventral surgical exposure problems. In light of the above, cervicothoracic laminectomies often necessitate fusion and stabilization. Traditional dorsal crossed-rod strategies may be successfully used in this region. In general, it is not considered prudent to terminate a long construct in this perilous junctional region.

D Thoracic Spine

The thoracic spine is characterized by larger vertebral bodies that are protected by the rib cage and a relatively smooth bend at each segmental level. Deformities often have elements in each of the fundamental planes—namely, kyphotic, scoliotic, and rotational components. This complexity is attributable to the phenomena of coupling. It occurs when one deformation obligates a second deformation such as lateral bending and rotation about the long axis of the spine. Failure to understand and factor this concept into the correction scheme can lead to disastrous results.

Deformity correction often may require a "loosening of the spine" in order to achieve adequate correction. Release procedures may be combined with a ventral interbody fusion (including cages) to help maintain the deformity correction and to increase the arthrodesis rate.

The utilization of the McCormack, Karaikovic, and Gaines load-sharing classification scheme can be helpful in the decision-making process for evaluating trauma patients (7). This is particularly so for the determination of the adequacy of ventral weight-bearing structures. It provides insight into the assessment of the ability of an injured spine to eventually reestablish ventral weight-bearing ability.

1 Coronal Plane Deformities

Ventral strategies typically use segmental screws and rods (e.g., Kaneda) that are placed through a "traditional thoracotomy" or an extrapleural thoracotomy. The

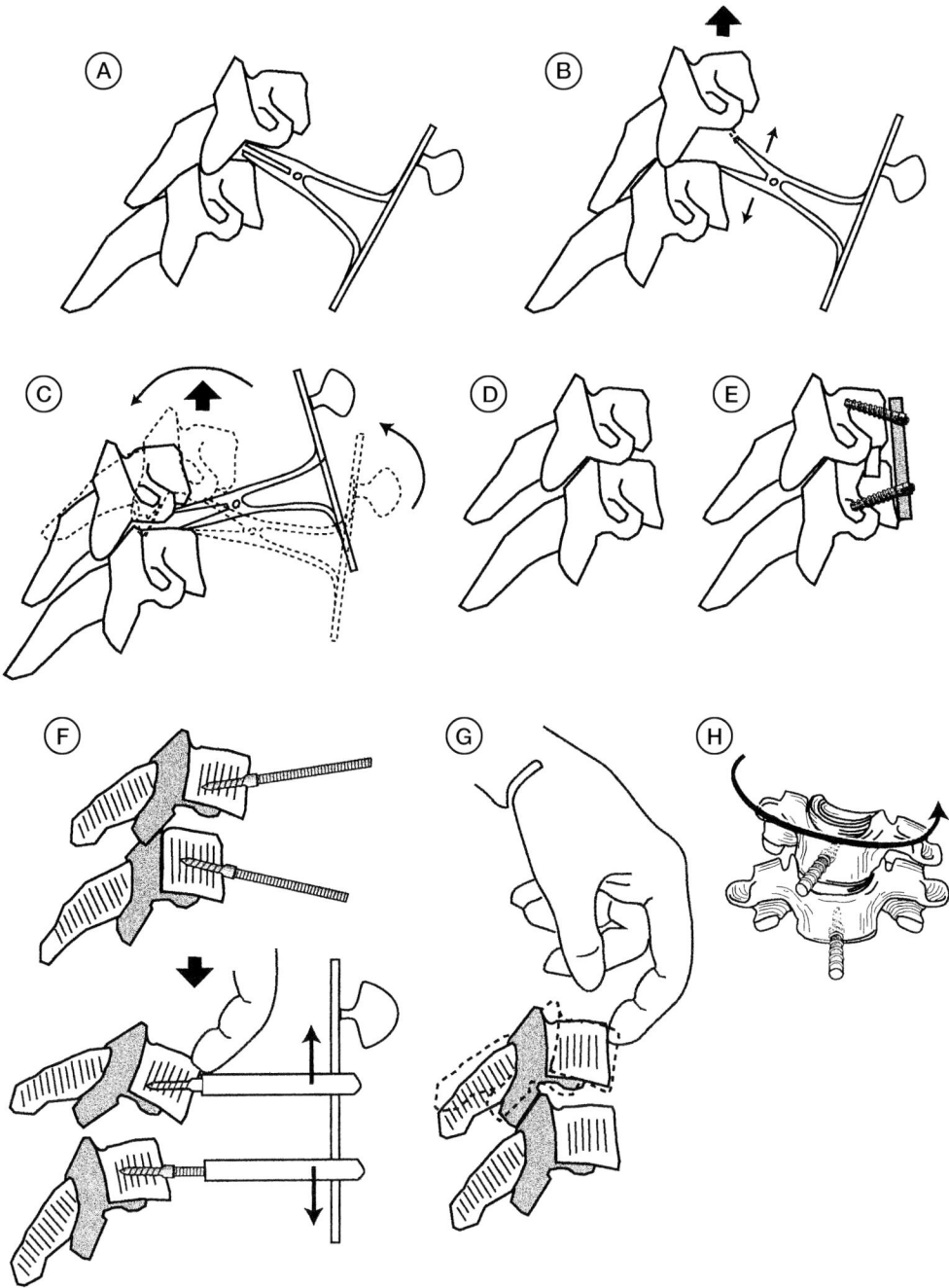

Figure 2 (A) Locked facets may be approached ventrally with a diskectomy followed by utilizing a disk interspace spreader first to (B) distract, then (C) dorsally rotate, achieving (D) a normal alignment. (E) Fixation and fusion may then be accomplished.

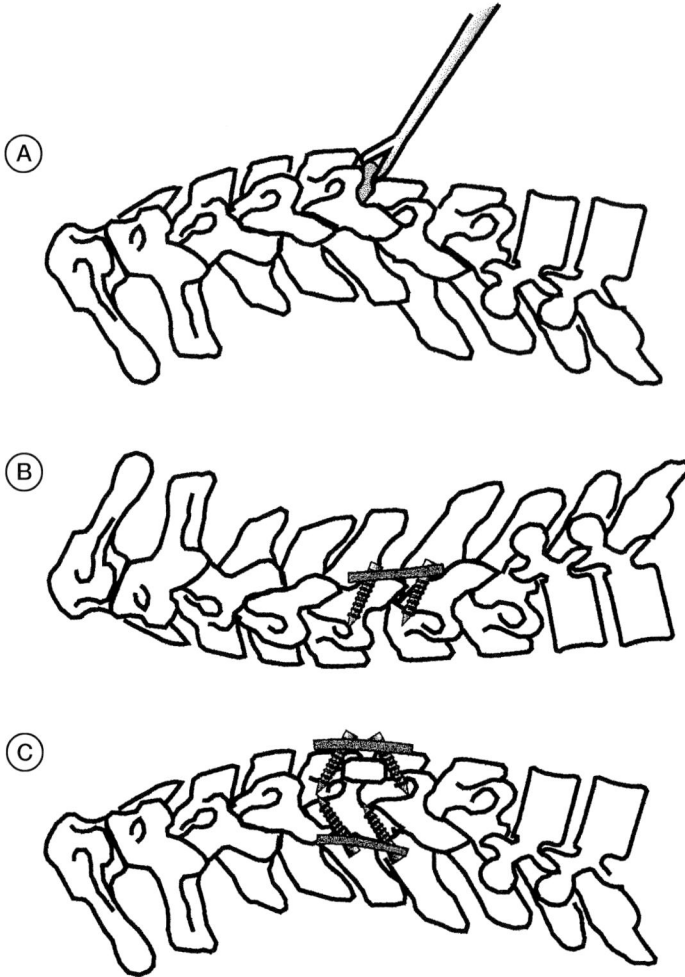

Figure 3 A 540° operation achieves decompression, reduction, and stabilization through (A) ventral decompression, (B) dorsal reduction, and (C) ventral stabilization and fusion, respectively.

screws are placed on the convex side of the scoliotic curve from neutral vertebra to neutral vertebra. The neutral vertebra is that which has no angulation at its rostral and caudal disk interspaces and is typically at the transition between adjacent curves. The result is typically a shorter construct than that achievable through a dorsal strategy. A comprehensive strategy commonly employs either one or a combination of compression and distraction, the crossed-rod technique, and/or the derotation maneuver.

Dorsal strategies rely on the same basic technique of derotation. The rods may be affixed to the spine via hooks, screws, cables, or wires. Because dorsal attempts at derotation tend to be less efficacious and precise, longer constructs are usually required and often must be supplemented with additional concave distraction and convex compression (8). Longer constructs often lead to a higher incidence of rod fracture and acceleration of end-fusion degenerative changes. Strategies to combat these include cross-fixation, using larger diameter rods, and external immobilization (9).

2 Sagittal Plane Deformities

The first step in correcting kyphotic deformities is quantification. This may be accomplished by measuring the angle from the superior endplate of the vertebral body one level above the involved vertebral body to the inferior endplate of the vertebral body one level below. The correction itself begins with the crossed-rod technique supplemented with ventral interbody distraction as necessary (Fig. 1A,B) (10). Longer constructs are generally more effective due to the larger bending moment that can be generated through the longer moment arm. In situ rod bending can be added to make final adjustments, but one must always be cognizant of the additional stresses that this strategy can place on the implant, as well as the spine (11).

E Thoracolumbar Junction

The same strategies described above for coronal and sagittal plane deformities in the thoracic region may be applied to this transitional zone. Ventral release procedures, via open or endoscopic techniques combined with interbody structural struts provide substantial deformity reduction and maintenance of reduction ability (12).

Coronal plane deformities in this region are typically complex, often being composed of two or more curvatures. This often necessitates long dorsal fixation. Two important, but less obvious, issues must be addressed. First, when determining the length of the fusion, the impact of the limitation of motion can be substantial at the level of L4 and below (13). Second, coronal plane balance, which is often overlooked (compared to sagittal plane balance), must not be forgotten.

F Lumbar Spine

The above-mentioned strategies for the thoracic and thoracolumbar spine are likewise applicable to this region. A majority of deformities have a significant translation component that requires careful consideration of sagittal plane balance. An important factor in the attainment and maintenance of lordosis is intraoperative positioning. Surgical beds or frames that foster lordosis by encouraging extension of the spine and hips are optimal. Pelvic flexion during surgery can result in inadequate lordosis acquisition. The correction of a flat back may require aggressive osteotomy and/or ventral load-bearing adjuncts.

G Lumbosacral Region

This region is notoriously biomechanically complex. The correction process begins with an assessment of instability, typically with flexion and extension radiographs. Although this is commonly attained while the patient is standing, the lateral decubitus position off-loads the spine, thus minimizing pain and allowing a more accurate assessment. Spondylolisthesis may require aggressive surgical strategies with accompanying lumbar, sacral, and pelvic fixation. An accurate assessment of the likelihood of deformity progression is critical. A fusion is not always beneficial and the same may be said of instrumentation, if a fusion is performed. Long moment arms that pass ventral or caudal to the lumbosacral pivot point are often required to achieve adequate correctional bending moments (Fig. 4). Finally, while deformity correction is the ultimate goal, strategies that do not involve reduction or that attain an incomplete reduction may still be desirable, even when a decompression operation is performed.

III   SPECIAL TECHNIQUES

There are a few specialized techniques that are very helpful in certain circumstances. Spondylectomy involves removal of a vertebral body and reconnection of the vertebral body above to the vertebral body below, usually with some form of interbody spacer (Fig. 5). As always, one must be cognizant of sagittal balance.

Another tool for correction of sagittal plane deformities is osteotomy. Although the technique is applicable throughout the spine, risk of injury to the spinal cord

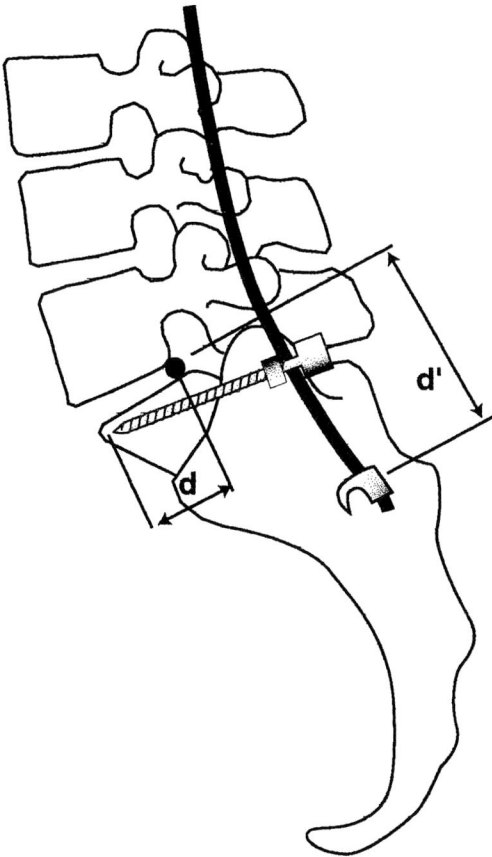

Figure 4   Long moment arms (d and d′) that pass ventral and caudal to the lumbosacral pivot point (dot) may be required to achieve adequate correctional bending moments.

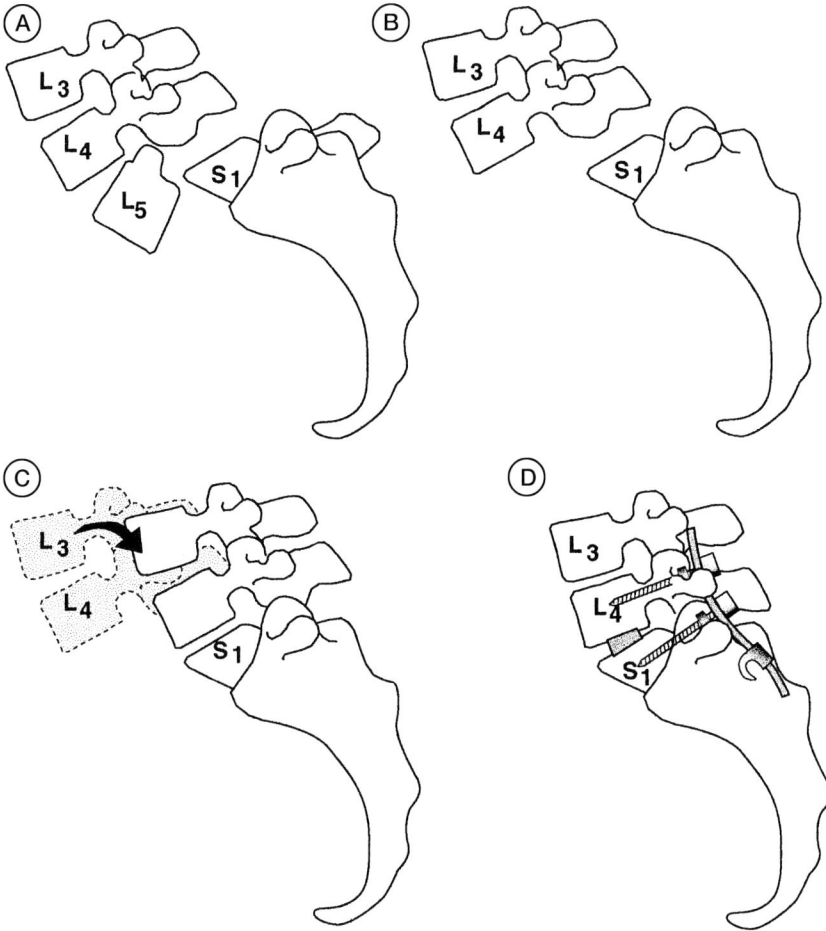

Figure 5 L5–S1 (A) spondylolisthesis can be managed with an (B) L5 corpectomy and (C) reduction and the docking of L4 on S1. An interbody fusion may be used as a spacer and for fusion acquisition. (D) Dorsal instrumentation maintains fusion.

finds this technique most often utilized in the upper thoracic and lumbar regions. The first step is to identify the axis about which the spine is deformed. The axis is perpendicular to the long axis of the spine and lies in the coronal plane. The ventral-to-dorsal location of the axis determines the amount of bone removal and the end result (Fig. 6). For a lordosing procedure, the axis is located near the posterior longitudinal ligament. A dorsal wedge or eggshell osteotomy is more appropriate when the axis is near the anterior longitudinal ligament.

Osteotomies are most effective when performed at the apex of a curve. Local factors such as the presence of neural elements (e.g., cervical spinal cord) may override the above preference. Of historical interest is that pelvic osteotomies were once used to achieve the same goal of sagittal balance.

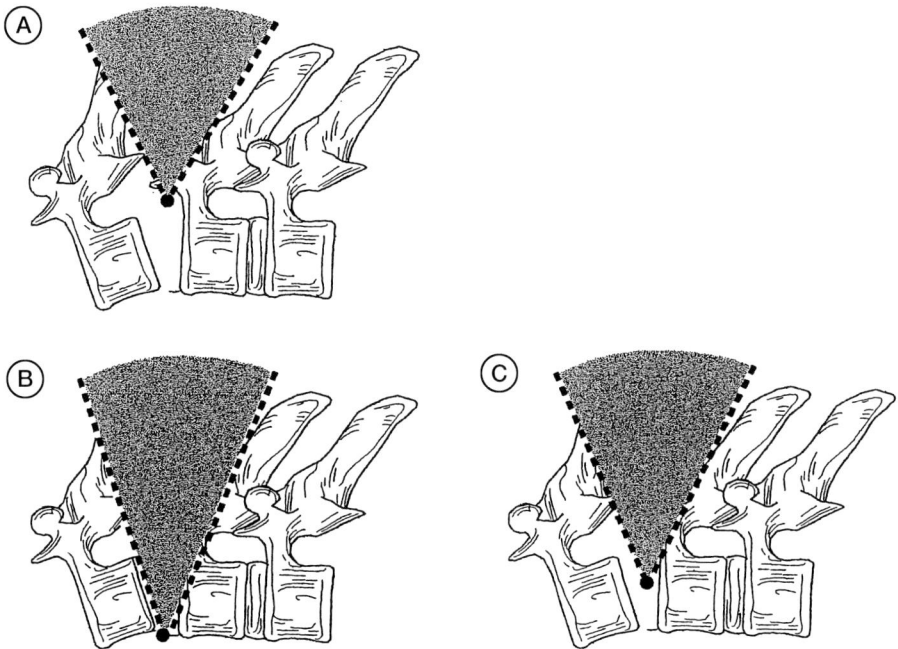

Figure 6 The axis for sagittal plane correction (axis about which correction occurs) is perpendicular to the long axis of the spine axis (dot). It is usually located in the region of the posterior longitudinal ligament (A). This axis could be located ventrally, in the region of the anterior longitudinal ligament, for dorsal wedge osteotomies (B) or in the interbody region for combined ventral and dorsal osteotomies (C).

IV   CONCLUSIONS

The correction of deformity may be achieved by a variety of methods, each with its own advantages and disadvantages. Understanding the biomechanical principles involved facilitate the clinical decision-making process, thus enabling the surgeon to optimize patient outcome. The ultimate goal is to provide a biomechanically sound environment, thus facilitating a nonpathological relationship between the neural elements and the surrounding bony and soft-tissue confines.

REFERENCES

1.   Abel R, Gerner HJ, Smit C, Meiners T. Residual deformity of the spinal canal in patients with traumatic paraplegia and secondary changes of the spinal cord. Spinal Cord 1999; 37:14–19.
2.   White AA, Panjabi MM. Clinical Biomechanics of the Spine, 2nd ed. Philadelphia: Lippincott, 1990:30–342.
3.   Goto S, Mochizuki M, Kita T, Murakami M, Nishigaki H, Moriya H. Transoral joint release of the dislocated atlantoaxial joints combined with posterior reduction and fusion for a late infantile atlantoaxial rotatory fixation. A case report. Spine 1998;23:1485–1489.

4. Matsunaga S, Sakou T, Nakanisi K. Analysis of the cervical spine alignment following laminoplasty and laminectomy. Spinal Cord 1999;37:20–24.

5. Berrington N. Locked facets and disc herniation. J Neurosurg 1994;80:951 (letter).

6. Ordonez BJ, Benzel EC, Naderi S, Weller SJ. Cervical facet dislocation: techniques for ventral reduction and stabilization. J Neurosurg: Spine 2000;92:18–23.

7. McCormack T, Karaikovic E, Gaines RW. The load sharing classification of spine fractures. Spine 1994;19:1741–1744.

8. Betz RR, Harms J, Clements DH, Lenke LG, Lowe TG, Shufflebarger HL, Jeszenszky D, Beele B. Comparison of anterior and posterior instrumentation for correction of adolescent thoracic idiopathic scoliosis. Spine 1999;24:225–239.

9. Johnston CE, Ashman RB, Sherman MC, Eberle CF, Herndon WA, Sullivan JA, King AGS, Burke SW. Mechanical consequences of rod contouring and residual scoliosis in sublaminary segmental instrumentation. J Orthop Res 1987;5:206–216.

10. Akbarnia BA. Transpedicular posterolateral decompression in spinal fractures and tumors. In: Bridwell KH, DeWald RL, eds. *The Textbook of Spinal Surgery*, 2nd ed. Philadelphia: Lippincott-Raven Publishers, 1997:1925–1933.

11. Voor MJ, Roberts CS, Rose SM, Glassman SD. Biomechanics of in situ rod contouring of short-segment pedicle screw instrumentation in the thoracolumbar spine. J Spinal Disord 1997;10:106–116.

12. Wall EJ, Bylski-Austrow DI, Shelton FS, Crawford AH, Kolata RJ, Baum DS. Endoscopic discectomy increases thoracic spine flexibility as effectively as open discectomy. Spine 1998;23:9–16.

13. Winter RB, Carr P, Mattson HL. A study of functional spinal motion in women after instrumentation and fusion for deformity or trauma. Spine 1997;22:1760–1764.

51

Surgical Complications Related to the Management of Traumatic Spinal Injuries

ALEXANDER J. GHANAYEM

Loyola University of Chicago, Maywood, Illinois, U.S.A.

ALEXANDER R. VACCARO and JUSTIN P. KUBECK

Thomas Jefferson University Hospital and the Rothman Institute, Philadelphia, Pennsylvania, U.S.A.

OREN G. BLAM

Thomas Jefferson University Hospital, Philadelphia, Pennsylvania, U.S.A.

Complications related to the surgical treatment of spine fractures can occur during the intraoperative period, as well as the early and late postoperative period. Intraoperative complications include problems associated with particular approaches to the spine used at the time of surgery, issues related to patient positioning on the operating table and neurological deterioration. Postoperative complications fall into four broad categories, including general medical complications, problems related to specific surgical approaches, postoperative infection, and loss of internal fixation. This chapter will review these potential complications and include strategies helpful in both prevention and management of these problems.

I NEUROLOGICAL COMPLICATIONS

Neurological deterioration during and after the surgical treatment of a spine fracture can be one of the most devastating complications facing patients, the patient's family, and the spine surgeon. "First do no harm" applies very well to this category. Prevention is a concept that must be applied continuously throughout the intraoperative period.

Patients undergoing surgical treatment for fractures involving neurological deficit, such as incomplete spinal cord lesions, or with the potential for neurological deficit, are probably at greatest risk for neurological deterioration. One issue that is clearly controversial and well beyond the scope of this chapter is the timing of surgical intervention related to patients with neurological deficits. There is general agreement that patients with progressive deficits should undergo early surgical intervention. Beyond that, the debate continues as to whether early or late surgical intervention is safer for avoiding neurological complications. Regardless of the timing of surgery, other guiding principles need to be enforced. Patients with spinal cord lesions, or the potential for cord deficits, need to maintain adequate blood flow to the spinal cord throughout the surgical procedure. Therefore, hypotension should be avoided during the intraoperative period. This requires careful monitoring on behalf of the anesthesiologist, but also clear communication from the surgeon as far as expectations, anticipated blood loss, and the duration of surgery.

In the intraoperative period, spinal cord monitoring can be used to help monitor neurological function. One should be aware that while spinal cord monitoring can be sensitive to changes in spinal cord function, these changes may occur anywhere from 5 to 20 min prior to their detection. A change in monitoring should prompt a search for reversible causes, including the use of certain anesthetic agents, oxygenation of the patient, lead placement on the patient, changes in spinal alignment either from positioning, exposure, traction, manipulation, or placement of spinal instrumentation around the neurological elements. Hopefully, searching for these reversible causes will result in correction and normalization of monitoring signals (Fig. 1). In some cases, no identifiable cause can be found. This may represent an intraoperative vascular insult to the spinal cord. Despite technical perfection, removing bone or disk fragments that were causing cord compression can allow sudden arterial reflow into the spinal cord resulting in vascular congestion and the onset of neurological compromise. This is probably one of the most helpless situations facing the spine surgeon. There is essentially nothing to do other than finish the operation, provide supportive care, and perhaps add high-dose steroids. Recovery from this complication is variable.

II SPINAL INSTRUMENTATION

The use of spinal instrumentation has greatly helped a surgeon's ability to treat patients with spinal fractures. These tools require that the surgeon be familiar with their indications and proper use. Preoperative planning in terms of the type of instrumentation to be used including which levels to be instrumented, the size of implants to be used, and an alternative plan should an unrecognized fracture be encountered, all help prevent problems with the use of spinal instrumentation. Posterior stabilization systems should avoid the use of sublaminar wires around any compromised neurological level and hooks should never be placed at the injury level. Image-guided systems or routine fluoroscopy can be used to aid the surgeon in proper placement of lateral mass screws in the cervical spine and pedicular screws at the cervicothoracic junction and the thoracic and lumbar spines. Iatrogenic neurological injury from surgical intervention approaches 1% in the management of spine trauma

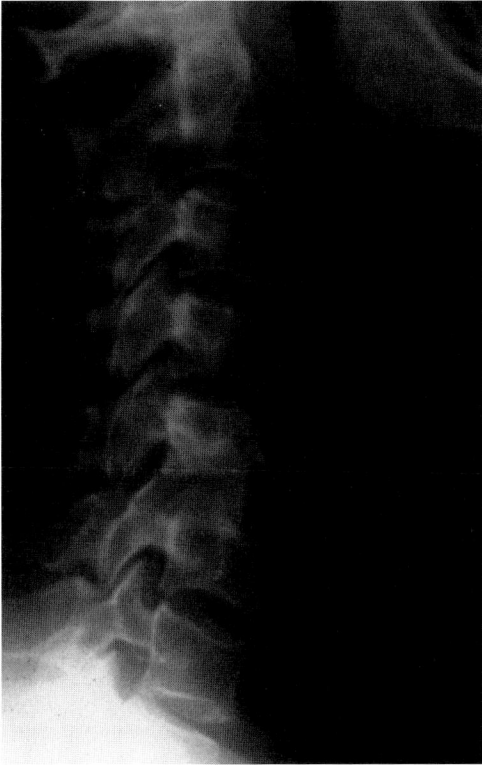

Figure 1 A lateral plain x-ray of the cervical spine film revealing intrusion into the spinal canal by the bone graft due to overimpaction of the graft. The patient underwent surgery for removal of a traumatic disk protrusion following an anterior diskectomy and open reduction of a unilateral facet dislocation. Spinal cord monitoring during impaction of the graft revealed a sudden drop in somatosensory evoked potential (SSEP) conduction. At this point, the graft was removed and the signal returned to normal.

and is usually related to the insertion of spinal instrumentation. This complication is more frequent with posterior instrumentation systems, especially in the setting of overdistraction or compression. Once again, intraoperative spinal cord monitoring can help prevent these complications. A wake-up test may also be helpful when reliable spinal cord monitoring is not available or when changes are detected in reliable monitoring readings.

Accurate anterolateral plating systems require preoperative templating and maintaining the patient in a strict lateral decubitus position to ensure appropriate screw insertion in the coronal plane. Anterior cervical plating using a unicortical system rarely results in any neurological complications unless midline orientation is confused. Surgeons using bicortical screws need to template and carefully measure screw lengths prior to insertion.

Finally, fixation of the posterior occipital cervical junction requires an accurate assessment of the anatomy, including calvarial thickness, especially if occipital screw fixation is anticipated. The bony anatomy must be of the appropriate size and dimension to safely accommodate a C2–C1 transarticular screw or a C2 pedicle or isthmus screw if these implants are chosen for insertion. The course of the vertebral artery must be clearly delineated to avoid injury to that structure.

Current spinal instrumentation systems allow the surgeon to essentially "move" the spine in any direction. This may introduce the potential for iatrogenic deformity. Extension of distraction instrumentation into the lower lumbar levels or sacrum may result in the creation of an iatrogenic flatback deformity (Fig. 2). Distraction instrumentation in the lumbar region may also result in localized lumbar kyphosis. Posterior instrumentation systems have the strength to stabilize the spine using shorter constructs. If the cephalad end of a construct ends at or just inferior to the apex of the normal thoracic kyphosis, a junctional kyphotic deformity can be induced above the construct. Extending the constructs a few more segments beyond the apex can avoid this complication.

III SPINAL FLUID LEAK

Spinal fluid leak can occur after anterior or, more commonly, posterior surgical procedures. Iatrogenic durotomies should be primarily repaired. This can be technically difficult in an anterolateral decompressive procedure and may require the use of a fascial patch and/or lumbar cerebrospinal fluid drain. Traumatic tears should be suspected when lamina fractures are noted on preoperative imaging studies in the presence of a neurolgical deficit and should be repaired when encountered (Fig. 3).

IV POSTOPERATIVE COMPLICATIONS

A Medical Complications

Patients with spine fractures may also have associated skeletal appendicular injuries. Mobilization of a multisystem trauma patient is important to prevent pulmonary dysfunction, skin breakdown, deep vein thrombosis, and pulmonary embolus. A team approach is extremely important in mobilizing these patients to avoid many of these complications. These patients in the presence of a spinal cord injury are often given high-dose steroids and require some sort of gastric ulcer prophylaxis to avoid the complication of gastric mucosal breakdown.

B Surgical Approaches and Patient Positioning

Patient positioning, while sometimes left to the less-experienced staff, is an important part of the surgical procedure to avoid the potential for further spinal segment displacement. Performing a successful posterior reduction and stabilization of a unilateral cervical facet dislocation does not help the patient if he awakens with a brachial plexus or peripheral nerve lesion in the upper extremity secondary to improper positioning. In prone cases, the upper extremities need to be padded at the wrist and elbow and the weight of the shoulder should not allow traction to be placed on the brachial plexus. Care should also be taken to pad the peroneal nerve at the level of the fibular neck. In the lateral position, the downside peroneal nerve is clearly at risk and should be padded. The upside peroneal nerve should not be forgotten as supporting straps may pass over that region causing a compression neuropathy. An axillary roll must also be placed as well. In supine cases, care must be taken once

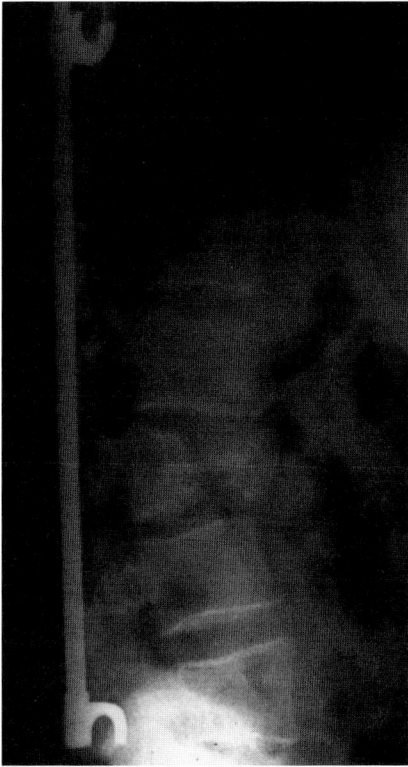

Figure 2   A lateral x-ray revealing evidence of an iatrogenic flatback deformity with localized kyphosis at the fracture site (L3). This was the result of excessive distraction, through the use of instrumentation, at the thoracolumbar junction extending into the lumbar region. Despite healing of the fracture, the patient developed symptoms of back pain (flat back syndrome) due to the resultant deformity.

again to pad around the ulnar nerves at the elbows, avoid extreme positions of the wrists, and pad around the peroneal nerves at the level of the fibular neck. Finally, and most importantly, care must be taken to appropriately protect the face in the prone positioning to avoid skin breakdown or undue pressure around the eyes resulting in visual defects. The entire surgical team needs to take responsibility for this issue and reassess the position of the patient throughout the operative period.

During the anterior exposure of the cervical spine, injuries to the trachea, esophagus, or carotid sheath structures are often related to retraction and, in some cases, are unavoidable. In lengthy procedures, retraction of the soft tissues should be released at specific time intervals to allow soft-tissue relaxation. The use of high-speed burrs should be carefully regulated with starting and stopping of the burr done only within the confines of a disk space or vertebral trough to avoid injury to the anterior soft tissues. Finally, the recurrent laryngeal nerve is thought more commonly at risk during a right-sided anterior approach to the cervical spine, but may also be injured in the left-sided approaches within the trachealesophageal groove due to pressure retraction.

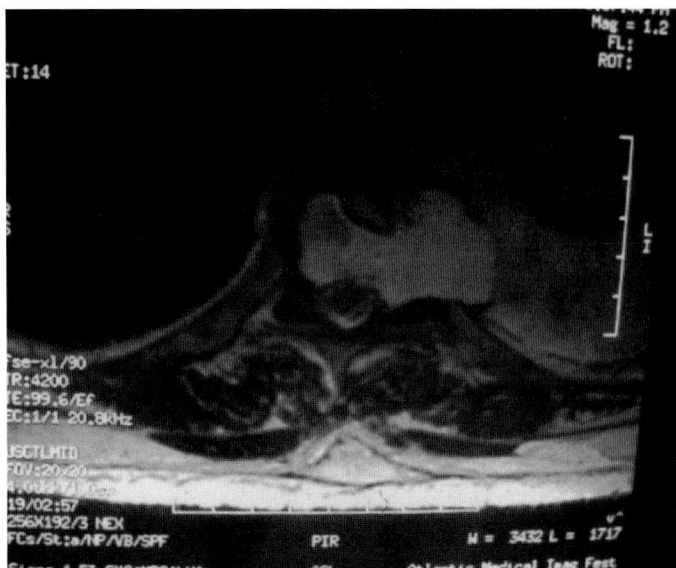

Figure 3 Sagittal MRI of the cervical spine revealing evidence of prevertebral soft-tissue swelling with fluid (abscess) collection. This was due to an iatrogenic esophageal perforation during an anterior cervical approach for a symptomatic traumatic disk herniation following a closed reduced unilateral facet dislocation.

In the thoracic and thoracolumbar spine, surgical exposure complications may involve the creation of a neuroma from injury to the intercostal nerve in the thoracic spine or sensory nerves in the thoracolumbar spine. Meticulous exposure and closure may prevent the occurrence of a hernia during anterior thoracolumbar exposures.

C Infection

Postsurgical spine infections are, in general, less common than infections after surgery in other regions of the musculoskeletal system. The vertebral column has an advantage in that it is well enveloped in soft tissue and the vascular supply is excellent. Infections after posterior surgical approaches generally are more common than after anterior approaches.

Infections following posterior surgical procedures may be minimized through meticulous handling of the soft tissues. This includes relaxing the paraspinal muscle retractors in long cases to allow adequate blood flow into the paraspinal musculature. Irrigation on a regular basis may also be helpful in washing away any wound contaminants. A diagnosis of a perioperative infection requires a high index of suspicion. Postsurgical purulent drainage should be considered as the result of a deep infection until proven otherwise. Early irrigation and debridement is the mainstay of treatment. Spinal instrumentation may be left in place during the phase of serial debridements provided adequate irrigation and debridement is employed, the implants remain well fixed, and postsurgical antibiotics are administered.

Infections after anterior cervical procedures also require a high index of suspicion. Wound drainage, difficulty swallowing, and unexplained fever are usually the early signs of anterior cervical postsurgical infection (Fig. 4). Once again, early irrigation and debridement is the mainstay of successful treatment of this complication. Well-fixed spinal implants may be left in place and postsurgical antibiotics should be administered. Infections after anterolateral procedures in the thoracic and thoracolumbar spine are very common. Usually they involve the superficial soft tissues. Deep wound infections are difficult to diagnose and may only be realized after a prolonged period of unexplained constitutional symptoms. Postsurgical CT scan imaging may demonstrate the presence of an abscess at the operative site. Early irrigation, debridement and appropriate antibiotic selection are the hallmarks of successful treatment.

D   Internal Fixation Failure

Internal fixation failure can occur prior to healing of the fracture and fusion construct (Fig. 5). Postoperative bracing may help minimize this complication. The use of internal fixation, however, is designed to minimize postoperative bracing requirements and to improve patient mobility and functional recovery. Therefore, brace requirements should be tailored to fit the individual patient.

Factors placing the patient at risk for loss of fixation include the presence of osteoporosis, inadequate conferred biomechanical stability from the chosen form of internal fixation, misapplied internal fixation, or the development of an unstable pseudoarthrosis.

In patients with osteoporosis, multiple levels of spinal fixation improve overall fixation strength and minimize the potential for instrumentation migration. Significant anterior column deficiencies, especially in the thoracolumbar spine, associated with

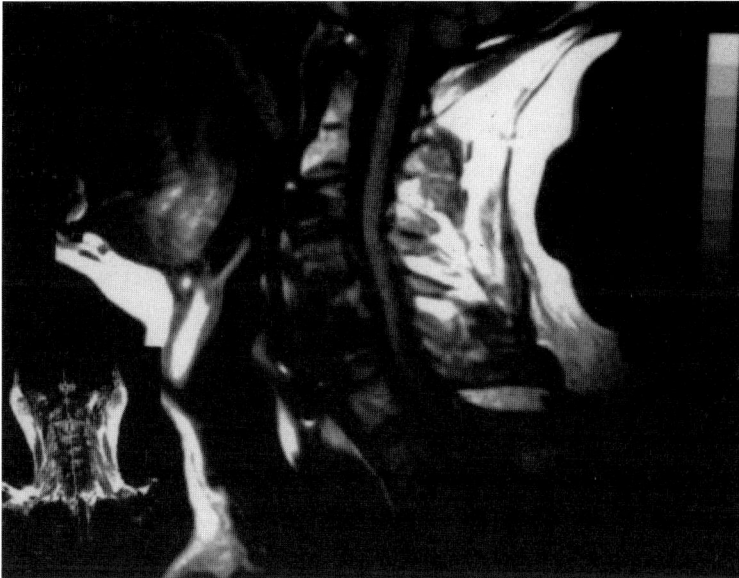

Figure 4   Axial plane MRI of the T9 vertebral level revealing evidence of a significant cerebral spinal fluid leak due to traumatic disruption of the dura noted at the time of corpectomy for a T9 burst fracture.

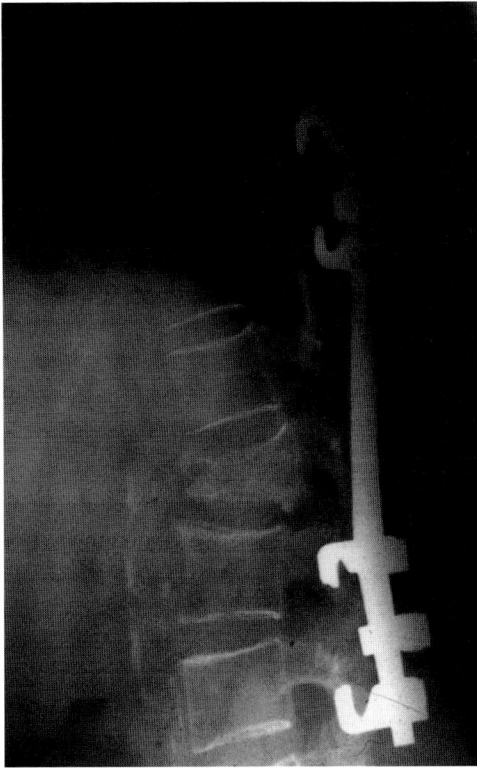

Figure 5 A lateral plain x-ray revealing superior hook-and-rod displacement with loss of spine reduction following surgical stabilization of a L2 burst fracture.

posterior instability may be better stabilized with an anterior and posterior reconstruction procedure as opposed to a single approach. The use of methlymethacrylate is not recommended in spinal trauma reconstruction aside from osteoporotic compression fractures and is associated with tension fatigue failure especially with posterior applications. Interbody spacers such as mesh cages or bulk allografts are effective in reconstructing the anterior weight-bearing column of the spine.

Once the loss of fixation is noted on postoperative radiographs, the surgeon should take immediate steps to prevent further implant or spinal alignment displacement. This may include reoperation at the same site with revision of the instrumentation and/or stabilizing the spine from another (usually opposite) surgical approach.

V   CONCLUSION

Surgical complications associated with spine trauma can have minimal to devastating long-term complications to the patient's well being and overall functional outcome. Understanding these complications, as well as the strategies used to prevent them, can significantly improve the quality of care of the spinal trauma patient. In many cases, complications related to the surgical care of spinal trauma are entirely unavoidable and therefore treatment strategies to care for these occurrences should become part of the basic training of a well-educated spinal surgeon.

52

Rehabilitation After Traumatic Spinal Cord Injury

CHRISTOPHER S. FORMAL

Magee Rehabilitation Hospital, Philadelphia, Pennsylvania, U.S.A.

MICHAEL F. SAULINO and JOHN F. DITUNNO, Jr.

Thomas Jefferson University, Philadelphia, Pennsylvania, U.S.A.

I INTRODUCTION

"Will I be able to walk again?" The concerns foremost in the minds of persons with traumatic spinal cord injury (SCI) mirror those of the rehabilitation team. Prolonged survival after SCI is now the rule, and thus prevention of secondary disease, optimization of function, and reintegration of the person into the community are paramount (1).

Spinal fracture and SCI are impairments—abnormalities of body structure and function—and always require management by a surgeon. A functional deficit, such as inability to walk, is a disability, and disruption of a societal role, such as loss of a job, is a handicap. Disability and handicap are addressed by the rehabilitation team, which also has responsibility for minimizing secondary problems such as pressure ulcer and urinary tract infection.

The rehabilitation team has several members. A physical therapist can address lower extremity function and problems with mobility. An occupational therapist can facilitate upper extremity function and performance of activities of daily living. Nursing staff handle issues including bowel and bladder function, and pressure ulcer treatment. The rehabilitation team functions under the direction of a physiatrist—a specialist in rehabilitation medicine—or a physician with subspecialty certification in spinal cord medicine. While each team member has primary responsibilities, any member of a properly functioning interdisciplinary team can contribute to the resolution of any problem.

II   COMMON MEDICAL PROBLEMS

A   Morbidity

Persons with SCI are at particular risk for certain types of morbidity, with some differences between problems in the acute and chronic phases. Prevention and treatment of these problems are considered in later sections.

Morbidity during the acute rehabilitation phase (which follows the initial acute hospitalization) includes pressure ulceration, which occurs in about 25% of patients treated in Model Systems centers in the United States (2). The most common location is over the sacrum. Atelectasis and/or pneumonia occur in 13%. Deep vein thrombosis (DVT) is found in 10% of patients acutely, and pulmonary embolus (PE) occurs in 3%. This incidence of DVT and PE is lower than that noted historically, probably because of improved vigilance and prophylaxis. Autonomic dysreflexia occurs in about 8% initially, and in 29% of those with complete tetraplegia. Urinary tract infection is common acutely.

A study of persons with chronic SCI followed in England for many years revealed an annual incidence of 23% for pressure ulcer and 20% for urinary tract infection (3). Pressure ulcer was also noted to be the most common morbidity in a study of patients followed in United States Model Systems, occurring in 15% of patients during the first postinjury year, and increasing in subsequent years (4). Autonomic dysreflexia, urinary tract problems, and pneumonia/atelectasis were also noted to be common.

B   Thromboembolic Disease

Thromboembolic disease is common after SCI. Approximately 40% of unprophylaxed patients develop DVT during the acute phase (5). The risk of death from PE during the first year after SCI is more than 200 times that for the general population. DVT most commonly occurs in the weeks after SCI, with a much lower risk in persons with chronic injury.

The increased risk of thromboembolism is likely due to venous stasis and hyercoagulability. Classic symptoms of DVT, such as calf tenderness, may be lacking, because of sensory loss, and symptoms of PE, such as shortness of breath, may be wrongly attributed to concurrent problems such as atelectasis. DVT can present fever of unknown origin, and PE can cause sudden death.

The high incidence and unreliable presentation of DVT suggest that screening studies should be considered. Daily physical examination by physician and nurse can be supplemented by, for example, weekly venous imaging by ultrasound for the first several weeks when the incidence is highest.

A prophylactic strategy can address venous stasis and hypercoagulability. Pneumatic compression devices can be used for the first 2 weeks, followed by compression hose. Unfractionated heparin 5000 units subcutaneously q 12 h, or a low-molecular-weight heparin, such as enoxaparin 30 mg subcutaneously q 12 h, can be administered for 2 to 3 months after injury. In cases with multiple risk factors (such as lower limb fracture, history of DVT, cancer, heart failure, obesity, age over 70), or in the presence of a high, complete cord lesion, placement of a caval filter can be considered.

C Autonomic Dysfunction

High thoracic and cervical SCI can cause loss of supraspinal control of sympathetic activity with dysregulation of functions normally impacted by sympathetic mechanisms (6). Baseline sympathetic activity after SCI is low, although there may be hyperresponsiveness of peripheral sympathetic receptors, perhaps as an adaptive response. Clinical problems result from inappropriately low or high sympathetic responses—the former during the acute phase, the latter in the subacute and chronic phases. Problems are most common in those with levels of T6 and above, as such levels isolate the sympathetic outflow to the splanchnic vascular bed.

Resting blood pressure is low with higher cord lesions. This is asymptomatic. Orthostatic blood pressure changes can cause weakness, lightheadedness, and fainting. Management includes gradual mobilization, liberal sodium intake, compression hose, and abdominal binder (7). Fludrocortisone acetate 0.1 mg per os daily can expand intravascular volume, and thus is helpful. Midodrine, titrated upward from a dose of 5 mg per os bid or tid daily, may be helpful. This agent can cause supine hypertension, and presumably may exacerbate any tendency toward autonomic hyperreflexia.

Bradycardia is common soon after injury, and usually resolves after several weeks. Tracheal suctioning can exacerbate bradycardia, and can cause asystole, perhaps through a reflex increase in vagal output. Symptomatic bradycardia can be treated with intravenous atropine, or by a transvenous, external, or implanted pacemaker.

Autonomic hyperreflexia (AH) is an acute, potentially lethal complication peculiar to those with spinal levels above T7. Presenting symptoms include severe headache, and presenting signs include hypertension. The pathophysiology appears to involve an unmoderated sympathetic response, below the level of the lesion, to a noxious stimulus, commonly a blocked bladder catheter. Adrenoceptor hypersensitivity (AH) below the level of the lesion contributes, and may be essential, to accounting for the observation that AH does not occur acutely after injury, but only later when such hypersensivity has had a chance to develop. Headache may be due to intracranial arterial dilatation, which occurs as part of attempts by the parasympathetic system to adjust for the hypertension. Management includes placement of the patient in a sitting position, which causes a decrease in intracranial blood pressure; a check for an inciting stimulus, such as a distended bladder; and, if necessary, administration of medications, such as topical nitroglycerin. Prophylaxis can be achieved with alpha-blocking agents, such as terazosin (8).

D Neuropathic Pain

Neuropathic, "spinal" pain after SCI is perceived at or below the level of injury. Descriptors often involve temperature ("hot," "burning," "sunburned," "frost-bitten") and electricity ("like an electric shock"). Pain can exist apart from any external stimulus (rest pain), or can result from a stimulus that would not, under normal conditions, cause any pain (allodynia), or can be excessive in response to a painful stimulus (hyperalgesia). These may result from changes in central neuronal function, including increased spontaneous activity and reduced thresholds of response (9).

Evaluation of neuropathic pain after SCI must include consideration of the possibility of a treatable underlying condition, such as an unstable spine, or post-traumatic cystic myelopathy. A change in an established pattern of neuropathic pain may be induced by an unrelated disease process such as a renal stone.

Patients are relieved to be told that their pain need not reflect any active problem, and need not cause them to curtail their activities. Indeed an increased level of activity may decrease suffering. Medicinal treatment includes the use of anticonvulsants and antidepressants (10). Anticonvulsants may be particularly useful in cases of lancinating, "electrical" pain. Gabapentin, beginning at a dose of 100 mg per os tid and gradually titrating upward, is typically used, with precautions for sedation. Tricyclic antidepressants may be useful for more constant, diffuse pain. Amitryptiline, beginning at a dose of 10 mg per os q hs and gradually titrating upward, is one of several agents. Precautions must be taken for its anticholinergic effects. Patients should be told that relief with these agents may not be immediate, as the initial dose may require modification, and, in any case, the medication's effect may not be apparent for days or weeks.

E   Neurogenic Bladder Dysfunction

SCI is typically followed by a period of bladder flaccidity. With suprasacral injury, reflexes eventually return. However, these may be unable to cause efficient voiding due to the tendency of reflex sphincter activity to directly oppose reflex detrusor contraction. This occurs because of the isolation of the urinary tract apparatus from higher centers, which normally coordinate reflex activity. This problem is called detrusor–sphincter dyssynergy.

Acute bladder management is by in-dwelling catheter, as the bladder is likely to be flaccid. Intermittent catheterization is not practical during the initial phase, when urine output cannot be controlled, and is likely to be high, because of the administration of intravenous fluids.

Long-term management has several objectives (11,12). Patients require a drainage method that is socially acceptable, and that will avoid wetting the skin. Bladder emptying should be complete, avoiding high residual volumes. Storage and drainage of urine should occur under low intravesicle pressure, as pressures over 40 cm H_2O have been found to correlate with renal deterioration. Chronic use of an in-dwelling catheter should be avoided, where possible, because it can cause various soft tissue problems, renal problems, and possibly bladder cancer.

Selection of a bladder drainage method occurs ideally after urodynamic evaluation. A method available to those with good hand function, or skilled attendants, is clean, intermittent catheterization. The patient is instructed to limit fluid intake, and catheterization is performed every 4 to 6 h. Reflex bladder contractions, which could cause high storage pressure and incontinence between catheterizations, can be inhibited by agents such as oxybutinin 5 mg per os tid, or tolterodine 2 mg per os bid. An option available to men with reflex bladder contractions is reflex voiding into a condom catheter. Problems can include urinary retention or high intravesicle voiding pressure because of detrusor–sphincter dyssynergy. Voiding pressure can sometimes be decreased by alpha-blocking agents such as terazosin, which is titrated upward from a dose of 1 mg per os q h, or tamsulosin 0.4 mg per os q d. More definitive control of voiding pressure can be obtained by sphincter-defeating surgery, such as sphincterotomy or placement of a urethral stent. A woman with high tetraplegia (and lack of skilled attendants) will often elect to use a chronic in-dwelling catheter. This, as noted, frequently leads to soft tissue problems, or renal problems, and necessitates eventual intervention such as a ureteral diversion. Recently bladder management by electrical stimulation has become available.

In the past, renal disease was a frequent cause of death for those with chronic SCI. It is now unusual. However, significant problems such as urinary tract calculi and hydronephrosis still occur (Figs. 1 and 2). Thoughtful planning of bladder management can avoid this. Annual surveillance of the urinary tract may detect subclinical problems and allow modification of the bladder regimen before significant complications occur. A testing regimen that will evaluate the anatomy and function of the upper and lower tracts includes a renal ultrasound, renal nuclear scan, cystogram, and urodynamic examination.

F   Neurogenic Bowel Management

Neurogenic colonic dysfunction is a particularly distressing and limiting impairment for a substantial proportion of those with SCI (13,14). Lower motor neuron dysfunction, as with cauda equina and conus medullaris injury, causes constipation with slow colonic transport and incontinence due to a flaccid sphincter mechanism. Upper motor neuron dysfunction also causes constipation with slow colonic transit, and stool retention due to spasticity of the sphincter apparatus. With upper motor neuron injury, however, reflexes allowing defecation may remain functional and can be exploited in establishing a bowel program. The bowel program is a regimen, repeated on a daily or every other day basis, which can include diet, specified fluid intake, oral medication, medication per rectum, timing, and positioning. The goals of the program are continence and convenience.

The steps involved in establishment of a bowel program are evaluation, preparation of the patient, trials of a specific bowel program, and finally adjustment of the program.

Evaluation includes a thorough history to determine any preinjury problems or patterns. Neurological assessment, with examination of the bulbocavernosus and anocutaneous reflexes, can suggest the presence of upper or lower motor neuron bowel dysfunction. Patients presenting with problems, including diarrhea, are often impacted, and this can be suggested by physical examination and confirmed by x-ray. Patients may be taking medications, such as antibiotics, that can have unintended effects upon the bowel, such as diarrhea. Evaluation may include testing of a stool specimen for *C. difficile* toxin.

Preparation of the patient includes education about the anticipated program. Complicating problems, such as impaction and *C. difficile* infection, must be treated before the program can succeed.

The specific program may include several measures. A typical problem is stool that is too hard because of the prolonged colonic transport time, which leads to drying of the stool. Intervention includes maintenance of adequate intake of fluid and fiber, with fiber acting as a sponge to hold moisture within the stool. Docusate sodium 100 mg per os bid can increase the ease with which water enters the stool. Patients with lower motor neuron dysfunction may experience greater continence with stool that is firmer than would be optimal for upper motor neuron dysfunction. A second problem is prolonged colonic transit time. Intervention includes maintenance of adequate stool bulk, which stimulates contractions of the colon. Again, fiber

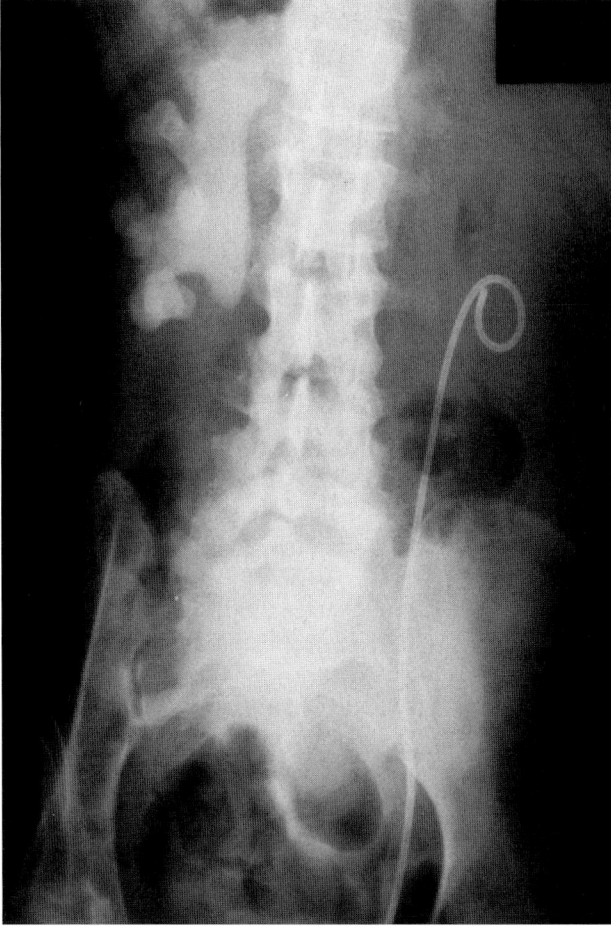

Figure 1   Right renal staghorn calculus in a patient with chronic SCI. Recurrent urinary tract infections likely contributed to its development.

is helpful with this. A bowel stimulant, such as two senna tablets per os daily, can be effective. These are typically taken 8 h before planned bowel evacuation. As these measures decrease bowel transit time, stool consistency may become softer. A third problem is incontinence. The goal is to establish a set time for daily bowel evacuation, ideally after a meal, to take advantage of any gastrocolic reflex that may be present. Specific evacuation strategies may differ for upper and lower motor neuron problems. With upper motor neuron injury, defecation can be triggered with application of an irritant to the anorectal area, such as stimulation with a gloved finger, or application of a bisacodyl enema or suppository. With lower motor neuron bowel dysfunction, evacuation may be by use of Valsalva and digital removal. In either case emptying is facilitated by a seated position on a commode, as opposed to side-lying in bed.

Adjustment of the bowel routine over time is commonly needed, usually with a good eventual result. For those with persistent difficulty, use of a pulsed-irrigation

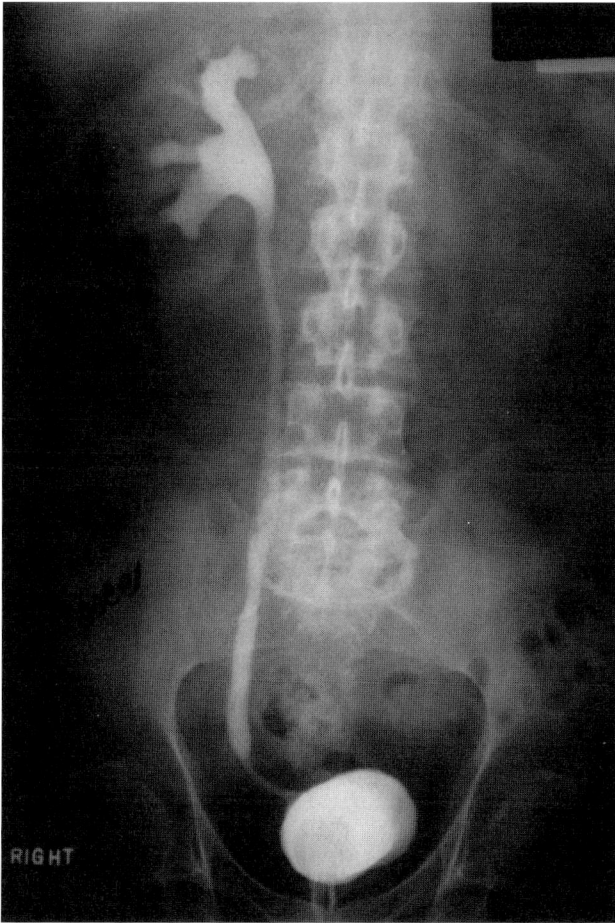

Figure 2 Cystogram, performed by the instillation of contrast into the bladder, in a person with chronic SCI. Reflux is observed from the bladder up to the dilated collecting system on the right. This sort of problem can complicate chronic use of an indwelling catheter, or a bladder regimen with high intravesicle pressure.

enhanced evacuation device can be used, and colostomy can be considered. In the future, bowel control may be achieved (as with bladder control) by electrical stimulation.

G Heterotopic Bone Formation

Heterotopic ossification is the formation of new bone in soft tissue planes surrounding a joint. It can occur subsequent to various types of injuries, including spinal cord injury, after which it most commonly involves hips. Presentation can include some combination of generalized or localized lower extremity swelling, loss of hip range of motion, fever, and elevated alkaline phosphatase level. It may occur subclinically and be noted incidentally on x-rays. Laboratory examination includes serum alkaline phosphatase, x-ray, and bone scan. Bone scan may be positive before x-ray changes are noted.

The main clinical problem (apart from distinguishing it from other problems, such as deep vein thrombosis, which can present similarly) is the loss of range of motion (Fig. 3) Loss of hip motion may complicate bed and chair positioning, and can make dressing and bathing difficult. Range-of-motion exercises can be used in an attempt to limit eventual loss of joint range, despite concern over possibly exacerbating the underlying process of ossification.

Measures possibly to limit the eventual amount of bone mass formed include use of etidronate, nonsteroidal anti-inflammatory drugs, and irradiation (15). Etidronate can be given 20 mg/kg/day per os for 2 weeks, followed by 10 mg/kg/day for at least 10 weeks. An intraveous preparation is also available for acute use. Indomethacin 25 mg per os tid can also be given. Low-dose irradiation can also be applied.

Severe loss of range can be treated surgically (16). The possibility of recurrence may be limited by use of medications and irradiation as described above.

H Pressure Ulceration

Pressure ulceration can be the most limiting seqeula of SCI, and can confine an otherwise independent individual to bed rest. An annual incidence of nearly 25% for those with chronic SCI pairs it with urinary tract infection as the most common complications (3).

Pressure to soft tissue above capillary pressure is the principal cause. Shear, which here refers to prolonged displacement of soft tissue relative to the underlying bone, can distort interposed blood vessels and can also lead to tissue breakdown. Shear can occur over the sacral area when a person sits at an angle in bed, with the bed surface fixing the skin at one point, and gravity causing descent of the underlying sacrum. Whether SCI makes tissue more sensitive to pressure is uncertain.

Evaluation includes an assessment of the ulcer's depth. Destruction of tissue is often more extensive beneath the surface, and indeed breakdown may begin here rather than at the skin level. The location provides information about cause. Ischial ulcers are typically due to sitting; trochanteric ulcers are due to sidelying. Sacral ulcers, if high, may be due to supine lying. Lower ulcers, in the intergluteal area, may relate to sitting up at an angle.

Prophylaxis involves limiting pressure, and the time over which pressure is applied. Wheelchair and bed cushions are available that limit pressure in any one area by distributing it evenly over the available body surface. Weight shifting while in a wheelchair and turning in bed reduce the time of exposure to pressure. Sophisticated bed surfaces use baffles that are alternately inflated and deflated, avoiding exposure long enough to damage tissue. These surfaces are expensive, although not as expensive as a pressure ulcer.

Treatment of an established ulcer involves limiting or eliminating pressure to the area. This effectively confines a person with an ischial ulcer to bed rest. Local care includes removal of necrotic tissue by sharp debridement and topical enzymatic debriders. Cleansing is accomplished with normal saline solution, with topical antibiotics used only for foul wounds. Dressing selection depends in part upon the amount of drainage present. Gauze can wick away excessive wetness. However, a

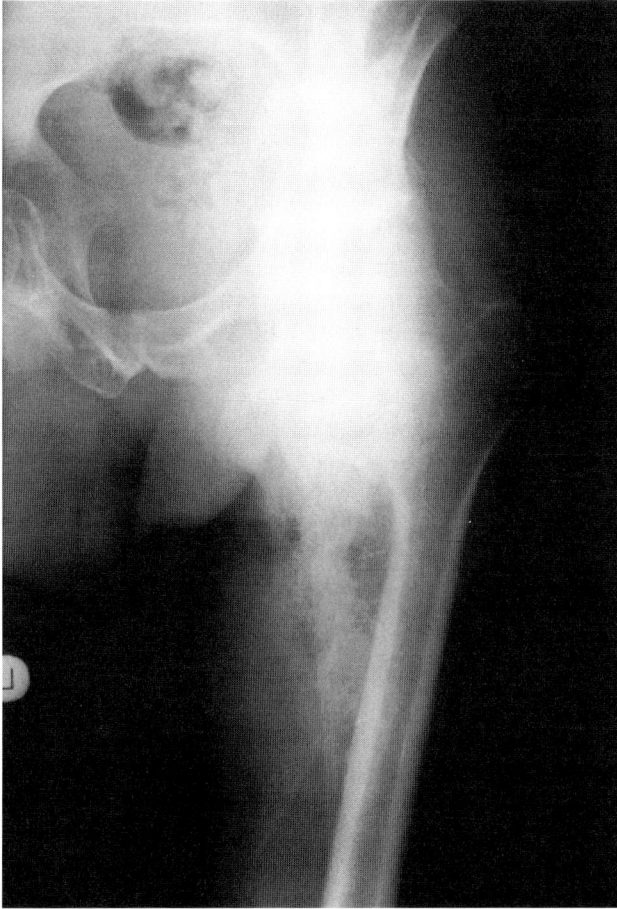

Figure 3 Heteropic ossification after SCI. The right hip is ankylosed.

relatively dry wound may benefit from dampened gauze, or the use of an occlusive or semiocclusive dressing, because a moist wound bed fosters healing more so than a dry environment. Little healing can be expected in the absence of proper nutrition, including adequate provision of calories, protein, vitamin C, and zinc. Smoking slows healing.

Deep ulcers can be treated surgically with debridement and repair by myocutaneous flap. Surgery is best deferred until nutritional status is adequate. Postsurgical care is prolonged and crucial.

I Spasticity

Spasticity is a velocity-dependent increase in muscle tone. It occurs commonly after SCI and other types of upper motor neuron injury. There is resistance to passive motion of the limbs, exaggerated deep tendon relexes, clonus, and involuntary co-contraction of muscle groups. Spasticity occurs after complete and incomplete cord injuries. SCI is usually immediately followed by a period of flaccidity, with spasticity developing over subsequent weeks.

Spasticity has desirable and undesirable effects. It can be used to assist with mobility, especially by those with incomplete injuries. It can improve circulation, and may be useful for decreasing the risk of deep vein thrombosis and osteoporosis. Spasticity can also interfere with positioning, mobility, and hygiene, and spasms can be painful. A decision to intervene must consider both the positive and negative aspects of a patient's spasticity.

Intervention can occur in stages (17) (Table 1). The bedrock of treatment is the elimination of exacerbating factors and regular muscle stretching. Several medications, which can be used in concert, are available (Table 2). Peripheral invasive intervention, such as botulinum toxin injection, is particularly useful in cases where only one or a small number of muscles are problematic. An implanted pump for delivery of intrathecal baclofen is an involved, effective, nondestructive treatment.

J Mortality

The life expectancy of those who survive SCI long enough to reach a hospital has improved over the past decades, although it is below normal. The 18-year cumulative survival for those treated at a Model System is 75%, compared to 92% for the general population (18). Persons sustaining paraplegia at age 20 have an average subsequent life exectancy of 44 years, compared to 57 years for the general population (19). Mortality after SCI is highest in the first year after injury, after which rates decline. Despite encouraging morbidity and mortality for many subsets of SCI, mortality remains high for the elderly. It is hoped that those injured today will have a better prognosis than that noted above, which is from retrospective data.

The causes of death have changed. In the past, urinary tract disease and renal failure were leading causes of mortality. At present, renal failure in those with SCI is unusual. The leading cause of death at present is pneumonia, and the risk for a person with SCI far exceeds that for the general population. Nonischemic heart disease ranks second, and sepsis ranks third. Pulmonary embolus is one of the leading causes of death for younger patients, a leading cause for those with paraplegia, and a leading cause in the first year after injury, when its frequency far exceeds that in the general population.

Table 1 Hierarchy of Interventions to Reduce Spasticity

Central ablative procedures such as rhizotomy and myelotomy
Peripheral procedures including neurolyis and contracture release
Intrathecal baclofen delivered by an implanted pump
Botulinum toxin injection (useful for treatment of problems caused by specific muscle
   groups)
Oral medication (see Table 2)
Regular muscle stretching and joint range of motion
Prevention and treatment of noxious stimuli—pressure ulcer, urinary tract infection, urinary
   tract stone, ingrown toenail

Interventions at the bottom of the tier are less invasive and are typically employed before the higher measures.

Table 2 Oral Pharmacological Agents for the Treatment of Spasticity

Drug	Daily dosage range	Common side effects
Baclofen	5–200 mg (in divided doses)	Hypotonia Sedation/confusion Withdrawl syndrome
Tizanidine	2–36 mg (in divided doses)	Fatigue Dry mouth Sedation Elevated LFTs
Clonidine*	0.2–0.6 mg (in divided doses)	Orthostatic hypotension
Diazepam	5–40 mg (in divided doses)	Sedation Cognitive effects Tolerance Dependence
Gabapentin	200–3200 mg (in divided doses)	Sedation/fatigue Ataxia Dizziness
Dantrolene	25–400 mg (in divided doses)	Weakness Elevated LFTs

LFTs: liver function tests.
*Transdermal delivery available.

III FUNCTIONAL REHABILITATION

A Major Areas of Function

The rehabilitation team is concerned with areas of function, including mobility, activities of daily living, and management of bowel and bladder function. Patients may be independent in performance of an activity, with or without specialized equipment, or may require varying levels of supervision or assistance.

B Neurological Recovery

The early neurological examination can predict later neurological status (20,21). Deterioration is unusual. However, the majority of those with complete injuries remain complete. Those with initial ASIA Impairment Scale grade of B have about a 31% chance of improving to D at 1 year follow-up, while those with initial grades of C have a 67% likelihood (Table 3). Patients with cervical injuries, and at least 2/5 strength in the zone of injury, are likely to eventually gain functional strength at the next neurological level. Initial sparing of sacral pin sensation suggests a favorable prognosis for eventual ambulation.

In addition to physical examination, MRI examination of the spinal cord can provide information regarding future recovery. The appearance of hemorrhage within the cord suggests a poor prognosis, with a gradually improved prognosis suggested by contusion, edema, and a normal appearance of the cord, respectively (22).

Improvement after SCI may be mediated in part by recovery of partially damaged neurons. In addition, recovery at the level of injury may occur because of peripheral sprouting of spared neurons. Distal recovery after incomplete lesions may

Table 3   Correlation of Admission and One-Year
Follow-Up Frankel Grades

Admission Frankel Grade	One-year follow-up Frankel grade			
	A	B	C	D
A	84	8	5	3
B	10	30	29	31
C	2	2	25	67
D	2	1	2	85

Frankel grades closely correspond to ASIA Impairment Scale
grades. Figures are percentages. Rows need not sum to 100 as
Frankel E grades are not included. Note that "admission" here
refers to admission to a Model SCI center, which may have
occurred up to seven days after injury.
Source: Ref. 20.

be mediated by receptor up-regulation, and by an expanse of synaptic fields, allowing
an increase in the influence of spared pathways (22). A similar mechanism may
underlie the development of spasticity. It is possible that early use of spared descending pathways, by exercise and weight bearing, may lead to increased recovery by
favoring the development of new synapses between spared axons and denervated
distal motor neurons (23).

C   Expected Levels of Function

While goals must be individualized, there are certain expectations, according to level,
for healthy individuals with SCI who have received rehabilitation training (24). A
person with tetraplegia above the level of C5 is dependent upon others for activities
such as feeding, dressing, and bathing, and requires the availability of an attendant
at all times. However, a powered wheelchair offers such a person independence in
mobility, in an accessible environment, and independence in weight shifting. Persons
with levels of C5 and C6 have increased functional capacity, but still require physical
assistance for activities such as dressing, bathing, and transfers. A person with a level
of C7 may be independent, with the proper equipment, in all these areas, requiring
only some help with bowel management. Paraplegia is compatible with total independence at a wheelchair level. However, even such individuals may require the
assistance of a homemaker.

D   Gait

Some degree of ambulation may be possible for persons with thoracic-level, complete
paraplegia, and no lower extremity function (24). However, bilateral knee-ankle-foot
orthoses, and a walker or crutches are required. Coming to a standing position is
laborious, the gait is in a swing-to rather than a reciprocal pattern, and velocity is
slow. Such a pattern cannot match wheelchair mobility and is useful for exercise
only. Most patients with no lower extremity function are not trained in gait. With a
level of L2, active hip flexion and reciprocal gait become possible. With a level of

L3, ambulation with ankle-foot orthoses, rather than knee-ankle-foot braces, is possible. However, the hips remain unstable, due to the lack of active hip abduction and extension, and so bilateral canes or crutches, or a walker, must be used. This gait may be sufficient for community ambulation, but is still laborious, and a wheelchair may be preferred by some patients.

Functional ambulation may become possible for patients admitted with ASIA B tetraplegia (23). Sparing of sacral pin sensation may indicate a good prognosis in such patients. A majority of those admitted with ASIA C tetraplegia achieve some level of functional gait. Knee extensor strength of at least 3 out of 5 on one side by 2 months after injury suggests a good prognosis for this group. A central cord or Brown–Sequard pattern also is associated with eventual ability to ambulate.

Persons with spastic, incomplete SCI tend to walk at a low velocity, and have characteristic changes in gait pattern partly because of spasticity (25). Knowledge of the effects of antispasticity treatment upon gait in these subjects is incomplete, but evidence suggests that improvement is possible. Animal and human studies have shown that externally induced stepping movements, applied to a subject with complete paraplegia suspended over a treadmill, can bring about rhythmic, locomotor-like responses (26). This has been taken to suggest not only the presence of a central pattern generator located within the lumbar spinal cord, but also the potential for a training effect. A multicenter study is in progress to determine whether treadmill training initiated after incomplete SCI can lead to subsequent improved ambulatory capacity compared to conventional treatment. The use of functional neuromuscular stimulation is considered below.

E Upper Extremity Reconstructive Surgery

"Tendon transfer" surgery offers the opportunity to utilize an innervated but non-essential muscle to provide a lost function (27). Such surgery is usually not considered until a year after injury. Candidates must be willing to tolerate several weeks of postoperative immobilization, during which previously gained abilities may be lost. Techniques are well developed for the upper limb, but not the lower.

A person with a spinal level of C5 may have good shoulder control and strong elbow flexion. Active elbow extension is lacking, making overhead activity impossible. Such a person may benefit from a transfer procedure to the triceps tendon. One of the muscles available for transfer is the posterior deltoid. A person with a level of C6 may lack effective lateral pinch, and may benefit from transfer of a muscle, such as the brachioradialis, to the tendon of the flexor pollicis longus. Other procedures are available to provide active finger flexion and extension. Functional neuromuscular stimulation is described below.

F Functional Neuromuscular Stimulation

Electrical stimulation of intact peripheral nerves can bring about contraction in muscles paralyzed by upper motor neuron injury (28). Stimulation can be by transcutaneous, percutaneous, or implanted electrodes. Such stimulation can be useful for exercise and for function.

Functional neuromuscular stimulation (FNS) can be used in the upper extremity to provide lateral pinch and palmar grasp to persons with, for example, C5 and C6 tetraplegia. A totally implantable system is available, with control by the position of the contralateral shoulder. Upper extremity FNS is often combined with tendon transfer surgery.

Patterned lower extremity FNS by external electrodes can allow a stationary bicycle exercise program, with beneficial cardiopulmonary, soft tissue, and psychological effects. As with the general population, benefits are only obtained with the patient's commitment to the exercise regimen. FNS, combined with lower extremity orthoses and a walker, can allow gait. Control is by switches placed on the walker. The performance of such a system is not sufficient to substitute for a wheelchair. It can be useful for specific limited mobility.

IV   LIFE IN THE COMMUNITY

A   Residence

The great majority of those with traumatic SCI are discharged to private residences in the community (29). Community disharge is a goal of the rehabilitation process, and occurs in well over 90% of patients treated with the Model Systems. Community discharge can place a significant burden upon the patient's support system, but is usually preferable to a custodial care facility, where the population is typically older, and where procedures may not be geared to fostering the resident's function.

B   Marriage

While those married at the time of SCI have an increased rate of subsequent separation and divorce, over 75% of such marriages that survive the first year following injury remain intact 5 years after injury (29). Persons with SCI subsequently marry at a rate below that of the general population, perhaps because of the poverty in which many of them live, as well as a decrease in the amount of social contact. Nearly 90% of those single at the time of SCI are still single 5 years after injury, compared with an expected figure of 65% in the absence of SCI.

C   Employment and Education

Persons with SCI may, in many instances, have a need to improve their educational level in order to find employment. While the average educational level at 5 years after injury is below that of the general population, at 10 and 15 years it exceeds that average. Those with tetraplegia, as a group, achieve a higher educational level than those with paraplegia, and those with complete injuries reach a higher level than those with incomplete injuries (29).

About 59% of persons sustaining traumatic SCI are employed at the time of injury (30). The rate of employment declines immediately after SCI, but increases over subsequent years. It does not reach the level of the general population. Caucasian race, young age at time of injury, and years of education are associated with a greater chance of employment. Severity of injury correlates inversely.

D   Sexual Physiology After SCI

Sexual drive persists after SCI, though sexual physiology may be altered. In men with upper motor neuron syndromes, erections in reponse to local stimulation ("reflex" erections) are common, while erections in response to cortical stimuli such as thoughts and sights ("psychogenic" erections) are lost (31). Reflex erections, while common, may not persist long enough for sexual activity. Those with lower motor neuron syndromes do not demonstrate reflex erections, but, when sympathetic outflow from the lower thoracic and upper lumbar segment is spared, may have psychogenic erections.

Management of erectile dysfunction can include exploration of sexual expression not involving erection. Most men are also interested in options for improving erectile function. Sildenafil has proven effective in cases of upper or lower motor neuron injury. It is taken orally 20 to 60 min prior to the time of desired erection. The use of nitrate-containing medications is an absolute contraindication to sildenafil use because of the possibility of a fatal response. Patients must be educated regarding this, as nitrates are used by some to control episodes of autonomic hyperreflexia, in addition to their use in cardiac disease. Patients with known cardiac illness should be evaluated by a cardiologist prior to sildenafil use.

Other options for improving erectile function after SCI include intracavernosal injection of papaverine or prostaglandin E1. Priapism and penile fibrosis are possible. Prostaglandin E1 can also be applied transurethrally using a catheter device. Hypotension is a possible side effect, although the risk can be decreased by the use of a venous constrictive band at the base of the penis. Vacuum tumesence devices are effective. Precautions must be taken for local tissue injury. Implantation of a penile prosthesis carries several risks, including extrusion, probably because of the lack of local protective sensation.

A substantial proportion of women retain the capacity for orgasm after SCI, regardless of severity of injury (32). After SCI, vaginal vasocongestion can occur in response to local stimulation. Women with complete injuries above T6 do not, however, demonstate vaginal vasocongestion in response to psychogenic stimulation alone, because of the isolation of the brain from the sympathetic outflow to the genitals (33).

E Fertility

Men can be infertile after SCI due to ejaculatory dysfunction and problems with the quantity and quality of sperm. The coordination of events leading to ejaculation—seminal emission, bladder neck closure, and perineal muscle contraction—is disrupted. The reasons for poor sperm quality are unclear. Systemic endocrine changes, histological abnormalities in the testis, seminal abnormalities, urinary tract infection, and local factors such as increased scrotal temperature may play a role.

Techniques are available to induce ejaculation in men with SCI who are otherwise anejaculatory. The semen can then be used for in vitro fertilization. External vibratory stimulation involves the use of a vibrator over the glans and frenulum to induce an ejaculatory reflex. Electroejaculation is the rhythmic delivery of current, using a rectal probe, to sympathetic efferent fibers. These techniques carry the risk of autonomic hyperreflexia.

Women with SCI typically experience amenorrhea for up to a year after injury (34). Periods then begin again, and fertility returns. SCI does not contraindicate pregnancy (35). However, the risk of certain SCI-related problems such as urinary tract infection and pressure ulcer may increase with pregnancy. Persons with SCI often take medications for various problems, and some of these should be avoided during pregnancy. In addition, a woman with SCI may not sense the usual indicators of labor, which raises the possibility of an unattended preterm delivery, suggesting that surveillance be maintained as the pregnancy advances, perhaps by hospitalization, or by the use of a home uterine contraction monitor.

F Psychological Adjustment and Life Satisfaction

There is no characteristic pattern of adjustment typical of those with SCI. Theories of stages through which patients pass have not been supported empirically. Many of those with SCI are able to respond constructively to the enormous stressors with which they are faced. Group and individual psychological treatment, including a cognitive behavioral approach, may be conducive to positive adjustment (36). Significant depression occurs occasionally, and may require pharmacological intervention (37). Persons with SCI have an increased risk of death from suicide, particularly in the years immediately following injury. After 10 years, the rate of suicide approaches that of the general population (29).

Most long-term survivors of SCI feel fortunate to be alive (3). Even among patients with a high level of injury, including in many cases of ventilator dependence, quality of life has been found to be acceptable, and most have a clear desire to live (38). Quality of life after SCI is less influenced by neurological status than by the degree to which the person is able to resume roles in society (39). While research pursues the goals of preventing and reversing neurological deficit, we must continue to work to remove barriers impeding the return of persons with SCI to active roles in the community.

ACKNOWLEDGMENTS

Supported in part by the Regional Spinal Cord Injury Center of Delaware Valley Model SCI Systems grant to Thomas Jefferson University from the National Institute for Disability Research and Rehabilitation #H133N950021.

REFERENCES

1. Ditunno JF Jr, Formal CS. Chronic spinal cord injury. N Engl J Med 1994;330:550–556.
2. Chen D, Apple DF Jr, Hudson LM, Bode RK. Medical complications during acute rehabilitation following spinal cord injury—current experience of the Model Systems. Arch Phys Med Rehabil 1999;80:1397–1401.
3. Whiteneck GG, Charlifue SW, Frankel HL, Fraser MH, Gardner BP, Gerhart KA, Krishnan KR, Menter RR, Nuseibeh I, Short DJ, Silver JR. Mortality, morbidity, and psychosocial outcomes of persons spinal cord injured more than 20 years ago. Paraplegia 1992;30:617–630.
4. McKinley WO, Jackson AB, Cardenas DD, DeVivo MJ. Long-term medical complications after traumatic spinal cord injury: a regional model systems analysis. Arch Phys Med Rehabil 1999;80:1402–1410.
5. Consortium for Spinal Cord Medicine. Prevention of Thromboembolism in Spinal Cord Injury. Washington, DC: Paralyzed Veterans of America, 1997.
6. Teasell RW, Arnold JMO, Krassioukov A, Delaney GA. Cardiovascular consequences of loss of supraspinal control of sympathetic nervous system after spinal cord injury. Arch Phys Med Rehabil 2000;81:506–516.

7. Staas WES Jr, Formal CS, Freedman MK, Fried GW, Schmidt Read ME. Spinal cord injury and spinal cord injury medicine. In: DeLisa JA, Gans BM, eds. Rehabilitation Medicine: Principles and Practice, Third Edition. Philadelphia: Lippincott-Raven, 1998: 1259–1291.

8. Consortium for Spinal Cord Medicine. Acute Management of Autonomic Dysreflexia: Adults with Spinal Cord Injury Presenting to Health-Care Facilities. Washington, DC: Paralyzed Veterans of America, 1997.

9. Eide PK. Pathophysiological mechanisms of central neuropathic pain after spinal cord injury. Spinal Cord 1998;36:601–612

10. Bryce TN, Ragnarsson KT. Pain after spinal cord injury. Phys Med Rehab Clin North America 2000;11:157–168.

11. Nygaard IE, Kreder KJ. Urological management in patients with spinal cord injuries. Spine 1996;21:128–132.

12. Lightner DJ. Contemporary urologic management of patients with spinal cord injury. Mayo Clin Proc 1998;73:434–438.

13. Stiens SA, Bergman SB, Goetz LL. Neurogenic bowel dysfunction after spinal cord injury: clinical evalaution and rehabilitative management. Arch Phys Med Rehabil 1997; 78:S-86–S-102.

14. Consortium for Spinal Cord Medicine. Neurogenic Bowel Management in Adults with Spinal Cord Injury. Washinton, DC: Paralyzed Veterans of America, 1998.

15. Freebourn TM, Barber DB, Able AC. The treatment of immature heterotopic ossification in spinal cord injury with combination surgery, radiation therapy and NSAID. Spinal Cord 1999;37:50–53.

16. Stover SL, Niemann KMW, Tulloss JR. Experience with surgical resection of heterotopic bone in spinal cord injury patients. Clin Orth Rel Res 1991;263:71–77.

17. Meythaler JM. Spastic hypertonia. Phys Med Rehab Clin North Am 2001;12:725–977.

18. DeVivo MJ, Stover SL. Long-term survival and causes of death. In: Stover SL, DeLisa JA, Whiteneck GG, eds. Spinal Cord Injury: Clinical Outcomes from the Model Systems. Gaithersburg, MD: Aspen, 1995:289–315.

19. DeVivo MJ, Krause JS, Lammertse DP. Recent trends in mortality and causes of death among persons with spinal cord injury. Arch Phys Med Rehabil 1999;80:1411–1419.

20. Marino RJ, Ditunno JF Jr, Donovan WH, Maynard F Jr. Neurologic recovery after traumatic spinal cord injury: data from the Model Spinal Cord Injury Systems. Arch Phys Med Rehabil 1999;80:1391–1396.

21. Ditunno JF Jr. Predicting recovery after spinal cord injury: a rehabilitation imperative. Arch Phys Med Rehabil 1999;80:361–364.

22. Kirshblum SC, O'Connor KC. Predicting neurologic recovery in traumatic cervical spinal cord injury. Arch Phys Med Rehabil 1998;79:1456–1466.

23. Little JW, Ditunno JF Jr, Stiens SA, Harris RM. Incomplete spinal cord injury: neuronal mechanisms of motor recovery and hyperreflexia. Arch Phys Med Rehabil 1999;80:587–599.

24. Consortium for Spinal Cord Medicine. Outcomes Following Traumatic Spinal Cord Injury: Clinical Practice Guideline for Health-Care Professionals. Washington, DC: Paralyzed Veterans of America, 1999.

25. Barbeau H, Ladouceur M, Normal KE, Pepin A, Leroux A. Walking after spinal cord injury: evalaution, treatment, and functional recovery. Arch Phys Med Rehabil 1999;80: 225–235.

26. Pinter MM, Dimitrijevic MR. Gait after spinal cord injury and the central pattern generator for locomotion. Spinal Cord 1999;37:531–537.

27. Waters RL, Sie IHS, Gellman H, Tognella M. Functional hand surgery following tetraplegia. Arch Phys Med Rehabil 1996;77:86–94.

28. Chae J, Triolo RJ, Kilgore K, Creasey GH. Functional neuromuscular stimlulation. In: DeLisa JA, Gans BM, eds. Rehabilitation Medicine: Principles and Practice, 3rd ed. Philadelphia: Lippincott-Raven, 1998:611–631.

29. Dijkers MP, Abela MB, Gans, Gordon WA. The aftermath of spinal cord injury. In: Stover SL, DeLisa JA, Whiteneck GG, eds. Spinal Cord Injury: Clinical Outcomes from the Model Systems. Gaithersburg, MD: Aspen, 1995:185–212.

30. Krause JS, Kewman DK, DeVivo MJ, Maynard F, Coker J, Roach MJ, Ducharme S. Employment after spinal cord injury: an analysis of cases from the Model Spinal Cord Injury Systems. Arch Phys Med Rehabil 1999:80:1492–1500.

31. Monga M, Bernie J, Rajasekaran M. Male infertility and erectile dysfunction in spinal cord injury: a review. Arch Phys Med Rehabil 1999:80:1331–1339.

32. Sipski ML, Alexander CJ, Rosen RC. Orgasm in women with spinal cord injuries: a laboratory-based assessment. Arch Phys Med Rehabil 1995;76:1097–1102.

33. Sipski ML, Alexander CJ, Rosen RC. Physiological parameters associated with psychogenic sexual arousal in women with complete spinal cord injuries. Arch Phys Med Rehabil 1995;76:811–818.

34. Sipski ML. The impact of spinal cord injury on female sexuality, menstruation and pregnancy: a review of the literature. J Am Paraplegia Soc 1991;14:122–126.

35. Baker ER, Cardenas DD. Pregnancy in spinal cord injured women. Arch Phys Med Rehabil 1996;77:501–507.

36. North NT. The psychological effects of spinal cord injury: a review. Spinal Cord 1999: 37:671–679.

37. Consortium for Spinal Cord Medicine. Depression Following Spinal Cord Injury: A Clinical Practice Guideline for Primary Care Physicians. Washington, DC: Paralyzed Veterans of America, 1998.

38. Hall KM, Knudsen ST, Wright J, Charlifue SW, Graves DE, Werner P. Follow-up study of individuals with high tetraplegia (C1-C4) 14 to 24 years postinjury. Arch Phys Med Rehabil 1999;80:1507–1513.

39. Dijkers M. Quality of life after spinal cord injury: a meta analysis of the effects of disablement components. Spinal Cord 1997;35:829–840.

Index